Vertebrate Anatomy and Physiology for Veterinary Technician Students

First Edition

Bassim Hamadeh, CEO and Publisher
John Remington, Managing Acquisitions Editor
Carrie Baarns, Senior Manager, Revisions and Author Care
Gem Rabanera, Senior Project Editor
Laureen Gleason, Production Editor
Jess Estrella, Senior Graphic Designer
Kylie Bartolome, Licensing Associate
Natalie Piccotti, Director of Marketing
Kassie Graves, Senior Vice President of Editorial
Jamie Giganti, Director of Academic Publishing

Cover image copyright © 2020 iStockphoto LP/101cats.

Printed in the United States of America.

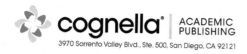
cognella® | ACADEMIC PUBLISHING
3970 Sorrento Valley Blvd., Ste. 500, San Diego, CA 92121

Vertebrate Anatomy and Physiology for Veterinary Technician Students

First Edition

Boris Zakharov

LaGuardia Community College

cognella®

SAN DIEGO

Contents

CHAPTER 15   The Cardiovascular System   429

CHAPTER 16   The Circulatory System II: Blood Vessels   459

Chapter 1

Introduction to Anatomy and Physiology

LEARNING OBJECTIVES

This chapter will introduce you to the basic concepts of vertebrate anatomy and physiology. First of all, you will find a general definition and outline of vertebrates. This chapter contains information on both anatomy and physiology and their basic concepts that encompass these scientific disciplines. It is expected that when you finish reading this chapter, you will be able to:

1. Describe what characteristics are common to all vertebrates.

2. Discuss the evolution of vertebrates.

3. Discuss the subject and methods of anatomy and physiology.

4. Describe the principles of vertebrate body organization and functioning.

5. Use basic terminology of these scientific disciplines.

INTRODUCTION

Anatomy and physiology are two of the oldest scientific disciplines, known from ancient times. This is not surprising. The interest in our own body and its normal functioning as far as the bodies of other animals is an intrinsic part of human curiosity. Despite its ancient origin, anatomy remains a powerful tool for understanding the body's organization. Comparative anatomy explains the basic principles of body design, helps reveal evolutionary relations among organisms, and find forces that drive animals' historical development. A special relation exists between structural body organization and its normal functioning. This relation was formulated as correspondence between structure and function. Thus, anatomy was forever bound with physiology—a scientific discipline that studies function. That is why this course includes both disciplines. Anatomy allows us to understand the basic principles of body organization, while physiology helps us understand how the body works.

This chapter will introduce you to basic concepts of animal body organization and important anatomic terminology. It will familiarize you with the most fundamental principles of the functioning of living organisms and, in a few particular examples, will demonstrate how these principles work. But first you will find a brief description of vertebrates and their evolution.

1.1   Survey of Vertebrates

Brief Description of Vertebrates

Vertebrates are animals with an endoskeleton. Their most significant characteristic, which gives them their name, is a vertebral column. Their bilaterally symmetric body is organized around a vertebral column that creates a main body axis, which supports, protects, and serves as an attachment for muscles and internal organs. Vertebrates include fishes, amphibians, reptiles, and mammals. All these animals are grouped in the subphylum Vertebrata. Together with cephalopods (amphioxi, or lancelets) and urochordates (tunicates, or sea squirts), they constitute the phylum Chordata (fig. 1.1). Instead of the vertebral column, the cephalopods and urochordates have chorda—a rodlike structure made of cartilage. The tunicates and lancelets are sometimes called **protochordates**. They possess all three typical chordate structures in the larval and/or adult forms. These animals link vertebrates to the rest of the animal kingdom. Vertebrata is the biggest chordate group. Currently, the subphylum includes more than 66,000 species. Animals of this phylum have following three basic characteristics at some period of their life:

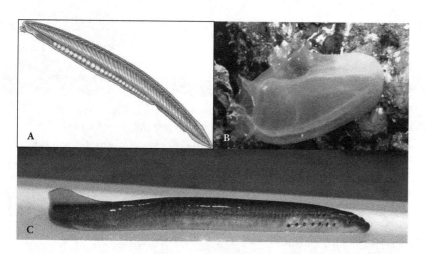

FIGURE 1.1   Chordates. A. Lancelet; B. Sea Squirt; C. Lamprey.

1.   A supporting dorsal rod called a **notochord**, which in adult animals is replaced by the vertebral column.
2.   A dorsal tubular nerve cord with a central canal filled by cerebrospinal fluid.
3.   Pharyngeal pouches or gill clefts (slits). In fishes, water from the mouth passes to the pharynx and goes out through the gill slits, which are supported by gill bars and used for gas exchange. In terrestrial vertebrates, gill slits present only in the embryo.

Other characteristics shared among vertebrates are:

1.   A closed circulatory system, where a ventral two- to four-chambered heart facilitates blood movement; blood vessels form a continuous system of tubes, where red blood cells circulate.
2.   The digestive system of vertebrates consists of the gastrointestinal tract, an extensive tube extending from the mouth to the anus. The system includes the digestive glands, liver, and pancreas.
3.   The kidneys are excretory and water-regulating organs that conserve or remove water.
4.   All vertebrates with jaws have an extraordinarily complex immune system.

TABLE 2.1   Four Major Groups of Biological Macromolecules

	Examples	Functions	Monomer (building block)
Carbohydrates	Starch, glycogen (polysaccharides)	Energy storage, cell surface marker, cell signaling	Simple sugars (glucose, galactose)
Proteins	Hemoglobin, enzymes, collagen	Catalyze reactions, physical structure, cell signaling	Amino acids (glycine, cysteine)
Nucleic Acids	DNA, RNA	Store genetic information, gene expression	Nucleotides (A, C, G, T)
Lipids	Triacylglycerol, cholesterol	Energy storage, cell membranes, hormones	Fatty acids and glycerol

CHECK YOUR UNDERSTANDING

- Describe the three components of a nucleotide.

- What are the principal differences between DNA and RNA?

- What role do ATP molecules have?

CHAPTER SUMMARY

- The atom is the smallest structure of matter that retains the properties of the chemical element. It is built of three subatomic particles: **protons, neutrons,** and **electrons**. Protons are positively charged particles. Together with neutrons, they constitute the **atomic nucleus**. Electrons are negatively charged particles. They rotate around the nucleus and constitute the **electron shell**. The weight of atomic particles and atoms is measured in subatomic units (au). The weight of the proton and neutron is almost equal and is roughly 1 au. The weight of the electron is negligible. Almost all atom mass (99.95 percent) is concentrated in the nucleus.

- Atoms are electrically neutral. The nucleus carries all positive electric charge, and the electron shell carries all negative electric charge. The positive charge of the proton is +1 and the negative charge of the electron is –1. In an electrically neutral atom, the number of protons in the nucleus is equal to the number of electrons in the electron shell. The number of neutrons varies. The varying number of neutrons in the nucleus results in the existence of isotopes: atoms that are identical in the number of protons and electrons, but different in the number of neutrons. Because every neutron has a mass of 1 au, isotopes have a different atomic mass.

- Electrons move around the nucleus on orbits organized in shell layers. The first shell layer accommodates a maximum of 2 electrons. The second shell holds up to 8 electrons. The third shell holds 18 electrons. The nucleus occupies a very small space in the total volume of an atom. When two atoms create chemical bonds, they interact by their outer electron shells, but not by their nuclei.

- A group of atoms with similar chemical properties is called a **chemical element**. The number of protons in the nucleus corresponds to the **atomic number**. Chemical elements undergo periodic transformation of their physical and chemical properties, which allows them to be organized in the periodical table of chemical elements. Every chemical element occupies a position in this table according to its atomic number.

- The number of chemical bonds created by a particular element is called the **valence** of this element. Chemical bonds are formed only by electrons from the outermost electron shell. This electron shell is called a **valence shell**, and electrons on this shell are called **valence electrons**. Atoms follow the octet rule: an atom reaches a stable state when it has eight electrons in the outer shell. Atoms from the first line (hydrogen and helium) become stable when their only electron shell has two electrons. Atoms are neutral, because they have an equal number of protons and electrons. When an atom loses or gains electrons, it becomes electrically charged. The electrically charged atom is called an **ion**. When the atom loses electrons, it becomes a positively charged **cation**. When the atom gets additional electrons, it becomes a negatively charged **anion**. According the octet rule, atoms in columns 1 and 2 in the periodic table tend to lose electrons from their outermost electron shell. When an atom from the first column loses its one outermost electron, it gets an electric charge +1. Atoms in the second column have two electrons in their valence shell, and when they lose them, these atoms get a charge +2. Atoms in column 17 have seven electrons in the valence shell. These atoms easily accept additional electron to satisfy the octet rule. When they accept an additional electron, they gain a negative charge –1. Chlorine, fluoride, and iodine all tend to take one electron from other atoms. Oxygen and serum from column 16 have six valence electrons, and they accept two additional electrons and become –2. The opposite electrically charged atoms attract each other and form **ionic** chemical bond.

- Chemical bonds created through equally sharing valence electrons between atoms are called **covalent bonds**. When two atoms create a covalent bond by sharing one electron from one atom and one electron from another atom, they create one covalent bond. Thus, one covalent bond is made of two electrons that rotate around both atoms. A double covalent bond has four electrons: two electrons from one atom and two from the other. A triple covalent bond is made of three electron pairs: three electrons from one atom and three from another; and four covalent bonds are formed by eight electrons: four from each atom. Elements from column 14 (carbon, silicon, germanium, indium) have four electrons on their valence electron shell. When a carbon atom shares its electrons with another carbon atom, both atoms get eight electrons on their outermost electron shell, which makes both of them stable.

- Atoms do not attract electrons with equal force. The force with which an atom pulls electrons is called **electro-negativity**. Oxygen and nitrogen are among the most electronegative elements. When they create a covalent bond with other elements, they pull shared electrons on themselves and strip an electron cloud from other atoms. An unequal distribution of electrons causes development of a small negative charge around oxygen and makes the opposite atom lightly positively charged. This electrically charged covalent bond is called a **polar covalent bond**.

- Polarized molecules create bonds that hold atoms by weak electric interactions that are called **hydrogen bonds** (or **H-bonds**).

- Weak interactions between atoms and molecules caused by correlations in the fluctuating polarizations of nearby atoms are called van der Waals forces. These attractions are not chemical bonds. Van der Waals forces quickly vanish with increasing distance between interacting molecules.

- Hydrogen atoms in water molecules do not have enough strength against highly electronegative oxygen, and electrons tend to stay near oxygen. As a result, the water molecule is lightly positively charged at its hydrogen ends and negatively charged at the oxygen end. Molecules with a partial negative charge at one end and a positive charge at the other are called **dipoles**. A dipole water molecule forms hydrogen bonds with four other water molecules.

- Hydrogen bonds hold water molecules together and create a water lattice. The lattice gives water some very important properties: 1) liquid water is denser than ice; 2) water has a shifted boiling point that stabilizes body temperature; 3) the resistance of water molecules to separation, known as **cohesion**, holds water molecules together and creates phenomena such as **surface tension** and water molecule **adhesion**; and 4) polar water molecules easily separate molecules and ions, which makes water a good solvent.

- Molecules that easily dissolve in water are called **hydrophilic**. Molecules that do not mix with water and cannot be dissolved are called **hydrophobic**. Molecules that have hydrophobic and hydrophilic regions are called **amphiphilic**. When mixed with water, amphiphilic molecules turn their hydrophilic part toward water and turn the hydrophobic region away from water.

- The process of movement of water across a semipermeable membrane is called **osmosis**. A semipermeable membrane is a membrane that allows some substances to pass but stops others. The force that drives osmosis is called **osmotic pressure**. The solution with a higher solute concentration has greater osmotic pressure. In osmosis, water molecules move from a solution with lower osmotic pressure to a solution with higher osmotic pressure. The comparative measure of osmotic pressure is called **tonicity**. A solution with higher osmotic pressure is called **hypertonic**. A solution with lower osmotic pressure is **hypotonic**. When solutions have the same osmotic pressure, they are called **isotonic**.

- Water molecules split into cation hydrogen (H^+) and anion hydroxide group (OH^-). The proportion of dissociated into H^+ and OH^- water molecules is small, only 1 molecule out of 10,000,000 (1×10^{-7}). Solutions with increased concentration of H^+ are called **acids**. Solutions with increased concentration of OH^- are called **bases**. Pure water is neutral; that is, it is not acidic nor basic. To describe the acidity of the water solution, a numerical scale called the **pH scale** was developed: $pH = -\log_{10} [H^+]$. Neutral pure water has $pH = -\log_{10} [1 \times 10^{-7}] = -[-7] = 7$. The number 7 is the midpoint of the pH scale. Solutions with pH below 7 are acidic. Solutions with pH above 7 are basic or alkaline.

- Chemical substances that resist pH changes are called **buffers**.

- Complex macromolecules built of carbon atoms are called **organic molecules**, as opposed to simple molecules called **inorganic molecules**. Carbon creates four covalent bonds and can organize in long chains or rings. All organic molecules are built from smaller compounds or building blocks called **monomers**. Monomers bind together into a **polymer**. The process of polymer construction is called **polymerization**. Organic molecules are grouped in four classes: **carbohydrates**, **proteins**, **lipids**, and **nucleic acids**.

- Carbohydrates serve as a fuel for production of chemical energy, structural elements, and signaling molecules. Monomers of carbohydrates are called **monosaccharides**. Monosaccharides are soluble in water. Monosaccharides can exist in linear form, but pentoses and hexoses usually fold in rings.

- Carbohydrates that are made of two monosaccharides are called disaccharide. The chemical bond that links two monosaccharides is called a **glycosidic bond**. The most important disaccharides are sucrose, a simple table sugar; maltose, a sugar in germinating seeds; and lactose, a sugar in milk. Polysaccharides are the macromolecules formed by polymerization of monosaccharide by a dehydration reaction. Common polysaccharides are starch and cellulose in plants, and glycogen and chitin in animals.

- Proteins have very diverse functions. Structural proteins build and support cellular structures. Extracellular structural proteins support organization of tissues. Enzymes regulate chemical reactions. Transport proteins carry substances. Proteins also play a role as signaling molecules, like the hormones insulin and thyroxin. Immunoglobulins protect organism from pathogens.

- Monomers of proteins are called **amino acids**. There are 20 amino acids that constitute the whole diversity of existing proteins. Animal organisms can synthesize some amino acids, but there is a group of amino acids that cannot be synthesized. These amino acids are called **essential amino acids**, and they have to be received by an organism from food.

- Polymers of amino acids are called **polypeptides**. Polypeptides are made of ten or more amino acids. Protein is a macromolecule containing one or more polypeptides. The sequence of amino acids in a protein molecule is unique and creates a **primary protein structure**. This primary protein structure may be folded in an **alpha helix** or a **beta-pleated sheet**. Both types of folds are created by hydrogen bonds. The alpha helixes and beta-pleated sheets are folded again in a **tertiary structure**, also created and stabilized by hydrogen bonds and ionic interactions inside the polypeptide chain. Proteins, which are made of a few polypeptide chains, have a **quaternary structure**. The quaternary structure is created by special chemical bonds between polypeptides, such as sulfur bridges: – S – S –.

- Fat molecules, or lipids, constitute all membranes of the cell. Lipids also play a significant role as an energy source. A special group of ring-structured lipids called steroids serve as hormones. Cholesterol has a structural role in the organization of cellular membranes. Lipids are classified in two groups: **triglycerides** and **steroids**.

- Triglycerides are made of a **glycerol** and three **fatty acid** molecules. Fatty acid is a carbohydrate molecule with a carboxyl group on one end. Three fatty acids are attached to glycerol by an ether bond through the dehydration synthesis.

- Triglycerides have much fewer oxygen atoms than carbohydrates, and their molecules are not polarized. That makes triglycerides hydrophobic. The length of the carbon chain varies, but usually it has 15 to 18 carbons. Fatty acids where all carbon atoms bind together by a single covalent bond are called **saturated**. Fatty acids that have double covalent bonds between carbon atoms are called unsaturated. Correspondingly, there are saturated and unsaturated fats. A single chemical bond in saturated fatty acid makes this molecule linear. In unsaturated fatty acid, a double bond between two carbon atoms creates a kink. When the carbon atoms next to the carbon atoms connected by a double bond lay on the same side of the double bond, this unsaturated fatty acid is called a **cis isomer**. When the next atoms are on different sides, it is called a **trans isomer**.

- The linear shape of saturated fatty acids allows molecules of saturated fats to come close to each other and make a dense package. At room temperature they are usually solid, like lard. The kink in unsaturated fatty acids does not allow them to be packed densely, and at room temperature they are liquid, like olive oil. Cis fats have kinks in their unsaturated fatty acids exposed on one side of the molecule, which makes this double bond accessible to digestive enzymes. In trans fats the double bond is hidden from digestion by enzymes.

- A special group of triglycerides is called **phospholipids**. In phospholipids one fatty acid is replaced by a **phosphate group** ($-PO_3$). A phosphate group has three atoms of oxygen and is highly polarized. The presence of a polarized group in a nonpolarized molecule makes it amphiphilic: it is hydrophilic on one side (head) and hydrophobic on the other (tail). When mixed with water, phospholipids self-organize in membranous films, in which phospholipid heads bind with water by H-bonds and tails turn away from it.

- Steroids are lipid molecules with four rings of carbons. The most common steroid is cholesterol. It is a precursor to most steroid molecules in the animal body. Cholesterol is also an important element of cellular membranes.

- Nucleic acids store and process genetic information. Monomers of nucleic acids are nucleotides. There are five nucleotides classified in two groups: **purines** and **pyrimidines**. There are two purines: **adenosine** and **guanine**; and three pyrimidines: **cytosine, thymine**, and **uracil**. Every nucleotide has three components: 1) a nitrogenous base, 2) a five-carbon (pentose) sugar, and 3) a phosphate group. The nitrogenous base contains a nitrogen atom, which is strongly electronegative and polarizes the nucleotide molecule. Polarization of the nucleotide facilitates development of hydrogen bonds with other polarized nucleotides. Nucleotides also have other roles. Adenosine triphosphate (ATP) is a major source of energy for most body processes.

- There are two types of nucleic acids: **deoxyribonucleic acid (DNA)** and **ribonucleic acid (RNA)**. DNA consists of two polynucleotide strands held together by hydrogen bonds between nitrogenous bases. The development of hydrogen bonds follows the complementary principle: when a particular purine nucleotide binds only with a particular pyrimidine nucleotide. In this way, adenine (A) binds with thymine (T), and guanine (G) binds cytosine (C). Both DNA strands correspond to each other in that the nucleotide sequence in one strand is complementary to the nucleotide sequence in the other strand.

- The term *RNA* relates to a diverse class of nucleic acids. Their common properties are 1) all RNAs have a single poly-nucleotide strand; 2) in all RNA thymine (T) is replaced by uracil (U); and 3) DNA has deoxyribose sugar, while in RNA it is ribose. RNAs function as messenger molecules between DNA and the cytoplasmic biochemical machinery for proteins' synthesis, transport, and regulatory molecules.

CHECK YOUR KNOWLEDGE

LEVEL 1. CHECK YOUR RECALL

1. Building blocks of organic molecules are known as:
   A. Electrolytes
   B. Polymers
   C. Monomers
   D. Enzymes
   E. Functional groups

2. The monomer of a carbohydrate is:
   A. Fatty acid
   B. Amino acid
   C. Nucleotide
   D. Monosaccharide
   E. Glycerol

3. Select the simplest sugar:
   A. Sucrose
   B. Glycogen
   C. Lactose
   D. Glucose
   E. Starch

4. What is the building block of a lipid?
   A. Glucose
   B. Fatty acid
   C. Glycogen
   D. Nucleotide
   E. Amino acid

5. Water molecules have _____ bonds and because of that create _____ bonds between each other.
   A. ionic/covalent
   B. polar covalent/hydrogen
   C. covalent/ionic
   D. hydrogen/covalent
   E. polar covalent/hydrogen

6. Diffusion of water molecules through a semipermeable membrane is called:
   A. Active transport
   B. Osmosis
   C. Hydrolysis
   D. Filtration
   E. Pinocytosis

7. Which term includes all others in the list?
   A. Monosaccharide
   B. Disaccharide
   C. Starch
   D. Carbohydrate
   E. Polysaccharide

8. Choose the pair of terms that correctly completes this sentence:
   Glucose molecules are to _____ as _____ are to proteins.
   A. carbohydrates; amino acids
   B. amino acids; fatty acids
   C. amino acids; monosaccharides
   D. glycoside linkages; polypeptide bonds
   E. nucleic acids; fatty acids

9. Which of the following is the most abundant inorganic substance in a cell?
   A. Oxygen
   B. Carbon dioxide
   C. Water
   D. Carbohydrates
   E. Proteins

10. Cholesterol is an organic molecule classified as:
    A. Lipid
    B. Protein
    C. Nucleic acid
    D. Carbohydrate
    E. Glycolipid

11. Substances that dissolve in water include all of the following **except**:
    A. Proteins
    B. Salts
    C. Glucose
    D. Nucleic acids
    E. Lipids

12. How do unsaturated fats differ from saturated fats?
    A. Unsaturated fats have two glycerol molecules in their structure, whereas saturated fats have only one.
    B. Unsaturated fats have double bonds between carbon atoms, whereas saturated fats have only single bonds.

13. Neutrons have _____, whereas protons have _____.
    A. no electric charge; positive electric charge
    B. positive electric charge; no electric charge
    C. negative electric charge; positive electric charge
    D. positive electric charge; negative electric charge
    E. no electric charge; negative electric charge

14. Calcium (Ca) has atomic number 20. Calcium has _____ protons and _____ electrons.

    A. 10; 10
    B. 40; 40
    C. 20; 20
    D. 20; 18
    E. 10; 18

15. Oxygen's atomic mass is 16, and its atomic number is 8. An oxygen nucleus has _____ protons and _____ neutrons.

    A. 16; 8
    B. 8; 16
    C. 16; 16
    D. 8; 8
    E. 12; 12

16. Carbon has four valence electrons, and oxygen has six valence electrons. Carbon's valence is _____, and oxygen's valence is _____.

    A. 4; 4
    B. 6; 6
    C. 2; 2
    D. 2; 4
    E. 4; 2

17. True or false: Hydrophobic molecules dissolve in any amount of water.
18. True or false: Saturated fats have double chemical bonds in fatty acids.
19. True or false: Cis fats are much more easily digestible than trans-fat molecules.
20. Match the term with its description:

    _____ Amino acid   a. A weak bond between two polarized molecules
    _____ Monosaccharide   b. A monomer of protein molecules
    _____ Nucleotide   c. A chemical bond formed by shared electrons
    _____ Polymer   d. A building block of polymer molecules
    _____ Monomer   e. A monomer of polysaccharide molecules
    _____ Hydrogen bond   f. A molecule constructed by repeated monomers
    _____ Covalent bond   g. A monomer of nucleic acids

LEVEL 2. CHECK YOUR UNDERSTANDING

1. Explain in your own words why fluorine creates a single ionic bond with potassium.
2. What will happen if protein loses its 3-D shape?
3. Explain why digestion of fat takes much more time and is more complicated than digestion of proteins or carbohydrates.

4. Explain why carbohydrates are hydrophilic, whereas fat molecules are hydrophobic, even though both are made of carbon, hydrogen, and oxygen.

LEVEL 3. APPLY YOUR KNOWLEDGE TO REAL LIFE

1. Can eating or drinking highly acidic food or drink cause acidosis of the blood?
2. Explain the mechanism of maintaining a stable pH of the blood by buffers. Is this homeostatic mechanism based on positive or negative feedback?

Chapter 3

The Cell

Basic Structural Element of Life

LEARNING OBJECTIVES

The cell is a fundamental element of life. All organisms, from bacteria to blue whales, are made of cells. The mammalian body is composed of trillions of cells. An exploration tour inside the cell will help you better understand the primary principles of body organization and function. After reading this chapter, you will understand:

1. The major components of cell structure.

2. The structure and role of cell membranes.

3. The transport of substances across cell membranes.

4. The classification of organelles and their functions.

5. The cytoskeleton and junctions between cells.

6. The major events of cell division.

INTRODUCTION

The cell is a fundamental unit of living organisms. There are trillions of cells classified into more than 600 different cell types. Nevertheless, there are several basic processes common to all cells. These processes are cell metabolism, transport of substances, communication among cells, and cell reproduction.

The complete set of all reactions inside the cell is called **cell metabolism**. Based on the result of chemical reactions, they are classified in three groups: **anabolic**, **catabolic**, and **oxidation-reduction reactions**.

Anabolic reactions are reactions of synthesis resulting in production of more complex molecules than the initial components. Polymerization reactions are anabolic reactions. Synthesis of polysaccharides, polypeptides, triglycerides, and nucleic acids all are anabolic reactions. Polymerization of macromolecules is always a dehydration synthesis reaction accompanied by release of water.

In catabolic reactions, complex macromolecules are degraded to simple components. Chemical bonds that bind monomers into polymers are ruptured, and monomers are released. These reactions are the opposite of dehydration synthesis. The breakdown of chemical bonds is controlled by enzymes. For example, the enzyme amylase catalyzes destruction of glycosidic linkage in polysaccharides. One of the glycosidic linkage covalent bonds that binds an oxygen atom with both carbon rings (see chapter 2, page 33) ruptures and frees one vacant valence in the oxygen atom, which is immediately occupied by hydrogen, and another vacant valence gets a carbon atom in the ring. It binds with the hydroxyl group. Thus, breaking one glycosidic linkage between two monosaccharides requires one water molecule. Catabolic reactions are usually hydrolysis reactions that consume water.

Oxidation-reduction reactions are characterized by transfer (or just a shifting) of electrons from one atom to another. For example, when oxygen binds with two hydrogen atoms, the hydrogens' electrons shift toward oxygen. This transfer of electrons releases energy, because rotating electrons close to oxygen requires less energy to hold them on their orbit than on the orbit close to hydrogen. The creation of ionic bond is also an oxidation-reduction reaction. The released energy may dissipate in the form of heat. That is why many oxidation-reduction reactions are accompanied by a significant increase in temperature. Most oxidation-reduction reactions in a cell are located in the mitochondria. A series of mitochondrion enzymes organizes the flow of electrons from one atom to another, step by step. The last atom that receives these electrons is oxygen, because it is the strongest electronegative element in the cell. Now you understand why living organisms need oxygen. Of course, there are many organisms that receive energy through other chemical reactions without oxygen. But transfer of electrons to oxygen releases maximum energy. Organisms that use oxygen for energy generation have much higher metabolism and more competitive. This chain of reactions is called the electron transport chain. In the electron transport chain, energy is released in small amounts, which increases the efficiency of its conversion into new chemical bonds. The oxidation-reduction reaction between the glucose molecule and oxygen releases a significant amount of energy that accumulates in the molecules of ATP. The ATP molecules are used as a storage site for energy, which they release to activate most processes in the cell.

Every cell has an "infrastructure" for storage and transport of substances inside and outside. This system includes special transport molecules, "railroads" made of cytoskeleton, and membranous vesicles for storage. As a matter of fact, substances inside and outside the cell do not move accidentally by diffusion. They are anchored to membranes or the cytoskeleton and can move only along the surface of these structures. This makes their movement precise and fast.

Every cell "knows" its position in the body and what it has to do. Each cell monitors 1) its own state, 2) the state of the environment, 3) and the state of other cells of the body. The major means through which a cell can do this monitoring are special signaling molecules, such as prostaglandins or hormones, and electrical interactions, such as nerve impulses. All these factors are means of intercellular communication.

Every multicellular organism begins its life from a single cell: an egg fertilized by sperm, called a zygote. Growth and development of an organism is not possible without cell division, which leads to an increase in the total number of cells. Some cells in the body are permanent, and their life span lasts the whole life of the organism. Nerve and cardiac muscle cells belong to this group. On the other hand, there are many cells that have a comparatively short life. For example, epithelial cells that line the stomach survive only a few days and have to be regularly replaced. There are two types of cell division: **mitosis** and **meiosis**. Mitosis is a division characteristic of somatic cells (somatic cells are all cells of the body except gametes: sperm and egg cells). Gametes are produced through meiosis.

CHECK YOUR UNDERSTANDING

- What is the difference between anabolic and catabolic reactions?

- What is the role of oxidation-reduction reactions?

- Why are animals that use oxygen to generate energy dominant on earth?

3.1 Overview of Cell Structure and Function

The Cell—A Fundamental Unit of Life

Studies of living organisms with microscopes in the 18th century showed that the bodies of all organisms, from plants to animals, are made of cells. This discovery was formulated in a most broad and fundamental biological concept called **cellular theory**. Cellular theory states:

1. Only cells, but not subcellular structures, possess all properties characteristic of living organisms.
2. All organisms are made of cells.
3. All cells that exist now originated from preexisting cells.

Chapter 1 discussed levels of organization of living organisms. A cell is constructed of many structural elements: water molecules; a huge diversity of macromolecules that perform multiple tasks in cell organization and function; different membranous, fibrous structural elements; and many organelles, some of which are responsible for protein synthesis, others for energy production, others for intracellular digestion, and so on. But none of these subcellular structures possesses all properties necessary for living organisms to survive, develop, and evolve. Only the cell combines all characteristics of living organisms and makes life on earth possible.

All organisms are made of cells. Even the smallest organisms, like bacteria and protists (amoebas or paramecium), are unicellular organisms, where the organism is a cell. The only exclusion from this rule is viruses. A virus body is a virion: a capsule made of proteins with nucleic acid that carries viral genetic information inside. Viruses lack most properties of living organisms. For example, they do not have their own metabolism and cannot reproduce. For that, they invade a host cell and use its biochemical machinery. Many scientists doubt whether viruses should be counted as living organisms.

All cells in every organism originate from a zygote. All cells of future organisms will contain cells, which will develop from a future zygote. This future zygote will originate from the fusion of sperm and egg cells produced by organisms from a previous generation. There is a continuous chain of cells from generation to generation. In the 18th century, before the development of cell theory, naturalists believed that life spontaneously emerged in a favorable environment. French scientist Felix Pouchet stated that air could cause spontaneous generation of living organisms in liquids. In the late 1850s, he performed experiments and claimed that they were evidence of spontaneous generation. He made a bullion in a chemical flask and left it exposed to air for some time. After a few days the bullion was populated with fungi and bacteria. This event is probably familiar to you. In a series of simple, absolutely decisive, and beautiful classic experiments, Louis Pasteur closed the discussion about spontaneous generation of life. In the first experiment he placed boiled liquid in flasks and let hot air enter the flask. One flask he closed and demonstrated that no organisms grew in it. Another group of flasks he opened and let dust enter. As a result, in some flasks he observed the growth of organisms. He also showed that in flasks that were open at high altitude, organisms grow much slower. This demonstrated that air at high altitudes contains less dust and fewer microorganisms that can contaminate liquid in a flask. In the second series of experiments, Pasteur used swan neck flasks containing a fermentable liquid (fig. 3.1). Air was allowed to enter the flask via a long, curving tubular neck. A long, curved tube stops dust particles from reaching sterile liquid. Nothing grew in the broths unless the flasks were tilted, making the liquid touch the contaminated walls of the neck. This showed that the living organisms that grew in such broths came from outside, on dust, rather than spontaneously generating within the liquid or from the action of pure air. For these experiments in 1862 Pasteur won the Alhumbert Prize from the French Academy of Science. Today the technique of heating food in closed, isolated containers to preserve it is called pasteurization.

Pasteur's experiments demonstrate that no new cells emerge from nonliving matter. However, they do not answer the question of where the first cell came from: a cellular Eve? The theory of the origin of life from nonliving matter is called **abiogenesis**. The transition from nonliving to living entities was not a single event but a gradual process of increasing complexity. In a series of classic experiments in 1952, Miller and Urey demonstrated that most amino acids can be synthesized from inorganic compounds under conditions that existed on prehistoric earth.

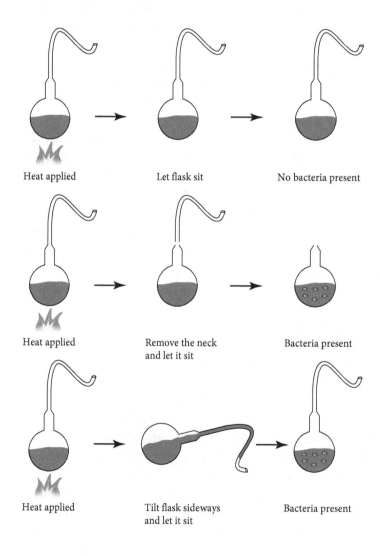

FIGURE 3.1   Louis Pasteur's Experiment.

Cell Diversity

Cells are very diverse in their shape, internal organization, and role in an organism. In the mammalian body there are more than 600 different types of cells. The size of cells varies from 6 to 8 μm in diameter (red blood cells) to 9 cm (many mammalian eggs). The shape of cells is also very diverse and varies from oval or rounded, like adipocytes, to highly branched, like neurons, or very long, like skeletal muscle cells. The structural diversity of cells corresponds to their functional differences based on differences in their metabolisms. These metabolic differences develop together with the organism. After fertilization, the zygote represents the whole organism. The zygote divides, and after a series of divisions it creates a ball of identical cells called blastomeres. The further divisions of blastomeres at some point result in the appearance of cells with different properties. The process that leads to the emergence of cells with different structural organization and different metabolism is called **differentiation**. Segments of DNA called genes contain genetic information. Since all cells in an organism originate from one single zygote, all cells in the organism possess identical genetic makeup. In this situation, how do cells become so different? It happen because 1) every cell in the body "exactly knows" its position and receives complete instructions on what it has to do from the organism; 2) each cell controls its metabolism through activation and inhibition of genes: the phenomenon called **gene expression**; and 3) in different cells, different genes are expressed. For example, adipocyte (a fat-containing cell) has genes for synthesis of hemoglobin (a protein that carries oxygen molecules in red blood cells), but these genes are inhibited (not expressed). On the other hand, adipocyte synthesizes the hormone leptin, which controls appetite. Red blood cells also have a gene that codes production of leptin, but in red blood cells this **db gene** is inactive.

Even being different, all cells share a number of common features. Every cell is surrounded by a semipermeable membrane called the **plasma membrane**, which protects the cell and maintains its integrity and functions. The plasma membrane is only one part of a very complex membranous network. Inside the cell this network creates the so-called **endoplasmic reticulum (ER)**. The ER penetrates through the whole cell body and separates the internal space into compartments. In the center the ER associates with the **nuclear envelope**: a membrane that separates the nucleus from other cell structures. The contents of the cell between the plasma membrane and the nuclear envelope is called **cytoplasm**. Cytoplasm is composed of a liquid medium with varying viscosity called **cytosol** and structural elements called **organelles**. A network of tubular and filamentous threads called the **cytoskeleton** is responsible for cell shape maintenance and transport of substances (fig. 3.2).

CHECK YOUR UNDERSTANDING

- What process leads to the development of differences among cells of the body?

- Name three major components of an animal cell.

- What constitutes cytoplasm?

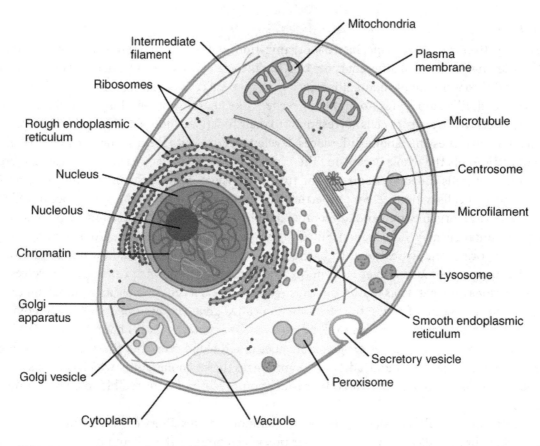

FIGURE 3.2   A Generalized Model of an Animal Cell.

3.2   Overview of Cell Structure

The Plasma Membrane (Phospholipid Bilayer; Fluid Mosaic Model of the Plasma Membrane)

The plasma membrane is the phospholipid bilayer that surrounds a cell. Its organization and role are a perfect illustration of the relationship between form and function. The plasma membrane separates the cell's interior from the external environment. It protects and secures cell integrity. At the same time, through the plasma membrane the cell receives all necessary nutrients and oxygen for cellular respiration, removes waste materials and carbon dioxide, and communicates with other cells in the organism.

Two major components make the plasma membrane: phospholipids and proteins. Phospholipid molecules are amphiphilic (see chapter 2, page 38). They have two regions, which have a different "attitude" toward water molecules. Their fatty acid tails are hydrophobic and avoid any contact with water molecules, whereas their heads contain a phosphate group and are hydrophilic; that is, they "love" to create hydrogen bonds with water molecules. Thanks to these properties, phospholipid molecules demonstrate the phenomenon of self-organization in water. They create two types of structures in water solutions: 1) micelle and 2) bilayer membranes (fig. 3.3).

Dipole water molecules create hydrogen bonds among each other. Polar molecules like glucose easily break down hydrogen bonds between water molecules and establish new hydrogen bonds between themselves and water molecules. That is why these molecules easily dissolve in water. Nonpolar hydrophobic molecules do not create hydrogen bonds with other molecules at all. They cannot break hydrogen bonds between water molecules and create their own hydrogen bonds. That is why water molecules that are connected to each other by hydrogen bonds eject nonpolar molecules. When amphiphilic phospholipid molecules contact water, they turn in such a way that their polarized heads create hydrogen bonds with bipolar water molecules and keep their hydrophobic tails away. This is possible in two cases:1) when phospholipids create a bubble with the heads oriented out toward water and tails hidden from water inside the bubble; 2) when phospholipids organize in a bilayer with the heads looking outside and have contact with water and the tails hidden from water inside

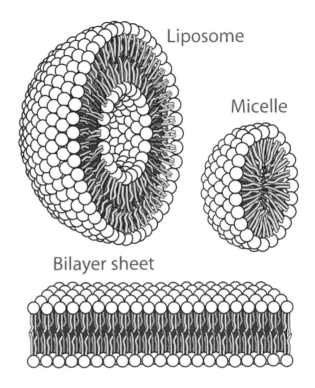

FIGURE 3.3   Micelle, Liposome or Lipoprotein Complex (Lpc), and Bilayer Membrane Created by Phospholipid Molecules in Water Solutions.

two layers, like in a sandwich. Alternatively to the formation of a micelle or bilayer, phospholipids can create a monolayer film at the air-water border, with the phospholipid heads toward the water, and the fatty acid tails faced toward air.

In a bilayer phospholipid, molecules can move only horizontally and cannot flip-flop from one layer to the other. For such a layer change, a phospholipid molecule has to turn and its head has to break hydrogen bonds with water molecules. At the same time, its hydrophobic tail has to turn toward water. Both events for a phospholipid molecule are hardly possible, and phospholipid molecules move only inside the same layer. The ability of phospholipid molecules to move generates the phenomenon of membrane fluidity. Membrane fluidity depends on the type of fatty acids that constitute the phospholipid molecules. Saturated fats with straight fatty acid tails, as a rule, are packed more densely than unsaturated fats. As a result, membranes that contain more unsaturated fats have a higher fluidity than membranes dominated by saturated fats. The fluidity of the membrane is an important characteristic. The fluidity identifies The plasma membrane's permeability for substances. The membrane with unsaturated fats is leaky and permits substances to pass through more easily. The membrane with saturated fats is much denser and usually is less permeable (fig. 3.4). Cholesterol easily penetrates the phospholipid bilayer and, like other fat molecules, occupies space among hydrophobic fatty acid tails. It increases membrane fluidity. Cholesterol plays an important role in the control of plasma membrane permeability.

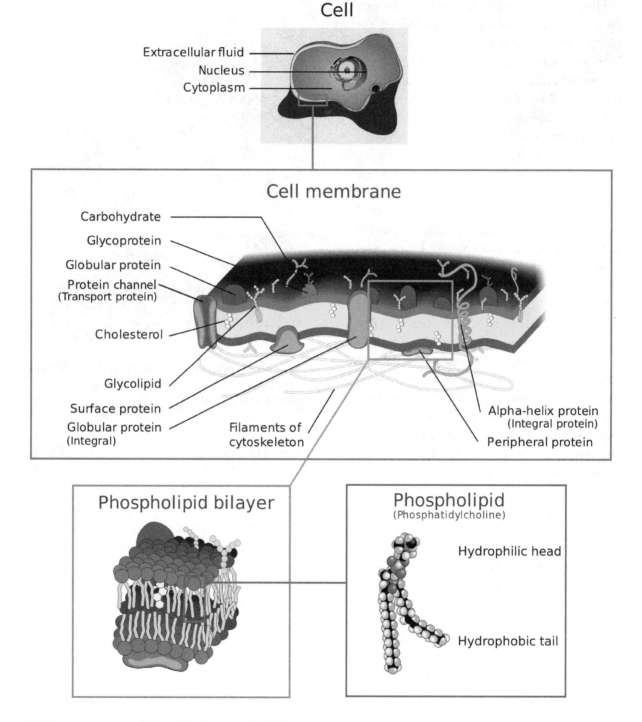

FIGURE 3.4   Permeability of the Phospholipid Bilayer.

It is obvious that the phospholipid bilayer creates an impermeable barrier for big macromolecules such as proteins and polysaccharides. Small inorganic molecules have more chance to pass through this membrane, but ions and polarized molecules, like water, cannot penetrate the hydrophobic internal layer. Only small and electrically neutral molecules, like molecules of oxygen or carbon dioxide, can pass easily. For transport of ions, electrically charged, and big organic molecules there are special transport proteins built into the phospholipid bilayer.

Proteins are the second component of cell membranes, especially the plasma membrane. Proteins are responsible for transporting substances across membranes. Special proteins that create reversible chemical bonds with signaling molecules, such as hormones and prostaglandins, are called **receptor proteins**. Proteins on the plasma membrane surface participate in intercellular connections and self-recognition. Depending on their type and role in construction of the plasma membrane, all proteins are divided into two classes: **transmembrane** or **integral proteins** and **peripheral proteins**. Integral proteins penetrate through both phospholipid layers and are as exposed inside as outside of the cell. Peripheral proteins occupy a position from one or the other side of the membrane. Protein molecules are scattered over the phospholipid bilayer. In some areas of the plasma membrane, the population of proteins may be dense, whereas in other areas there may be very few proteins. Together with phospholipid molecules, proteins are in constant motion. Because the plasma membrane is made as a mosaic of phospholipids and proteins that are constantly in motion, the model that describes the organization of the plasma membrane is called the **fluid mosaic model** (fig. 3.5).

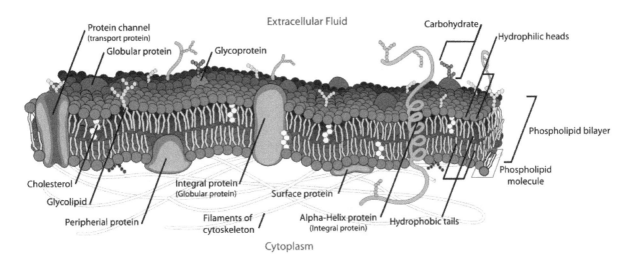

FIGURE 3.5   Fluid Mosaic Model of the Plasma Membrane.

Transport across the Plasma Membrane

Only small and nonpolar molecules, like oxygen and carbon dioxide, can easily pass the plasma membrane. The movement of these molecules across the plasma membrane follows a simple rule of diffusion: these molecules move from a place of high concentration to a place where their concentration is lower.

Ions and polarized and big molecules cannot cross the membrane. They need special pathways or tunnels to cross the plasma membrane from one side to the other. A group of integral proteins called **channel proteins** plays the role of these pathways. Some channel proteins are like tunnels. They simply permit molecules to pass through the membrane. **Aquaporin** is an example of such a protein. An aquaporin molecule has a canal that exactly fits the size and shape of water molecules. Thus, dipole water molecules can come inside and outside of the cell through channels made of aquaporin molecules. The movement of water through this channel is similar to a simple diffusion. Aquaporin facilitates diffusion of water molecules. This type of diffusion is called **facilitated diffusion**. Both simple and facilitated diffusion take place by themselves where there is an inequality in the concentration of molecules. Application of energy is not required for molecules' movement. For that reason, this movement of substances across the plasma membrane is called **passive transport**. In passive transport, substances can move in both directions by following their gradient of concentration. Because channel proteins for passive transport facilitate the movement of molecules all the time and in both directions, they also are called **leaking channels**.

Another type of substances movement across the plasma membrane is called **active transport**. Active transport requires energy to move substances from one side of membrane to the other side. Passive transport happens by itself without the cell spending energy, and you may compare it with a wheel rolling or with water flowing down a hill. Active transport needs energy and may be compared with movement up the hill. In active transport, a substance creates weak reversible chemical bonds with the transport protein. When chemical bonds are created, the transport protein changes its confirmation (a 3-D shape) and the substance occurs on the other side of the membrane (fig. 3.6). After changing confirmation chemical bonds with substance breakdown, the substance is released and the transport protein returns to its original confirmation, ready to bind again with another substance molecule.

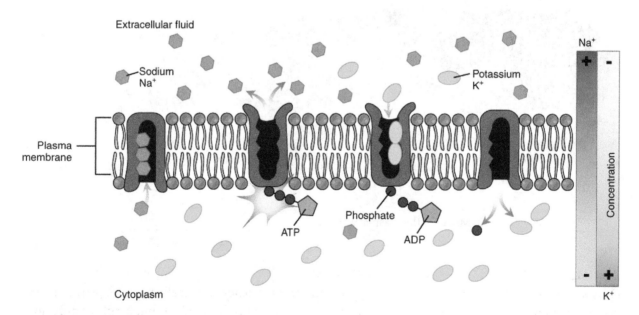

FIGURE 3.6   Active Transport across the Plasma Membrane.

Active transport does not depend on the concentration of transported molecules and may be continued even if the concentration of the substance on the side where it is transported is much higher. Thus, when passive transport equalizes molecules' concentration across the membrane, active transport increases the difference in substance concentration across the membrane. Active transport proteins are often called **pumps**, because like pumps, they move substances "against their will" from a place with low concentration to a place with high concentration.

A classic example of such a protein is a **sodium-potassium ATP-dependent pump**. You probably already have an idea what this pump does—it pumps ions of sodium and potassium across the membrane, and to be able to do that, it uses ATP molecules as an energy source. The sodium-potassium pump transports sodium ions out of the cell and potassium ions inside the cell. The Na^+/K^+ pump creates unequal distribution of these ions across the plasma membrane: the concentration of Na^+ outside the cell may become ten times higher than inside the cell. At the same time, the concentration of K^+ inside the cell may be seven times higher than outside.

There are three types of pumps: **uniports**, **simports**, and **antiports**. Uniports are pumps that drive a single substance across the membrane in one direction. An example of this uniport transport is the calcium (Ca^{2+}) pump in muscle cells. Simports move two or more substances together across the membrane in the same direction. This way, for example, cells drive molecules of glucose inside together with Na^+. Antiport pumps drive two or more substances together through the membrane in opposite directions, as already described for the Na^+/K^+ pump. Transport of two or more substances across the plasma membrane is also called **cotransport** (fig. 3.7).

Transport proteins are very effective in driving selective molecules and ions across the plasma membrane, but they are limited by the size or amount of transported material. Transport proteins cannot drive very big macromolecules or a large amount of organic material. For transporting a large amount of material or a solid organic body—for example, bacteria—a cell uses special membranous vesicles called **endosomes**. The walls of endosomes are made of phospholipid bilayers similar to the plasma membrane. They easily incorporate in the plasma membrane or separate from it. The membrane surrounds the area that contains a large amount of materials or an organic body and drives the vesicle inside or outside the cell. The vesicular transport inside the cell is called **endocytosis**. Transport outside the cell is called **exocytosis**. Both types of the vesicular transport are classified in three groups: **phagocytosis**, **pinocytosis**, and **receptor-mediated transport**.

Endocytosis. Phagocytosis is a process of ingesting of big chunks of food or a pathogenic organism, like bacteria. A group of white blood cells called phagocytes specialize in ingesting pathogen agents or damaged and dead cells. When a phagocyte contacts with, for example, bacteria, receptor proteins in the plasma

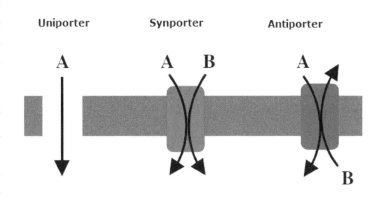

FIGURE 3.7 Three Types of Pump Transport Mechanisms.

membrane bind with antigen molecules on the bacteria surface. The wall around the contact area extends and embraces the bacteria. The membranous extensions are called **pseudopodia**. Pseudopodia merge and enclose bacteria inside the membranous vesicle. The vesicle detaches from the plasma membrane and drives inside the cell, where bacteria will be digested by proteolytic enzymes from a special organelle called a **lysosome**.

Pinocytosis is a process of ingesting liquid droplets. Liquid that fills the space between cells is called **interstitial fluid**. Solute molecules dissolved in interstitial fluid bind with receptor proteins in a shallow groove on the surface of the plasma membrane. The creation of chemical bonds among solute and receptors causes an increase of groove fold inside the cell. The borders of the fold fuse, and a vesicle with enclosed fluid pinches from the plasma membrane and drives inside the cell. Inside the cell, the vesicle fuses with another vesicle called an **endosome**. In the endosome, substances in fluid are sorted and modified for further processing.

VETERINARY APPLICATION

Hereditary Spherocytosis. Hereditary spherocytosis (HS) is an autosomal dominant form of hemolytic anemia. The disease is characterized by an abnormal spherical shape of red blood cells and increased permeability to sodium ions. These abnormalities result from the defects in the erythrocyte plasma membrane protein spectrin, which normally supports and stabilizes the phospholipid bilayer. Red blood cells progressively lose membrane when they circulate through the narrow capillary system of the spleen. Depleted of membrane, the cells become spherical. Spherocytes have a diameter approximately two-thirds the diameter of normal red blood cells. Spherocytes with multiple defects are easily destroyed by an animal's immune system. As a result, the animal develops hemolytic anemia. Anemia may be mild, moderate, severe, or not present at all. Severe hemolytic anemia requires animal hospitalization and red blood cell transfusions. The animal will have an enlarged spleen. In golden retrievers, the disease is inherited. Nonhereditary spherocytosis can be caused by genetic mutations, nutritional deficiencies, or toxins such as acetaminophen, methylene blue, daily intravenous injections of propofol in cats, phenothiazines, and dried red maple leaves. The overall mortality rate associated with spherocytosis is high: approximately 50 percent.

Receptor-mediated endocytosis is similar in many ways to pinocytosis. It consists of selective transport of particular substances; cholesterol or iron, for example. The substance of interest binds with the receptor protein, located in a protein-coated pit. The development of chemical bonds between the receptor protein and the target substance causes an increase in pit depth. Its borders fuse and create vesicle pinches from plasma membrane. The freed vesicle fuses with the endosome for further processing (fig. 3.8).

Exocytosis is a vesicular transport from a cell. In general, exocytosis may be regarded as the reverse of the endocytosis process. The substances that have to be removed or released are enclosed in the endosome. The endosome drives toward the plasma membrane. The endosome membrane fuses with plasma membrane and substance occurs outside the cell.

A special transport that consists of endocytosis and exocytosis together, when the substance first drives inside and then outside of the cell, is called **transcytosis**. For example, oxygen is processed in red blood cells through transcytosis. At the first step of the process, it incorporates in the hemoglobin molecule. The second step consists of releasing oxygen into the interstitial fluid.

Endocytosis

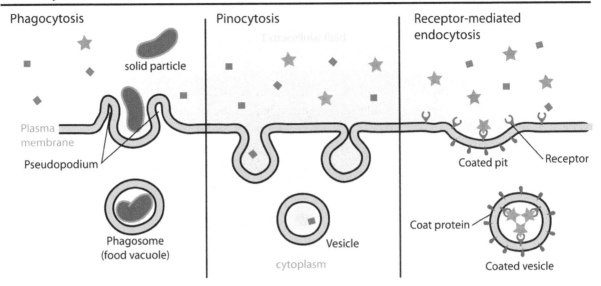

FIGURE 3.8   Three Types of Endocytosis.

Often, cells have extensions of the plasma membrane. Depending on their length and function, extensions are classified in three groups: **microvilli**, **cilia**, and **flagella**. Microvilli are characteristic of cells that specialize in absorption, such as epithelia cells in the small intestine or kidney. Microvilli are short extensions that increase the surface area of the plasma membrane of these cells up to 40 times. Cilia are much longer than microvilli. Inside, cilia contain a cytoskeleton associated with motor proteins. This organization of cilia makes them moveable. Cilia movement has many functions, depending on the type of cell. In respiratory epithelium and vas deferens cilia, movement facilitates sweeping of mucous from respiratory canals and propels sperm cells toward the exit. Structurally, flagella are very similar to cilia. Both contain a ring of nine pairs of microtubules surrounding two central microtubules. Both move via motor protein actions. In vertebrates, flagella are found only in sperm cells, where the flagella drive sperm to meet the egg.

CHECK YOUR UNDERSTANDING

- How do phospholipids organize in water solutions? Explain why.

- List the five major functions of plasma membrane proteins.

- What do diffusion and facilitated diffusion have in common? How are they different?

- Explain the difference between phagocytosis and receptor-mediated transport.

Organelles

An organelle is a structure in cytoplasm that is specialized on a particular function. Organelles are classified in two groups: 1) organelles enclosed in membrane: mitochondria or membrane-bound organelles (endoplasmic reticulum, lysosomes, and peroxisomes); and 2) organelles not enclosed in membrane, or non-membrane-bound organelles (ribosomes and centrosomes).

The **endoplasmic reticulum** is one continuous membranous network made of a phospholipid bilayer. It is continuous with the plasma membrane on one side and the nuclear envelope on the other. The membrane encloses a fluid-filled space called the **ER lumen**. The first electron microscope studies of the endoplasmic reticulum demonstrated that there are two types of membranes on electron images. One type of membranes has a wavy rough surface, and the other type of has a flat, smooth surface. The system of endoplasmic reticulum membranes with a wavy surface is called the **rough endoplasmic reticulum (RER)**. The system of ER membranes with a flat surface is called the **smooth endoplasmic reticulum (SER)** (fig. 3.9). It was found that the RER surface is rough because of ribosomes attached to the membrane.

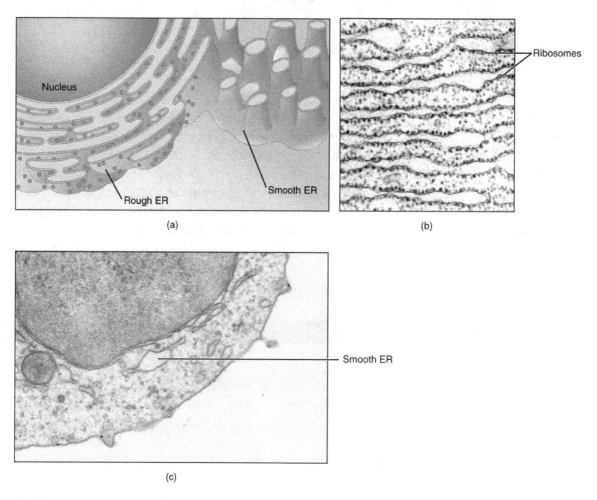

FIGURE 3.9   Endoplasmic Reticulum.

Smooth endoplasmic reticulum has no ribosomes, and its surface remains smooth. When it was discovered that ribosomes are the organelles responsible for protein synthesis, it was concluded that for synthesis of proteins, ribosomes have to attach to the RER. Now it is known that there are active ribosomes that do not associated with the RER. However, it is true that the RER is a major area for protein synthesis. The intensity of RER development is a good sign of metabolic activity of the cell. The RER lumen contains proteins called **chaperons**. Ribosomes on the surface of the RER bind amino acids in polypeptide chains; that is, create a primary protein structure. Functionally active protein has to be folded into tertiary and quaternary structures. Chaperons fold polypeptide chains into functionally active proteins. A new polypeptide chain synthesized by ribosomes is transported into the RER lumen, where chaperon designs the protein's final shape.

For a long time it was believed that the SER, as far as it has no connection with ribosomes, is an inactive part of the ER. Later it was found that the SER is very active and performs many vital functions. The SER is a place for synthesis of lipids, phospholipids, cholesterol, and steroids. Cells that are responsible for the synthesis of these compounds as a rule have a very developed SER. Another vital SER function is cell detoxification. It collects various toxins, drugs, and harmful substances, and before removing them from the organism, converts them into less harmful compounds. Studies show that in a situation of drug abuse, the size of the SER increases more than two times above the norm. Hepatocytes—cells of the liver that play a primary role in detoxification of an organism from drugs—as a rule have a very intensively developed SER. Some specialized cells, like skeletal and cardiac muscle cells, use SER lumen for Ca^{2+} storage. The SER lumen of these cells is enlarged and called a **cisterna**.

The **Golgi apparatus** is another membranous network located between the RER and the rest of the cytoplasm. It consists of a system of flattened and piled membranous sacs. The sacs are separated from each other and from the ER. Internally, they are filled with cytosol. Every sac has its own particular role. The Golgi apparatus receives new, just-synthesized proteins from the RER packed in endosomes. In the Golgi apparatus, these proteins are stored, modified for use, and labeled for further transport to their destination. Thus, the Golgi apparatus plays the role of the storage and shipping department of the cell (fig. 3.10).

Mitochondria are organelles surrounded by two membranes. The outer membrane is smooth. The inner membrane is very extensively folded. The folds of inner membrane are called **cristae**. Cristae significantly increase the total surface of the inner membrane and contain a system of special proteins collectively carrying the **electron transport chain**—an essential part of **oxidation-phosphorylation reactions**, a type of oxidation-reduction reaction. The goal of these reactions is to release energy from carbohydrates' chemical bonds and accumulates it in ATP molecules. These reactions are only a part of the process called **cellular respiration**. Cellular respiration is a principal mechanism of energy production in the cell. Cellular respiration can be divided into two steps. The first step takes place in the cytoplasm. It is called **anaerobic respiration** because it proceeds without oxygen. The second step takes place in mitochondria and is called **aerobic respiration**. This step proceeds only in the presence of oxygen, which plays the role of the electrons' acceptor (see oxidation-reduction reactions, page 64). That is why the mitochondrion is often also called the "power plant" of the cell (fig. 3.11).

Mitochondria have unique properties. The outer membrane structurally is very similar to a bacterial cellular wall. Mitochondria have their own DNA organized in a ring, like it is organized in bacteria. Thanks to DNA, mitochondria reproduce by themselves independent from cellular division. All these

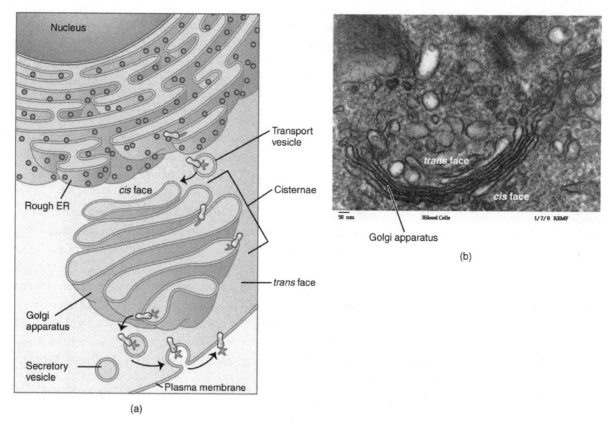

(a)

(b)

FIGURE 3.10   Golgi Apparatus.

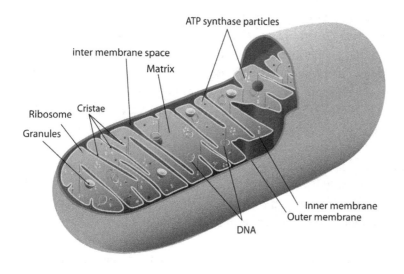

FIGURE 3.11   Mitochondrion.

specific characteristics suggest to scientists that originally mitochondria were independent living organisms like bacteria. This led to the development a **theory of symbiogenesis**, according to which eukaryotic cells originally had no mitochondria. At the beginning of evolution, mitochondria were bacteria, which tend to parasitize on eukaryotic cells. This parasitism was not severe, and the host cell had a good chance of surviving. With time, eukaryotic cells learned how to get benefits from parasitic mitochondria. They learned to provide parasitic mitochondria with monosaccharides and receive from them energy stored in ATP molecules. On that step of mutual evolution (so-called coevolution), the relationship among mitochondria and host cells was changed from parasitism to symbiosis. Finally, this symbiotic relationship became so strong and important for both partners that nowadays neither of them can survive without the other. This theory found support among scientists, and now the origin of some other organelles—chloroplasts, for example—is explained as a result of symbiogenesis (fig. 3.12).

Lysosomes are membrane-bounded organelles. They are sacs that contain very strong enzymes that can degrade all organic molecules. The membranous wall of lysosome holds these enzymes inside the lysosome and does not allow the enzymes to go out into the cytosol, where they can create serious damage to the cell. The principal functions of lysosomes are intracellular digestion of nutrients and degrading of pathogenic invaders and dam-

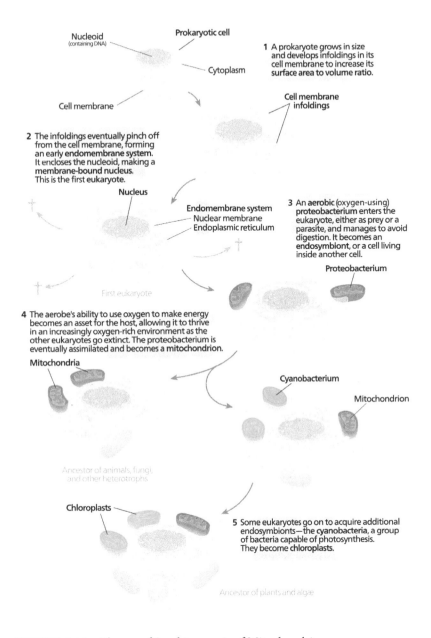

FIGURE 3.12   Theory of Symbiogenesis of Mitochondria.

aged cellular structures. Lysosome enzymes are active only in an acidic environment. That is why the pH of fluid inside the lysosome is around 5.0. If damaged lysosome spills its enzymes into the cytosol, whose pH is 7.2, the enzymes lose their activity. The nutrients are delivered inside the cell inside endosomes through the endocytosis. When the endosome appears inside the cell, lysosome approaches it. Membranes of the food vacuole and lysosome fuse, and enzymes of lysosome mix with nutrients inside the endosome.

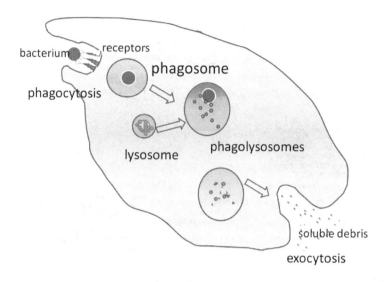

FIGURE 3.13   Phagocytosis.

The macromolecules of the food break down to monomer molecules. Monomers cross the membrane of the food vacuole into the cytosol and may be reused for synthesis of new molecules (fig. 3.13).

Peroxisomes got their name from the major reaction they perform. They oxidize and strip hydrogen off certain organic molecules to produce hydrogen peroxide (H_2O_2). Hydrogen peroxide then is used for:

1. Oxidizing toxic substances, such as alcohol and drugs. Oxidation reactions convert toxic compounds into less toxic compounds for their further removal from the body. That is why peroxisomes are very numerous in liver and kidney cells, which carry a major burden in removing toxins from an organism.
2. Breaking down fatty acids. Most such breakdown reactions take place in the peroxisomes. The products of these reactions are simple sugars. They are transported into cytosol and used in synthesis of new fatty acids or as a fuel in oxidation-phosphorylation reactions in mitochondria for production of ATP molecules.
3. Participating in synthesis of phospholipids. Phospholipids are essential components of all membranous structures of the cell.

VETERINARY APPLICATION

Metabolic Enzyme Deficiency. Metabolic enzyme deficiencies cause specific lysosomal storage diseases. The type of disease depends on which lysosome enzyme a dog loses. The absence of a particular enzyme in lysosome results in the cell's inability to digest specific molecules, and these molecules begin to accumulate. Accumulation of substances in the cell changes the osmotic pressure in cytoplasm. The cell swells, loses normal functions, and may burst. Genetic metabolic enzyme deficiencies manifest soon after birth. Lysosomal storage diseases progress rapidly, and affected dogs usually die between four and six months of age, as there is no cure. **Ceroid lipofuscinosis** is caused by the lack of an enzyme that breaks down lipids. Lipids accumulate in nerve cells and organs such as the spleen, liver, and kidneys. It affects border collies, chihuahuas, cocker spaniels, dachshunds, English setters and salukis. Specific symptoms include diminished eyesight, behavioral changes, dementia, seizures, and ataxia (loss of muscle coordination).

Ribosomes are non-membrane-bounded organelles. They are tiny structure consisting of two subunits. Each unit is a complex assemblage of proteins and a so-called ribosomal RNA (rRNA). When they are inactive, ribosomal subunits are separated from each other, but in the presence of the messenger RNA (mRNA) that delivers genetic information about protein construction, they organize into a protein synthesizing complex. Active ribosomes may exist in two forms: bound with RER or free form floating in cytosol. Bounded ribosomes synthesize proteins that are used by other membrane-bounded organelles, such as lysosomes, peroxisomes, or mitochondria, or participate in organization of cellular membranes. Free ribosomes synthesize proteins that mostly are used in cytosol (fig. 3.14).

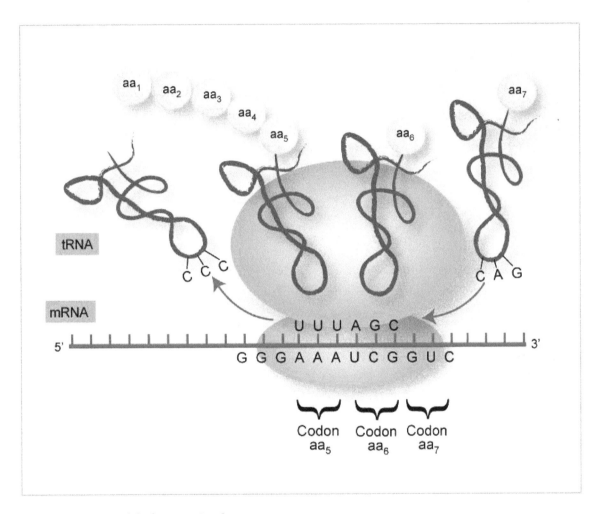

FIGURE 3.14   Model of Protein Synthesis.

The Cytoskeleton

The cytoskeleton consists of three principal types of protein assembles: **actin filaments**, **microtubules**, and **intermediate filaments**. The cytoskeleton runs through the cytoplasm from the nuclear envelope to the plasma membrane. The cytoskeletal matrix is a dynamic structure capable of rapid growth or disassembly, depending on the cell's requirements at a certain point in time (fig. 3.15).

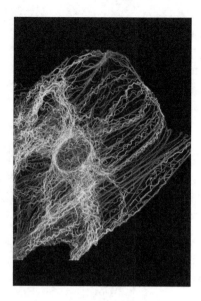

FIGURE 3.15   Cytoskeleton of Fibroblast.

Actin filaments were discovered in muscle cells, where they are responsible for cell contraction. Later it was found that actin is an inalienable part of all cells and constitutes 5 to 30 percent of the total protein in a cell. The actin molecules in nonmuscle cells is different from that found in skeletal muscle. There are six forms of actin found in animal cells. Actin filaments are the principal element of muscle cells' contractile mechanism. In nonmuscle cells, actin filaments are responsible for contraction, as in the myoepithelial cells of lactiferous tubules of the mammary glands. During cell division, in cytokinesis of the telophase, an actin contractile ring forms a cleavage furrow. The ring contracts and (like a belt fastened tightly around the waist) forms a deep groove between two cells. The process of cell division is finished when the cleavage furrow separates into two daughter cells. In fibroblasts, actin filaments create stress fibers that counteract external forces that pull apart body tissues and, thus, protect the organism's integrity.

VETERINARY APPLICATION

Duchenne Muscular Dystrophy. Duchenne muscular dystrophy (DMD) is a hereditary disease caused by a recessive mutation in the X chromosome. Golden and Labrador retrievers, German short-haired pointers, Weimaraners, and corgis are at risk. The location of the mutated gene on the X chromosome means that male dogs inherit the disease from mothers. Female dogs usually are carriers but also can have the disease if they are homozygous on this mutation. Mutation results in an abnormal structure of the transmembrane protein dystrophin. This protein links the extracellular matrix to actin molecules within the cytoskeleton. The abnormal dystrophin does not complete this transmembrane linkage. Membrane stability fails, and muscle fiber develops necrosis.

Dogs with DMD have progressive muscle weakening starting at about eight weeks of age. Symptoms can range from a change in the dog's gait to widespread muscle atrophy, and include thickening of the tongue, coughing spasms, difficulty swallowing, poor growth, general weakness, skeletal muscle atrophy, slow heart rate, pelvic limb weakness, and loss of appetite. There hasn't been much help available for dogs with DMD. It is considered a fatal disease. Less than half of affected dogs live beyond six weeks of age. Dogs with DMD shouldn't be bred, which isn't a problem, since affected dogs usually do not reach reproductive age. All dogs that carry this mutation and their offspring should be sterilized to prevent further transmission of this hereditary disease.

Intermediate filaments (IFs) primarily play a structural role. IFs create a frame that resists and protects from mechanical stress placed on the cell. IFs are essential elements of Z disks of adjacent myofibrils in skeletal muscle cell. Special connections between epithelial cells called desmosomes also contain IFs. In opposition to actin microfilaments and microtubules, IFs are composed of heterogeneous monomers.

Microtubules are polymers composed of the protein tubulin. Tubulin is a dimer of two monomers: α- and β-tubulin. Microtubules have a variety of functions. Microtubules make the internal frame of cilia of ciliated epithelial cells and fla-gellum of sperm cell. Microtubules are part of the mitotic and meiotic spindle apparatus responsible for chromosomes' movement. They also constitute the inter-cellular transport system. Ribosomes and membrane-bound organelles, as a matter of fact, do not freely float in cytosol. All of them are attached to microtubules. This attachment facilitates organelles' location, activity, and transport (fig. 3.16).

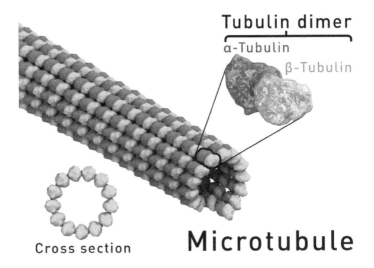

FIGURE 3.16   Microtubules.

The Nucleus

The nucleus is the biggest organelle in the cell. It contains chromosomes that carry genetic information. The nucleus is sepa-rated from the rest of the cell by a **nuclear envelope**. The nuclear envelope is continuous with the ER and consists of a phospholipid bilayer and special proteins. A large protein complex in the nuclear envelope creates so-called **nuclear pores**. Nuclear pores are tunnels designed for transport of giant macromolecules such as mRNA from the nucleus, where they are synthesized, to the cytoplasm, where they are used for protein synthesis. Inside, the nuclear envelop is filled with a fluid called the **nucleoplasm** (fig. 3.17).

Genetic information is coded by the sequence of nucleotides in DNA. A sequence of three nucleotides, or a trip-let, corresponds to one amino acid in a polypeptide chain. A sequence of triplets that carries a complete information about the primary structure of protein molecule is called a **gene**. This classic definition of the gene as a piece of DNA that codes pro-tein's primary structure was expressed in a popular molecular genetics statement: **One gene—one protein**. This definition, as a matter of fact, has many exclusions and is rarely cited nowadays. For example, proteins with a quaternary organization, such as hemoglobin, are made of few polypeptide chains (hemoglobin is made of four polypeptide chains: two α- and two β-globin chains). Each polypeptide

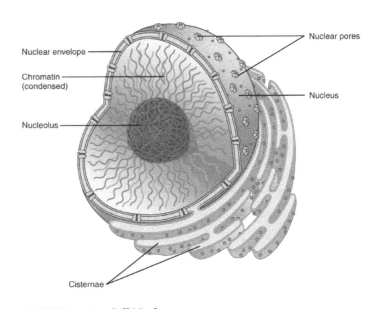

FIGURE 3.17   Cell Nucleus.

chain of these proteins has its own gene. So hemoglobin protein is coded by two genes. On the other hand, immunoglobulins are very diverse proteins, but all are coded by a comparatively smaller number of genes. The diversity of these proteins results from processes of reorganization of the nucleotide sequences in mRNA molecules. The original immunoglobulin mRNA is cut into many pieces, and then these pieces are bound together in varying sequences. Genes are just a small piece of a DNA molecule. As a rule, they have a very particular location on DNA, which is called a **locus**. DNA molecules associate with a number of different proteins. Some of these proteins play a structural role. They create a frame for spatial packaging of DNA molecules. The other proteins control and regulate DNA transcription, or repair damage. The complex of a DNA molecule with structural and regulatory proteins is called **chromatin**. Chromatin makes up chromosomes (fig. 3.18). Different species have different set of chromosomes. All cells in the body of a sexually reproducing organisms have two sets of chromosomes. One set of chromosomes came from the mother, and the other set from the father. Thus, every chromosome with a particular set of genes on the particular loci from the mother has a partner chromosome with exactly the same set of genes at the same loci from the father. These pairs of chromosomes are called **homologous chromosomes**.

A functionally active nucleus usually has one or more small, rounded dark bodies called **nucleoli** (single **nucleolus**). A nucleolus is not a solid body. It is just an area in the nucleus with a highly concentrated aggregate of proteins, DNA, and RNA. It is a factory of ribosome synthesis. Ribosomes have two subunits: one large and one small. The nucleolus is the place where these subunits are produced. They are produced separately and in this decomposed state transported to the cytoplasm through the nuclear pores.

The process of protein synthesis is divided into three principal steps: **transcription**, mRNA transport and processing, and **translation**:

$$\text{DNA} \xrightarrow{\textbf{Transcription}} \text{RNA} \xrightarrow{\textbf{Translation}} \text{protein}$$

Transcription is a process of copying the nucleotide sequence in a gene into the nucleotide sequence of mRNA. The genetic code of the DNA is similar to RNA, except DNA thymine is replaced by uracil in

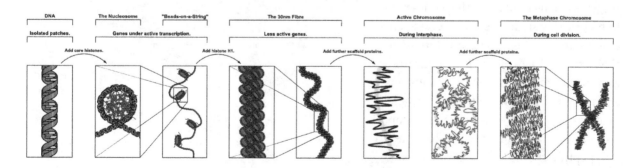

FIGURE 3.18   Chromatin and Chromosomes.

RNA (see chapter 2, page 52). The nucleotide sequence from a DNA molecule is rewritten (transcribed) into the nucleotide sequence of the mRNA. A special protein RNA polymerase synthesizes mRNA by copying a DNA strand. Only one DNA strand is copied. This strand is called the template strand. To begin synthesis of mRNA, RNA polymerase has to "know" what gene has to be copied, where to begin, and where to end copying of the gene. A special complex of proteins called transcription factors controls the process of gene copying. Transcription factors bind to a special sequence of nucleotides on the DNA template strand called the promotor. A protein helicase unwinds the double helix DNA molecule and exposes the template strand for copying. RNA polymerase "recognizes" transcription factors and binds to their proteins and to the DNA sequence following the promotor. This step of transcription is called transcription initiation.

After RNA polymerase creates chemical bonds with the initial sequence of nucleotides of the gene, it catches nucleotides that freely float in nucleoplasm and catalyzes formation of hydrogen bonds between complementary nucleotides and the template strand. Nucleotides of a new molecule of RNA polymerase are bound together by covalent bonds. RNA polymerase moves along the template strand and one by one adds nucleotides, binds them by hydrogen bonds to the complementary nucleotides on the DNA template strand, and creates covalent bonds to bind nucleotides in a new strand. This step of transcription is called elongation.

Elongation continues until the RNA polymerase reaches a special triplet at the end of the gene that functions as the landmark of the gene end. This sequence is named the terminator. When the RNA polymerase reaches the terminator, it detaches from the DNA and releases a finished single strand of pre-mRNA molecule. This last step is called termination. Thus, transcription proceeds in three steps: initiation, elongation, and termination (fig. 3.19).

Eukaryotic genes have a very complex organization. In addition to the promotor at the beginning and terminator at the end, they have inclusions of nucleotide sequences that do not carry information about protein structure. These "senseless" sequences are called introns, as opposed to informative regions of the gene called exons. Introns are transcribed together with other nucleotides into pre-mRNA and have to be removed from pre-mRNA before using it for protein synthesis. The process of removal of senseless introns is called mRNA processing. It includes cutting pre-mRNA at both ends of all introns, removing introns, and binding (splicing) remained exons by covalent bonds (fig. 3.20).

Translation got its name by analogy with translation from one language to another; for example, from English to Spanish. In biochemical translation, the language based on the alphabet of nucleotides is translated into the language based on the amino acid sequences. Processed mRNA is transported from

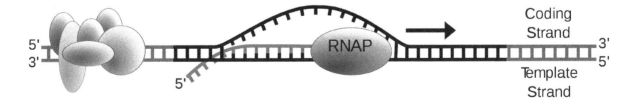

FIGURE 3.19   Transcription.

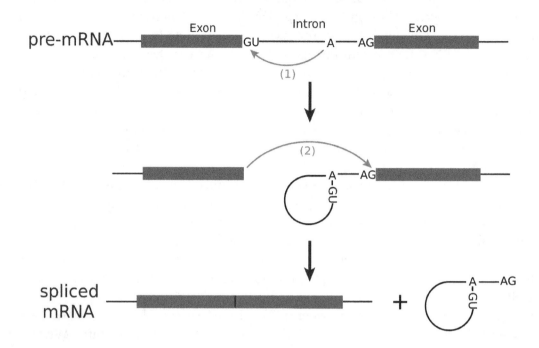

FIGURE 3.20   mRNA Processing.

the nucleus through the pores in the nuclear envelop to the cytoplasm. In cytoplasm mRNA associates with a large ribosome subunit. After that, a complex of mRNA and the large ribosome subunit binds with a small ribosome subunit. One more active agent of the translation process is the so-called transfer RNA (tRNA). There are a number of tRNAs. Every tRNA specifically binds with only one of 20 amino acids that constitute protein molecules (some amino acids may be bound by a few tRNAs). tRNA finds corresponding amino acid in the cytosol and transports it to the site of protein synthesis. Every amino acid is coded by a sequence of three nucleotides called a triplet. Some amino acids are coded by two or even three triplets. In mRNA these triplets are called codons. The first codon is called the start codon, and it always codes the amino acid methionine. The ribosome subunits assemble around this start codon. tRNA has the shape of a cloverleaf. One site of this molecule specifically binds with the corresponding amino acid. The opposite side of tRNA has a triplet of nucleotides complementary to this amino acid. This triplet on the tRNA is called the anticodon. The anticodon of tRNA searches for a complementary codon on the mRNA and binds with it via a hydrogen bond. It is the methionine tRNA loaded with methionine amino acid that binds first to the start codon. The attachment of methionine tRNA to the start codon causes the ribosome to take one step ahead and prepare the next codon for binding with the next tRNA. When the next tRNA loaded with new amino acid binds with this anticodon, the ribosome catalyzes synthesis of the peptide bond between the first and second amino acids. At that time, the ribosome takes the next step and prepares the next codon to bind with the new tRNA's anticodon. The attachment of the third tRNA weakens the hydrogen bond between the first codon of mRNA and the anticodon of the first tRNA. The first tRNA has already lost its amino acid cargo, and now it is released back into the cytosol for the next load. The ribosome continues step by step to move along the mRNA and binds amino acids to each other, until it reaches the stop codon. At that time, the stop codon is already bound with a special protein called release factor. When the ribosome run upon the release factor at the stop codon, the synthesis of the polypeptide

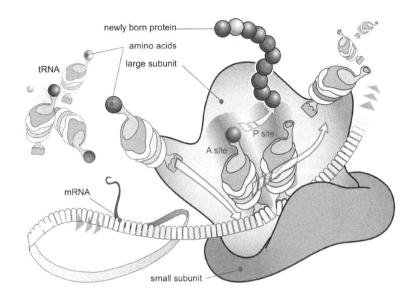

FIGURE 3.21   Translation.

chain is terminated. The ribosome disassembles into mRNA, large and small ribosomal subunits, and releases a new synthesized polypeptide chain. Finally, the polypeptide chain is processed by a special protein called chaperon that folds the polypeptide into a tertiary structure (fig. 3.21).

CHECK YOUR UNDERSTANDING

- Which organelle detoxifies chemical such as alcohol?

- Which organelle degrades molecules and organisms ingested via endocytosis?

- Where in the cell is the majority of cholesterol synthesized?

- What is the relation between a codon and a triplet?

3.3   Cell Cycle and Cellular Division

The adult animal body of average size is composed of approximately 100,000 trillion cells. The above mentioned cell theory states that cells do not spontaneously emerge from nowhere. All of them came from already existing cells. All cells in an animal body originate from a zygote: a single fertilized egg cell. In adult organisms, there are always a population of cells that continuously divide or are able to divide to replace dead or somehow lost cells. Between divisions, the cell has to maintain its life, participate in some organism activities, and prepare itself for the next division. The period of cell life from its emergence in a previous division to the end of the next division, when cell disappears, is called the **cell cycle**. The period of cell division is comparatively short. It may continue from minutes to a couple of hours, and as a rule, it is much shorter than the period of cell life between divisions. The period of cell life between two divisions is called **interphase**. In some cells, interphase is comparatively short, just a few hours, whereas in others it may continue the rest of the cell's life. Permanent cells, such as neurons and cardiac muscle cells, do not divide again and stay in interphase up to the end of their life. In this case, we say that they are in G_0 phase of interphase. Many cells of the organism retain the ability for cellular division, but they divide only in special situations. For example, hepatocytes—liver cells—do not divide. However, when the liver is damaged, some hepatocytes divide and replace damaged cells.

The first period of interphase that follows immediately after the last cell division is called **G_1 phase**. G_1 phase is characterized by fast cell growth and often specific reorganization to perform particular tasks. The letter G here stands for "gap." At G_1 phase, the cell synthesizes proteins, multiplies organelles, and "decides" if it is going to divide again or has to turn to G_0 state.

If the cell "decides" to divide, from G_1 phase it transits to next step of interphase called **S phase**. The letter S stands for "synthesis." A cell at S phase begins preparation for the upcoming division. It synthesizes and multiplies molecules and structures that have to be equally divided between two daughter cells when the cell splits. First of all, the cell duplicates all DNA molecules. Originally, every chromosome contains one double helix of DNA molecule. In S phase this single DNA doubled, and at the end of S phase, every chromosome has two identical DNA molecules. That is why when chromosomes condense and become visible in a light microscope, you can see that every chromosome has two chromatids (which look like the letter X). Both chromatids contain identical DNA molecules, because one molecule is an exact copy of the other.

Duplication of DNA in S phase is performed by an enzyme DNA polymerase. The process begins by an enzyme helicase that unwinds the double helix and separates DNA strands. The enzyme called primase attaches a short sequence of nucleotides called primer to unwind the free ends of the DNA. DNA polymerase can bind with DNA only when a short primer is already attached. DNA polymerase adds new nucleotides to the primer and elongates a new chain until it reaches the end of the copied DNA molecule (fig. 3.22). Because new nucleotides are added according a complementary principle, new strands are exact copies of the old DNA molecule. Both DNAs associate with proteins and create their own chromatin that, because both are exact copies of the original DNA molecule, are called **sister chromatids**. Sister chromatids at that time remain bound in one chromosome by a special protein complex called the **centromere**.

Beside duplication of DNA, cells also double centrosome—an organelle needed during cell division—and multiply other organelles. The following S phase period of interphase is called **G_2 phase**. In the second gap phase, the cell is already determined to divide and is ready for that. It accumulates materials and creates storage of energy, which it will use during the cellular division. The point when the cell "decides" that it is ready to divide is called the checkpoint. There are five checkpoints in the cell cycle: two in G_1 phase, one in S phase, one in G_2 phase, and one during the division. These checkpoints are controlled by cyclin and cyclin-dependent proteins. When the concentration of cyclin reaches a particular level, the cell initiates division (fig. 3.23). There are two types of cellular division: **mitosis** and **meiosis**. Cumulatively, all cells of the body except sperm and egg cells are called **somatic cells**. Somatic cells divide by mitosis, and gametes (sperm and eggs) divide by meiosis.

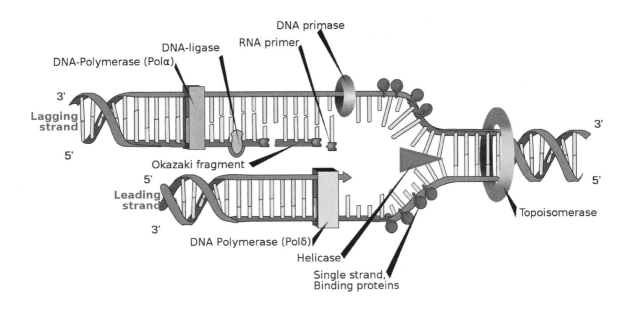

FIGURE 3.22   Process of DNA Duplication.

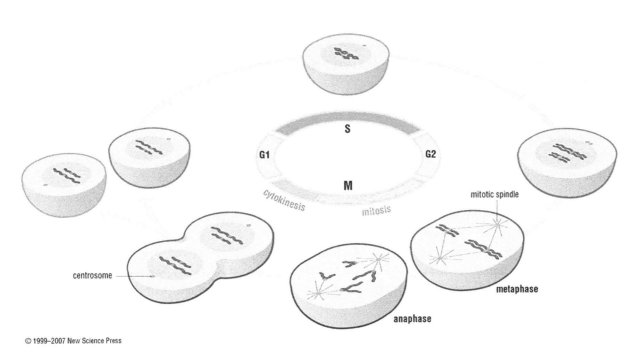

FIGURE 3.23   Cell Cycle.

Mitosis

Mitosis, or M phase, of the cell cycle is a division of somatic cells. It is a continuous process. But for analysis, it was subdivided in four steps or phases: **prophase**, **metaphase**, **anaphase**, and **telophase**.

Prophase is the first step of cellular division, and it begins with chromosomes condensation. Chromatin, which constitutes chromosomes, folds many times. As a result of that, chromosomes become shorter and thicker. At some point they become clearly visible in a light microscope, and one can see that every chromosome contains two sister chromatids bound together at a centromere. Other structures that become clearly visible in prophase are **centrosomes**. Centrosomes are tubular structures, the major component of which is the protein tubulin. Centrosomes begin movement in opposite directions and spread **spindle fibers** to create an **aster**. The nuclear envelop disintegrates and nucleoli disappear.

Metaphase is the longest phase of mitosis. In metaphase, centrosomes occupy positions in opposite sites (poles) of the cell. Spindle fibers reach maximum growth. They bind centrosomes with centromeres of chromosomes. Chromosomes line the plane in the middle distance between cell poles called the **metaphase** or **equatorial plate**. The centromere of every chromosome at this point is bound by spindle fibers with both centrosomes.

In **anaphase** every chromosome splits at the centromere and two sister chromatids become separated. The length of the spindle fibers decreases, and sister chromatids move apart toward opposite poles of the cell. From this moment sister chromatids become independent and are called chromosomes.

Telophase is the final step of mitosis. In telophase chromosomes associate around two new centers near cell poles. Two nuclear envelopes develop around two groups of chromosomes. Spindle fibers disintegrate, and centrosomes again become invisible. Chromosomes also become thin and invisible. The phase is terminated by the division of cytoplasm and separation of two daughter cells. The cytoplasm division is called **cytokinesis**. It begins with development of a ring groove on the cell surface called a **cleavage furrow**. The cleavage furrow deepens toward the cell center and finally splits the cell in two halves. From this very moment, the two daughter cells begin their independent, individual life. They begin their individual life with G_1 phase of interphase. The final sequence of events in mitosis is next: **prophase → metaphase → anaphase → telophase** (fig. 3.24).

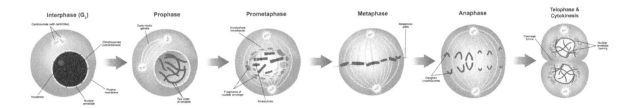

FIGURE 3.24   Mitosis.

CHECK YOUR UNDERSTANDING

- Describe the total sequence of events in mitosis.

- How many DNA molecules contain every chromosome in prophase?

- What will happen if a cell accomplishes mitosis without cytokinesis?

CHAPTER SUMMARY

- A complete set of all reactions inside cell is called **cell metabolism**. Metabolic processes are classified in three groups: **anabolic**, **catabolic**, and **oxidation-reduction reactions**. Anabolic reactions involve synthesis, which produces more complex molecules than the initial components. Synthesis of polysaccharides, polypeptides, triglycerides, and nucleic acids all are anabolic reactions. In catabolic reactions, complex macromolecules are degraded into simple components. Oxidation-reduction reactions are chemical reactions associated with a transfer of electrons from one atom to the other. This transfer of electrons is accompanied by transfer of energy and conversion of this energy in a new form.

- The cellular theory states: 1) only cells, and not subcellular structures, possess all properties characteristic of living organisms; 2) all organisms are made of cells; 3) all existing cells originate from preexisting cells.

- Cells are very diverse in their shape, internal structural organization, and role in the organism. In the mammalian body there are more than 600 different types of cells. The process of development of structurally different cells is called **differentiation**. Differentiation is based on 1) the ability of a cell to identify its position and receive complete instructions from the organism about what it has to do, and 2) the ability to control metabolism through **gene expression**.

- Cells are surrounded by the **plasma membrane**. The content of the cell between the plasma membrane and the nuclear envelope is called the **cytoplasm**. The cytoplasm consists of liquid media with varying viscosity called **cytosol** and structural elements called **organelles**. A network of tubular and filamentous structures called the **cytoskeleton** maintains the cell's shape and transports substances.

- The plasma membrane is a phospholipid bilayer that surrounded a cell. It protects and secures cell integrity by separating its interior from the external environment. Two major components constitute the plasma membrane: phospholipids and proteins.

- In a bilayer phospholipid, molecules can move only horizontally and cannot flip-flop from one layer to the other. The ability to move or fluidity of phospholipids in the membrane depends on the type of fatty acids. Saturated fats are packed more densely than unsaturated fats. As a result, membranes that contain more unsaturated fats have higher fluidity than membranes where saturated fats dominate. The fluidity of the membrane identifies its permeability for substances. A membrane with unsaturated fats is leaky and permits substances to pass through much more easily. The membrane with saturated fats is much denser and usually is less permeable. Cholesterol can penetrate the bilayer and increase membrane fluidity.

- Proteins are the second component of cellular membranes. They are responsible for transporting substances across membranes. Proteins create reversible chemical bonds with signaling molecules, such as hormones and prostaglandins, called **receptor proteins**. Proteins on the plasma membrane surface participate in intercellular connections and self-recognition. Proteins are divided in two classes: **transmembrane** or **integral proteins** and **peripheral proteins**. Together with phospholipid molecules, proteins are in constant motion. Because the plasma membrane is made as a mosaic of phospholipids and proteins, which are in motion, the model that describes this organization of plasma membrane is called the **fluid mosaic model**.

- Only small and nonpolar molecules, like oxygen and carbon dioxide, can easily pass the membrane. They move across the plasma membrane by simple diffusion.

- Ions, polarized, and big molecules cannot cross membranes. A group of integral proteins called **channel proteins** provides pathways for movement of these substances. Some channel proteins simply permit molecules to pass through the membrane by diffusion. This type of diffusion via channel proteins is called **facilitated diffusion**. Both simple and facilitated diffusions are called **passive transport**. In passive transport, substances can move in both directions following their gradient of concentration.

- Active transport requires energy to move a substance from one side of the membrane to the other. Active transport proteins are called **pumps**, because they move substances "against their will" from a place with low concentration to a place with high concentration.

- There are three types of pumps: **uniports**, **simports**, and **antiports**. Uniports drive a single substance across the membrane in one direction. An example of this uniport transport is the calcium (Ca^{2+}) pump in muscle cells. Simports move together two or more substances across the membrane in the same direction. This way, for example, cells drive inside molecules of glucose together with Na^+. Antiports drive together two or more substances through a membrane in opposite directions. A Na^+/K^+ pump drives Na^+ out and K^+ inside the cell. Transport of two or more substances across the plasma membrane is also called **cotransport**.

- Movement of a large amount of dissolved molecules or solid materials across the plasma membrane performed inside special membranous bubbles is called **endosomes**. The vesicle membrane surrounds macromolecules or big pieces of substances and drives them inside or outside the cell. Vesicular transport directed inside the cell is called **endocytosis**. Transport outside the cell is called **exocytosis**. Both types of the vesicular transport are classified in three groups: **phagocytosis**, **pinocytosis**, and **receptor-mediated transport**.

- A special transport that consists of endocytosis and exocytosis together, when the substance first drives inside and then outside of the cell, is called **transcytosis**.

- Extensions of plasma membrane are classified in three groups: **microvilli**, **cilia**, and **flagella**. Microvilli are short extensions that increase the surface area of the plasma membrane of these cells up to 40 times. Cilia are much longer than microvilli. Inside, cilia contain the cytoskeleton associated with motor proteins. This organization of cilia makes them moveable. Cilia movement has many roles, depending on the type of cell. In respiratory epithelium, cilia movement facilitates sweeping of mucous from respiratory canals. Structurally flagella are similar to cilia. Both contain a ring of nine pairs of microtubules surrounding two central microtubules. Both move via motor protein actions. In vertebrates, flagella are found only in sperm cells.

- Organelles are classified in two groups: 1) organelles enclosed in a membrane: mitochondria, endoplasmic reticulum, lysosomes, and peroxisomes; and 2) organelles not enclosed in membrane: ribosomes and centrosomes.

- The **endoplasmic reticulum** is a continuous membranous network made of a phospholipid bilayer. It is continuous with the plasma membrane on one side and the nuclear envelope on the other. The membrane encloses a fluid-filled space called the **ER lumen**. There are two types of ER: **rough endoplasmic reticulum** and **smooth endoplasmic reticulum**. RER provides a surface for ribosome attachment and is a site of proteins synthesis. The intensity of the RER development is a sign of synthetic activity of the cell. The lumen of the RER contains proteins called **chaperons**.

- The SER is a place for synthesis of lipids, phospholipids, cholesterol, and steroids. The SER removes toxins from the cytoplasm. It collects various toxins, drugs, and harmful substances and converts these to less harmful compounds. Skeletal and cardiac muscle cells use the SER lumen for Ca^{2+} storage. The SER lumen of these cells is enlarged and is called **cisternae**.

- The **Golgi apparatus** consists of a system of flattened and piled membranous sacs. The sacs are separated from each other and from the ER. The Golgi apparatus receives new synthesized proteins from the RER packed in endosomes. In the Golgi apparatus these proteins are stored, modified for use, and labeled for further transport to the destination place.

- **Mitochondria** are organelles with two membranes. The outer membrane is smooth. The inner membrane is extensively folded. These folds are called **cristae**. Cristae increase the surface of the inner membrane and contain a system of special proteins collectively carrying the **electron transport chain**, an essential part of **oxidation-phosphorylation reactions**. The goal of these reactions is to release energy from carbohydrates' chemical bonds and accumulate it in ATP molecules. These reactions are only a part of the process called **cellular respiration**. Cellular respiration is a principal mechanism of energy production in a cell. Cellular respiration can be divided in two steps. The first step takes place in the cytoplasm. It is called **anaerobic respiration** because it proceeds without oxygen. The second step takes place in the mitochondria and is called **aerobic respiration**, because it occurs only in the presence of oxygen as a final acceptor of electrons.

- **Lysosomes** are sacs containing strong enzymes for digestion of organic molecules. The principal function of lysosomes is intracellular digestion of nutrients and degrading of pathogenic invaders and damaged cellular structures.

- **Ribosomes** consist of two subunits. Each unit is a complex assemblage of proteins and ribosomal RNA (rRNA). When they are inactive, ribosomal subunits are separated from each other, but in the presence of the messenger

RNA (mRNA), they organize into a protein synthesizing complex. Active ribosomes may exist in two form: bound with the RER or free form floating in cytosol.

- The cytoskeleton consists of three types of protein assembles: **actin filaments**, **microtubules**, and **intermediate filaments**. The cytoskeleton penetrates the cytoplasm from the nuclear envelope to the plasma membrane.

- The nucleus contains chromosomes. It is surrounded by the **nuclear envelope**. A large protein complex in the nuclear envelope creates **nuclear pores**. Nuclear pores are tunnels for transporting giant macromolecules, such as mRNA.

- Genetic information is coded by the sequence of nucleotides in DNA. A sequence of nucleotides that carries complete information about the primary structure of protein molecule is called a **gene**. As a rule, genes have a particular location on DNA called the **locus**. DNA molecules associate with a number of different proteins. Some of these proteins play a structural role. They create a frame for spatial packaging of DNA molecules. The other proteins control and regulate DNA transcription, or repair damage. The complex of a DNA molecule with its structural and regulatory proteins is called **chromatin**. Chromatin constitutes chromosomes. Cells of a sexually reproducing organisms have two sets of chromosomes. One set of chromosomes came from the mother and the other from the father. Every mother chromosome with a particular set of genes on the particular loci has a partner chromosome with exactly the same set of genes at the same loci from the father. These pairs of chromosomes are called **homologous chromosomes**.

- The process of protein synthesis is divided in three principal steps: **transcription**, mRNA transport and processing, and **translation**.

- The period of a cell's life from the first cellular division to the end of the next division is called the **cell cycle**. The period of a cell's life between two divisions is called **interphase**. Permanent cells do not divide and stay in interphase to the end of their life. These cells are in G_0 phase of interphase.

- The first period of interphase that follows immediately after the last cell division is called G_1 **phase**. G_1 phase is characterized a fast cell growth and often specific reorganization to perform particular tasks. At G_1 phase the cell synthesizes proteins, multiplies organelles, and "decides" whether it is going to divide again or has to turn toward G_0 state.

- At S phase the cell synthesizes and duplicates molecules and structures that have to be divided between daughter cells, first of all DNA molecules. Originally, every chromosome contains one double helix DNA molecule. In S phase this single DNA doubled, and at the end of S phase, every chromosome has two DNA molecules called sister chromatids.

- The phase following S phase period of interphase is called G_2 **phase**. The cell accumulates materials and creates energy storage that it will use during cellular division. The point when the cell "decides" that it is ready to divide is called the checkpoint. There are five checkpoints in the cell cycle. These checkpoints are controlled by cyclin and cyclin-dependent proteins. When the concentration of cyclin reaches a particular level, the cell divides. There are two types of cellular division: **mitosis** and **meiosis**. Somatic cells divide by mitosis; gametes (sperm and eggs) divide by meiosis.

- Mitosis or M phase of the cell cycle is a division of somatic cells. It is subdivided in four steps or phases: **prophase**, **metaphase**, **anaphase**, and **telophase**. The sequence of events in mitosis is **prophase → metaphase → anaphase → telophase**.

- Prophase begins with chromosomes condensation. Chromatin that constitutes chromosomes folds many times, and chromosomes become shorter and thicker. Centrosomes move apart and spread **spindle fibers** to create **aster**. The nuclear envelop disintegrates, and nucleoli disappear.

- In metaphase centrosomes occupy positions in opposite poles of the cell. Spindle fibers bind centrosomes with centromeres of chromosomes. Chromosomes line the plane in the middle distance between cell poles called the **metaphase** or **equatorial plate**. The centromere of every chromosome at this point is bound by spindle fibers with both centrosomes.

- In **anaphase** every chromosome splits, and two sister chromatids are separated. The length of the spindle fibers decreases, and sister chromatids move apart toward cell poles. From this moment sister chromatids become independent and are called chromosomes.

- **Telophase** is the final step of mitosis. Chromosomes integrate around two new centers and two nuclear envelopes develop around them. Spindle fibers disintegrate, and centrosomes become invisible. Chromosomes also become invisible. The phase is terminated by the division of cytoplasm called cytokinesis and separation of daughter cells.

CHECK YOUR KNOWLEDGE

LEVEL 1. CHECK YOUR RECALL

1. The major functions of a cell membrane are:
   A. Maintain the wholeness of the cell
   B. Control the entry and exit of various substances in and out of the cell
   C. Create a membrane potential for excitable cells
   D. Provide self-recognition for the cell to the body immune system
   E. All of the above

2. Mitochondrion is:
   A. An organelle that functions as a storage space for molecules that are not in use
   B. An organelle that generate energy for the cell by synthesis of ATP
   C. An organelle that is responsible for the synthesis of proteins
   D. An organelle that is responsible for intercellular digestion by its digestive enzymes
   E. A membranous structure that participates in intercellular transport

3. The two major components of the cell membrane are:
   A. Lipids and carbohydrates
   B. Proteins and carbohydrates
   C. Lipids and proteins
   D. Carbohydrates and nucleic acids
   E. Nucleic acids and lipids

4. Which of the following describes a lysosome?
   A. A double-membrane organelle that generates energy for the cell
   B. A complex network of membranes that participate in protein synthesis
   C. A nonmembranous organelle that is responsible for protein synthesis
   D. A single-membrane vesicle with powerful digestive enzymes
   E. A small single-membrane vesicle used by the cell for food transportation

5. The Golgi apparatus is an organelle that functions in:
   A. Synthesis of carbohydrates
   B. Decomposition (detoxification) of toxins and free radicals
   C. Storage and shipping department of the cell
   D. Production of energy for cellular needs
   E. Intracellular food digestion

6. Smooth endoplasmic reticulum participates in _____ synthesis, whereas rough endoplasmic reticulum participates in _____ synthesis.
   A. nucleic acids; proteins
   B. proteins; carbohydrates
   C. proteins; lipids
   D. lipids; proteins
   E. DNA; RNA

7. S phase is a period of the cell cycle characterized by:
   A. DNA duplication
   B. Chromosome line the equatorial plate
   C. Fast growth of a cell
   D. Chromosomes move to opposite cell poles
   E. Cleavage furrow splits cell in two daughter cells

8. Synthesis of complex compounds from simple molecules is called:
   A. Catabolic metabolism
   B. Anabolic metabolism
   C. Oxidation-reduction reaction
   D. Oxidation-phosphorylation reaction
   E. Hydrolysis

9. Movement of glucose molecules together with Na^+ is an example of:
   A. Diffusion
   B. Facilitated diffusion
   C. Passive transport
   D. Uniport transport
   E. Simport transport

10. A sodium/potassium pump is an example of:
    A. Passive transport
    B. Untiport transport
    C. Uniport transport
    D. Simport transport
    E. Facilitated diffusion

11. The period of the cell cycle when chromosomes line the equatorial plate is:
    A. G_1 phase
    B. S phase
    C. Prophase
    D. Metaphase
    E. Anaphase

12. Before DNA polymerase begins synthesis, the DNA strand has to be separated by _____,
    and _____ has to attach an initial nucleotide sequence.
    A. helicase; primase
    B. primase; helicase
    C. cyclin; transcription factors
    D. transcription factors; termination factors
    E. cyclin; helicase

13. Telophase follows _____ and is characterized by _____.
    A. prophase; decomposition of nuclear envelop
    B. metaphase; chromosomes line the equatorial plate
    C. anaphase; development of two nuclear envelopes around two sets of chromosomes
    D. S phase; fast cell growth
    E. metaphase; separation of sister chromatids and their opposite movement

14. Interphase together with _____ constitutes the _____ cell cycle.
    A. G_1 phase; sperm
    B. S phase; egg
    C. meiosis; somatic
    D. mitosis; sperm
    E. mitosis; somatic

15. Chaperon is responsible for _____ after _____.
    A. primary protein structure development; transcription is finished
    B. primary protein structure development; RNA splicing is finished
    C. primary protein structure development; translation is finished
    D. tertiary protein structure development; transcription is finished
    E. tertiary protein structure development; translation is finished

16. True or false: Transcription is a process of DNA duplication.
17. True or false: Chromatin is a complex of DNA and proteins.
18. True or false: Sexually reproducing organisms get chromosomes from both parents.
19. True or false: Actin microfilaments are a major component of desmosomes.
20. Match the term with its description:

_____ Microtubules   a. Organelles responsible for protein synthesis
_____ Actin microfilaments   b. Transport of substances in and out of a cell
_____ Ribosomes   c. Responsible for deepening the cleavage furrow
_____ Peroxisomes   d. Responsible for intercellular transport
_____ Gene   e. Extension of plasma membrane
_____ Aerobic respiration   f. DNA segment that codes protein structure
_____ Cilia   g. Production of hydrogen peroxide
_____ Transcytosis   h. Production of ATP for energy purposes

LEVEL 2. CHECK YOUR UNDERSTANDING

1. Explain the difference between facilitated diffusion and active transport.
2. Why is synthesis of mRNA called transcription, whereas synthesis of proteins is called translation?
3. Can an oxidation-reduction reaction be an anabolic reaction? Explain your answer.
4. Explain why water molecules cannot easily cross the plasma membrane.
5. Why do the hepatocytes of alcoholics often have an abnormally increased smooth endoplasmic reticulum?

LEVEL 3. APPLY YOUR KNOWLEDGE TO REAL LIFE

1. The drug **nocodazole** blocks polymerization of tubulin into microtubules. Predict what effect this drug will have on the respiratory system. What effect will this drug have on mitosis?
2. The drug **arylsulfonamide** blocks some types of aquaporin molecules. Explain what will happen with the cells when treated with this drug.
3. Red blood cells called erythrocytes have no nucleus. How do red blood cells divide: by mitosis or meiosis? Explain your answer.

Chapter 4

Tissue

The Next Level of Body Organization

LEARNING OBJECTIVES

Tissues are groups of cells organized for specific functions. Tissue includes not only constituting cells but also the extracellular environment. The extracellular environment is a media in which cells may express their properties. This chapter describes four main types of tissues, their structural organization, functions, and most common locations in the animal body. When you finish reading this chapter, you will be able to answer these questions:

1. What is tissue, and what are the major principles of cell organization in tissue?

2. What is the structure and role of epithelial tissue?

3. What is the structure and role of connective tissue?

4. What is the classification of muscular tissue?

5. What is the structure and role of nervous tissue?

INTRODUCTION

The body of an adult animal contains millions of cells organized in groups according their role in the organism. These groups of cells that have a similar internal structure and function are called **tissue**. Each tissue has special characteristics and plays a specific role in the organism. At the same time, there are some common principles of tissue organization. First of all, tissue consists not only of cells but also of intracellular materials and structures cumulatively called the **matrix** or **extracellular matrix**. The matrix is a complex combination of fibers embedded into homogeneous media of varying consistency. The extracellular matrix is as important in tissue organization and function as the cells that constitute it.

4.1   Overview of Tissues

Four Major Types of Tissues

Depending on the types of cells and extracellular matrix, tissues are classified in four main groups: **epithelial**, **connective**, **muscular**, and **nervous**.

Epithelial tissues always occupy a position on the border. Epithelial tissue covers the body and is a major component of the integumentary system. It covers cavities and lumens of hollow organs, such as the small intestine and trachea. A special type of epithelial tissue called endothelium lines tubular organs, such as blood vessels. The borderline position suggests that the primary function of epithelial tissue is protection. To be able effectively protect underlying tissues and organs, epithelial cells are densely packed and leave no room for the matrix. This makes epithelial coverage impermeable for foreign agents. On the other hand, the epithelium has to be a gate for the exchange of gasses, nutrients, and waste products between the organism and the environment. Thus, the epithelium facilitates diffusion of gases in the lungs and capillaries, and transport of substances in the digestive tract and kidneys. Secretory epithelial cells produce and release a large number of substances called **secrets**. Single or organized in groups, secretory epithelial cells form glands.

Connective tissues are the most diverse tissue type. They are made of many different types of cells. The matrix is also very diverse in terms of fibers and ground substance. The matrix consistency varies from solid and strong, as in bones, to liquid, as in blood. The matrix constitutes a significant portion of connective tissue. Cells are widely separated, and the matrix may constitute a major part of the tissue by volume. As the name implies, connective tissue underlines all other tissues and organs and connects, supports, and protects them. Connective tissues also provide storage and transport substances in the organism.

Muscular tissues are characterized by the ability of muscle cells to contract and extend. Their primary function is movement. Contraction of muscle cells moves the body, propels food in the digestive tract and sperm in reproductive organs, and creates blood pressure that forces blood to flow inside the blood vessels. Muscular tissue has much less matrix between cells compared to connective tissues. Cells of these tissues are highly specialized and in most cases are permanent; that is, do not divide.

Nervous tissue has the most complex organization. The cellular component of the tissue is presented by structurally and functionally diverse **neurons** and supporting **neuroglia cells**. The extracellular matrix of nerve tissue is gelatinous and contains special glycoproteins. Recent studies demonstrate that the matrix plays a very important role in nerve tissue development and regeneration after damage. The primary role of nervous tissue is to be a principal structural component of sensory organs and the nervous system, which collects, analyzes, and executes responses in changes in internal organism conditions and the external environment. In short, the role of the nervous system may be formulated as an integrative function.

CHECK YOUR UNDERSTANDING

- Describe the four main tissue types.

- Which two main components constitute tissue?

Major Components of Tissue

Each type of tissue has two main components: cells and the extracellular matrix (ECM). The balance between these two components varies significantly. Epithelial tissues have a minimal amount of ECM. Cells in epithelial tissues are organized in cell sheets and are bound by cell junctions. Connective tissue, on the other hand, contains a large amount of matrix, which widely separates cells. Cells of connective tissues rarely form permanent cell junctions with each other. The ECM is a product of tissue resident cells secreted into interstitial space via exocytosis. The ECM has two components: 1) fibrous proteins and 2) **ground matter** or **ground substance**. The fibrous proteins create an interlocking mesh with the space filled by ground substance: a solution of polysaccharides and composite glycoprotein molecules.

Glycoproteins have a net negative charge. Negatively charged glycoproteins in the ECM bind positively charged sodium ions (Na^+), which attracts water molecules via osmosis. Water molecules held in the ECM by hydrogen bonds with Na^+ keep tissue and resident cells hydrated.

Chondroitin sulfate molecules contribute to the tensile strength of cartilage, tendons, ligaments, and aortic walls. Keratin sulfates are present in the ECM of eye cornea, cartilage, bones, and horns. **Hyaluronic acid** is another ECM component that absorbs a significant amount of water and swells. ECM swelling creates turgor force that resists external pressure and keeps tissues expanded. Hyaluronic acid is a major component of the ECM of connective tissues in load-bearing joints. It is also a chief component of the interstitial gel.

Collagen is the most abundant fiber protein in the animal body. It accounts for 90 percent of bone matrix. Collagens give structural support to resident cells. Protein **elastin** gives tissue elasticity and makes it extensible like rubber. These properties are very important for tissues in organs such as lungs, blood vessels, and skin. A structural fibrous protein **reticulin** is a special type of collagen molecule called collagen type 3. It is found together with other types of collagen and elastin in sperm cell flagellum and mammalian skin. Fibronectins are glycoproteins that connect cells to the ECM collagen fibers and help platelets stick to each other during blood clotting and cell movement (migration of neutrophils and fibro-blasts, for example) during wound healing.

CHECK YOUR UNDERSTANDING

- What are the two main ECM components?

- What role do fiber proteins play in tissue?

- What macromolecules constitute ground substance?

Cell Junctions

Different tissues have different relations among resident cells. In connective tissue, cells are rarely bound to each other. Usually they are separated by a significant amount of matrix, and most of their communication goes through messenger molecules and the ECM. On the other side are epithelial cells. They form continuous protective sheets. Cells may simply adhere to each other by glycoprotein molecules in the ECM or may be bound by integral proteins in cell membranes that form **cell junctions**. Cell junctions are classified in three groups: 1) **tight junctions**, 2) **desmosomes**, and 3) **gap junctions**.

Tight junctions are formed by integrin proteins in the plasma membranes of adjacent cells. Two cells stick to each other by plasma membranes and interwoven integrin molecules. Like a zipper, they lock cells tightly together. This junction does not leave space between cells, and big macromolecules cannot pass this cell barrier. This type of cell junction is common for epithelium that line a surface where leakage is not desirable. For example, tight junctions bind cells that line blood vessels (fig. 4.1).

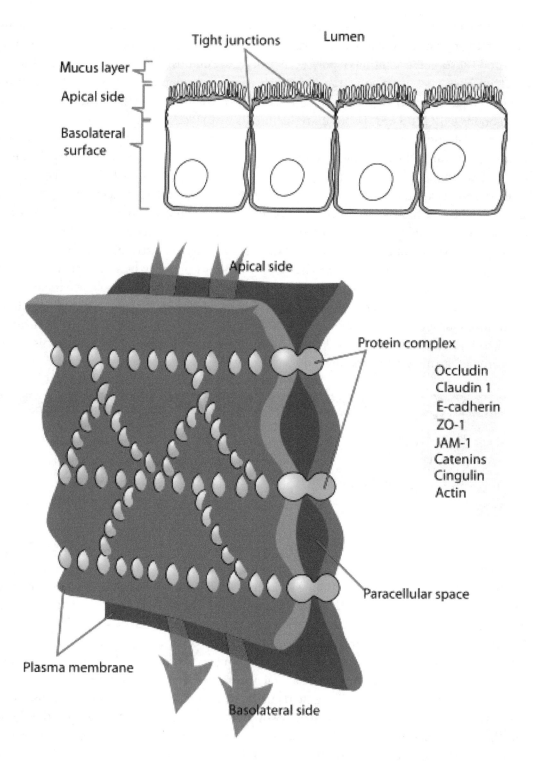

FIGURE 4.1   Tight Junction among Epithelial Cells of the Mucus Membrane That Line the Respiratory System and Part of the Digestive System.

Desmosomes are composed of desmosome-intermediate filament complexes (DIFC). This complex is made of a network of cadherin proteins, linker proteins, and keratin intermediate filaments. The DIFCs are subdivided into three regions: the extracellular core region, or desmoglea; the outer dense plaque, or ODP; and the inner dense plaque, or IDP. Desmosomes hold cells at approximately 34 nm distance and permit movement of some molecules. Desmosomes are the strongest cell junctions and are found in tissue that experiences intense mechanical stress, such as cardiac muscle, urinary bladder, gastrointestinal mucosa, and epithelium of the skin (fig. 4.2).

Gap junctions are formed by special membrane proteins called connexons. Connexons are transmembrane proteins that pass through plasma membranes of adjacent cells and create pores. Proteins hold cells together tightly, and pores connect cytoplasm of adjacent cells. Depending on the confirmation of connexons, pores may be open or closed. Open pores permit free movement of substances, ions, and electric impulses between adjacent cells. This type of junction is common among muscle cells but is found in all types of tissues (fig. 4.3).

As a matter of fact, cell adhesion and all three types of cell junctions can be found in different combinations in the same cells.

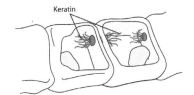

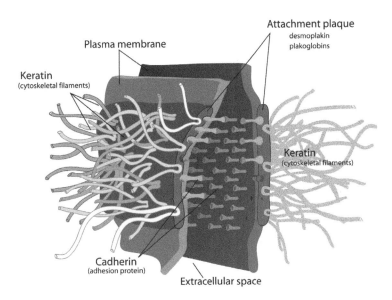

FIGURE 4.2   Desmosomes.

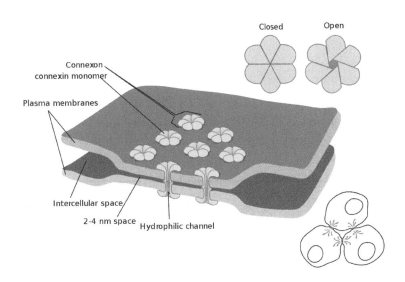

FIGURE 4.3   Gap Junction.

CHECK YOUR UNDERSTANDING

- Describe three types of cell junctions.

- What would happen if cell junctions—for example, between epithelial cells of the skin—are damaged?

- What proteins form a gap junction?

VETERINARY APPLICATION

Pemphigus is a general designation for a group of autoimmune skin diseases. The immune system attacks desmosomes and destroys desmosomes' complex protein desmoglein 1. Destruction of protein in desmosomes disrupts cell junctions between epithelial cells. This causes ulceration and crusting of the skin, as well as the formation of fluid-filled sacs and cysts (vesicles) and pus-filled lesions (pustules). Some types of pemphigus can also affect the epithelium of the gums. The hallmark sign of pemphigus is a condition called acantholysis, where the skin cells separate and break down. There are three types of pemphigus that affect cats: pemphigus foliaceus, pemphigus erythematosus, and pemphigus vulgaris.

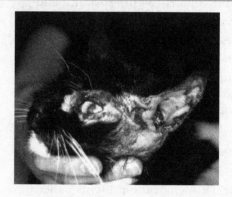

IMG 4.1   Pemphigus Foliaceus in Cat.

4.2   Epithelial Tissue

Major Characteristics of Epithelial Tissue

Epithelial tissues occupy a borderline position in the body. They form skin, line the digestive system and other tubular structures in the body, such as ureters and urinary bladder, and form the endothelium of blood vessels. This borderline position suggests that epithelial tissue has to perform the following functions:

1. **Protection.** Epithelial tissue creates a continuous impermeable shield against harmful chemicals and pathogens. Layers of epithelial cells protect underlying structures from mechanical stress and extremal temperatures. Specialized epithelial cells of the skin accumulate the hydrophobic protein **keratin**. Cells loaded with keratin form a waterproof skin surface that protects the body from dehydration in dry air and keeps underlying structures moist and soft.

2. **Transport control.** The epithelium not only protect the organism from pathogens and harmful substances, it also controls and facilitates transport of nutrients, oxygen, and removal of waste products. The mucous lining of the digestive tract is the only surface for absorption of nutrients from the small intestine into the blood flow for their further distribution in the body, and retention of water in large intestine. The epithelial lining of the lungs is the only pathway for oxygen and carbon dioxide. Gasses are transported passively by diffusion through the epithelial lining of the lungs. Most nutrients, especially fats, drive from the small intestine lumen into body fluids by active transport.

3. **Immune defense.** The epithelium of skin creates a physical barrier for pathogenic organisms. Keratinized epithelial cells form a thick layer of dead dry cells, which creates a trap for many viruses, bacteria, and fungi. Besides that, there are specialized phagocytes called dendritic cells that create a nonspecific immune reaction against pathogen agents and cancerous cells.

4. **Secretion.** Secretory epithelial cells produce and release substances called secrets. Secrets are very diverse chemically and in the role they play in an organism. Secretory cells may be single or create clusters. A single secretory cell forms a unicellular gland. They have no ducts and secrete their products directly on the free surface of open body cavities, and thus are considered exocrine. The most common unicellular exocrine glands are the goblet cells found in the epithelium of the trachea and the digestive tube. Secretory cells clustered in a group form a multicellular gland. There are two type of glands: 1) exocrine glands release their secrets on the open body surface or into tubes that open on the body surface; 2) endocrine glands release their secrets, called hormones, into the interstitial space or directly into the blood flow.

5. **Sensation.** As far as epithelial tissues directly contacting external and internal environments, they carrying special receptors to monitor changes in these environments. Through receptors in the skin, the organism receives information about air temperature and humidity, texture of objects, and vibrations. Receptor cells in the walls of blood vessels inform about blood pH and pressure. Modified epithelial cells form the hearing receptors of the organ of Corti and taste buds.

Taking into consideration all these functions, it becomes clear why these cells usually are bound by tight junctions and desmosomes. Their protective role requires that epithelial cells usually have to be very densely packed. The dense packaging of epithelial cells does not leave a room for other tissues and structures. That is why epithelial tissues are avascular. They have no blood vessels inside the tissue. All blood supply the epithelium receives from other nearby tissues. This absence of a direct blood supply results in epithelium thickness. The epithelium cannot be very thick. With an increase in thickness, apical cells experience a progressive decrease of oxygen and nutrient supplies. Apical cells are subjected to continuous harmful environmental pressure. Their life span is short, and new cells have to replace dead ones. That is why epithelial cells, as a rule, regularly divide.

Epithelial tissue cells that directly contact the open environment have one side of the cell surrounded by an open space. The cell surface that contacts the open space is called a **free** or **apical surface**. The free surface of epithelial cells often have extensions: microvilli or cilia (see chapter 3, page 75). Cells with cilia are called **ciliated epithelium**. Ciliated epithelium is found in respiratory organs, such as the trachea and bronchi, in ducts that transport sperm and egg cells, and so on. Microvilli significantly increase the free cell surface and are characteristic of small intestine mucosa, where they are responsible for absorption of nutrients. The side opposite to the free surface side of epithelial cell lies on underlying body tissues. This cell side is called

basal. The basal side of epithelial cell rests on a glue-like substance called the **basement membrane**. The basement membrane is composed of two layers: **basal lamina** and underlying **reticular connective tissue**. The underlying connective tissue attaches to the basal lamina by collagen fibers. The basement membrane is produced by epithelial cells and firmly holds together the epithelial layer with underlying tissues.

CHECK YOUR UNDERSTANDING

- Describe the major functions of epithelial tissue.

- What is the difference between the apical and basal sides of an epithelial cell?

- What is the role of the basement membrane?

Classification of Epithelial Tissues

Epithelial tissues are classified according to the shape of cells and number of cellular layers. By the shape, epithelial cells are divided in three classes: **squamous**, **cuboidal**, and **columnar**. Squamous epithelial cells are flat. Their nuclei are squeezed between plasma membranes. Cells are tiny and, as a rule, form thin cellular layer like a tile. A single layer of squamous cells is easily permeable by gasses and small nonpolar molecules. In cuboidal epithelium, cells have the shape of a cube. The nucleus of these cells occupies a central position. In columnar epithelium, cells are long; they are much longer than they are wide. The nucleus in these cells usually is located close to the basal area. In many cases, the cell's free surface carries cilia. The epithelium with cilia on the cells' apical surface is called **ciliated columnar epithelium** (fig. 4.4).

According to the number of cell layers, epithelial tissues are divided in two groups: **simple** and **stratified epithelium**. Simple epithelium consists of one single layer of tightly joint cells. These cells can be squamous, cuboidal, or columnar. Thus, there are three types of simple epithelium: **simple squamous**, **simple cuboidal**, and **simple columnar epithelium** (fig. 4.4). Stratified epithelium refers to epithelial tissue with more than two cellular layers. As a rule, the deepest layer of this epithelium consists of cuboidal or rare columnar cells, whereas apical cells can be squamous, cuboidal, or columnar. According to the shape of the cells in the apical layer, stratified epithelium is classified as **stratified squamous**, **stratified cuboidal**, and **stratified columnar epithelium** (fig. 4.4).

In addition to these six types, there are two more types of epithelial tissues: **pseudostratified** and **transitional**. Pseudostratified epithelium got its name from the fact that this epithelium creates one single cellular layer and, thus, has to be called simple, but it looks as if it has two cell layers. The cells that constitute this epithelium are columnar, but they have different heights. Some cells are longer than others. All cells rest on basement membrane, but not all of them reach the free surface. Nuclei of these cells are also located a different distance from the basement membrane and, as a rule, are organized in two lines, which creates the illusion of two cellular layers (fig. 4.5).

Transitional epithelium is characterized by the ability of resident cells to change their shape from cuboidal to squamous. This type of epithelium is characteristic of organs that experience regular extensions and collapses, like a urinary bladder (fig. 4.6).

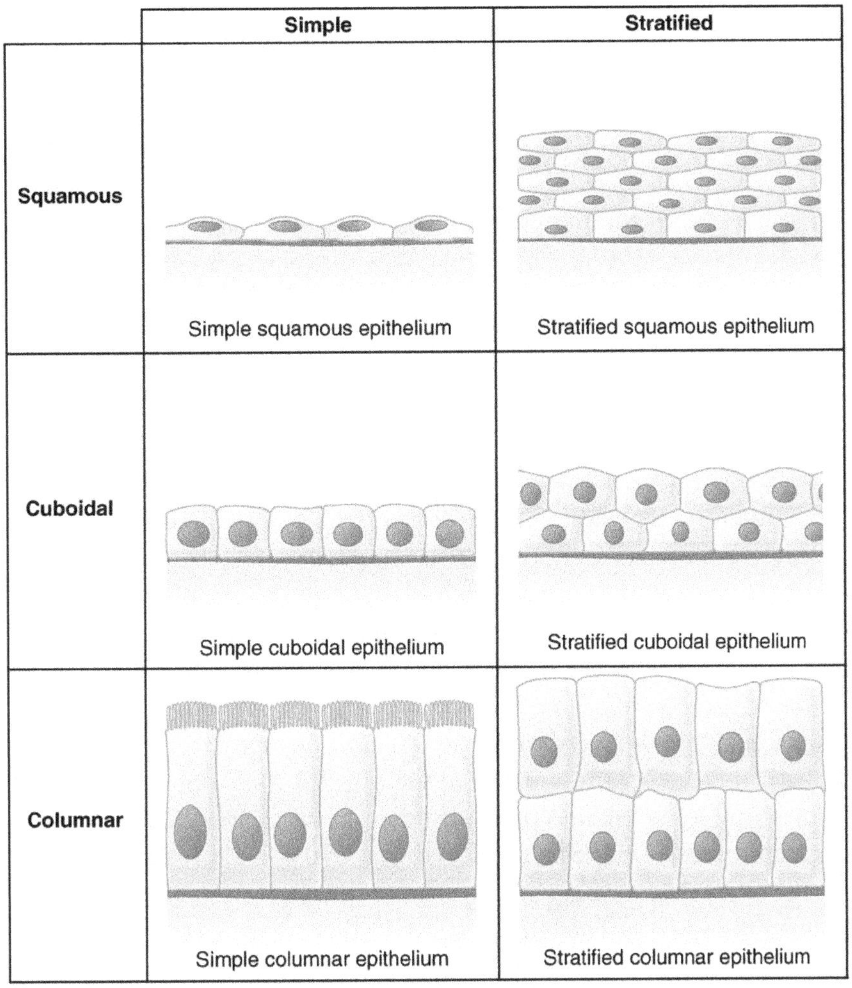

	Simple	Stratified
Squamous	Simple squamous epithelium	Stratified squamous epithelium
Cuboidal	Simple cuboidal epithelium	Stratified cuboidal epithelium
Columnar	Simple columnar epithelium	Stratified columnar epithelium

FIGURE 4.4   Six Types of Epithelium.

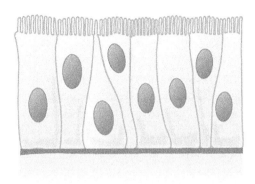

FIGURE 4.5   Pseudostratified Columnar Epithelium.

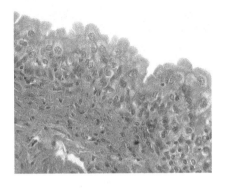

FIGURE 4.6   Transitional Epithelium.

So, together with **glandular epithelium**, there are nine basic types of epithelial tissues that participate in organization of different organs and have different functions.

CHECK YOUR UNDERSTANDING

- What is the name of epithelium that is one cell thick?

- What type of epithelium participates in skin formation?

- Where does pseudostratified epithelium get its name?

- Name all nine types of epithelium.

The Role of Epithelial Tissue in Body Organization

Simple squamous epithelium has ideal characteristics to form tiny membranes and easily permeable surfaces. Layers of squamous cells look like tiles in a bathroom. Gasses such as oxygen and carbon dioxide easily diffuse through a single layer of flat cells. That is why simple squamous epithelium forms respiratory surface of lungs. Simple squamous epithelium also creates endothelium of blood vessels. In capillaries simple squamous epithelium facilitates movement of gasses, nutrients, and waste materials through capillary walls.

Simple cuboidal epithelium is less permeable, but it is more protective compared with simple squamous epithelium. In kidneys, it creates walls of nephron tubules and collecting ducts. It is not desirable that urine produced in nephron leak back into the body fluids. Movement of substances through the layer of cuboidal cells is easy to control. This helps regulate urine content and prevent return of waste and toxic material back into the blood flow.

Simple columnar epithelium is located in organs where there is a need to thoroughly control incoming substances. Columnar cells protect underlying tissues and transport only needed to organism substances. This type of epithelium creates lining most of digestive tract and uterus.

Pseudostratified columnar epithelium is found in the respiratory system. Columnar cells of this epithelium have cilia on apical surface. Because this epithelium is mostly found in the respiratory system, it also is called **respiratory epithelium**. Together with columnar cells, respiratory epithelium has secretory cells that produce mucus. Mucus-producing cells are called **goblet cells**. Goblet cells are scattered along the respiratory epithelial lining. Produced mucus covers internal walls of air pathways and traps airborne bacteria, spores, dust, and other contaminants. Mucus with trapped particles are swept away by a wave-like beating of cilia. This continuous movement of mucus with trapped particles out of the respiratory system is called the mucus conveyer.

Stratified squamous epithelium forms thick membrane-like structures that cover and protect body. As a rule, cells of this epithelium are organized in multicellular layers called strata (the singular is *stratum*). The deepest layer (stratum) located close to the basement membrane consists of epithelial stem cells that regularly divide and replace dead cells. This layer is called the **stratum germinativum** or **stratum basale**. There are two types of membrane-like structures made of stratified squamous epithelium: **keratinized cutaneous membrane** and **nonkeratinized mucous membrane**. Keratinized membrane is a principal part of skin, whereas nonkeratinized membranes line body cavities that are open outside the body: mouth, vagina, and anus.

Stratified cuboidal epithelium consists of a few cell layers. Only the apical layer has really cuboidal cells. This epithelium is protective. It lines walls of sweat glands, mammary glands, ceruminous glands, and salivary glands.

Stratified columnar epithelium is a very rare type of epithelium. It consists of two layers. The apical layer has columnar cells, whereas the basal layer is made of cuboidal cells. Stratified columnar epithelium is found in the ducts of certain glands, including salivary glands, part of the male urethra, and cornea of the eye.

Transitional epithelium consists of multiple layers of epithelial cells that can contract and expand as needed. This type of epithelial tissue is found in urothelium—a lining of the urinary system, including renal pelvis, urinary bladder, ureters, some regions of urethra, and prostatic and ejaculatory ducts of prostate (fig. 4.7).

CHECK YOUR UNDERSTANDING

- Why are the walls of lung alveoli composed of simple squamous epithelium?
- Which cells of columnar epithelium produce mucus?
- In which hollow organs does the internal lining consist of transitional epithelium?
- What factors restrict the thickness of stratified epithelium?

Glandular epithelium consists of cells whose major role is manufacturing and releasing secrets. Cells of glandular epithelium form secretory glands. Glands are divided in two principal classes: **endocrine glands** and **exocrine glands**. The secrets of endocrine glands are called hormones. Endocrine glands release hormones into the surrounding ECM or into the blood flow. Exocrine glands secrete their products into the ducts or directly on the open surface. Through these ducts secret is transported outside of the body, like sweat glands do, or into the lumen of a body organ, like gastric glands release gastric juice into the lumen of the stomach. A gland that consists of only one cell is called a **unicellular gland**. Goblet cells are an example of a unicellular gland (fig. 4.8).

A gland that consists of more than one cell is called a **multicellular gland**. Multicellular exocrine glands are classified according to the shape of the gland and its duct. Thus, glands that have the shape of a tube are called **tubular**. A gland that has the shape of a ball or sphere is called **alveolar** or **acinar gland**. A gland with a single not branched duct is called **simple**, and a gland with a branched duct is called **compound**. Very often, glands have a combination of these features, and their names include all these characters (fig. 4.9).

Another classification of exocrine glands is based on the way they produce and release secrets. According to this approach, exocrine glands are divided in three groups: **merocrine**, **apocrine**, and

Cells	Location	Function
Simple squamous epithelium 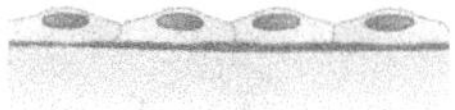	Air sacs of lungs and the lining of the heart, blood vessels, and lymphatic vessels	Allows materials to pass through by diffusion and filtration, and secretes lubricating substance
Simple cuboidal epithelium 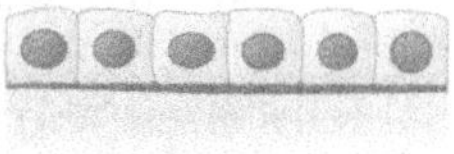	In ducts and secretory portions of small glands and in kidney tubules	Secretes and absorbs
Simple columnar epithelium 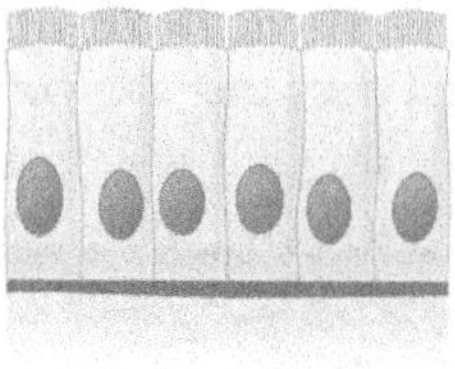	Ciliated tissues are in bronchi, uterine tubes, and uterus; smooth (nonciliated tissues) are in the digestive tract, bladder	Absorbs; it also secretes mucous and enzymes
Pseudostratified columnar epithelium 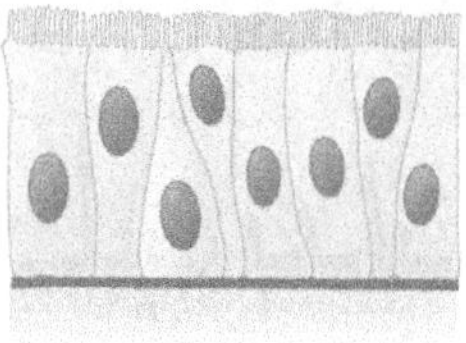	Ciliated tissue lines the trachea and much of the upper respiratory tract	Secretes mucus; ciliated tissue moves mucus
Stratified squamous epithelium 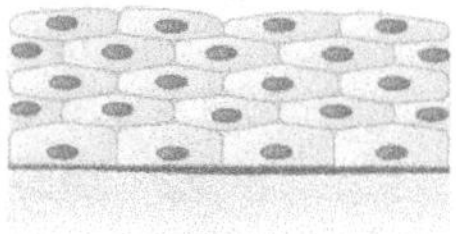	Lines the esophagus, mouth, and vagina	Protects against abrasion
Stratified cuboidal epithelium 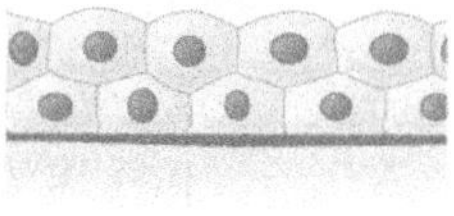	Sweat glands, salivary glands, and the mammary glands	Protective tissue
Stratified columnar epithelium 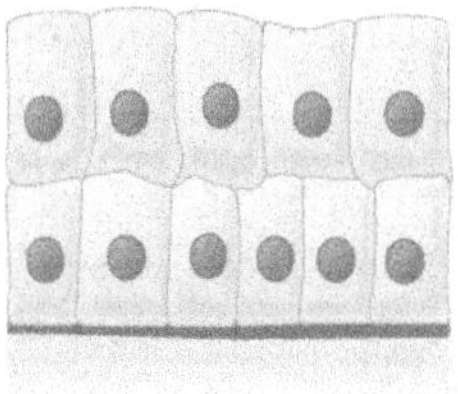	The male urethra and the ducts of some glands	Secretes and protects
Transitional epithelium 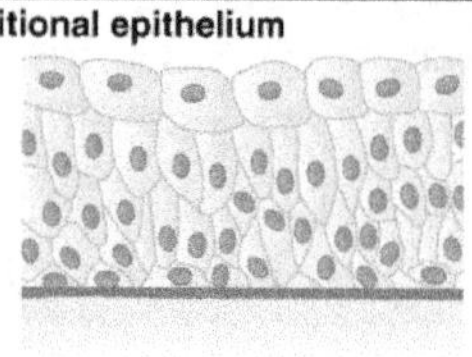	Lines the bladder, uretha, and the ureters	Allows the urinary organs to expand and stretch

FIGURE 4.7   Epithelial Tissues, Their Location, and Function.

holocrine glands. Merocrine glands continuously manufacture secrets, pack them in membranous sacs, and release them outside the cell via exocytosis. The cell during this process does not experience significant changes and may continue to produce secrets. Eccrine sweat glands are this type of exocrine glands. In opposite to merocrine glands, holocrine glands do not release secretes but accumulate them inside the cell. The process of secret manufacturing continues until the cell is ruptured and releases, together with secret, the entire cell content. The ruptured cell dies and has to be replaced by a new cell. Two examples of a holocrine gland are the sebaceous glands in the skin and melbomian (tarsal) glands in the eyelids. The mode of manufacturing secrets in apocrine glands is intermedium to that of merocrine and holocrine glands. Apocrine glands manufacture secrets and accumulate it in apical area of the cell close to free surface. When some significant amount of secret is accumulated, an apocrine cell releases it together with the apical part of the cell. The cell is damaged but does not die. It takes some time for the cell to repair the damage and restore activity. Mammary glands are an example of true apocrine glands (fig. 4.10).

Secretions of exocrine gland are of three types: **serous**, **mucous**, and **mixed secretions**. Serous secretion is a pale yellow transparent fluid composed of proteins and water. Serous fluid is very slippery. It creates a thin film that lubricates internal membranes, such as

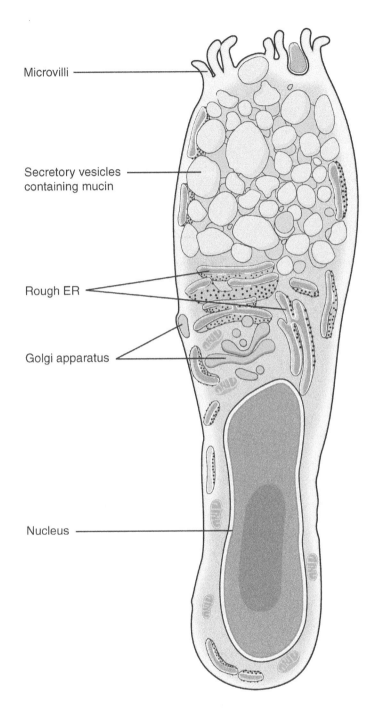

FIGURE 4.8   Goblet Cell, a Unicellular Exocrine Gland.

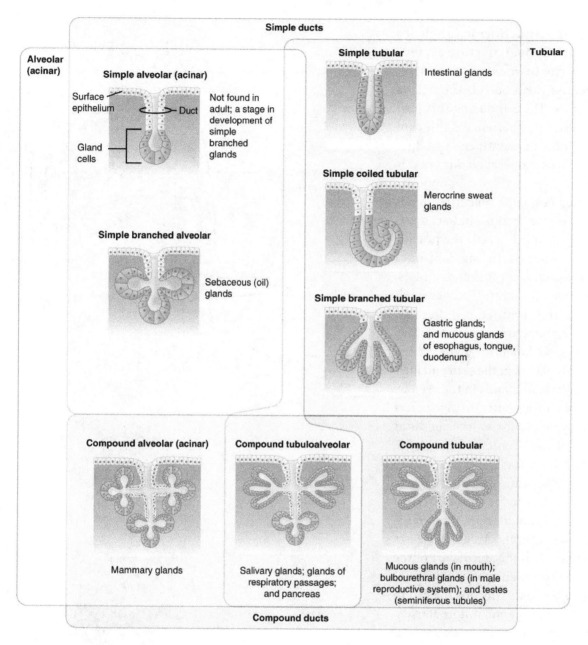

FIGURE 4.9   Different Types of Multicellular Glands.

pleural membranes, for smooth frictionless movement of internal organs. Mucous secretion contains thick viscous mucus and is found in the lumens of many internal tubular organs, where it creates a protective coverage. Mixed secretions are characterized by combination of serous and mucous fluids. Saliva of the salivary glands is an example of such mixed secretion.

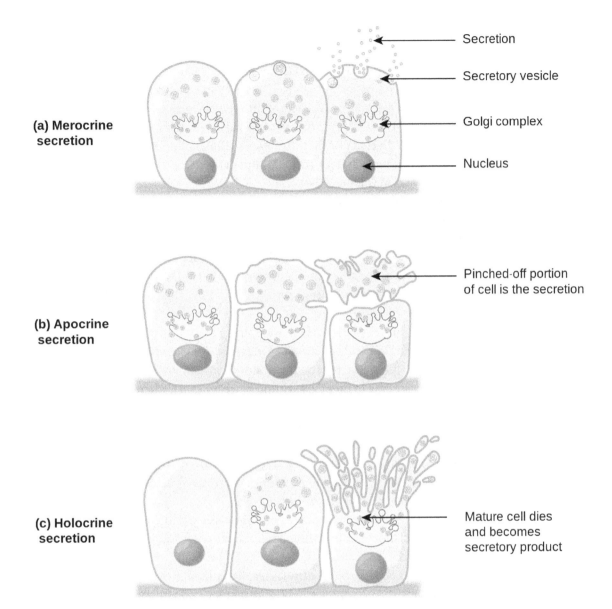

(a) Merocrine secretion

Secretion

Secretory vesicle

Golgi complex

Nucleus

(b) Apocrine secretion

Pinched-off portion of cell is the secretion

(c) Holocrine secretion

Mature cell dies and becomes secretory product

FIGURE 4.10   Three Types of Exocrine Secretions.

CHECK YOUR UNDERSTANDING

- What is the difference between exocrine and endocrine glands?

- How do you classify goblet cells? Explain your answer.

- What is the difference between merocrine and holocrine glands?

- Describe the difference between acinar and tubular compound glands.

4.3   Connective Tissue

Major Characteristics of Connective Tissue

In connective tissue, cells are separated by substantial distances. The space among cells is filled by matrix. Connective tissue is the most diverse type of tissue. Cells of different shape, size, and function constitute connective tissues. The matrix (ECM) is also very diverse and varies from solid to liquid. The diversity of connective tissues corresponds to diversity of their functions. There are four functional categories of connective tissue cells: 1) defense (immune system cells); 2) support (skeletal system cells); 3) storage (fat cells); and 4) transport and distribution (blood cells).

The major common cells of connective tissues are **fibroblasts**. Fibroblasts form most types of connective tissues. Fibroblasts manufacture ground matter and fibers of ECM and create structural framework (stroma) of animal tissues. Unlike the epithelial cells, fibroblasts do not form flat monolayers. They are evenly distributed in tissue and do not form permanent cell junctions. Fibroblasts maintain the ability to divide and also can slowly migrate over the substratum. Thanks to that ability, they first fill space where cells were injured; that is, they play a critical role in wound healing. The life span of a fibroblast, as measured in chick embryos, is 57, plus or minus 3 days.

Connective tissue cells of the immune system include wandering phagocytes and sedentary cells. The wandering immune system cells by origin and function fall in two major classes: **macrophages** and **neutrophils**. In general, for these cells it is characteristic move slowly in search of pathogenic agents, dead cells, and contaminating substances. Some of them finally find place to reside, where they spend the rest of their life. Sedentary cells spend their whole life in the place of their forming, such as **mast cells**. Mast cells are the largest cells of connective tissue. Mast cells associate with blood vessels and nerves, particularly in the skin, digestive tract, lungs, mouth, and nose. The cytoplasm of these cells contains granules with inflammatory mediators, such as heparin and histamine. In response to a pathogenic agent's stimulation, these cells release their inflammatory mediators and generate a protective inflammation reaction. In the case of a false response, they may develop allergy or anaphylaxis.

Support cells of connective tissues include osteocytes of bone tissues and chondrocytes of cartilage tissues. Both types of cells have the characteristic ability to manufacture specific matrix (bone or cartilage matrix) and live inside a closed space called a lacuna.

The most important storage cells are fat cells, or **adipocytes**. Body tissues that predominantly contain adipocytes are called **adipose tissues**. Adipocytes not only store fat molecules, they also play multiple roles in many vital functions. Adipose tissue cushions internal organs and prevents their damage. This tissue forms an insulating layer beneath the skin to prevent water loss and helps maintain stable body temperature. Adipocytes manufacture a number of hormones, such as leptin. Leptin suppresses the hunger center in the hypothalamus and controls appetite. Production of leptin by adipocytes is controlled through the classic homeostatic negative feedback. Adipocyte manufactures leptin as a reaction on additional depositions of fat molecules. The more fat deposited in adipocyte, the more leptin adipocyte produces. Leptin inhibits appetite, and when its level reaches some critical point, the animal loses its appetite. Without appetite, the animal does not eat. The level of fat in body fluids decreases, and the organism consumes adipocyte's fat storage. Depletion of fat storage decreases production of leptin, and the animal again gains appetite. Adipocytes convert the male hormone androgen into estrogen. In female organisms, this adipocyte activity help maintain some minimal level of estrogen for normal female organism functioning and normal reproductive cycles. Low adipose tissue caused by malnutrition may cause disturbances in the reproductive cycle.

Transport and distribution cells, first of all, are red blood cells, or erythrocytes. Erythrocytes transport and distribute oxygen and partially transport carbon dioxide.

The ECM of connective tissues is very diverse, but three major fibrous components prevail. These three components are collagen, elastin, and reticulin (see page 101). The ground substance varies from liquid in blood, to gel in cartilage, and to solid in bone. The ground matter substance/fibers ratio also varies significantly. In fibrous connective tissues, such as tendons, there are much more collagen fibers than ground substance, whereas in hyaline cartilage, the ECM mostly consists of gel ground matter and very little fibers.

VETERINARY APPLICATION

Feline cutaneous asthenia is a rare inheritable skin disease of cats characterized by abnormal elasticity, stretching, and improper healing of the skin. Pendulous wing-like folds of skin form on the cat's back, shoulders, and haunches. Even stroking the cat can cause the skin to stretch and tear. A recessive autosomal form of feline cutaneous asthenia has been identified in Siamese cats and related breeds. In the homozygous state, it is lethal. Cats with cutaneous asthenia cannot be grasped by the scruff, as this may tear away. Cats may also have slipping joints. There are two genetic traits linked to feline cutaneous asthenia. One comes from a dominant allele, while the other comes from a recessive. Both result in similar pathology. Mutation results in abnormal collagen fibers packaging. Abnormal collagen is soft and easily stretches. It cannot maintain skin tension. Skin becomes overly stretchable and may be easily torn apart. Even normal scratching and playing with other cats will begin to cause tears in the skin, usually starting at around eight weeks of age. Injuries often heal rapidly, leaving scars. In heterozygous cats, normal and abnormal fibrils often exist inside the same collagen fiber. Homozygous cats are not likely to survive for very long.

Classification of Connective Tissues

Connective tissues are very diverse, and it is difficult at first glance to say why so many very different tissues are identified as connective tissues. One reason is principles of structural organization: a comparatively small amount of separated cells and large amount of ECM. The second fundamental reason is its roots in the common origin of all connective tissues, embryonic tissue known as a mesenchyme. Mesenchyme is a derivative of embryo mesoderm: one of three primary embryo leaflets. These embryonic cellular layers are ectoderm, mesoderm, and endoderm. Ectoderm gives rise to epithelial and nervous tissues. Endoderm forms the columnar lining of the digestive tract and organs associated with digestion, cells of lungs, and the thyroid and pancreatic glands. Mesoderm occupies a position between ectoderm and endoderm. It develops in connective and muscular tissues.

Connective tissues are classified into two big classes: **connective tissue proper** and **special connective tissue**. Connective tissues proper are divided in two groups: **loose connective tissues** and **dense connective tissues**. There are three major types of loose connective tissues: **areolar**, **adipose**, and **reticular**. Areolar connective tissue is the most generalized type of connection tissue. The principal cells of this tissue are fibroblasts. The ECM contains gel ground substance and all three major fiber types: collagen, elastin, and

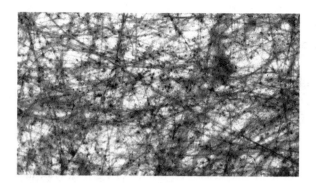

FIGURE 4.11   Areolar Connective Tissue.

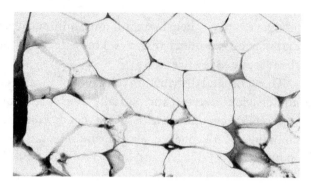

FIGURE 4.12   Adipose Tissue.

reticulin. Collagen gives this tissue tensile strength. Elastin and reticulin make it extensible, elastic, and flexible. This tissue is found everywhere. It underlines skin and attaches it to internal organs, muscles, and bones. Areolar tissue forms external coverage of all internal organs and all serous membranes (fig. 4.11). This tissue has a good blood supply and is quick to grow and to repair after injury.

Adipose tissue mostly contains adipocytes (fig. 4.12). When we think about fat tissue, we usually imagine something that is loaded with fat and inert. As a matter of fact, adipose tissue is very active. Fat deposition in adipocytes is dynamic and constantly in use and restoration. In addition to adipocytes, adipose tissue contains the stromal vascular fraction of cells including preadipocytes, fibroblasts, vascular endothelial cells, and a variety of immune cells such as adipose tissue macrophages. The two types of adipose tissue are white adipose tissue, which stores energy, and brown adipose tissue, which generates body heat. Adipose tissue is derived from preadipocytes. Tissue development is controlled in part by the adipose gene. Recent studies demonstrate that mutation in this gene causes obesity and may constitute a risk factor promoting the development of insulin resistance and type 2 diabetes. This tissue has a well-developed network of blood vessels. A good blood supply guarantees a high metabolic activity of adipose tissue.

Reticular connective tissue is named for the reticulin fibers, which are the main structural element of this tissue ECM. The cells that make the reticular fibers are fibroblasts called reticular cells. Reticular connective tissue forms a scaffolding for other cells in several organs, such as lymph nodes and bone marrow. Reticular connective tissue is never found alone. There are always some other cells scattered among the reticular cells and reticular fibers (fig. 4.13). Reticular connective tissue has an intimate association with blood and lymph vessels; that is, it is highly vascularized.

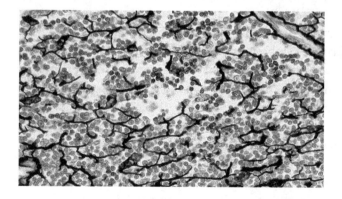

FIGURE 4.13   Reticular Connective Tissue.

Dense connective tissues are of three types: **regular**, **irregular**, and **elastic connective tissue**. The basic difference among these tissues are ECM fibers. Cellular component of the regular dense connective tissue are fibroblasts.

Fibroblasts deposit collagen fibers in an increased amount. This collagen in regular dense connective tissue is deposited in a regular way, side by side in one direction, and finally fills almost all space in the ECM. As a result, this creates structures that are very flexible, strong for tension, and resistant to extension, such as tendons (fig. 4.14). The increased amount of parallel oriented collagen fibers does not leave room for blood vessels, and this tissue is counted as avascular. As a result of poor blood supply, tissue is slow to grow and heal after injuries. For example, tendons, which are mostly regular dense connective tissue, repair after injury slower than bones.

Irregular dense connective tissue differs from regular by the deposition of collagen fibers. In irregular dense connective tissue, collagen fibers are not parallel to each other (fig. 4.15). The irregular directions of collagen make this tissue less strong and resistant to extension. On the other hand, this tissue is more flexible and can resist extension forces from different directions. This property is important in organs that experience tensions from many directions, like skin. Besides that, irregular dense connective tissue has a well-developed blood vessel network, which supplies not only this tissue, but also other nearby tissues; for example, epithelium. Skin dermis is mostly made of this tissue. Capsules that cover many organs, such as liver, kidney, and blood vessels, contain irregular dense connective tissue combined with other tissues.

Elastic dense connective tissue contains more elastin than collagen fibers. Elastin fibers make this tissue more stretchable than regular or irregular tissues. This tissue prevails in ligaments (fig. 4.16).

There are three types of special connective tissues: **cartilage**, **bone**, and **blood**. Blood ECM is a liquid called blood plasma. Blood plasma has very complex and varying ground matter containing gasses (oxygen, carbon dioxide, nitrogen, etc.), nutrients (carbohydrates, amino acids, and fats),

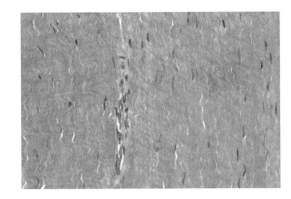

FIGURE 4.14   Regular Dense Connective Tissue.

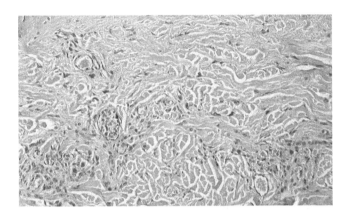

FIGURE 4.15   Irregular Dense Connective Tissue.

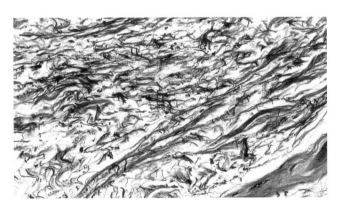

FIGURE 4.16   Elastic Dense Connective Tissue.

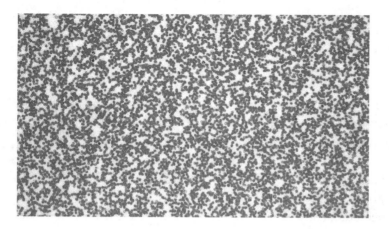

FIGURE 4.17   Blood.

electrolytes, and proteins (albumins, immunoglobulins, transport proteins, etc.). Blood ECM contains special water-soluble fiber proteins, such as fibrinogen. The cellular component of blood includes erythrocytes, white blood cells, and cellular fragments called platelets or thrombocytes. Together they constitute formed elements of blood. The major functions of blood are transport and distribution of gasses, nutrients, and waste materials; maintenance of tissues' osmotic pressure, and defense from pathogens (fig. 4.17).

The principal cells of cartilage are **chondrocytes**. They are found in all types of cartilage tissues. Chondrocytes reside in ECM spaces filled with interstitial fluid and surrounded by matrix of different consistency. All cartilages are avascular. Their blood supply is poor. That is why cartilage is a slow-growing and slow-healing tissue. The basic difference among the three cartilages are the amount and type of fibers in the ECM. Hyaline cartilage has almost no fibers. Its ECM is a clear transparent gel. The gel in hyaline cartilage is resilient, slippery, and creates a protective coverage of movable joints between bones. This cartilage also is called **articular cartilage**. Hyaline cartilage may be found in many structures. As a rule it is always associated with bones and joints. For example, costal cartilage binds sternal bones with ribs. An embryo skeleton originally is made of hyaline cartilage. During the organism's development, embryo hyaline cartilage is replaced by bones in a process called **ossification**.

Elastic cartilage has elastin fibers, which makes this tissue flexible. Its major role is to provide support and maintain the shape of the body structure. Elastic cartilage forms earlobes (pinna) and epiglottis of larynx.

Fibrocartilage is a tough strong tissue with high resistance to external forces. This tissue got its name because of a high amount of collagen in the ECM. Collagen fills the ECM and leaves almost no room for ground substance. In addition to chondrocytes, it has fibroblasts, which produce collagen and some amount of elastin fibers. This composition of the ECM gives fibrocartilage great tensile strength and elasticity. Fibrocartilage is found in the symphysis pubis, annulus fibrosus of intervertebral discs, menisci in knee joints, and some elements of the temporomandibular joint (TMJ) (fig. 4.18).

There are two types of bone tissues: **compact** and **spongy bones**. The difference between these two types is in the ECM structural organization. In compact bones the ECM is composed of very dense ground substance consisting of calcium phosphate salts that constitute 65 percent of bone mass and collagen. Calcium and collagen are deposited in concentric circles called lamellae organized around a central canal. Lacunae with osteocytes are located in these lamellae. A central canal carries blood vessels that nourish bone tissue. To transport oxygen and nutrients to osteocytes, all lacunae are connected by a network of tiny channels called **canaliculi**. This structure is called **osteon**. Spongy bone has no osteons. Bone tissue

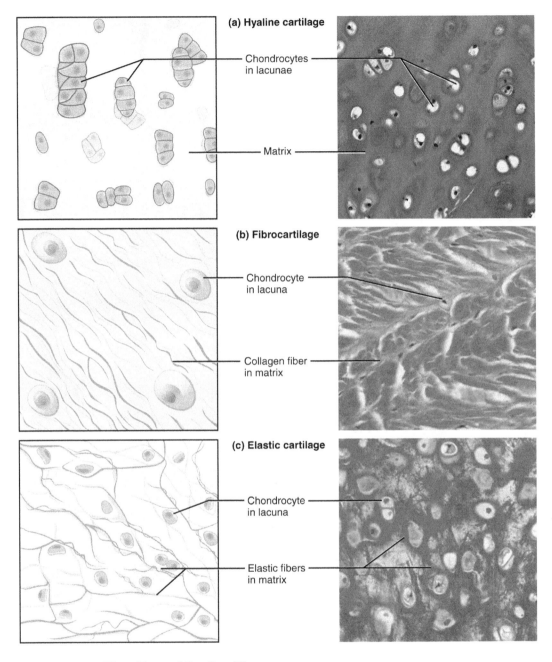

FIGURE 4.18 Three Types of Cartilage Tissues.

forms a network of spicules with lacunae and osteocytes. Spicules of spongy bone leave empty spaces that are filled with red bone marrow—a blood-producing (hematopoietic) tissue (fig. 4.19).

There are three cell types in both bone tissues. Bone-building cells are called **osteoblasts**. Osteoblasts are young osseous cells that produce the ECM. They absorb calcium from the interstitial fluids, form

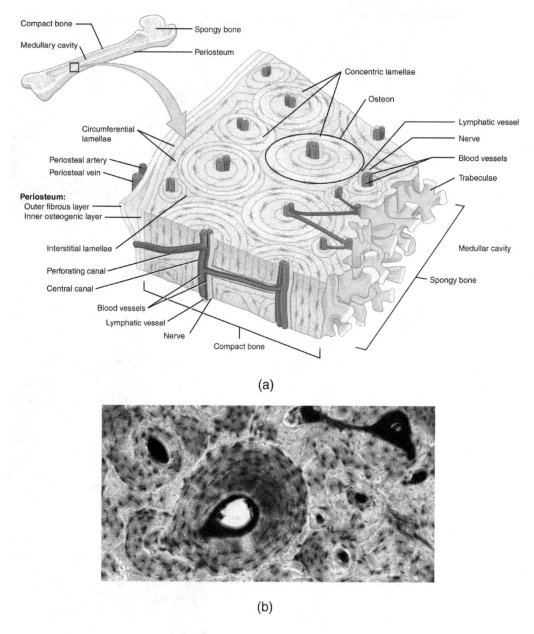

FIGURE 4.19   Two Types of Bone Tissue.

calcium salts, and deposit these salts in ECM. They also produce collagen, which forms a mesh network that holds calcium salts together. Calcium salts held together by collagen fibers fill space between cells. Only a small space around the osteoblast, called the **lacuna**, remains free of calcium and contains some amount of interstitial fluid. Osteoblast trapped in the lacuna transforms into the mature bone cell called **osteocyte**. Osteocyte remains inside the lacuna. Its major function is to maintain healthy bone tissue with a proper ratio of organic and inorganic substances. The third type of bone cells are **osteoclasts**. Osteoclasts originate from microphages' line of white blood cells. The cytoplasm of these cells contains granules with very strong hydrolytic enzymes. When released into bone tissue, these enzymes break down organic components of the ECM and release calcium into the blood flow; that is, they destroy bone tissue.

The total result of this review of connective tissues is presented in table 4.1.

TABLE 4.1   Classification of Connective Tissues

Connective Tissue Proper		Special Connective Tissue		
Loose Connective Tissue	**Dense Connective Tissue**	**Cartilage**	**Bone**	**Blood**
1. Areolar	1. Regular	Hyaline	Compact	
2. Adipose	2. Irregular	Elastic	Spongy	
3. Reticular	3. Elastic	Fibrocartilage		

CHECK YOUR UNDERSTANDING

- What is the main characteristic of connective tissue?

- What are the functions of adipose tissue?

- Describe the difference between cartilage and bone.

- What is the difference between regular and irregular dense connective tissues?

- Name three major fibers in connective tissue ECM. Describe their differences.

The Role of Connective Tissues in Body Organization

Connective tissues have many functions. In three words, these may be described as: connection, protection, and transportation. Areolar connective tissue is found everywhere. It is elastic, stretchable, and soft. It underlines skin, forms serous membranes, and connects other tissues. Adipose tissue maintains fat storage and participates in manufacturing of steroids. Brown fat generates heat. Adipocytes control appetite and maintain a balance of energy production. Reticular tissue form scaffolds for other tissues. Particularly, reticular tissue plays a very important role in the organization of lymphatic organs. All types of dense connective tissues, first of all, are structural elements of organs where elasticity and strong tension resistance is needed.

Hyaline cartilage is a primary structural material of vertebrate embryo skeleton. Later it is replaced by bone tissue, but it persists in joints. Elastic cartilage is a structural material of flexible organs, such as earlobes, the nose, and some parts of the larynx. Fibrocartilage is a strong material resistant to pressure and tension. It creates stress resistant structures such as intervertebral discs and symphysis joints.

Degenerative joint disease (DJD) is relatively common in horses as they age. Large-sized horses may have a higher risk of developing DJD over time. DJD is when the cartilage in a horse's joints deteriorates or thins. This cause the horse to be in pain or discomfort when walking or being ridden. Articular cartilage is hyaline in nature. Along with elasticity and shock-absorbing functions, it provides a smooth gliding surface for joint motion. Cartilage is an avascular tissue and, because of that, has very poor regenerative ability. DJD is characterized by degeneration of cartilage and hypertrophy of bone, which tries to compensate hyaline cartilage degeneration. This processes markedly affect soft tissues of joint synovial membrane. The synovial membrane inflames and develops edema. As the disease progresses, ankyloses (stiffness) occurs and changes in joints become irreversible.

The most common factor that initiates DJD, especially in a young thoroughbred, is trauma. A minor trauma of articular cartilage may persist for a long time, because of the poor regenerative ability of cartilage tissue. The joints that are most often involved are the carpus and the fetlock. The average racehorse after a brief morning workout spends the rest of the day standing in its stall. Often a horse races unprepared without warming up before the race, which may lead to injury. A minor injury may remain unnoticed, and often the horse may race despite the injury. Veterinarian practitioners relieve developing joint pain with drugs, such as phenylbutazone and corticosteroids. All of these lead to cartilage injury and worsening untreated injury, which leads to DJD development.

Blood transports oxygen, carbon dioxide, nutrients, and waste materials. White blood cells, as a part of the immune system, protect the organism from pathogen agents and harmful substances.

Bones create a frame of the body that holds the body's shape and protects internal organs, such as the brain inside the cranium. Bones provide a place for muscle attachment. Together they create a system of levers that moves the body. Bones store calcium and play an important role in calcium homeostasis. Red bone marrow produces all types of blood cells.

4.4   Muscular Tissue

Classification of Muscles

There are three classes of muscular tissue: **skeletal**, **cardiac**, and **smooth muscles**. Muscular tissue has a very small amount of ECM. The major difference among these three tissues is in the different types of muscular cells. Muscle cells are permanent and do not divide, and even the blood supply of muscular tissues as a rule is pretty good. Skeletal muscle cells are long and multinuclear, with well-visible light and dark stripes. This striation is a result of internal organization of contractile myofilaments made of actin and myosin fibers. That is why these muscles are also called striated muscles. Another important characteristic of skeletal muscles is smooth endoplasmic reticulum developed into cisternae for calcium storage. Skeletal muscle cells' contraction is activated by cortex regions of the brain. Because in humans the cortex is responsible for consciousness, these muscles are also called voluntary, meaning they are controlled by the conscious mind. It is difficult to say how conscious the behavior of an animal is, but traditionally in vertebrates these muscles are also called voluntary muscles.

Cardiac muscles are also striated. These cells are comparatively short; they have only one nucleus and are branched. Cardiac muscle cells are bound by intercalated discs. An intercalated disc is a complex combination of tight junctions, desmosomes, and gap junctions. A combination of desmosomes and tight junctions guarantees a strong connection between cells. Gap junctions provide continuous and fast transport of cytoplasm components and transmission of electrical impulses from one cell to another. Cardiac muscles are not under voluntary control. These cells are able to generate contractile impulse and spread this impulse to all cardiac cells. This ability to generate a wave of muscle cells contraction is called self-excitability.

Smooth muscle cells are comparatively short and spindle shaped. These cells have only one nucleus, located in the cell center. They have no striation. This means that smooth muscle cells' contractile fibers are organized differently than in cardiac and skeletal muscle cells. The contraction of these muscles is controlled by autonomous nervous system; that is, is out of "conscious" control from the brain. These cells also often demonstrate self-excitability, like cardiac muscles (see fig. 8.1, chapter 8).

The Role of Muscles in Body Organization

Skeletal muscles are associated with the skeleton. Together, they create a system of levers that move the body. Skeletal muscles generate heat and play an important role in regulation of body temperature. Skeletal muscles stabilize joints between bones and protect internal organs. Contraction of muscles surrounding veins and respiratory muscles (diaphragm and internal intercostal muscles) facilitates blood circulation.

Cardiac muscles are the major muscles of the heart. The ability of these muscles to generate waves of muscle contractions is a basic requirement for continuous unstoppable blood circulation. Special properties of these muscles make the heart a principal never-tired engine for blood movement.

Smooth muscles line the walls of all tubular and hollow organs: from blood vessels to the digestive tract. Contractions of these muscles propel food in the stomach and small intestine, push urine out of the body, and maintain blood pressure in the circulatory system. Smooth muscles can hold tension for a long time. On this property of smooth muscles is based a locking mechanism of most sphincter muscles, such as the internal anal sphincter, the pyloric sphincter between the stomach and duodenum, or the lower esophageal sphincter.

CHECK YOUR UNDERSTANDING

- Describe the difference between cardiac and skeletal muscles.

- What role do intercalated discs play in organization of the myocardium? Predict what will happen with cardiac muscles if the intercalated discs fail.

- What kind of muscle is responsible for contraction of the walls of the birth canal during delivery?

4.5 Nervous Tissue

Major Characteristics of Nervous Tissue

Nervous tissue is made of the most specialized cells in the vertebrate body—neurons. The principal characteristics of these cells are the ability to generate nerve impulse (an action potential) and to conduct these impulses on long distances without decreasing their intensity. On these characteristics of neurons are based their ability to collect, combine, and transmit vital information for control of all body functions. Neurons are permanent cells, and if a neuron dies, it cannot be replaced by another neuron. The characteristics of neurons are described in more detail in chapter 10. Besides neurons, the cellular component of nervous tissue includes neuroglia or just glia cells. There are six classes of neuroglia cells. Every type of neuroglia has its special characteristics and particular function in organization of the nervous system (fig. 4.20).

The ECM of nervous tissue constitutes a significant total volume of nervous tissue. It is a three-dimensional network that surrounds the cells. It acts as a biological scaffold for the structure of the CNS and controls the diffusion and availability of molecules for biochemical signaling and communication. The regenerative capacity of tissues is also directly related to the ECM. Disorders of the ECM cause a loss of the regenerative ability of the tissue and cells. Moreover, a proper immune and toxic response to infections, as we know now, depends on the correct equilibrium in the ECM components. In the nervous system, the ECM are synthesized and secreted by both neurons and glia. An astonishing number of extracellular matrix glycoproteins are expressed in dynamic patterns in the developing and adult nervous system. Neural stem cells, neurons, and glia express receptors that mediate interactions with specific extracellular matrix molecules. Functional studies in vitro and genetic studies in mice have provided evidence that the extracellular matrix affects virtually all aspects of nervous system development and function.

CHECK YOUR UNDERSTANDING

- What two types of cells constitute nervous tissue?

- Describe three main properties of neurons.

- What is the role of nervous tissue?

The Role of Nervous Tissue in Normal Body Function

Nervous tissue is a principal tissue of the nervous system. The fundamental role of the nervous system is control over activity of all organs of the body, uniting their activities into a harmonious functioning organism. The nervous system plays a crucial role in maintaining body homeostasis and regulation of all vital body functions. It controls skeletal and smooth muscle contractions, and manufacturing and release of secrets by body glands. It controls blood pressure and oxygen level in body tissues, monitors and regulates electrolytes' level in body fluids, and many other vital functions. Nervous tissue is a material foundation of the highest functions of organisms expressed in their behavior and social organization.

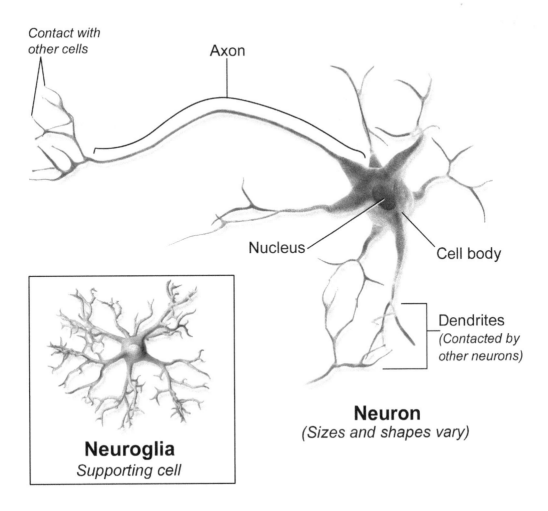

Neural Tissue

FIGURE 4.20   Nervous Tissue.

CHAPTER SUMMARY

- Structurally and functionally similar group of cells are called **tissue**. Each tissue has special characteristics and plays a specific role in organism. Tissue consists of cells and intracellular materials called the **matrix** or the **extracellular matrix** (ECM). The matrix is a complex combination of fibers embedded into homogeneous media of varying consistency called ground substance or ground matter. Depending on the types of cells and extracellular matrix, tissues are classified in four main types: **epithelial**, **connective**, **muscular**, and **nervous tissues**.

- **Epithelial tissue** covers the body and is a major component of the integumentary system. It covers cavities and lumens of hollow organs, such as the small intestine and trachea. A special type of epithelial tissue called endothelium lines tubular organs, such as blood vessels. The primary function of epithelial tissue is protection. Epithelial cells leave no space among cells for the ECM.

- **Connective tissues** are the most diverse tissue made of different cells. The matrix is also diverse and constitutes a significant portion of connective tissue. Connective tissue underlines other tissues and organs; connects, supports, and protects them; and transports substances.

- **Muscular tissues** are contractile, extensible, and elastic. Contraction of muscle cells moves the body, propels food in the digestive tract and sperm in reproductive organs, and creates blood pressure that forces blood to flow in blood vessels. Muscular tissue has much less matrix between cells compared to connective tissues. Cells of these tissues are highly specialized and do not divide.

- **Nervous tissue** is the most specialized tissue. The cellular component is presented by structurally and functionally diverse **neurons** and **neuroglia cells**. The extracellular matrix is gelatinous and contains special glycoproteins. The primary role of nervous tissue is to be a principal structural component of sensory organs and the nervous system, which collects, analyzes, and executes responses to changes in the internal and external environment.

- The ECM is a product of cells secreted into interstitial space via exocytosis. It has two components: 1) fibrous proteins and 2) **ground matter** or **ground substance**. Negatively charged glycoproteins in the ECM bind positively charged sodium ions (Na^+), which attracts water molecules via osmosis. Water molecules held in the ECM by hydrogen bonds with Na^+ keep tissue and resident cells hydrated. ECM swelling creates turgor force that resists external pressure and keeps tissues expanded. Protein **collagen** structurally supports resident cells. Protein **elastin** gives tissue elasticity and makes it extensible and elastic. A fibrous protein **reticulin** is found together with collagen and elastin in sperm cells' flagellum and mammalian skin.

- There are three types of cell junctions: 1) **tight junctions**, 2) **desmosomes**, and 3) **gap junctions**. Tight junctions are formed by integrin proteins in plasma membranes of adjacent cells. Cells stick each other, and integrin molecules lock them together. This junction does not leave space between cells, and macromolecules cannot pass the cell barrier. Desmosomes are composed of desmosome-intermediate filament complexes (DIFC). Desmosomes hold cells approximately at 34 nm distance and permit limited movement of some molecules. Desmosomes are the strongest cell junctions and are found in tissues that experience intense mechanical stress, such as cardiac muscle, urinary bladder, gastrointestinal mucosa, and skin epithelia. Gap junctions are formed by proteins connexons. Connexons are transmembrane proteins that pass through the plasma membranes of adjacent cells and create pores in them. Pores of gap junctions permit free movement of substances, ions, and electric impulses between adjacent cells.

- Epithelial tissue has to perform 1) protection, 2) transport, 3) immune defense, 4) secretion, and 5) sensation. Secretory epithelial cells may be single or create clusters called glands classified in two groups: 1) exocrine glands release their secrets on the open body surface or into tubes that open on the body surface; 2) endocrine glands release their secrets. called hormones, into the interstitial space or directly in the blood flow.

- Epithelial cells have two spatially and functionally different sides. One side that contacts with open space is called **free surface**. The free surface of epithelial cells often has extensions: microvilli or cilia. Cells with cilia are called **ciliated epithelium**. Microvilli significantly increase free cell surface and are a characteristic of small intestine mucosa. Ciliated epithelium is found in respiratory organs, such as the trachea and bronchi, and in ducts that transport sperm and egg cells. The opposite side of epithelial cell is covered by glue-like substance (an ECM of the epithelial tissue) called the **basement membrane**. The basement membrane is composed of two layers: **basal lamina** and underlying **reticular connective tissue**. The underlying connective tissue attaches to the basal lamina by collagen fibers. The basement membrane is produced by epithelial cells and firmly held together by the epithelial layer with underlying tissues.

- Epithelial tissues are classified according the cells' shape: **squamous**, **cuboidal**, and **columnar epithelium**; and number of cellular layers: **simple** and **stratified epithelium**.

- Multicellular exocrine glands are classified according the shape of the gland and its duct. Glands that have the shape of a tube are called **tubular**. When a gland has the shape of a ball or sphere, it is called **alveolar** or **acinar gland**. Glands with a single not branched duct are called **simple**, and glands with a branched duct are called **compound**.

- Another classification of exocrine glands is based on how the gland releases secrets. Merocrine glands continuously manufacture secret and release it via exocytosis. The cell is not damaged and may continue to produce secrets. Holocrine glands do not release secretes but accumulate them inside the cell. The process of secret manufacturing continues until the cell is ruptured and releases entire cell content. The ruptured cell dies and is replaced by a new cell. The apocrine glands produce secret and accumulate it in the apical area of the cell. When some significant amount of secret is accumulated, the cell releases it by detaching the apical part of the cell. The cell is damaged but does not die. It takes some time for the cell to repair the damage, and the cell may continue to manufacture a new portion of secret. Secretions of exocrine glands are of three types: **serous**, **mucous**, and **mixed secretions**.

- Connective tissue cells fall into three functional groups: 1) defense, 2) support, and 3) storage and distribution.

- The most common cells of connective tissues are **fibroblasts**. Fibroblasts manufacture ground matter and fibers of the ECM and create the structural framework (stroma) of animal tissues. They are evenly distributed in tissue and do not form permanent cell junctions. Fibroblasts maintain the ability to divide and can slowly migrate over substratum.

- Protective connective tissue cells include wandering phagocytes and sedentary cells. The wandering immune system cells by origin and function fall in two classes: **macrophages** and **neutrophils**. For these cells it is characteristic to move slowly in search of pathogenic agents, dead cells, and contaminating substances. Sedentary cells spend their life in the place of their forming.

- Three are three major fibrous components in the ECM of connective tissues: collagen, elastin, and reticulin. The ground substance varies from liquid in blood, to gel in cartilage, and to solid in bone. The ground substance/fibers ratio also varies significantly. In fibrous connective tissues, such as tendon, there are much more collagen fibers than ground substance, whereas hyaline cartilage ECM mostly consists of gel ground matter and very few fibers.

- Connective tissues fall in two classes: **connective tissue proper** and **special connective tissue**. Connective tissues proper are divided in two groups: **loose connective tissues** and **dense connective tissues**. There are three types of loose connective tissues: **areolar**, **adipose**, and **reticular**. Areolar connective tissue is the most generalized type of connection tissue. The principal cells of this tissue are fibroblasts. The ECM contains gel ground substance and three types of fibers: collagen, elastin, and reticulin. Collagen gives this tissue strength. Elastin and reticulin make it extensible, elastic, and flexible. This tissue underlines skin and attaches it to internal organs, muscles, and bones. Areolar tissue forms external coverage of all internal organs and all serous membranes. Adipose tissue mostly contains adipocytes. Adipose tissue is very active; its fat deposition is dynamic. The main structural part of reticular connective tissue is reticulin fibers. Reticular connective tissue forms a scaffolding for other cells in several organs, such as lymph nodes and bone marrow.

- There are three classes of dense connective tissues: **regular**, **irregular**, and **elastic**. Cells of the regular dense connective tissue are fibroblasts. Fibroblasts produce collagen in increased amount. This collagen has a regular side-by-side orientation and fills all space in the ECM. This creates structures that are very flexible, strong for tension, and resistant to extension, such as tendons. In irregular dense connective tissue, collagen fibers are not parallel. The irregular directions of collagen make this tissue less strong and resistant to extension, but more flexible and resistant to extension forces from different directions. Elastic dense connective tissue contains more elastin fibers. Elastin fibers make this tissue stretchable. It prevails in ligaments.

- There are three types of special connective tissues: **cartilage**, **bone**, and **blood**. Blood ECM is a liquid called blood plasma. Blood plasma has a very complex and varying content. It contains gasses (oxygen, carbon dioxide, and nitrogen), nutrients (carbohydrates, amino acids, and fats), electrolytes, and proteins (albumins, immunoglobulins, and transport proteins). Blood ECM contains water-soluble fiber proteins such as fibrinogen. The cellular component of blood includes erythrocytes, white blood cells, and cellular fragments called platelets or thrombocytes. Major functions of blood are transport and distribution of gasses, nutrients, and waste materials; maintenance of tissues' osmotic pressure; and defense from pathogens.

- The cells of cartilage are **chondrocytes**. Chondrocytes reside in lacunae filled with interstitial fluid and surrounded by matrix of different consistency. The basic difference among the three type of cartilages is the amount and type of fibers in the ECM. Hyaline cartilage has no fibers. Its ECM is a clear transparent gel. It is resilient, slippery, and creates a protective coverage of bone joints. Elastic cartilage has elastin fibers, which makes this tissue flexible. Its major role is to provide support and maintain the shape of body structures.

- There are two types of bone tissues: **compact** and **spongy bones**. In compact bones the ECM is composed of hard ground substance consisting of calcium phosphate salts that constitute 65 percent of bone mass and collagen. In spongy bone the dense ECM leaves an empty space filled with red bone marrow—a blood-producing (hematopoietic) tissue. The three principal cell types are **osteoblasts**, **osteocyte** and **osteoclasts**.

- There are three classes of muscular tissue: **skeletal**, **cardiac**, and **smooth**. This tissue has a small amount of ECM. Skeletal muscle cells are long and multinuclear with visible light and dark stripes. This striation is a result of internal organization of contractile myofilaments made of actin and myosin fibers.

- Cardiac muscles are striated. These cells are short. They have only one nucleus and are branched. Cells are connected by intercalated discs. Cardiac muscle cells are able to generate contractile impulse.

- Smooth muscle cells are comparatively short and fusiform shaped. These cells have only one nucleus, located at the center. Cells have no striation. Contractile fibers are organized differently than in cardiac and skeletal muscle cells. The contraction of these muscles is controlled by the autonomous nervous system. These cells often demonstrate self-excitability, like cardiac muscles, and may generate wave-like contractions called peristalsis.

CHECK YOUR KNOWLEDGE

LEVEL 1. CHECK YOUR RECALL

1. Injured tendons are slow to heal because the:
   A. Tissue is so hard
   B. Tissue is so fibrous
   C. Tissue has a small number of cells, which are so far apart
   D. Cells of this tissue do not divide
   E. Tissue has a very poor blood supply (avascular)

2. Which of the following is not one of the four basic types of body tissues?
   A. Epithelial tissue
   B. Connective tissue
   C. Muscles tissue
   D. Brain tissue
   E. Nervous tissue

3. The trachea and bronchi are lined by:
   A. Simple squamous epithelium
   B. Simple columnar epithelium
   C. Pseudostratified ciliated columnar epithelium
   D. Transitional epithelium
   E. Stratified columnar epithelium

4. Lungs' alveoli are composed of _____ , which best fits oxygen and carbon dioxide exchange.
   A. simple cuboidal epithelium
   B. transitional epithelium
   C. stratified cuboidal epithelium
   D. simple columnar epithelium
   E. simple squamous epithelium

5. The type of epithelial tissue that lines the urinary bladder is:
   A. Simple cuboidal epithelium
   B. Transitional epithelium
   C. Stratified cuboidal epithelium
   D. Simple columnar epithelium
   E. Glandular epithelium

6. The type of muscle found in the walls of blood vessels is:
   A. Cardiac
   B. Smooth
   C. Striated
   D. Skeletal
   E. Ciliated

7. Cartilage tissue is composed from cells called:
   A. Osteocytes
   B. Fibroblasts
   C. Chondrocytes
   D. Adipocytes
   E. Astrocytes

8. Which of these is **not** a connective tissue?
   A. Bone
   B. Cartilage
   C. Blood
   D. Tendon
   E. Myocardium

9. A general characteristic of connective tissue is that it:
   A. Consists of cells with much intercellular material among the cells
   B. Has no blood supply (avascular)
   C. Commonly is found lining body cavities and the body's surface
   D. Has cells usually tightly connected to each other; for example, by gap junctions

10. What type of protein fiber is commonly found in the extracellular matrix?
    A. Crystalline
    B. Collagen
    C. Keratin
    D. Fibrinogen
    E. Actin

11. What general tissue type binds, supports, and creates the immune protection of the body?
    A. Muscular
    B. Epithelial
    C. Nervous
    D. Connective

12. Tight junctions hold _____, whereas _____ is/are characteristic of cardiac muscle cells.
    A. skeletal muscle; desmosomes
    B. neurons; gap junctions
    C. mast cells; desmosomes
    D. smooth muscles; cell adhesion
    E. epithelial cells; gap junctions

13. The ECM of _____ contains collagen fibers, whereas the ECM of _____ has no collagen fibers at all.
    A. dense connective tissue; hyaline cartilage
    B. elastic tissue; fibrocartilage
    C. epithelial tissue; muscular tissue
    D. areolar tissue; bone tissue
    E. adipose tissue; blood

14. Goblet cells produce _____ and are an example of a(n) _____.
    A. serous fluid; unicellular endocrine gland
    B. mucus; unicellular exocrine gland
    C. mixed fluids; multicellular exocrine gland
    D. hormones; multicellular endocrine gland
    E. serous fluid; multicellular exocrine gland

15. Sebaceous glands are _____ and release secrets _____.
    A. merocrine glands; continuously without any damage to the cell
    B. apocrine glands; in big amounts together with some piece of the cell
    C. holocrine gland; only when they burst and die
    D. merocrine gland; in big amounts together with some piece of the cell
    E. apocrine gland; only when they burst and die

16. True or false: Cardiac muscle cells are striated multinucleated voluntary muscles.

17. True or false: Cells of the simple squamous epithelium in lungs' alveoli are bound to each other by gap junctions.

18. True or false: Mammary glands are an example of apocrine glands.

19. True or false: The walls of the urinary bladder are made of transitional epithelium.

20. Match the type of epithelium with its location:

    _____ Simple squamous epithelium   a. Urinary bladder and ureters
    _____ Stratified columnar epithelium   b. Trachea and bronchi
    _____ Simple cuboidal epithelium   c. Alveoli of the lungs
    _____ Stratified cuboidal epithelium   d. Skin
    _____ Simple columnar epithelium   e. Stomach and small intestine
    _____ Stratified squamous epithelium   f. Male urethra
    _____ Pseudostratified epithelium   g. Mammary glands
    _____ Transitional epithelium   h. Tubules of nephrons.

LEVEL 2. CHECK YOUR UNDERSTANDING

1. In your own words, explain why the procedures of cropping a dog's ear or piercing someone's nose usually do not cause bleeding (or almost no bleeding).

2. A microinfarction caused local death of cardiac muscle cells in the heart. Predict what kind of cells will replace the dead cardiac cells.

3. Vitamin C is required for collagen synthesis. Scurvy is characterized by vitamin C deficiency. Describe what changes will happen in the bones, ligaments, skin, and cartilage of an affected organism. What symptoms characterize this disease?

4. Most brain cancers are caused by carcinogenesis in neuroglia cells, but not neurons. Explain why this is so.

LEVEL 3. APPLY YOUR KNOWLEDGE TO REAL LIFE

1. The disease **arrhythmogenic cardiomyopathy** is a hereditary disease characterized by abnormal structure of connexin proteins in gap junctions, which affects the intercalated discs between cardiac muscle cells. Why does this disease cause cardiac failure?

2. The autoimmune disease **pemphigus foliaceus** results when an organism's own immune system attacks desmosomes in the epithelial cells of the skin. What changes in the affected person's skin do you expect to see?

3. In **pulmonary fibrosis**, elastin fibers of the lungs are replaced by collagen. How will this change influence breathing?

Chapter 5

Membranes and the Integumentary System

LEARNING OBJECTIVES

Upon completion of this chapter, readers should be able to:

1. Describe the simplest body organs—serous and mucous membranes.
2. Describe the structure of skin.
3. Explain the role and function of the integumentary system.
4. Describe accessory organs of the integumentary system, such as hair, claws, hoofs, antlers, horns, and different glands.

INTRODUCTION

The integumentary system is a group of organs whose major role is protection and maintenance of homeostasis in the body. The integumentary system includes skin, or integument—the largest and most extensive organ of the body. Skin covers the entire body and bears a number of accessary organs, such as claws, horns, sweat, and pheromone glands. The histological composition of the skin includes all four major types of tissues: epithelium, connective, muscular, and nervous. The integument creates a barrier for pathogens, parasites, toxic substances, and ultraviolet radiation. It helps maintain water balance and body temperature. The integument carries sensory organs that monitor environmental signals by touch, pressure, temperature, and so on.

The integument is exposed to harsh external environment and is frequently injured. The damage is decreased by external structures and skin layers composed of dead cells. At the same time a deep germinal layer regenerates and heals wounds. Histologically, the integument is classified as a cutaneous membrane. Thus, at first, we discuss what membrane is and explain classification of membranes.

5.1   Membranes of the Body

Organ—What Is That?

Membranes are the simplest organs of the body. Why do scientists consider a membrane to be an organ? Anatomists classify a structure of the body as an organ based on the following:

1. The organ is made of at least a few different tissues.
2. Tissues of the organ create a particular structure that has a specific position in the body.
3. The organ has a special role or function.
4. Every organ has a specific relationship with other organs.

Membranes—The Most Simple Organs of the Body

Now it is clear why a membrane is an organ. First of all, every membrane is made of a few tissues. For example, all serous membranes are made of secretory epithelium and areolar or loose connective tissue. Second, every membrane has a particular position in the body. For example, a pleural membrane is associated with the lungs and is located in the thoracic cavity. Third, every membrane has a specific role. For example, pericardial membrane protects and provides smooth movement of the heart. Every membrane is associated with nearby organs and with other membranes. For example, *greater omentum* covers and protects the intestines and is a part of a system of membranes, such as *lesser omentum* and *mesentery*.

Classification of Membranes

A membrane is a thin sheet of at least two tissues that lines the internal surface of a body cavity. Most membranes are made of a superficial layer of epithelial tissue and an underlying layer of connective, usually areolar tissue. Some membranes also may have a thin smooth muscle layer. Membranes anchor organs inside the body, provide organs smooth movement, create protective barriers for pathogens, and secrete various substances.

Membranes are classified in two groups: 1) true membranes and 2) membrane-like structures. The true membranes include **serous** and **synovial** membranes. The membrane-like structures are **mucous** and **cutaneous** membranes (table 5.1).

TABLE 5.1   Classification of Body Membranes

True Membranes		Membrane-Like Structures	
Serous Membrane	**Synovial Membrane**	**Mucous Membrane**	**Cutaneous Membrane**
Creates lining of closed body cavities	Creates lining of moveable joints	Creates lining of open body cavities	Creates coverage of body (skin)

Serous Membrane

Serous membrane, or **serosa**, lines completely closed body cavities and never has open contact with the external environment. All serous membranes are made of two cellular layers. One of these layers is a simple squamous epithelium, called **mesothelium**. This epithelial layer by the basement membrane binds to the second cellular layer made of areolar connective tissue. This double-layered membrane is folded in such a way that the simple squamous epithelial layer lines the internal walls of the fold and areolar tissue occupies the external walls of the folded membrane. One side of the serous membrane is attached to body walls (for example, to the walls of abdominal cavity). This side of the membrane is known as the **parietal layer**. The other side of the folded membrane binds to organs; for example, the small intestine. This layer is called **visceral** (fig. 5.1). Areolar connective tissue from both sides of parietal and visceral layers provides this connection. Faced inside, the fold mesothelium produces a thin, clear, watery fluid, known as **serous fluid**. This serous fluid fills the space between folds of the same membrane, known as a **cavity**. Inside the cavity serous fluid creates a lubricating film that provides a smooth frictionless movement of covered organs.

A particular serous membrane gets its name in correspondence with covered organ(s). Thus, serous membrane that covers the lungs is called **pleural membrane**, or **pleura**. The cavity of this membrane is known as a **pleural cavity**. The serous membrane in the abdominal cavity that covers the small intestine is called the **peritoneal membrane**, or **peritoneum**. The cavity of this membrane is the **peritoneal cavity**.

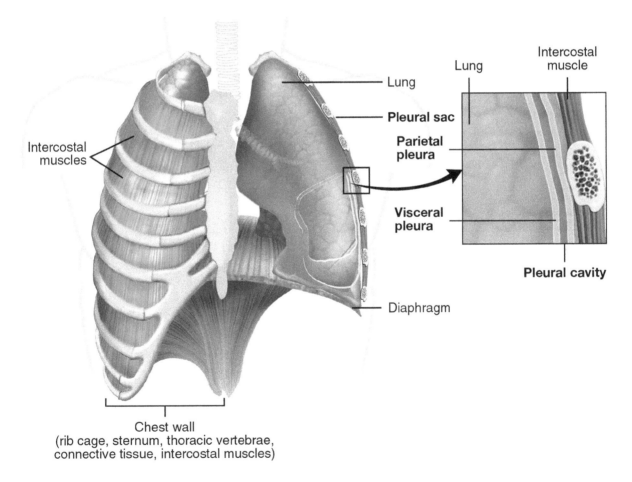

FIGURE 5.1   Serous Membrane (Pleura).

Synovial Membrane

The synovial membranes line and completely cover cavities of moveable joins, such as the shoulder, elbow, hip, and knee. Synovial membrane does not have a layer of epithelial cells. Both cellular layers of synovial membrane are made of connective tissue. The internal layer is made of special type fibroblasts called **synoviocytes**, and the external layer is made of a combination of areolar and irregular dense connective tissues. Synoviocytes secrete a lubricating watery **synovial fluid** that provides smooth frictionless movement of body joint.

Mucous Membrane

Mucous and cutaneous membranes are membrane-like organs. The mucous membranes, or **mucosa**, line cavities that open outside of the body: respiratory passages, nasal and mouth cavities, digestive tract, and male and female reproductive organs. The upper layer of mucosa is made of epithelium. The basement membrane of the epithelial layer binds it with a loose connective tissue called **lamina propria**. Very often lamina propria is underlined by a layer of smooth muscles. The epithelial layer has glands and goblet cells that secrete mucus. The mucus gives the name to this type of membrane (fig. 5.2).

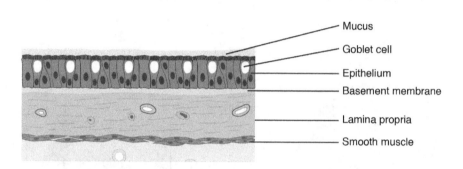

Mucus
Goblet cell
Epithelium
Basement membrane
Lamina propria
Smooth muscle

FIGURE 5.2   Mucous Membrane.

Cutaneous Membrane

The term *cutaneous membrane* refers to the coverage of the body. It is the biggest body membrane that creates the largest body organ: skin. Superiorly, skin is constructed of stratified squamous epithelium called **epidermis** and underlying **dermis** made of loose connective and irregular dense connective tissues. Epidermal cells accumulate waterproof protein, called **keratin**. The process of accumulation of keratin in epithelial cells is called **keratinization**. Keratinized cells die, and the upper layer of the epidermis, called the **stratum corneum**, contains only dead cells. This outermost layer of dead cells creates the perfect protective coverage of the body.

CHECK YOUR UNDERSTANDING

- Name the major types of membranes and membrane-like structures.
- What is the difference between serous and mucous membranes?
- What is the difference between parietal and visceral membranes?
- In your own words, give the definition of a pleural cavity.
- What is the principal role of synovial membrane?

5.2   The Integumentary System

The integumentary system consists of skin and accessory organs: hair, claws, nails, hoofs, horns, different glands, and so forth, collectively known as the **integument**. The integument protects the body from invasion of pathogenic agents, defends from predators, warms the body up in the winter and cools it down on hot summer days, helps retain water and remove wastes from body fluids, makes an animal "invisible" and camouflaged in its natural habitat, as well as makes an individual recognizable and attractive to the opposite sex.

Skin Structure and Function

The skin is an organ: 1) it is made of different tissues; 2) it has a species-specific shape and occupies a particular position in the body; 3) it has a characteristic physiology; 4) it has very special relations with other organs of the body; and 5) it plays a very particular role. The skin is the largest body organ. It makes up approximately 10 to 15 percent of the total body weight. Healthy skin is vital for effective maintenance of body homeostasis. Skin has two main components:

1. **Epidermis:** a superficial structure made of keratinized stratified squamous epithelium
2. **Dermis:** a deep structure made of areolar (loose) and underlying it irregular dense connective tissues

The epithelial basement membrane holds these two layers together like a glue (fig. 5.3).

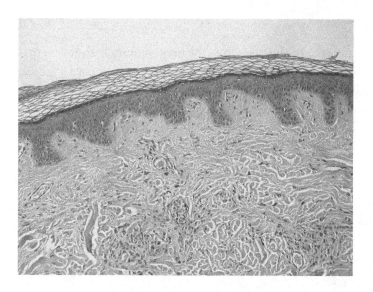

FIGURE 5.3   Cutaneous Membrane (Skin).

The Epidermis

The epidermis is made of keratinized stratified squamous epithelium. As you know from the previous chapter (see page 105), epithelium is an avascular type of tissue. It has no blood vessels, and it receives all oxygen and nutrients from the blood vessels of the underlying dermis. Another remarkable characteristic of epithelium is the absence of intercellular space and the fact that the cells are connected each other by tight junctions and desmosomes. Both characteristics facilitate the protective strength of the skin.

About 95 percent of the epidermis cells are **keratinocytes**—epithelial cells that manufacture and accumulate keratin. Keratin is a fibrous protein that is very tough and resistant to mechanical and chemical stress. Keratinocytes staffed with keratin create a perfect body protection against mechanical abrasion, pressure, and the effect of aggressive chemicals. Keratin fibers are hydrophobic, which helps maintain water balance in the body. Keratinocytes are linked by desmosomes that makes the epidermis strong and hardly permeable to pathogens. Other cells of the epidermis—**melanocytes**, **dendritic** or **Langerhans cells**, and **Merkel cells**—constitute about 5 percent or less of the epidermis.

Melanocytes are located at the very bottom of the epidermis in the basement membrane (fig. 5.4). Melanocytes produce pigment melanin that varies in color from orange-red to black. Melanocytes have long extensions that continue between keratinocytes. Pigment is produced in special membranous vesicles called **melanosomes**. Melanosomes produce, store, and transport pigment along the cytoplasmic extensions. From the melanocytes, the melanosomes may migrate into keratinocytes, where they are concentrated in regions most exposed to UV radiation. Thus, melanosomes create a shield that protects cells, especially the nucleus that contains DNA molecules, from damage. Pigment degrades in a few days, and new melanin molecules are continuously produced to maintain skin color. In general, skin color depends on 1) the color of produced melanin, 2) the amount of produced pigment, and 3) the distribution of melanosomes. When melanosomes are concentrated around the nucleus, the skin has a light color. When melanosomes move into cellular projections, pigmentation becomes more visible. Accumulation of melanosomes in keratinocytes creates a dark or black skin color (fig. 5.4). The production of melanin and movement of melanosomes is control by a **melanocyte-stimulating hormone (MSH)** produced by the intermediate lobe of the pituitary gland. Another factor that influence melanin synthesis and transport is exposure to UV radiation. Exposure to ultraviolet causes tanning or darkening of skin. That is why animals living at a high altitude, where UV radiation is high, often have dark fur.

Cancer is the most common cause of chronic disease and death in middle-aged and older dogs and cats. Thirty-three percent of cats and 50 percent of dogs over ten years of age die of cancer. Skin cancer is the most common type of canine cancer and the second-most common type of feline cancer.

Cancerous basal cell tumors are the most common skin cancer in cats. Middle-aged Persian and other long-haired cats are most susceptible to these tumors. Wirehaired pointing griffons, Kerry blue, and wheaten terriers are the most predisposed to basal cell tumors among dogs. Basal tumors grow from stratum basale. They may occur as a series of small nodular growths side by side on the back and chest of cats and as a single hairless lump on the head, neck, or shoulders of dogs. In most cases basal cell tumors are benign. Even if the dog or cat develops the cancerous form, basal cell carcinoma, the tumor usually can be removed without further problems.

Squamous cell carcinoma develops from mutant keratinocytes. Squamous cell carcinoma is most aggressive and deadly form of cancer. There are different types of squamous cell carcinomas, and different breeds of dogs are more susceptible to each type. Bloodhounds, Basset hounds, and standard poodles are at greatest risk for one type, while white-skinned, shorthaired breeds such as dalmatians, bull terriers, and beagles are prone to another type. Cats with white skin and hair are more likely to develop squamous cell carcinoma because they are more vulnerable to UV radiation. Squamous cell carcinoma may appear as a white or grayish ulcer, cauliflower-shaped lump, or a red bumpy area. These growths may include sores that do not heal and hair loss in the area. Most often the ulcers appear on the pet's belly since dogs and cats often take sun on their back.

Melanin has three major functions: 1) protecting DNA from damaging UV radiation, 2) decreasing the production of vitamin D in response to UV radiation, and 3) camouflaging an animal in its natural environment or signaling others about readiness to breed. At a first glance, it seems strange that an organism may need less vitamin D. Vitamin D increases absorption of Ca^{2+} in the small intestine and increases blood calcium. However, an excess of vitamin D can cause a calcium imbalance that may result in muscle cramps, heart problems, and kidney failure.

Dendritic or Langerhans cells are phagocytes—a part of the immune system. They protect an organism from invasion of pathogenic organisms through the skin. These cells originate from white blood cells known as monocytes. Monocytes tend to leave blood vessels, move into the interstitial space between cells, and transform into phagocytes. In the epidermis these phagocytes

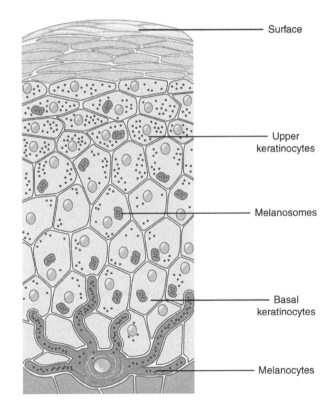

FIGURE 5.4   Melanocyte in Stratum Basale of Epidermis.

A group of invertebrate animals—cephalopods—which includes octopus, squid, and cuttlefish, are well known for their ability to change the color of their body, which they use for camouflage or to warn potential predators. These creatures have special pigment cells called chromatophores in their skin. These cells may change shape by muscular contraction. The change of cell shape causes a change of cell color. The muscular contraction is controlled by motor neurons that receive signals from photoreceptors. The cephalopods have well-developed color vision. Using their excellent eyesight and chromatophores, cephalopods camouflage themselves by creating color patterns that perfectly match their natural habitat.

Unlike the squid and octopus, chameleons do not modify their hues by accumulating or dispersing pigments within skin cells. Studies of *Furcifer pardalis*, a chameleon from Madagascar, show that this lizard has two superposed thick layers of iridophore cells—iridescent cells that have pigment and reflect light. The iridophore cells contain nanocrystals of different sizes, shapes, and organizations. The chameleons can change the structural arrangement of the upper cell layer by relaxing or exciting the skin, which leads to a change in skin color, as can be seen in the following image.

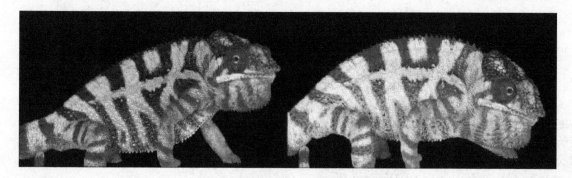

IMG. 5.1   This Male Chameleon Changed Color from Green to Yellow. Its Red Markings Also Became More Vibrant.

Credit: Michel Milinkovitch (https://www.livescience.com/50096-chameleons-color-change.html).

become dendritic cells. These cells develop cellular extensions that create a net that catches pathogens before they move deep inside the body.

Merkel cells have an oval shape. These cells are associated with dendrites of sensory neurons. Together with sensory neurons, these cells function to detect very light touch, fine texture, and shape.

Cells of the epidermis are organized into five layers, or **strata**. The deepest stratum rests on the basement membrane and is called the **stratum basale** or **stratum germinativum**. It is closest to the underlying dermis and blood supply. It consists of a single layer of constantly dividing cells. Nearby blood vessels from dermis provide cells of the stratum basale with oxygen and nutrients that make these cells metabolically and mitotically very active. All keratinocytes of the epidermis originate from these progenitor cells, and while this layer is not damaged epidermis can be regenerated. Melanocytes and Merkel cells are also located in the stratum basale.

The next superficial to the stratum basale is the **stratum spinosum**. It is the thickest layer. Keratinocytes of this layer are still close to blood vessels and are metabolically and mitotically active. This layer also contains dendritic cells that create a defense barrier against pathogens.

The middle layer is called the **stratum granulosum**. It consists of three to five cellular layers. Cells of this layer are characterized by special granules in the cytoplasm. These granules are of two types: one type contains keratin, and another contains lipid-based substances. The last granules release their contents by exocytosis in the interstitial space. Hydrophobic lipids coat superficial layers of the epidermis and prevent movement of water and water-soluble substances through the skin.

Superficial to the stratum granulosum is the **stratum lucidum**. It is a narrow, transparent layer of dead keratinocytes. This stratum presents only in thick skin and is absent in the thin skin of eyelids, for example (fig. 5.5).

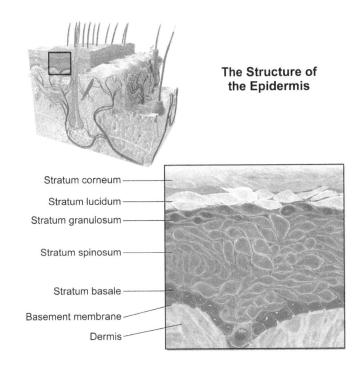

The Structure of the Epidermis

Stratum corneum
Stratum lucidum
Stratum granulosum
Stratum spinosum
Stratum basale
Basement membrane
Dermis

FIGURE 5.5   Structure of Epidermis.

The most superficial layer is called the **stratum corneum**. The stratum corneum consists of several layers of dead scaly keratinocytes, or what remain of them. Keratinocytes lose their internal structures and mostly contain keratin fibers. Cells lose their desmosomes and may be easily sloughed (fig. 5.5).

CHECK YOUR UNDERSTANDING

- Name the five strata of the epidermis from the bottom to the top.

- Describe the role of melanin and how it is distributed in the skin.

- Describe the cells of the epidermis and the keratinocyte life cycle.

- Can you explain the difference between thick and thin skin?

The Dermis

The dermis is another part of the skin located under the epidermis. The dermis is a vascularized component of the skin. It houses many receptors and is made of two types of connective tissues: **papillary** and **reticular layers**.

The papillary layer occupies a superficial position and accounts about 20 percent of the dermis. It is made of areolar (loose) connective tissue. The ECM of areolar tissue contains collagen and elastic fibers, which make this tissue strong, flexible, and stretchable to some degree. Collagen fibers of the areolar tissue penetrate into the basement membrane of the epidermis, interlace with collagen from the epidermis, and anchor the dermis in position. The most common cells of this tissue are fibroblasts and phagocytes.

The surface of the papillary layer, where it contacts with the epidermis, is folded. The projections of the papillary layer are known as **dermal papillae**. Dermal papillae help create a strong hold between the epidermis and dermis, and increase the strength of the skin. Small blood vessels known as capillaries create loops inside dermal papillae. Oxygen and nutrients from these capillary loops diffuse into the interstitial fluids of dermal papillae and from there move into the lower layers of the epidermis that lack blood vessels. Special tactile structures called **Meissner corpuscles** are also located in dermal papillae. These receptors are sensitive to a very light touch and are numerous in most body areas that are sensitive to touch (fig. 5.6).

The reticular layer is composed mostly of irregular dense connective tissue. Irregular dense connective tissue is characterized by the large amount of irregularly arranged collagen fibers. These fibers make skin

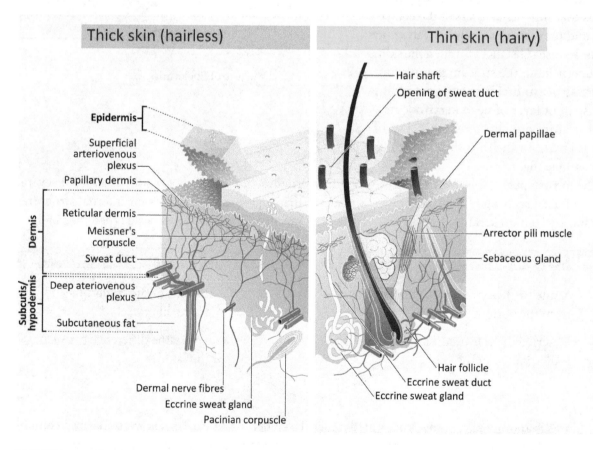

FIGURE 5.6   Skin Structure.

strong and prevent skin from being broken down by tension and extension. The layer is rich with blood vessels and nerve fibers. Accessory structures such as sweat glands, sebaceous glands, hair, and different sensory receptors are also housed in the reticular layer. The most common sensory receptors are called **lamellated** or **Pacinian corpuscles**. These receptors are sensitive to pressure and skin vibration (fig. 5.6).

CHECK YOUR UNDERSTANDING

- You have a light cut on your finger, but there is no blood in the wound. Can you explain why there is no blood?

- Describe the role of dermal papillae.

- Describe the difference between Meissner and Pacinian corpuscles.

5.3   Accessory Organs of the Skin

Accessory structures of the integument include different glands, hair, claws, nails, hoofs, horns, and antlers. These structures have many different functions.

Hair and Body Color

Hair or **pili** are small keratinized filamentous structures projecting from the skin of almost the entire body, except some regions with thick skin, lips, and parts of the external genitalia. A thick hair coverage or coat is called **fur** or **pelage** and is composed of **down hairs** and **guard hairs**.

Down or wooly hairs form an animal's undercoat. They are thin, soft, flat, and wavy. These hairs are usually short and very numerous. Down hairs are associated with numerous sebaceous glands. Sebum secreted by these glands covers skin and hair shafts, thus forming a waterproof coverage on an animal's body. Dense down hair coverage forms space for dry air, which creates thermal insulation of the animal body. In temperate regions with a cold winter, their number usually increases. The thickness of the undercoat varies among species. For example, huskies have a very thick coat, which guarantees they stay alive in hostile winter weather. In contrast, Dobermans almost have no undercoat and, because of that, cannot withstand cold weather.

Guard hairs are usually longer than down hairs. They form a coat of the animal's fur. These hairs have a long, coarse, straight shaft. Guard hairs are pigmented and usually carry the characteristics for the animal's color pattern, displayed for attraction or camouflage. Pigmentation of these hairs also protects the animal body from ultraviolet radiation and injuries. Animals with well-developed fur often have so-called **awn hairs**. These hairs combine properties of both down and guard hairs.

Specialized sensory hairs associated with sensory neurons around the snout of the animal are called **vibrissae** or "whiskers." This type of hair is especially well developed among nocturnal and burrowing mammals. Porcupines have stiff, strong, coarse hair called **quills** that protect the animal from predators.

The part of the hair hidden inside the skin is called the **root**. The remaining part that is exposed over the skin surface is called the **shaft**. Hair has an epidermal origin and is made of epithelial keratinocytes. When the keratinocytes of the root are alive, the cells of the shaft are completely keratinized and dead. In

Hair Follicles and Hair

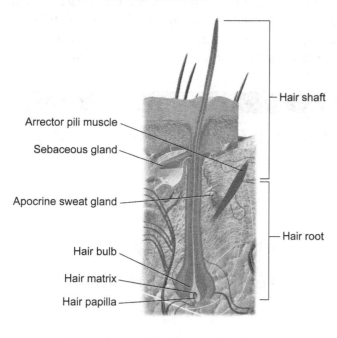

Hair shaft

Arrector pili muscle

Sebaceous gland

Apocrine sweat gland

Hair root

Hair bulb

Hair matrix

Hair papilla

FIGURE 5.7   Hair Structure.

cross section, the shaft has three layers: superficial scaly **cuticle**, the thick middle layer **hair cortex**, and the core with loosely spaced dead cells often with an air spaces between them called **hair medulla**.

The hair root is an epidermis that dips down into the dermis. At its end, hair root has a **hair follicle**. At the top of hair follicle dermis has projection known as **dermal papilla**. A single-cell layer of epithelial cells called **matrix cells** around the dermal papillae are those cells that produce all cells of the hair root and hair shaft. Capillaries in dermal papillae deliver oxygen and nutrients to germinal cells of the matrix and stimulate their proliferation. The hair shaft grows out of matrix cells in the hair follicle in cycles. The cycle of hair growth activity is made of three consecutive stages: growth, degeneration, and rest. The growth stage is characterized by an active proliferation of cells of the matrix. After the growth stage comes the degeneration stage, when cells become inactive and die. The last resting stage may continue for several weeks to a few months. During this period, stem cells of the hair papilla produce a new follicle, and a new hair cycle begins. At that time the old hair shaft falls out and is replaced by the new growing shaft. This cycle is driven by an intrinsic process, and cutting the hair has no impact on the rate of hair growth.

A group of smooth muscles that bind with hair follicles and are anchored in the dermis are called **arrector pili** muscles. These muscles make the hair stand erect in response to cold, fear, or anger. The pressure exerted by the muscle also forces sebum to move out the sebaceous gland along the hair follicle toward the skin surface (fig. 5.7).

Sebaceous and Sweat Glands

There are three major types of glands in the integument: sebaceous, eccrine, and apocrine. Scent, sweat, and mammary glands originate from them and may be considered as their derivatives.

Sebaceous glands are associated with hair roots and are absent in hairless body regions. They produce an oily secretion called **sebum** (fig. 5.7). This oily secretion is released into hair follicles and makes fur soft and waterproof. Sebaceous glands are not bound to hair follicles in areas around the mouth, on the penis, around the vagina, and on the nipples of mammary glands. The **wax glands** in the walls of the external auditory meatus that secrete earwax and the **tarsal glands** on the eyelids that produce oily film secretion on the eyeball surface both originate from sebaceous glands.

Some animals have specialized sebaceous glands. The glands are folds of the skin covered by fine hair and have numerous sebaceous glands. The secretion of the glands is a fatty yellow viscous fluid that dries and sticks to the skin. Sheep have three pairs of **sheep pouches**: 1) **infraorbital pouches** at the medial canthus of the eye, 2) **interdigital pouches** between the digits above the hooves, and 3) **inguinal pouches** in the groin. Goats have sebaceous **horn glands**, located caudal to the horn base. Secretion of these glands is increased during the breeding period and is especially pungent in bucks. Pigs have **carpal glands** on the mediopalmar surface of the carpus in both boars and sows.

    Eccrine glands produce thin watery fluids. They are not associated with hair follicles. In most mammals these glands are located on the soles. These glands function in thermoregulation and waste excretion.

    Apocrine glands produce a viscous fluid that is rich with lipids and like sebaceous glands associated with hair follicles. The secretion of these glands function in chemical signaling.

    Scent glands derivate from apocrine glands. Their secretions play a role in animal social communication: to mark territory, to identify an individual, and courtship. In rabbits and deer, scent glands are located on the chin. In antelopes and bats, they are on the face; in elephants, on the temporal region; in most carnivores, on the chest and arms; in rodents, dogs, cats, and mustelids, in their anal region; some animals, like a musk deer, on the belly; whereas kangaroo rats, peccaries, camels, and ground squirrels, on the back.

    Mammary glands are exocrine glands that produce milk. The evolutionary origin of mammary glands remains unclear, but most specialists agree that they most probably developed from apocrine sweat glands. The presence of these glands distinguishes mammalians from other animals. In some mammals, such as monotremes and marsupials, these glands are scattered over the ventral surface of the animal body. In other mammals, mammary glands are arranged into organs, such as breasts of primates, udders of ruminants, or dug of cats and dogs. Among females, mammary glands normally become active during lactation. However, lactation among males of the dayak fruit bat has been observed.

Tail Glands and Anal Sacs

Anal glands or **anal sacs** are group of small exocrine glands of different origin. In most mammals they are modified sebaceous glands, whereas in dogs they originate from apocrine sweat glands. In all cases, anal glands are small paired sacs located on both sides of the anus between external and internal anal sphincter muscles. Short ducts carry their secretions to the anal opening. During defecation, relaxed sphincter muscles and passing feces press on the glands and eject secretion onto the feces. The anal glands' secretions are liquids composed of fatty and serous materials with cellular debris. Often, these secretions have a foul smell, which acts as an individual identification label and/or territorial marker. Anal glands are found among carnivores including cats, bears, and sea otters. In skunks these glands tend to spontaneously empty when the animal is under stress and create a very sudden pungent odor. The opossum anal gland secretion has an odor of a rotting body, which the animals use to "play possum," or "play dead." Rabbits use secretions of these glands as a territorial marker.

    A sick animal with abnormally soft stool may not create enough pressure on the glands during defecation. As a result, the glands may fail to empty. They may accumulate their secretions and become swollen. Swollen glands press on the anus and create discomfort. Dogs, for example, with swollen anal sacs have difficulty sitting and standing. They often drag their posterior over the ground or lick or bite their anus. Cats with abstracted anal sacs may began to defecate everywhere in the house outside the litter box. Very often this uncontrollable defecation is wrongly interpreted as a behavioral abnormality,

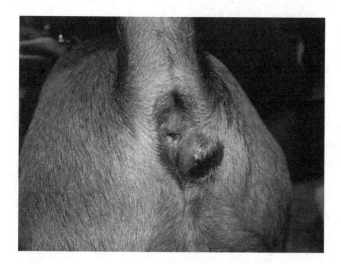

FIGURE 5.8   Abscess of Right Anal Gland in Dog.

whereas in reality it is caused by disease. The procedure that can relieve the discomfort is termed **anal sac expression**. It performed by gentle squeezing of the clogged anal sac to empty it. Fatty secretion of the anal sac is the perfect environment for different bacteria. The most common bacteria that inhabit anal sacs are *Escherichia coli*, *Enterococcus faecalis*, *Clostridium perfringens*, and different species of *Proteus* (fig. 5.8). Treatment of these infections includes usage of systemic antibiotics and frequent anal sac expression to release discomfort.[1]

The **violet** or **supracaudal gland** is a composite structure. It combines together modified sebaceous and apocrine sweat glands. These glands are found in the perineum, the dorsal surface of the animal tail, and the male prepuce. They are common among European badgers, canids (foxes, wolfs, and dogs), and felines, including domestic cats. The secretions of these glands contain steroid hormones and volatile molecules of terpenes that serve as pheromones. Thus, their principal functions are endocrine and pheromone signaling during the breeding period. Violet glands empty into special sweat glands with wide ducts that open at the base of guard hairs. In dogs both sexes have violet glands that usually are located in the area around the ninth caudal vertebra, but in some breeds they may be vestigial or absent (fig. 5.9). Foxes have a comparatively big violet gland that occupies up to a third of the upper surface of the animal's tail. They play a critical role in the metabolism of steroid hormones.[2]

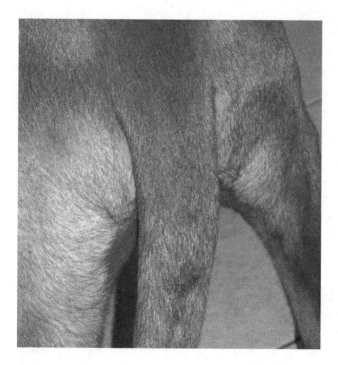

FIGURE 5.9   A Dark Spot on the Dorsal Surface of a Rhodesian Ridgeback Tail is a Violet Gland.

1   Stephen J. Ettinger and Edward C. Feldman, *Textbook of Veterinary Internal Medicine,* 4th ed. (Philadelphia: W. B. Saunders Company, 1995).

2   S. A. Shabadash and T. I. Zelikina, "The Tail Gland of Canids," *Biology Bulletin* 31, no. 4 (2004): 367.

Claws, Nails, and Hooves

Claws, nails, and hooves are made of tightly compressed, cornified keratinocytes of epidermis. **Claws** or **talons** are curved, compressed from the lateral side projections on the tips of digits. They are seen in some amphibians and most birds, reptiles, and mammals. A group of active dividing cells, called the **claw matrix**, is located at the claw base. These cells continually undergo mitosis and form a new claw at the claw base. The old claw cells, dead and heavily keratinized, are pushed toward the claw-free edge, where they are worn or broken. Primates are the only mammals that have **nails**. The nails have the shape of plates on the tips of fingers and toes. In general, nails grow the same way as claws (fig. 5.10).

VETERINARY APPLICATION

Declawing (Onychectomy). A cat's claw is part of the last bone (distal phalanx) in the cat's toe. The cat's claw arises from the unguicular crest and unguicular process in the distal phalanx of the paw. Most of the germinal cells that produce the claw are situated in the dorsal aspect of the ungual crest. This region must be removed completely, or regrowth remains possible. The only way to be sure all of the germinal cells are removed is to amputate the entire distal phalanx at the joint. Thus, onychectomy in the clinical definition involves either the partial or total amputation of the terminal bone.

Ungulates have **hooves** on the tips of their digits. The horse hoof has three parts: 1) hoof wall, 2) sole, and 3) frog. The hoof-like claws and nails are a product of integument. The hoof wall is open at the heel. It is U shaped and has few cellular layers, or strata. The superficial thin, shiny keratinized layer is known as the **stratum externa** or **tectorium**. The next layer is thickly keratinized and penetrated by coiled, tubular channels. It is called the **stratum medium**. The inner layer, the **stratum internum** or **lamellatum**, is a laminated, folded layer, whose projections (rete pegs) interdigitate with the dermis (corium). The hoof wall grows out from the base at a rate of about 6 mm per month. It takes 9 to 12 months to completely renew the hoof. The frog creates the bottom ground surface of the hoof. It is the heaviest keratinized part that fills the opening between the heel and the hoof wall. The sole fills the ground surface space between the wall and triangular frog. It consists of the epidermis and thickened dermis (the corium) of the sole. Deep in the sole is a fatty digital cushion or pad, a derivative of the hypodermis (fig. 5.11).

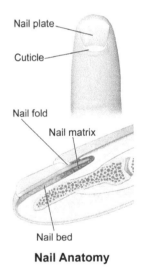

Nail Anatomy

FIGURE 5.10 Human Nail Anatomy.

Paw Pads

Many mammals have pads on their paws. In fig. 5.12 you can see pads on the dog's paw. The paw pad is a specialized anatomic structure on the sole. It is composed of hairless, heavily keratinized pigmented epidermis, underlined by adipose and irregular dense connective tissues. The dermis of the pad's skin carries multiple sweat glands that release perspiration fluids and, thus, plays an important role in the homeostasis of a dog's body temperature. Dogs have sweat glands only on the tongue and here, in the paw pads. This sweat gland distribution cools the dog's body and, at the same time, keeps

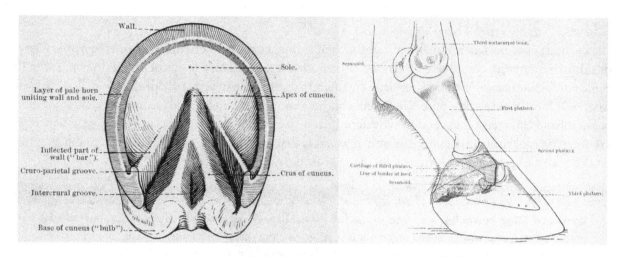

FIGURE 5.11   Anatomy of the Horse Hoof.

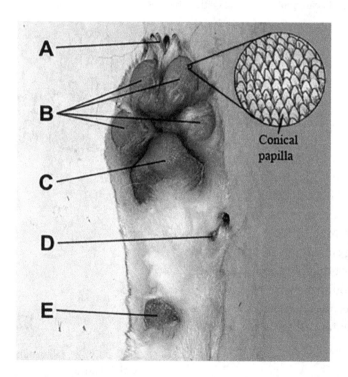

FIGURE 5.12   Dog's Paw. A. Claw; B. Digital Pads;
C. Metacarpal Pad; D. Dew Claw; E. Carpal Pad.

it dry. Secretions of these glands, like other sweat glands, is controlled by the sympathetic nervous system and some hormones, such as norepinephrine. Thus, a stressed dog can exude some fluids and leave a characteristic smelling footprint. The adipose tissue that underlines the skin of the pad insulates internal tissues from extreme temperature variations and protects the paws from injuries. Depending on the pad position, they are classified in three groups: 1) **carpal**, 2) **metacarpal** and **metatarsal**, and 3) **digital pads**. Skin on the external surface of the paw pads is intensively folded and forms so-called **pad conical papillae** (fig. 5.12), especially well developed on the carpal pads. These pads protect the dog's paws when walking on rough surfaces, particularly on slippery slopes. Thus, they function as brakes that allow the dog to keep its balance. The metatarsal, metacarpal, and digital pads, thanks to the especially thick adipose tissue layer, serve as shock absorbers. They prevent bones and joints of the foot from injuries during running and jumping.[3]

3   K. D. Budras, P. H. McCarthy, W. Fricke, and R. Richter, *Anatomy of the Dog* (Hanover, Germany: Schlütersche Verlagsgesellschaft, 2007).

Leprosy Among Armadillos. Leprosy (also known as Hansen's disease) is an infectious peripheral neurological disorder caused by *Mycobacterium leprae*. Nine-banded armadillos (*Dasypus novemcinctus*) are the natural host of *M. leprae*, and they may disseminate disease. Leprosy develops mainly in body regions with low temperature, including the skin and mucous membranes of the upper respiratory tract. The space between the conical papillae of paw pads of armadillos is the ideal place for *M. leprae*. When armadillos first became infected with *M. leprae* is still unclear. Leprosy was introduced to the New World at the time of colonization, and the animals must have acquired the infection from humans sometime in the last few hundred years. Nine-banded armadillos can transmit *M. leprae* zoonotically to humans in the South of the United States. Biomarkers of *M. leprae* infection have also been reported among wild armadillos in Brazil, Colombia, and Argentina.

The Planum Nasale

The planum nasale has a distinct cobblestone architecture. It is a pigmented, hairless surface on the top of the external nose, covered by a modified thick epidermis characterized by rete pegs (or rete processes, or rete ridges)—the epithelial extensions that project into the underlying dermis (fig. 5.13). The philtrum is the midsagittal groove in the nasal planum.

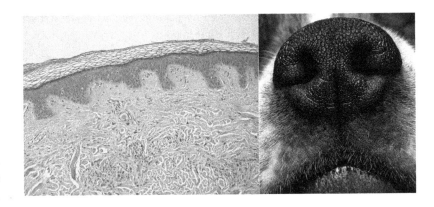

FIGURE 5.13   Planum Nasale of the Dog.

Ergots and Chestnuts

Ergots are normal growths on the legs of healthy horse (fig. 5.14B). The horse leg is a result of a long (about 50 million years) evolution from the extinct *Eohippus* that had five digits on its legs[4] to the modern *Eguus* with one single digit on which it, like a ballerina, runs. The rest of the digits during this long process were lost, but ergots as their vestigial remains remind us about the time when horses had more digits than the modern domesticated horse.

  Chestnuts are calluses on the inner sides of the legs. They are thickened skin that develops in places of frequent friction and pressure (fig. 5.14A). The skin thickens in the place that experiences continuous friction and pressure. The total number of layers increases, and additional stratum (stratum lucidum) develops. The underlying dermis increases collagen fiber deposition. These adaptations to abrasion and pressure result in the development of a protective callus on the legs of many animals. In horses these

---

4   Serge Legendre, *Les communautés de mammifères du Paléogène (Eocène supérieur et Oligocène) d'Europe occidentale: structures, milieux et évolution* (Munich: F. Pfeil, 1989), 110.

callosities (chestnuts) are located on the medial surface above the knee of the forelegs and below the hock on the hind legs. Their appearance and exact position are variable and characteristic to individual horse. That is why, in some horse breeds, they are used for horse identification and require photographing for horse registration.[5]

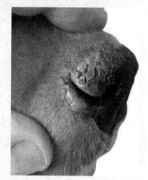

VETERINARY APPLICATION

Mucocutaneous Pyoderma. This condition affects dogs of any age and breed. German shepherds are predisposed. It affects the mucocutaneous junctions (MCJs) of the nose and lips most frequently, but other MCJs can also be affected. It is caused by bacterial infection (usually *S. pseudintermedius*). The first symptoms of the disease are erythema and swelling of the nose near the nasal sulci. Crusts then form followed by fissuring and erosion in some cases. A purulent discharge is often present, and the crusting can extend to the dorsal aspect of the planum nasalae.

Treatment with topical antibiotics such as mupirocin and topicals plus systemic antibiotics in more severe cases is highly effective. If recurrence is seen, topical mupirocin two or three times per week may be helpful for maintenance.

Horns and Antlers

Horns and antlers are derivatives of integument and underlying bones. In **horns** the integument produces a tough cornified sheath that covers the bony core of the horn. Horns never have branches. True horns are characteristic of Bovidae, including cattle, antelope, sheep, goats, and bison. Usually, both sexes have

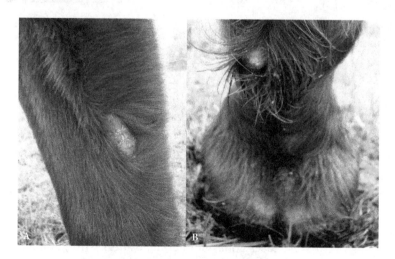

FIGURE 5.14   Chestnuts and Ergots. A. Chestnut; B. Ergot.

---

5   J. Warren Evans, Anthony Borton, Harold F. Hintz, and L. Dale van Vleck, *The Horse*, 2nd ed. (New York: Macmillan, 1990), 80.

horns, but in small species, such as sheep or goat, females may be hornless. Horn is a permanent structure and its growth continues throughout the animal's life.

In **antlers**, the overlying living skin, called **velvet**, creates the shape and provides vascular supply to the growing bone. Eventually, the velvet sheds away and only the bare bone remains. Antlers have a characteristic branched shape. Cervidae (deer, elk, and moose) have true antlers. Typically, only males have antlers, which are branched and shed annually. Caribou have antlers in both sexes. The annual cycle of antler growth and loss is controlled by luteinizing (LH) and follicle-stimulating hormones. Antlers grow, branch, and shed annually. By fall, sex hormones of the testes inhibit anterior pituitary gland production, and velvet on antlers dries and falls out. The bone part of the antlers also dries and finally dies. The continuous change in the hormonal state after the mating period leads to weakening antlers at the base where they are attached. The bone at the base breaks out, and the antlers fall down until the next spring (fig. 5.15).

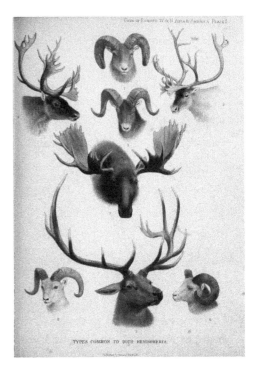

FIGURE 5.15   Horns and Antlers.

CHECK YOUR UNDERSTANDING

- Describe the types of hair and hair structure.

- Describe the difference between the hair root and hair shaft.

- Explain the process of claw growth.

- Describe the difference between eccrine and apocrine sweat glands.

- Describe the different types of sebaceous glands and their role.

CHAPTER SUMMARY

- A membrane is a thin sheet of cells that lines the internal surface of a body cavity. Most membranes are made of a layer of epithelial tissue and a layer of connective tissue. Some membranes also may have a thin layer of smooth muscles. Membranes anchor organs, secure smooth movement, create protective barriers for pathogens, and secrete various substances.

- Serous membrane or **serosa** lines closed body cavities and never contacts the external environment. It is composed of two layers: 1) a simple squamous epithelium, called **mesothelium**, and 2) an areolar connective tissue. This double-layered membrane is folded. One fold of the membrane binds to body walls and is called the **parietal layer**.

The other fold covers organs. It is called the **visceral** layer. Epithelial cells faced inside the fold produce a thin, clear, watery **serous fluid**. The serous fluid creates a lubricating film between membrane folds and guarantees a smooth frictionless movement of organ.

- The synovial membranes line cavities of moveable joins, such as the shoulder, elbow, hip, and knee. Both cellular layers of synovial membrane are made of connective tissue. The internal layer is made of special fibroblasts called **synoviocytes**, and the external layer is made of a combination of areolar and irregular dense connective tissues. Synoviocytes secrete a watery **synovial fluid** that provides smooth movement of a joint.

- Mucous membranes or **mucosa** line cavities that open outside of the body, such as respiratory passages, nasal and mouth cavities, and reproductive organs. The upper layer of mucosa is made of epithelium. The basement membrane of the epithelial layer binds it with a loose connective tissue called **lamina propria**.

- The cutaneous membrane is the biggest body membrane, which creates skin. Superiorly, skin is constructed of stratified squamous epithelium called the **epidermis** and the underlying **dermis** made of loose connective and irregular dense connective tissues. Epidermal cells accumulate waterproof protein called **keratin**. The process of accumulation of keratin in epithelial cells is called **keratinization**.

- Epidermis has five layers, or **strata**. The deepest stratum rests on the basement membrane and is called the **stratum basale** or **stratum germinativum**. It consists of a single layer of active dividing cells. **Melanocytes** and **Merkel cells** are also in this stratum. Superficial to the stratum basale is the **stratum spinosum**. It is the thickest layer. **Keratinocytes** of this layer are close to blood vessels and are metabolically and mitotically active. This layer also contains dendritic cells. The middle layer is the stratum granulosum, made of three to five cellular layers. Cells of this layer are characterized by granules in the cytoplasm. The granules are of two types: granules with keratin and granules with lipid-based substances. On top of the **stratum granulosum** lays the **stratum lucidum**: a narrow transparent layer of dead keratinocytes. This stratum presents only in thick skin and is absent in thin skin. The topmost layer is called the **stratum corneum**. It consists of several layers of dead scaly keratinocytes. Keratinocytes lose internal structures, contain keratin, and slough easily.

- The dermis is a vascularized part of the skin. It houses receptors and is made of two types of connective tissues: **papillary** and **reticular layers**. The papillary layer occupies the superficial position and accounts about 20 percent of the dermis. It is made of areolar (loose) connective tissue. An ECM of areolar tissue contains collagen and elastic fibers. The common cells are fibroblasts and phagocytes. The surface of the papillary layer has projections known as **dermal papillae**. Dermal papillae create a strong bond between the epidermis and dermis. Small capillary loops inside dermal papillae supply oxygen and nutrients to the epidermis. A tactile structure called **Meissner corpuscles** are also located in dermal papillae. The reticular layer is composed of irregular dense connective tissue. The layer is rich with blood vessels and nerve fibers. Accessory structures such as sweat glands, sebaceous glands, hair, and different sensory receptors are also housed in this layer.

- Hair or **pili** are small, keratinized filamentous projections of the skin. Hair forms animal coverage called **fur** or **pelage**. Fur has two components: an undercoat composed of **down hairs** and a coat made of **guard hairs**. Many mammals have hairs that combine characteristics of short, soft, curly down hairs and stiff, long, coarse guard hairs termed **awn hairs**. Specialized sensory hairs around snout are called vibrissae or whiskers. This type of hair is especially well developed among nocturnal and burrowing animals. Special stiff strong hairs of hedgehogs and porcupines are termed **quills**.

- The part of the hair hidden beneath the skin is called the **root**. The remaining part exposed over the skin surface is the **shaft**. The hair has an epidermal origin and is made of epithelial keratinocytes. When the keratinocytes of the root are alive, the cells of the shaft are dead. In cross section, the shaft has three layers: superficial scaly **cuticle**, the thick middle layer **cortex**, and the core with loosely spaced dead cell **medulla**. The hair root has a **hair follicle**. The hair follicle has dermal projection known as **dermal papilla**. A single-cell layer of epithelial cells called **matrix cells** around the dermal papillae produce all hair cells. Capillaries in dermal papillae deliver oxygen and nutrients to matrix cells. The hair shaft grows out of a hair follicle in cycles. The cycle has three consecutive stages: growth, degeneration, and rest. The growth stage is characterized by an active proliferation of cells in the hair papilla. During the degeneration stage, cells become inactive and die. The resting stage may continue from several weeks to a few months. A smooth muscle called **arrector pili** muscle makes the hair stand erect in response to stress.

- **Sebaceous glands** are associated with hair roots and are absent in hairless body regions. They produce an oily secretion called **sebum**. This oily secretion is released into hair follicles and makes fur soft and waterproof. The **wax glands** in the walls of the external auditory meatus that secrete earwax and the **tarsal glands** on the eyelids that produce an oily film secretion on the eyeball surface both originate from sebaceous glands. Sheep have special sebaceous glands organized in three pairs or **pouches**: 1) **infraorbital** at the medial canthus of the eye, 2) **inter-digital** between the digits above the hooves, and 3) **inguinal** in the groin. Goats have sebaceous **horn glands**, located caudal to the horn base. Pigs have **carpal glands** on the mediopalmar surface of the carpus in both sexes.

- **Eccrine glands** produce thin watery fluids. They are not associated with hair follicles. In most mammals these glands are located on the soles. These glands function in thermoregulation and waste excretion. **Apocrine glands** are associated with hair follicles. The secretions of these glands are viscous and function in chemical signaling.

- The **anal glands** are small exocrine glands composed of sebaceous and apocrine sweat glands. They are located on both sides of anus between internal and external anal sphincter muscles. Glands produce an oily liquid that serves for identification of individual members in an animal population, herd, or family.

- The **violet** or **supracaudal gland** has a dual function: 1) it participates in steroid hormones' metabolism, especially sex hormones; and 2) it produces volatile pheromones for communication between individuals of the same species, particularly between sexes. Violet glands are found on the dorsal side of canine and feline tails. They are most active during the breeding period.

- **Claws** or **talons** are curved, compressed from lateral side projections on the tips of digits. A group of cells in the **claw matrix** located at the claw base continually divides and forms a new claw at the claw base. The old claw cells, dead and heavily keratinized, are pushed toward the claw-free edge, where they are worn down or broken. Primates are the only mammals that have **nails**. The nails have the shape of plates on the tips of fingers and toes. In general, nails grow the same way as claws. Ungulates have **hooves** on the tips of their digits. A horse hoof has three parts: 1) wall, 2) sole, and 3) frog. The wall is open at the heel, U shaped, and has three layers, or strata. The superficial thin, shiny keratinized layer is known as the **stratum externa** or **tectorium**. The next layer is thick, keratinized, and permeated by coiled, tubular channels. This layer is called **stratum medium**. The inner layer is called **stratum internum** or **lamellatum**. Projections (rete pegs) of this layer interdigitate with dermis (corium). The frog creates the ground surface of the hoof. It is the heaviest keratinized part that fills the opening in the heel of the hoof wall. The sole fills the ground surface space between the wall and triangular frog. It consists of the epidermis and thickened dermis (the corium) of the sole. Deep in the sole is a fatty digital cushion or pad, a derivative of the hypodermis.

- Paw pads are classified as **digital**, **metacarpal**, and **carpal** pads. The pads protect animal legs when walking on rough surfaces. Paw pads have a thick layer of adipose tissue that insulates the inner tissues from extreme temperatures. The inner layer of skin on the paw has sweat glands that convey perspiration to the outer layer of skin. Paws also exude fluid when a dog is nervous or stressed.

- The planum nasale has a distinct cobblestone architecture. It is a pigmented, hairless surface on the top of the nose, covered by a modified thick epidermis characterized by rete pegs, the epithelial extensions that project into the underlying dermis.

- **Chestnuts** and **ergots** are growths on horse's legs. The ergots are what remain from horse's toes during their evolution. The chestnut is a thickened skin that develops in response to continuous friction and pressure located on the medial surface above the knee of the forelegs and below the hock on the hind legs.

- **Horns** and **antlers** are derivatives of the integument and the underlying bones. In horns the integument produces a tough cornified sheath that covers the bony core of the horn. Horns are permanent and never have branches. In antlers, the overlying living skin, called **velvet**, creates the shape and provides a vascular supply to the growing bone. Eventually, the velvet sheds away, and only the bare bone remains. Antlers are seasonal and have a characteristic branched shape.

CHECK YOUR KNOWLEDGE

LEVEL 1. CHECK YOUR RECALL

1. Skin, fur, claws, horns, and hoofs are parts of the:
   A. Lymphatic system
   B. Endocrine system
   C. Skeletal system
   D. Muscular system
   E. Integumentary system

2. Keratinocytes of the stratum corneum are dead because:
   A. They accumulate keratin and are too far from the blood supply in the dermis.
   B. Actually, they are living cells, not dead.
   C. All keratinocytes of the epidermis in all strata are dead.
   D. There are no keratinocytes in the stratum corneum.

3. Skin is another name for:
   A. Serous membrane
   B. Synovial membrane
   C. Cutaneous membrane
   D. Mucous membrane

4. The hair shaft core is called:
    A. Hair root
    B. Hair cuticle
    C. Hair medulla
    D. Hair cortex
    E. Hair follicle

5. The merocrine sweat glands:
    A. Cool the skin by evaporating sweat
    B. Excrete sweat that dilutes harmful chemicals and has antibacterial properties
    C. Excrete metabolites and waste products
    D. All of the above
    E. None of the above

6. Serous membranes are found lining the:
    A. Compartments of the ventral body cavity
    B. Compartments of the dorsal body cavity
    C. Digestive and reproductive tracts
    D. Joint capsules
    E. Exterior surface of the body

7. The cells in the epidermis that initiate an immune response against pathogens and cancer cells are:
    A. Dendritic cells
    B. Merkel cells
    C. Keratinocytes
    D. Melanocytes
    E. All of the above

8. Keratinocytes, Merkel cells, and melanocytes are found in the stratum:
    A. Germinativum (basale)
    B. Corneum
    C. Spinosum
    D. Granulosum
    E. Lucidum

9. The center of the hair that consists of soft keratin and that is not always present is the:
    A. Cuticle
    B. Medulla
    C. Matrix
    D. Cortex
    E. Follicular papillae

10. The layer that contains capillaries that supply the epidermis with oxygen and nutrients is:
    A.   Reticular layer of the dermis
    B.   Subcutaneous layer
    C.   Stratum corneum
    D.   Stratum basale
    E.   Dermal papille

11. True or false: Hair grows from matrix cells.
12. True or false: The pleural cavity is a space between the pleural membrane and body walls.
13. True or false: Sebaceous and eccrine seat glands are not associated with hair roots.
14. True or false: Melanocytes are the most numerous cells of the epidermis.
15. Match the term with its description:

    _____ Parietal membrane   a.   Internal part of skin made of connective tissue
    _____ Dermis   b.   Layer of dead cells found only in thick skin
    _____ Stratum basale   c.   Hairless branched bone outgrowth on head
    _____ Ergots   d.   Part of serous membrane attached to walls of body cavity
    _____ Horns   e.   Deep epidermal layer mostly of stem cells
    _____ Antlers   f.   Growths on the back of the fetlocks or ankle
    _____ Stratum lucidum   g.   Structure made of a tough skin sheath and bone core

LEVEL 2. CHECK YOUR UNDERSTANDING

1. Explain why anatomists consider membranes organs.
2. What are the major functions of the dermal papillae?
3. What makes it possible for hair on the neck to stand up when a cat is scared?
4. Explain the difference between horns and antlers.

LEVEL 3. APPLY YOUR KNOWLEDGE TO REAL LIFE

1. Manufacturers of shampoo for your pet often claim that their products contain vitamins that are necessary to keep the hair shaft healthy. Do hair shafts need vitamins?
2. Can you explain why many animals that live in a high mountain area have dark, often black fur?

Chapter 6

The Skeletal System

LEARNING OBJECTIVES

The skeleton creates a frame for an animal body. It harbors internal organs, anchors muscles, and stores calcium. This chapter describes the microscopic anatomy of compact and spongy bones and the gross anatomy of major bones—the organs of the skeletal system. When you finish reading this chapter, you will be able to:

1. Describe the functions of the skeletal system.

2. Explain the difference between compact and spongy bones.

3. Classify bones by their shape and role in the skeleton.

4. Describe the gross anatomy of major mammalian bones.

5. Explain the process of bone development and repair.

INTRODUCTION

The skeleton gives the vertebrate body shape, supports its weight, offers a system of levers that, together with muscles, produce movement, and protects soft organs. The skeleton develops deep within the body from the embryonic mesoderm. The skeletal system includes bones, cartilage, and joints. Bones are the primary organs of the skeletal system. Anatomists consider bone as an organ because 1) it is made of different tissues, 2) it has a particular location in the body, 3) it has a particular function, and 4) it has specific relations with other bones and body organs.

Bone tissue, or **osseous** tissue, is a main component of bones. However, there are also regular (tendons) and irregular (ligaments) dense connective tissues, blood vessels, and nerve fibers. Every bone has its special position in the body. For example, the femur is a part of the hind leg and is never found somewhere else. Every bone has a specific function. For example, the femur together with the muscles of the thigh form a lever for hind leg movement, whereas the frontal bone forms the cranium, which protects the brain. Both bones take part in hematopoiesis: a production of blood cells and platelets.

Together all bones have six functions:

1. **Protection.** Bones create protective structures. For example, the cranium protects the brain and the thoracic cage protects the heart and lungs. The vertebral column protects the spinal cord and the roots of spinal nerves.

2. **Support.** The skeleton forms the frame of the body. This frame forms the body's shape, helps hold body weight, and provides a surface for attachment of muscles and viscera.

3. **Movement.** Bones anchor muscles. Together, they form a system of levers for body movement.

4. **Mineral storage and acid-base homeostasis.** Bones are a major body storage site for minerals: calcium, phosphorus, magnesium, fluoride, and some others. These minerals are stored as salts in bone tissue ground matter. All salts are chemical compounds based on ionic bonds. Salt dissolved in the water of body fluids dissociates on ions. Water solutions with positive and negative ions conduct electricity. That is why these minerals are also called electrolytes (see chapter 2, page 38). Accumulation and release of these minerals by bone tissue is a decisive factor in acid-base balance regulation.

5. **Formation of blood cells.** Some bones harbor red bone marrow. Red bone marrow is the only hematopoietic tissue of adult mammals. It supplies blood flow with red and white blood cells, and platelets.

6. **Fat storage.** Yellow bone marrow in the medullary cavity of long bones consists of adipocytes. It stores triglycerides that are a source of energy. Every triglyceride molecule may release at least two times more energy than the same size carbohydrate molecule.

We begin our study of the skeletal system from bone's classification and gross anatomy. Then we discuss what tissues constitute healthy bone, and the processes of bone development and reparation. At the end of this chapter, you will find a brief description of cartilage and skeleton construction.

6.1   Bone Classification

Bone is an organ of the skeletal system. The number of bones in the body varies among different animals. In the same species their number also may be different. Even in the same organism, the number of bones varies with aging. Bones are different in size, shape, location, origin, and in many degrees in their function. For example, the femur and phalanx are both bones of the pelvic limb, but the femur plays a very important role in hematopoiesis in an adult organism, whereas the phalanx does not.

By origin, bones are classified in three groups: 1) bones that develop through the intramembranous ossification are called **intramembranous bones**; 2) bones that develop through cartilage ossification are called **endochondral bones**; and 3) bones that develop as a hardening inside dense connective tissues (tendons and ligaments) are called **sesamoid bones**.

The classification of bones by shape and size is the most convenient and widely used method by specialists. According to this approach, bones are divided in five classes: 1) **long**, 2) **short**, 3) **flat**, 4) **irregular**, and 5) **round bones**. As the name implies, long bones are much longer than they are wide. The femur, tibia, fibula, and other bones, mostly from limbs, belong to this class. Short bones have a length equal or almost equal to their width. Most phalanges are of this type bones. Flat bones form plates that cover and create a safe space for internal organs, like frontal, parietal, and temporal bones form the cranium for the

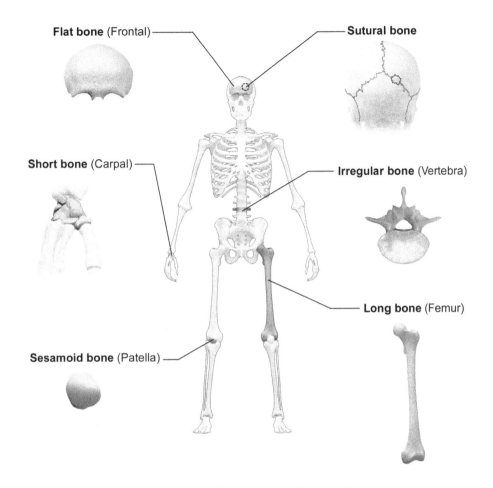

Flat bone (Frontal)

Sutural bone

Short bone (Carpal)

Irregular bone (Vertebra)

Long bone (Femur)

Sesamoid bone (Patella)

FIGURE 6.1   Classification of Bones of the Human Skeleton by Shape.

brain protection. By irregular bones, anatomists mean those bones whose shape is difficult to characterize by some particular geometric figure. Vertebra are classic example of such irregular bones. Round bones have an oval shape and a more or less smooth surface. They belong to sesamoid bones by their origin and, as a rule, develop in most heavy loaded joints, like a kneecap or patella (fig. 6.1).

VETERINARY APPLICATION

Wobbler syndrome is common among certain dog breeds, such as basset hounds, borzois, Doberman pinschers, and Great Danes. The disease also affects Thoroughbred horses. The cause(s) of the disease are still not clearly known. It results in narrowing of the spinal canal because of malformation of the vertebral canal in cervical vertebrae. The narrow vertebral canals of cervical vertebrae compress the spinal cord and cause slow, weak, and uncoordinated movement called **ataxia**. The name Wobbler syndrome came from the wobbly, uncoordinated gait. The disease may progress to complete paralysis. Medical treatment aims to decrease spinal cord compression and may include surgery.

6.2   Bone Gross Anatomy

The long bone has a long shaft called the **diaphysis**. On both ends of the bone there is a nub-shaped **epiphysis**. The epiphysis form joints with adjacent bones. They are covered by **articular cartilage**, which guarantees smooth, frictionless bone movement. Inside the diaphysis there is a hollow longitudinal space called the **medullary cavity** or **medulla**. The medullary cavity is filled with **yellow bone marrow**. Yellow bone marrow consists of bone major blood vessels and adipose tissue. The walls of the diaphysis are made of compact bone tissue. Compact bone tissue also forms the outer layer of the epiphysis. But inside, the epiphysis consists of **spongy** or **cancellous bone**. A space between the trabecula of spongy bone is filled by **red bone marrow**. Red bone marrow is a hematopoietic tissue. It consists of blood vessels and hematopoietic stem cells that produce blood cells. In adult mammals red bone marrow is the only hematopoietic tissue. In an aged animal red bone marrow continuously shrinks and is replaced by yellow bone marrow. Finally, red bone marrow remains only in the bones of the pelvis, the proximal epiphysis of the femur, and the humerus. With the decrease in the amount of red bone marrow, the production of blood cells also declines.

On the outside, the long bone is covered by the tough, glossy connective tissue membrane called the **periosteum**. The ECM of the periosteum has collagen type 1, which makes this membrane very strong. Collagen fibers of the periosteum intertwine on one side with collagen fibers of the tendons and on the other side with collagen fibers from the ECM of bone. These connections hold skeletal muscles firmly attached to bones. Inside the long bone diaphysis, the walls of the medullary cavity are covered by the **endosteum**. The endosteum is a delicate, tiny vascularized membrane. Blood vessels from the endosteum supply internal bone tissues and yellow and red bone marrow. Both membranes also harbor osteogenic cells and osteoblasts, which are crucial for bones' growth and repair (fig. 6.2).

Short, flat, irregular, and sesamoid bones have no diaphysis, epiphysis, or medullary cavity. As a rule, they have a capsule made of compact bone tissue and an internal core of spongy bone tissue. On the outside they are covered by the periosteum and inside, by the endosteum.

Bones have many external structures. Some of these structures provide a surface for muscle

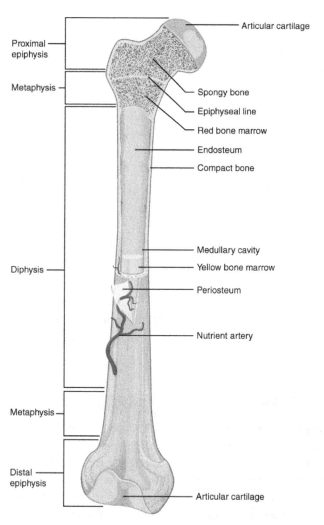

Proximal epiphysis

Metaphysis

Diphysis

Metaphysis

Distal epiphysis

Articular cartilage

Spongy bone

Epiphyseal line

Red bone marrow

Endosteum

Compact bone

Medullary cavity

Yellow bone marrow

Periosteum

Nutrient artery

Articular cartilage

FIGURE 6.2   Long Bone Structure.

attachment; others create a smooth surface for frictionless movement, and others have holes for blood vessels and nerves. All these structures can be combined in three major groups: 1) articular surfaces, 2) processes, and 3) holes and depressions.

1. **Articular surfaces.** An articular surface is a smooth area of compact bone shaped to form a joint with another bone. As a rule, it is covered by articular cartilage. A rounded articular surface is called the **head**. A small head is called the **capitulum**. A nub-shaped articular surface is called the **condyle**. A comparatively sharp articular surface is called the **facet**.
2. **Processes.** These are projections for attachment of tendons, ligaments, and membranes. These projections are classified according the shape and length. Most long projections are called **spinous projections**. The shorter projections are called **trochanters** and **tubercles**. Small numerous projections are known as **tuberosity**. Long ridge-like projections are called **spines**, **crests**, and **wings** or **ali**.
3. **Holes and depressions.** There are three types of holes: 1) comparatively big, round holes are called **foramen**; 2) comparatively small, narrow holes are called **canals**; and 3) irregularly shaped holes are called **fissures**. Types of depressions include 1) a shallow, broad depression called a **fossa**; 2) a small, rounded depression called a **fovea**; and 3) an indentation on the bone ridge called a **notch**.

CHECK YOUR UNDERSTANDING

- What are the two membranes associated with bone called?
- What is a long, tubular hollow space in a long bone called? What is inside of this space?
- What are the differences among the three types of holes in bones?
- What are the shaft and the end of a long bone called?

6.3 Bone Tissue

Histology of Bone Tissue

Bone or osseous tissue is a special type of connective tissue. Like all connective tissues, it consists of cells and a comparatively large amount of ECM between them (see chapter 4, page 120). Groups of four cell types form bone: **osteogenic cells**, **osteoblasts**, **osteocytes**, and **osteoclasts** (fig. 6.3). Besides these cells, bone also has blood cells, chondrocytes, and fibroblasts. ECM contains collagen fibers and solid ground matter made of inorganic compounds of calcium (bones contain 80 to 85 percent of all body calcium) and phosphate. Calcium and phosphate form different salts, mostly crystals of **hydroxyapatite**. Deposition of this salt in ECM makes bones hard, strong, and heavy. Besides hydroxyapatite, there are other salts, such as calcium bicarbonate, calcium fluoride, and so on. Collagen fibers in ECM form a mesh network, which holds salt crystals together and does not let them crumble like sand. An organic component of the ECM called **osteoid** is composed of collagen fibers and a number of organic molecules common in ECM, such

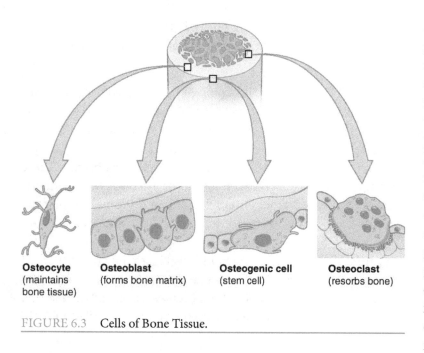

Osteocyte
(maintains
bone tissue)

Osteoblast
(forms bone matrix)

Osteogenic cell
(stem cell)

Osteoclast
(resorbs bone)

FIGURE 6.3   Cells of Bone Tissue.

as proteoglycans, glycosamino-glycans, and glycoproteins. In normal healthy bone, organic and inorganic components present in ratio: 35 percent of total bone weight consists of osteoid and 65 percent of inorganic component. Deviation from this ratio, as a rule, results in bone disease. For example, a decrease in organic component makes bone brittle and easy to break. A mutation in the gene that codes synthesis of collagen type 1 causes a hereditary bone disease known as **osteogenesis imperfecta**. On the other hand, a decrease in calcium salts in ECM makes bones soft and easy banded, as, for example, in **rickets**.

Both components of bone ECM are produced by osteoblasts and maintained in a normal healthy state by osteocytes. Osteoblasts are young bone cells. Osteoblasts have a cuboidal or columnar shape. They originate from flat **osteogenic cells**. Osteogenic cells are undifferentiated cells with a high mitotic activity; they are the only bone cells that divide. Osteogenic cells are located in the periosteum, endosteum, and walls of the osteon central canal. Osteogenic cells communicate through paracrine signaling molecules, such as prostaglandins, not only with other cells of the bone (osteoblasts, osteocytes, and osteoclasts) but also with cells of soft tissues, such as nervous tissue, tissues of the gut, muscles, adipose tissue, and testis. These signals control osteogenic cell division and development into osteoblasts. Osteoblasts are bone-building cells. They manufacture and deposit ECM around themselves. Osteoblasts are mostly concentrated in the periosteum and endosteum. From there they invade deep inside injured bone and restore it by building new bone tissue.

Trapped inside a small fluid-filled **lacuna**, osteoblasts transform into osteocytes. Osteocytes are permanent cells of bone tissue. They monitor the health state of the ECM. Osteocytes secrete paracrine-signaling molecules and through them control activities of osteoblasts and osteogenic cells.

Osteoclasts are large multinucleated cells. They originate from monocytes—white blood cells that give rise to all macrophages of the body. Osteoclast is formed by fusion of macrophages in a single cell. In contrast to free-moving macrophages, osteoclasts are sedentary. They reside on internal and external surfaces of bone. Their cytoplasm contains vesicles with strong hydrolytic enzymes. Osteoclasts also produce hydrogen ions. The release of hydrogen ions into ECM significantly increases ECM acidity. Acidic interstitial fluid dissolves inorganic components of the matrix (remember that it is made of salts, which are based on ionic bonds, and easily dissolves in acids). The enzymes released in ECM resorb organic components (first of all, collagen fibers). Thus, osteoclasts are bone-destroying cells. The process of bone destruction is called **bone resorption**. There are many factors that control osteoclasts' activity.

- What are the two main components of bone tissue?
- Describe four major cell types of bone tissue and their functions.
- What fibers constitute bone ECM?
- What substances constitute inorganic ground matter of bone ECM?

Compact Bone

As you already know (see chapter 4, page 120), there are two types of bone tissue: compact and spongy bone. As a rule, compact bone forms the shaft of long bones and creates epiphysis coverage. Compact bone is strong and heavy. Eight-five percent of this bone is ECM. Sixty-five percent of ECM consists of inorganic calcium salt crystals. That makes compact bone a very strong material that is able to hold body weight and withstand heavy pressure from outside. The structural unit of compact bone is the **osteon** or **Haversian system**. Osteons have the shape of a long tube with thick walls. Osteons are tightly packed side by side, like straws in broom. This packaging of osteons makes compact bone very strong and heavy.

At the center of the osteon is a central or Haversian canal. This central canal contains blood vessels and nerve fibers. It is a major provider of blood to the cells of osteons. Bone tissue is organized around the central canal in concentric rings called **lamellae**. Lacunae with osteocytes are located in these lamellae. Every lacuna is connected with other lacunae and the central canal by a network of tiny canals called **canaliculi**. Canaliculi form a system of tunnels in solid ECM to supply osteocytes inside lacunae with oxygen and nutrients. Central canals of adjacent osteons are bound by **perforating** or **Volkmann's canals**. Through these canals blood vessels and nerve fibers transit from one osteon to another. All of them receive blood from major blood vessels in the periosteum. Bone tissue is metabolically very active. It is constantly resorbed by osteoclasts and renewed by osteoblasts. The remnants of resorbed old osteons called **interstitial lamellae** fill the space between new osteons (fig. 6.4).

Spongy Bone

Spongy or cancellous bone forms the interior of long bones and most of the body of the epiphysis. Spongy bone has no heavy osteons. The ECM of spongy bone is organized in spicules or plates called **trabeculae**. Trabeculae form a network that leaves a space for red bone marrow, which fills all available space inside spongy bones. Trabeculae are covered by the periosteum and in cross section contain lamellae with osteocytes in lacunae. Lacunae of trabeculae are connected with red bone marrow for blood supply by short canaliculi (fig. 6.5).

Flat bones of the cranium on section look like a sandwich. From both sides they are covered by compact bone tissues. Inside the bone contains a thick layer of spongy bone, which is called **diploë** (fig. 6.6). Some bones have so-called **pneumatic diverticula**, or air sacs (frontal, ethmoid bones, and maxillae, for example). Pneumatic diverticula replace bone marrow with air sacs. The effect of the pneumatic diverticula is an overall reduction of body mass. The reduced body mass is an adaptation that allows pterosaurs and birds to fly, since the low body mass makes a big difference in keeping the animal aloft. The pneumatized vertebral column of sauropods reduces the animal's weight and makes it easier to support and move the massive neck.

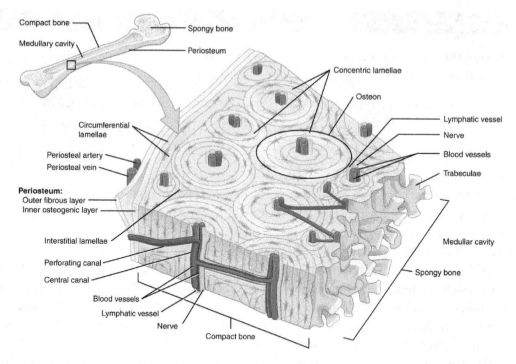

FIGURE 6.4   Compact Bone Structure.

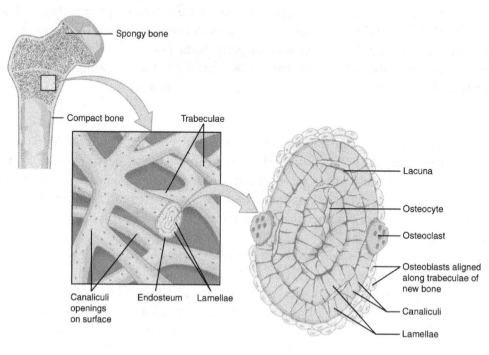

FIGURE 6.5   Spongy Bone.

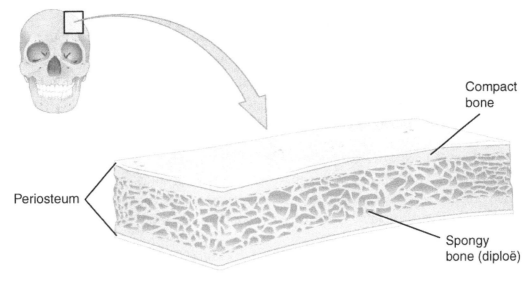

Periosteum

Compact bone

Spongy bone (diploë)

FIGURE 6.6   Spongy Bone of Cranial Flat Bones.

CHECK YOUR UNDERSTANDING

- What structural elements constitute compact bone?

- Are trabeculae structural elements of compact or spongy bone?

- What tissue fills the space inside spongy bone?

- What are lamellae and lacunae?

- What is the difference between a central canal and perforating canal?

- How do osteocytes get oxygen and nutrients?

Intramembranous Ossification

The process of bone formation is called **ossification** or **osteogenesis**. There are two major ways of bone formation: **intramembranous** and **endochondral**. The process that underlies development of the sesamoid bones is still unknown. To date, sesamoids are thought to develop inside tendons in response to mechanical stress from the attaching muscles. However, recent study in mouse embryos demonstrated that the patella initially develops as a bony process of the femur. Later, the patella is separated from the femur by a process of joint formation regulated by a mechanical load. At the end of this process, the patella becomes superficially embedded within the quadriceps' tendon.

Flat bones are flat because they are formed between two membranous sheets. Many bones of the skull and clavicles are formed this way. Membranes that form flat bone are part of an embryo tissue called mesenchyme. An embryonic mesenchyme is a connective tissue derived from the middle embryo cell layer called the mesoderm. Bones that develop from this tissue are called **primary bones**. They are temporal and after a while are replaced by the permanent **secondary bones**. In the process of intramembranous ossification, the internal content of a flat bone, which is a spongy bone, forms first. The two superficial layers of compact bone tissue, which cover the spongy bone core from the both sides, are formed later. The process begins at the area known as the **primary ossification center**. The sequence of events of intramembranous ossification is next:

1. Mesenchymal cells in the membrane intensively divide and form dense cell clusters called the **nidus**.
2. Cells of the nidus transform in osteogenic cells.
3. Osteogenic cells multiply through mitosis. Some osteogenic cells of the nidus develop into osteoblasts, and the nidus becomes a primary ossification center.
4. Osteoblasts of the primary ossification center secrete organic components of the bone ECM, first of all collagen type 1 fibers. Collagen fibers form a mesh network.
5. After production of some amount of collagen fibers, osteoblasts begin to accumulate calcium from the blood flow and interstitial fluids and deposit calcium salts inside the network of collagen fibers. This process is called **calcification**.
6. Osteoblasts enclose themselves in lacunae and reorganize into osteocytes.
7. Osteoblasts on the periphery of the primary ossification center continue to develop ECM and form trabeculae. Some of these trabeculae enlarge and merge forming larger trabeculae.
8. The spongy bone is growing in all directions from the primary ossification center. It also invades the periosteum. In the periosteum, cancellous bone reorganizes into osteons and forms compact bone tissue.
9. Vascular tissue fills the space between trabeculae and forms bone marrow (fig. 6.7).

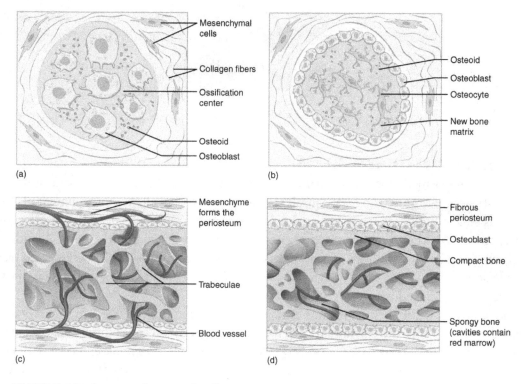

FIGURE 6.7   Intramembranous Ossification.

10. As a rule, there are multiple primary ossification centers. Flat bone is growing around all of these centers, until the growing pieces fuse and form a single bone. Often the ossification process continues after birth, and a newborn animal has soft, membranous not ossified areas between the cranial bones called **fontanels**.

CHECK YOUR UNDERSTANDING

- Which bones are formed through intramembranous ossification?

- What role do mesenchymal membranes play in intramembranous ossification?

- What are the soft, not ossified regions of the flat bones of a newborn called?

Endochondral Ossification

Endochondral ossification, as the term implies, takes place inside the embryonic cartilaginous model of the skeleton. The embryonic model consists of hyaline cartilage. On the outside, the model is covered by a connective tissue membrane called the **perichondrium**. Together with fibroblasts, the perichondrium contains cartilage stem cells called **chondroblasts**. Endochondral ossification begins during the fetal period and continues after birth. Endochondral ossification is a process of long bone formation, growth in length, and healing of fractures. Before ossification can take place, the cartilage model of the embryo skeleton has to be formed. The cartilage model grows in length by continuous division of chondrocytes and secretion of extracellular matrix. This process is called **interstitial growth**. The process of peripheral cartilage growth from the sides is called **appositional growth**. Chondroblasts form cartilage ECM. Chondroblasts completely enclosed in ECM transform into chondrocytes. There remains only a small free amount of ECM space around the chondrocyte, filled by interstitial fluid. The first site of ossification is called the **primary ossification center**. It is located in the middle of the cartilage model diaphysis. Then the following sequence of events takes place:

1. **The periosteum is formed.** Blood vessels grow inside the perichondrium, and chemical signals from blood trigger conversion of chondroblasts into osteogenic cells. Osteogenic cells develop in osteoblasts, and the perichondrium transforms into the periosteum.

2. **The bone collar is formed.** The osteoblasts from the periosteum secrete osteoid at the primary ossification center of the diaphysis of the cartilage model. This appositional growth of the bone ring around the cartilage model is called the **bone collar**.

3. **The matrix calcifies.** Chondrocytes in the cartilage of the primary ossification center begin to grow in size. This process is called **hypertrophy**. They stop secreting collagen and other proteoglycans and begin to secrete alkaline phosphate, an enzyme essential for mineral deposition. Production of alkaline phosphate triggers calcification of the cartilage matrix. Calcification of the cartilage matrix and development of the bone collar cuts off chondrocytes' blood supply, and eventually, they die. Their death leaves empty cavities.

4. **Blood vessels grow inside the emptied space, and osteoblasts replace chondrocytes.** Osteoclasts dissolve and clean the region with dead chondrocytes and create pathways for growing blood

vessels. Blood vessels grow inside the emptied area. Osteoblasts enter the cavity using the calcified matrix as a scaffold. Here osteoblasts find a lot of space and a good blood supply and begin to secrete osteoid. Osteoid deposition forms the early bone trabecula. Thus, the primary bone is a spongy bone. Osteoclasts, which continue their activity, break down spongy bone and form a medullary cavity. The process spreads from the primary ossification center toward both ends of the cartilage model.

5. **A secondary ossification center develops on both epiphyses.** As ossification progresses, the calcified cartilage is replaced by bone. Osteoclasts degrade most of the early spongy bone and clean the space to increase the medullary cavity. The medullary cavity immediately fills with bone marrow. About the time of birth in mammals, cartilage remains only in two locations in the epiphysis: an area deep inside the epiphysis called the **epiphyseal plate** and the area on the apical surface of the epiphysis called **articular cartilage**. A secondary ossification center appears in each epiphysis of long bones. Blood vessels grow inside the epiphysis. The epiphyseal plate includes all hyaline cartilage between the primary and secondary ossification centers. Chondrocytes of the epiphyseal plate continue to form new cartilage, and all bone growth happens only in the epiphyseal plate. This cartilage is replaced by bone in the same way as in the primary ossification center. The growth of new cartilage and its replacement by bone results in a bone growing in length. Growth continues until the cartilage in the epiphyseal plate is replaced by bone completely. The area of union of the primary and secondary ossification centers is called an **epiphyseal line**. The epiphyseal line is what remains from the epiphyseal plate. At this point, the organism's growth is terminated. The only cartilage that persists through the entire life span of an animal is an articular cartilage in joints between bones (fig. 6.8).

CHECK YOUR UNDERSTANDING

- Which structures and cells initiate endochondral ossification?

- What is the difference between primary and secondary ossification centers?

- Which cells form bone collar?

- What is the role of osteoclasts in endochondral ossification?

Bone Growth in Length

There are two different ways of bone growth: growth in length and growth in width. The growth of bone in length is called **longitudinal growth**. Longitudinal growth occurs in the epiphyseal plate, which consists of hyaline cartilage. Longitudinal growth is generated by mitotic divisions of chondrocytes, not by bone cells—osteoblasts. The epiphyseal plate has five zones corresponding the state of chondrocytes:

1. The zone closest to the epiphysis zone is called the **reserve cartilage zone**. The chondrocytes in this zone do not participate in bone growth. Their role is to maintain the hyaline cartilage of the epiphyseal plate and to provide reserve cells for cellular division.

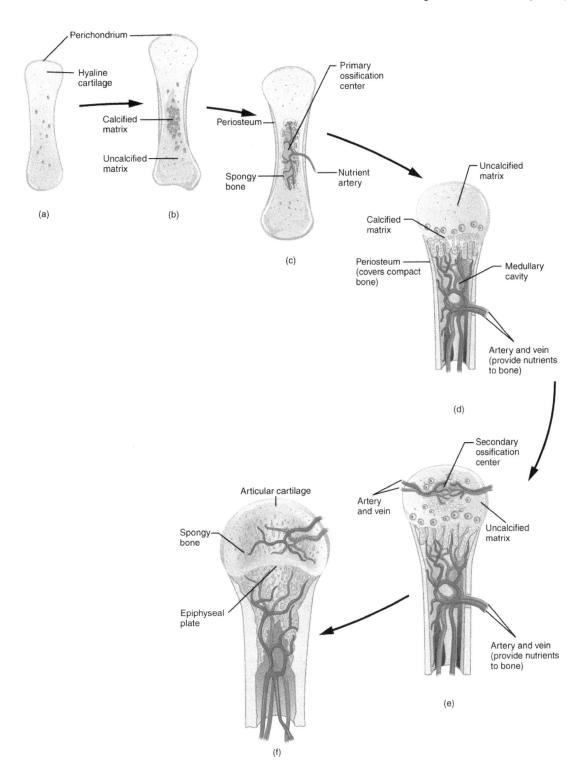

FIGURE 6.8   Endochondral Ossification.

2. The next zone following the reserve cartilage zone is the **proliferation zone**. Chondrocytes in this zone actively divide in their lacunae. This zone creates major longitudinal bone growth.
3. The next zone is called the **hypertrophy and maturation zone**. Chondrocytes of this zone grow above the regular chondrocyte size (hypertrophy) and become mature
4. The next zone is called the **calcification zone**. Chondrocytes in this zone stop growing and begin to deposit calcium salts in cartilage ECM. When ECM completely fills with calcium, chondrocytes die, suffocated by an absence of oxygen and nutrients.
5. The zone most distant from the epiphysis zone is called the **ossification zone**. This zone is populated by osteoclasts. Osteoclasts degrade dead chondrocytes and clean the space for the following osteoblasts. Migrated osteoblasts immediately begin secreting bone tissue. Eventually, cartilage is completely resorbed, and new bone replaces it.

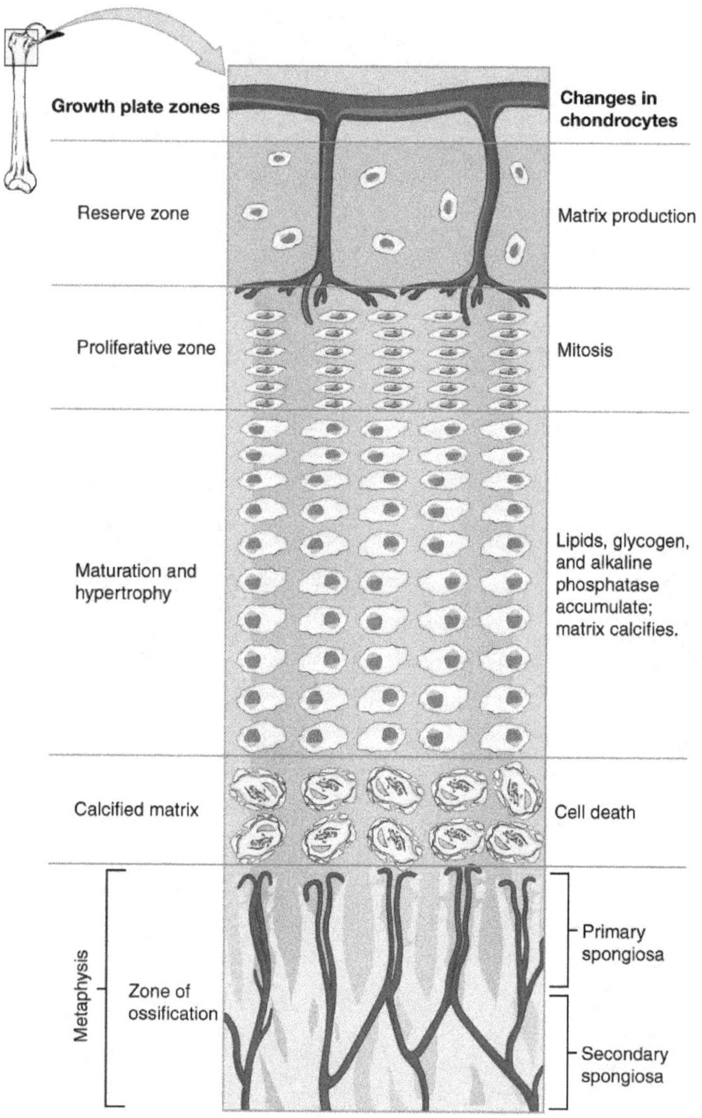

The whole process consists of the following sequence of events:

Chondrocytes divide in the proliferation zone → New chondrocytes are pushed from the proliferation zone to the hypertrophy and maturation zone → Hypertrophied chondrocytes change metabolism and move to the next zone → In the calcification zone, chondrocytes stop producing regular cartilage ECM and produce and deposit calcium salts → Chondrocytes trapped in calcified matrix die → Osteoblasts and osteoclasts invade the area with dead chondrocytes → Osteoblasts produce osteoid, and osteoclasts clean away the dead chondrocytes from the territory (fig. 6.9).

FIGURE 6.9   Longitudinal Bone Growth.

Cartilage is avascular tissue. It grows slower than bone tissue. As a result, proliferation and growth rate of the epiphyseal plate do not match the rate of ossification. With time epiphyseal plate thickness is decreased. The process of longitudinal bone growth continues until there are live chondrocytes that are able to divide in the epiphyseal plate. When the last chondrocytes die and are replaced by bone tissue, the epiphyseal plate closes. Only an epiphyseal line remains where the epiphyseal plate was. Development of the epiphyseal line signifies the end of longitudinal bone growth, which usually corresponds with the beginning of adulthood.

CHECK YOUR UNDERSTANDING

- What tissues constitute the epiphyseal plate?

- Name five zones of the epiphyseal plate, and describe what takes place in these zones.

- What is the difference between the epiphyseal plate and the epiphyseal line?

Bone Growth in Width and Remodeling

Bone growth in width is called **appositional growth**. It may happen at any time of an animal's life and is usually associated with physical stress experienced by the bone. Appositional growth is possible because the periosteum always contains some number of osteoblasts. Osteoblasts between the periosteum and bone deposit new bone tissue on the top of the old bone. The new layers of bone tissue have no osteons. They are simply circular bone tissue depositions that have the shape of a ring around an old bone. New layers are organized in concentric rings called **circumferential lamellae**. With formation of new circumferential lamellae, the old circumferential lamellae degrade and reorganize into osteons. As a result, the thickness of the compact bone increases. At the same time, osteoclasts from the endosteum resorb compact bone from the medullary cavity and transform it into spongy bone. Thus, with the increase of bone diameter, the diameter of the medullary cavity also grows.

Osseous tissue is very active. Even when bone growth is finished, it is constantly in a process of resorption and reconstruction. This resorption and reconstruction happen due to many physiological processes. Increase in physical stress on bone can cause its appositional growth. Low calcium in body fluids causes bone resorption and release of calcium in the blood flow. An excess of calcium in the blood causes deposition of new bone tissue. Reparation of bone fractures and replacement of old bone tissue with new tissue are also part of the remodeling process. Remodeling occurs through the activity of osteoclasts, which resorb old bone, and osteoblasts, which build new bone tissue (fig. 6.10). There are many factors that control osteoblast and osteoclast activity, from physical stress to nutrition and hormones. In general, there is a rule: in a young, fast-growing organism, osteoblast activity prevails over osteoclast activity. At that time, bones grow. In adult organisms, osteoblast and osteoclast activities are in dynamic equilibrium. In an aged organism, the activity of osteoblasts decreases, whereas the activity of osteoclasts remains almost at the same level. This often causes an observable decrease in bone mass in old organisms.

CHECK YOUR UNDERSTANDING

- What is the difference between longitudinal and appositional growth?

- What kind of cells are responsible for appositional growth, and where do they come from?

- What are the circumferential lamellae, and how do they develop?

- What is the relation between appositional growth and remodeling?

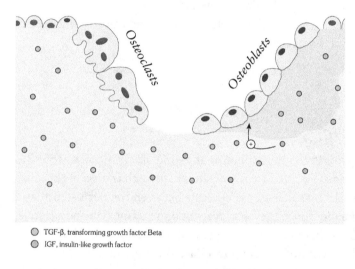

○ TGF-β, transforming growth factor Beta
○ IGF, insulin-like growth factor

FIGURE 6.10   Bone Remodeling.

The Role of Hormones in Bone Growth

There are many factors that influence bone growth, but hormones are among the main factors. First of all is the growth hormone, also known as somatotropin. The hormone is manufactured, stored, and released by lateral areas of the anterior pituitary gland. The hormone stimulates mitosis; that is, it actively promotes cell division. The effect of this hormone is obvious: it facilitates cell growth, division, and as a result of that, cell multiplication and growth of the body and individual organs. Insufficient growth hormone production or lack of sensitivity of target cells to it results in slow bone and cartilage growth, and dwarfism. An excess of this hormone in a young organism causes fast growth and gigantism. In an old organism, in which the epiphyseal plates are already closed, an excess of the growth hormone causes acromegaly, an abnormal growth of particular bones which have at least some amount of hyaline cartilage (for example, articular cartilage).

Two hormones play a very important role in regulation of blood calcium. Calcitonin stimulates activity of osteoblasts. Osteoblasts, stimulated by calcitonin, increase synthesis of ECM. They collect calcium, synthesize calcium salts, and deposit salts in bone matrix. Thus, calcitonin promotes bone growth. Another hormone is a parathyroid hormone (PTH), produced by the parathyroid glands as a reaction to a decrease of the blood calcium level below the norm. PTH stimulates osteoclast activity. Activated by PTH, osteoclasts increase bone resorption and release calcium in blood flow. Thus, both hormones regulate intensity of resorption and building of bones.

The sex hormones estrogen and androgen have a strong influence on the postnatal growth of bones and are responsible for characteristic sexual dimorphism among male and female skeletons. In addition, estrogen and androgen are important for the homeostasis of bone tissue during adulthood. A decline in the circulating levels of sex steroids leads to loss of bone mass and functional integrity. Deficiency of estrogen in females or both estrogen and androgen in males adversely affects skeletal development during growth and homeostasis during adulthood, and contributes to the development of osteoporosis in either sex.

Estrogen has a more potent effect on bone growth than testosterone. Estrogen promotes mitotic division of chondrocytes in the epiphyseal plate and causes fast growth of the female skeleton in puberty, when estrogen production rises. Because estrogen has a higher impact on bone growth, at the period of sexual maturation, females grow faster than males. The fast growth and ossification also cause early closing of the epiphyseal plate, and females stop growing earlier than males. Testosterone has less effect on bone growth. It causes slow growth of the male skeleton but increases the length of the growth period. That is why, in puberty, males grow slower than females, but their growth ends later. As a result, males usually have a bigger body. Testosterone has an effect not only on longitudinal but also appositional growth. That is why male bones are not only longer but also bigger in diameter. Castrated males that lack testosterone have longer bones. Their epiphyseal plate closes later. As a result, they are taller than males whose testosterone promotes ossification and closing of the epiphyseal plate.

CHECK YOUR UNDERSTANDING

- How does the growth hormone influence bone growth?

- What role do calcitonin and PTH play in bones?

- Why do mammalian females as a rule have a smaller skeleton than males?

Other Factors That Affect Bone Growth

Growth and health of bone tissue, as other tissues, depends on metabolism. Malnutrition and insufficient protein synthesis may result in a decrease in glycoproteins and collagen fibers in ECM. Bones become brittle and are easily fractured. Insufficient calcium causes a change in the organic and inorganic ratio in ECM toward an organic component. Bones with low calcium are soft and can bend and may develop rickets. Because the thyroid and parathyroid glands have a strong influence on the blood calcium balance, the health of these glands is very important for the health of bones.

VETERINARY APPLICATION

Parturient paresis (milk fever) is the result of low calcium in blood. The first milk produced by dairy cattle is called **colostrum**. Colostrum contains a high concentration of Ca^{2+}. To produce colostrum, a cow needs 3 g of Ca^{2+} per hour. When a cow has an insufficient calcium supply from food, she can develop milk fever within 72 hours following parturition. Symptoms include loss of appetite, muscle weakness, decrease of body temperature, labored breathing, and paralysis of hind legs. If left untreated, the cow can collapse into coma and die.

To prevent milk fever, cows should be given food fortified with sufficient amounts of calcium and vitamin D in the diet prior to parturition. If milk fever develops, cows are given an oral bolus of calcium carbonate.

Fat soluble (steroid) vitamins, **vitamin D, A**, and **K**, have a strong impact on the state of bones. A mammalian organism can synthesize vitamin D, but for that it needs ultraviolet (UV) light. The main effect vitamin D exerts is an absorption of food calcium in the small intestine. That is why veterinarians always prescribe food calcium supplement in combination with vitamin D. The vitamin also promotes calcium retention in kidneys, so the organism lose less calcium with urine. All these vitamin D effects help increase blood calcium and calcium availability for bone building. Farm cattle that lack direct sunlight exposure are also recommended to take a UV light bath to activate production of vitamin D. Vitamin A is needed for production of retinoic acid, which is an important hormone-like growth factor. It facilitates bone growth, and deficiency in vitamin A causes slow bone growth and a low ossification rate. In contrast, overdoses of vitamin A may cause bone overgrowth and ossification, which may cause abnormal skeleton development. Vitamin K play an essential role as a cofactor for synthesis of osteocalcin. Osteocalcin is a glycoprotein secreted by the osteoblasts. This glycoprotein is essential for binding calcium ions and formation of mineral ground substance in bone matrix.

Water-soluble **vitamin C** is required for collagen synthesis. Inadequate intake of vitamin C results in a decrease in collagen synthesis and, finally, in fragile bones. Because vitamin C is water soluble, organisms cannot store it long term, and this vitamin has to be taken in continuously with every meal in order to maintain a normal level of collagen production.

CHECK YOUR UNDERSTANDING

- What is the role of vitamin D in bone ECM balance?

- How does vitamin A affect bone growth?

- Why is vitamin C important for normal healthy bones?

Bone Repair

Bone injuries may be of different types and the result of many causes. The most devastating injury is a bone fracture. Bone may be fractured in many different ways. When tissues and organs that surround fractured bone stay unaffected, the fracture is called **simple**. **Compound fractures** involve nearby tissues and organs. If the broken bone does not penetrate the skin and is not exposed outside the body, the fracture is called **closed**. In contrast, an **open fracture** is characterized by exposure of the broken bone outside the body and profound bleeding. The bone may be broken on only one side, whereas the opposite side remains unbroken. This type of fracture is called a **greenstick fracture**. Greenstick fractures are the easiest to repair and heal. The most difficult fracture types include **oblique**, **spiral**, and **comminuted fractures** (fig. 6.11).

VETERINARY APPLICATION

Canine **hip dysplasia** is caused by malformation or abnormal development of the head of the femur. The malformed head does not fit to the acetabulum, and the femur "rattles around." The dogs most affected are puppies, especially from dysplastic parents. The loose movement of the head of the femur is painful and leads to degeneration of the hip joint. Definitive diagnosis of canine hip dysplasia requires pelvic radiography. Treatment ranges from weight reduction and restriction of the leg movement in the hip joint, to anti-inflammatory drugs, to different surgical interventions.

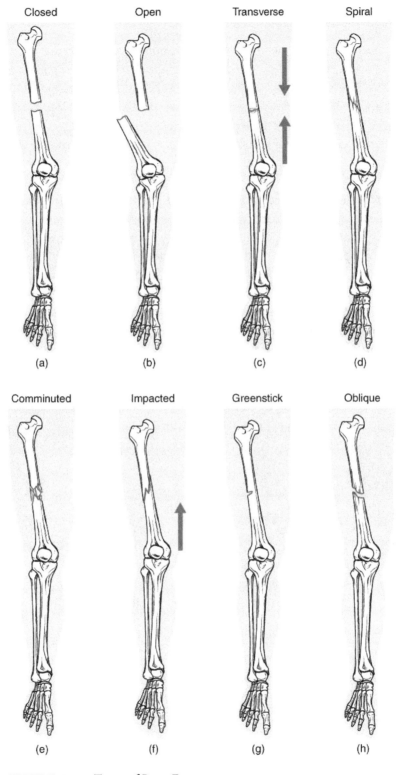

FIGURE 6.11   Types of Bone Fractures.

The process of a fracture healing has four major steps:

1. **Hematoma development.** Remember that bone is not only a bone tissue. Bone has a lot of blood vessels. That is why a bone fracture is usually accompanied by bleeding. Blood from the ruptured bone blood vessels fills the region of the bone fracture and forms a blood clot, or **hematoma**. The hematoma seals the broken blood vessels and stops the bleeding. Fibrous proteins in the blood clot seal the space between the bone's broken pieces.

2. **Formation of soft callus.** Fibroblasts from the periosteum invade the hematoma. Blood vessels also grow inside the hematoma. They deliver oxygen and nutrients to fibroblasts that migrated inside the hematoma. Fibroblasts secrete collagen fibers and form irregular dense connective tissue in place of the fracture. Irregular dense connective tissue binds together fractures of the broken bone. Osteogenic cells from the endosteum become chondroblasts that secrete hyaline cartilage. This complex of hyaline cartilage and irregular dense connective tissue is called soft callus.

3. **Bone callus development.** Osteoblasts from the periosteum secrete a collar of bone tissue around the soft callus. Building of the bone takes some time, during which osteoblasts migrate deeper and deeper inside the soft callus and replace it with bone tissue.

4. **Remodeling.** The primary bone of the bone callus is spongy bone. It is not very strong. Through the activity of osteoclasts and osteoblasts, it is replaced by secondary bone. Eventually, the primary bone callus is completely replaced by the secondary bone, and the bone regains its original shape and structure (fig. 6.12).

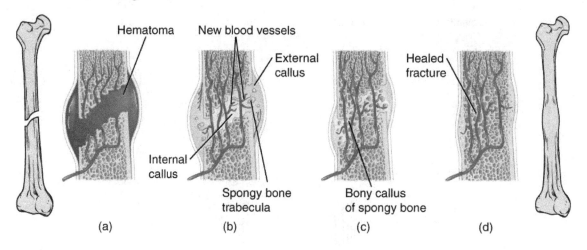

FIGURE 6.12   Bone Fracture Reparation.

CHECK YOUR UNDERSTANDING

- What tissues constitute soft callus?

- Where do osteoblasts that form bone callus come from?

- Where do osteoclasts come from, and what is their role in healing bone fractures?

6.4 Cartilage Tissue

Cartilage tissues play a very important role in vertebrate skeleton organization. There are big and evolutionarily very important groups of vertebrates whose skeleton is completely constructed of cartilage (Chondrichthyes—a class of cartilaginous fishes that includes sharks, rays, skates, and sawfishes). As a remnant of evolutionary history, all vertebrates during their individual development from an embryo to adult organism go through the stage in which their skeleton is made of hyaline cartilage.

Histology of Cartilage

There are three groups of cartilage tissues: **hyaline cartilage**, **elastic cartilage**, and **fibrocartilage** (see fig. 4.18). The principal cells of all three types of cartilage are **chondrocytes**. Chondrocytes originate from **chondroblasts**: young cartilage-built cells. Chondroblasts secrete cartilage ECM and, when ECM surrounds them completely, become chondrocytes. Chondrocytes reside in the fluid-filled lacunae, surrounded by ECM. The three types of cartilage differ by an organic component (osteoid) of the ECM. Hyaline cartilage has less fibrous proteins in ECM than other cartilages. That is why it is glossy and transparent. It is very resilient and slippery. In the skeletal system this cartilage forms the skeleton model of a developing fetus. In an adult organism it is present in joints as articular cartilage. Some joints, such as costal cartilage, are completely made of hyaline cartilage; in others, such as symphysis and vertebrate discs, it is an important structural element.

Elastic cartilage constructs the earlobes (pinna), eustachian (auditory) tube, and epiglottis of the larynx. Its matrix contains elastin protein fibers that have a yellow color. That is why this type of cartilage is also called yellow cartilage.

Fibrocartilage contains collagen fibers. It is a very strong shock-absorbing tissue. This type of cartilage forms very strong shock-absorbing joints, such as symphysis, intervertebral discs, fibrocartilage discs of the temporomandibular joint, and the menisci of the knee joint.

Cartilage Growth and Repair

Cartilage is an avascular tissue. It is supplied with oxygen and nutrients through the diffusion from other tissues. Diffusion through the cartilage ECM is a very slow process. This results in cartilage's slow growth and long repair period after injury. There are two methods of cartilage growth: **interstitial** and **appositional**.

Interstitial growth is a growth of the tissue from inside the tissue regions. Chondrocytes never lose the ability to divide. This makes possible division of chondrocytes deep inside the cartilage tissue. Divided chondrocytes may split their lacuna in two and secrete ECM between them. Thus, the total volume of cartilage tissue increases. Because cartilage is avascular and chondrocytes usually have a poor blood supply, they divide rarely and form ECM slowly.

Appositional growth is faster. It begins with chondroblasts in the perichondrium that covers the cartilage structure from outside. The perichondrium is close to blood vessels, and chondroblasts have a comparatively good blood supply. As a result, they grow fast, can frequently divide, and quickly build ECM. When the ECM locks them inside lacunae, chondroblasts become chondrocytes. This type of growth increases size on the periphery of cartilage structures.

Cartilage has limited repair capabilities. Chondrocytes are tied to lacunae and cannot migrate to the damaged area, and they have a poor blood supply. Therefore, cartilage damage is difficult to heal. As a rule, damaged hyaline cartilage is usually replaced by fibrocartilage scar tissue.

The Role of Hormones in Cartilage Growth

As for bone, growth hormone has major impact on cartilage growth. Growth hormone stimulates chondrocytes to proliferate and grow. Estrogen and testosterone also affect cartilage growth and ossification. Cortisol, a stress hormone secreted by the cortex of adrenal glands, reduces bone formation and prolongs cartilage life in the epiphyseal plate.

CHECK YOUR UNDERSTANDING

- What are the three types of cartilage tissue? What are the differences among them?

- Why is interstitial growth of cartilage tissue slow?

- When hyaline cartilage is damaged, what tissue grows in the damaged area?

- How does cortisol affect cartilage ossification?

6.5   A Brief Description of the Mammalian Skeletal System

Bones of the body form the skeleton, which naturally divides into three functional units: the **axial**, **appendicular**, and **visceral skeletons** (fig. 6.13). The principal differences among them are:

1. The axial skeleton forms the main body axis around which the whole animal body is organized. Thus, the axial skeleton provides attachment for other bones and viscera.
2. The appendicular skeleton forms the limbs of an organism. The girdle is the part of the appendicular skeleton that fixes limb position on the axial skeleton.
3. The visceral skeleton consists of bones and cartilaginous structures that form and support structural organization of the internal organs or viscera.

The Axial Skeleton

The axial skeleton forms the main body axis. It contains the skull, vertebral column, sacrum, bones of the hyoid apparatus, ribs, and sternum. All these structures are composite and are made of many bones.

The **skull** is the most complex part of the skeleton. In most domestic animals it consists of 37 or 38 bones. Most of these bones are bound by immovable joints called **sutures**. The only movable bone of the skull is the mandible. It is bound to the temporal bone by a synovial joint called the temporomandibular joint (TMJ). Skull bones are organized in three groups: 1) cranium bones, 2) ear bones, and 3) facial bones (fig. 6.14).

Cranial Bones

Frontal bones form the anterior wall of the cranium. In most mammals there are two frontal bones bound together by a **frontal suture** (fig. 6.17). In primates these bones are completely fused in a single bone. Anteriorly, frontal bones form the upper part of orbits. The anterior portion of the frontal bones

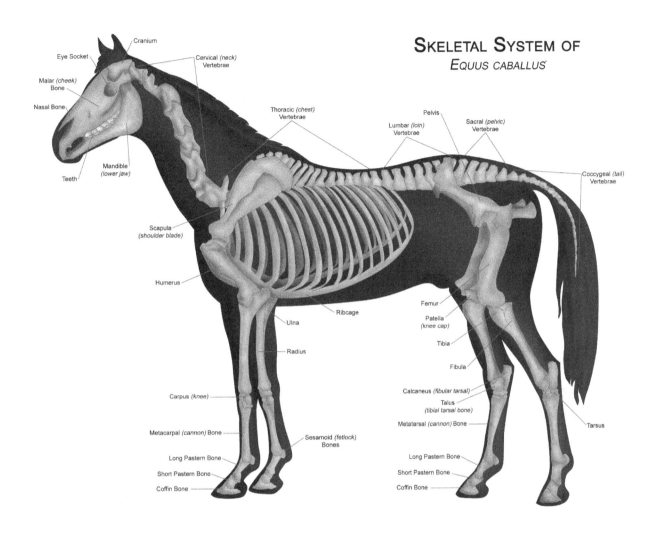

SKELETAL SYSTEM OF
EQUUS CABALLUS

FIGURE 6.13   Horse Skeletal System.

have large hollow chambers filled with air, called the **frontal sinus**. Posteriorly, frontal bones joint with parietal bones by a **coronal suture**.

Parietal bones form the roof of the cranium. These two bones are bound to each other along the midline by a **sagittal suture** or **sagittal crest**. Laterally, they are bound with temporal bones through the **squamous** or **temporal suture** and posteriorly with interparietal bones.

Interparietal bones are small bones between parietal and occipital bones. In many mammals they are not developed. Even among those animals that have interparietal bones, they are most clearly visible in young animals. In aged animals they often fuse with other bones and become indistinguishable (fig. 6.15).

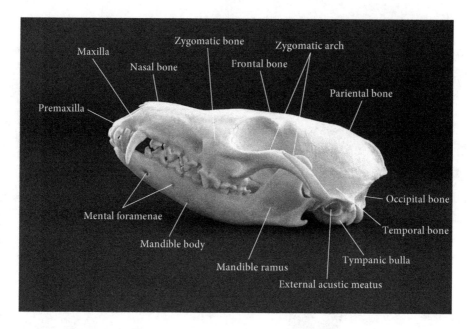

FIGURE 6.14   Fox Skull.

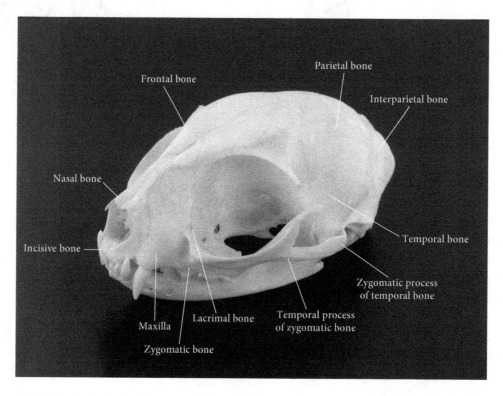

FIGURE 6.15   Cat Skull; Superio-Lateral View.

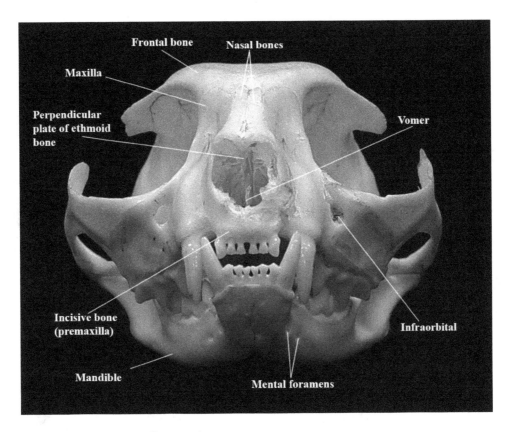

Frontal bone

Nasal bones

Maxilla

Perpendicular
plate of ethmoid
bone

Vomer

Incisive bone
(premaxilla)

Infraorbital

Mandible

Mental foramens

FIGURE 6.16   Cat Skull; Frontal View.

Occipital bone is a single bone that form the posterior wall of the cranium and part of the cranial floor. Ventrally, the bone has a big opening known as the **foramen magnum** (fig. 6.18). The foramen magnum is a passage in the cranium that binds the brain with the spinal cord. Laterally from the foramen magnum, there are two nub-shaped projections known as **occipital condyles**. Occipital condyles are part of the atlanto-occipital joint between skull and vertebral column. Laterally, occipital bones bind to temporal bones and anterio-ventrally to the basisphenoid bone.

Temporal or **squamous bones** form the lateral walls of the braincase (fig. 6.17). The geometry of these two bones is complex. From the lateral sides, bones have a hole called the **external acoustic meatus** or **external auditory canal** that leads inside the middle ear. Ventrally, the bone area that accommodates the middle and inner ears forms a spherical bone structure called the **tympanic bulla**. Anteriorly, temporal bones carry a long bone projection called the **zygomatic processes of the temporal bones**. The zygomatic processes of the temporal bones anteriorly fuse with the **temporal processes of the zygomatic bones** and form the so-called **zygomatic arch** that creates the cheeks' prominence. At the base of the ventral side of the zygomatic processes of the temporal bones there are grooves called **mandibular fossa**. Together with the condyloid process of the mandible, it forms the temporomandibular joint (TMJ).

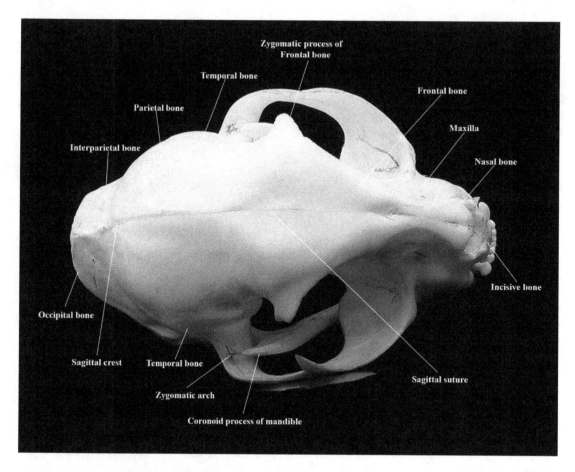

FIGURE 6.17   Cat Skull; Dorsal View.

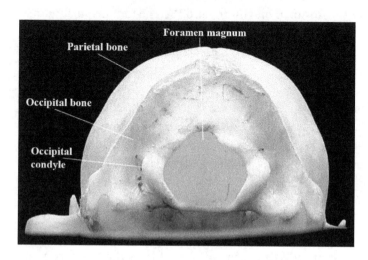

FIGURE 6.18   Cat Skull; Posterior View.

Sphenoid bone is irregular bone inside the cranium. Outside, only some parts of the bone are visible. The prominent part of the bone is the **sella turcica** or **pituitary fossa**. This structure accommodates and protects the pituitary gland.

Ethmoid bone is another single bone hidden inside the cranium. It forms the anterior portion of the cranial floor. Its sharp superior projection called **crista galli** provides attachment for the meninges. Ventrally, it continues into the **perpendicular ethmoid plate** that forms upper part of the nasal septum. Laterally on both sides from the crista galli are two **cribriform plates**.

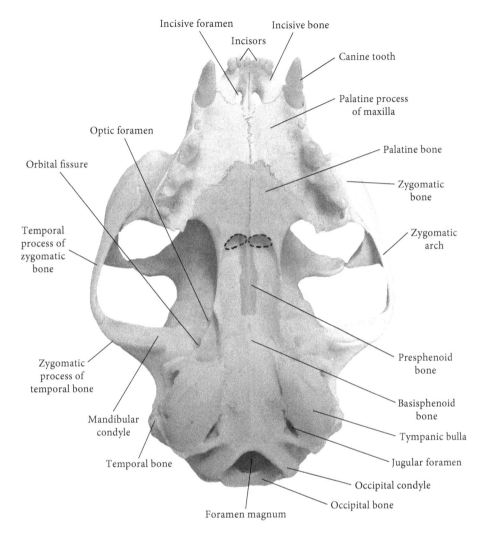

FIGURE 6.19   Cat Skull; Ventral View.

These plates have numerous tiny canals called **cribriform foramina**, which are passages of the axons of ophthalmic sensory neurons from the nasal cavity to the cranium (tab. 6.1).

Ear Bones

There are three pairs of ear bones (tab. 6.2). They are located inside the middle ear between the tympanic membrane and the oval window. These bones function to transmit air vibrations from the tympanic membrane to the oval window. The first bone that touches the tympanic membrane is the **malleus**. Vibrations from the malleus are transmitted to the **incus**, and from the incus to the **stapes**, which strikes the oval window.

TABLE 6.1   Cranial Bones

Bone	Number
Frontal bone	2
Parietal bone	2
Interparietal bone	2
Temporal bone	2
Occipital bone	1
Ethmoid bone	1
Sphenoid bone	1

TABLE 6.2 Ear Bones

Bone	Number
Malleus	2
Incus	2
Stapes	2

Facial Bones

Incisive bones or **premaxilla** are paired bones located at the most rostral part of the skull (fig. 6.16). These bones get their name from the fact that in most mammals, except ruminants, they carry the upper incisive teeth. Instead of incisors, ruminants (cattle, sheep, and goat) have a hard dental pad.

The maxilla makes up most of the upper jaw. It has a ridged area with sockets for canine and premolar teeth called **alveoli**. Superiorly, maxillae form lower ridges of orbits. Beneath these orbits, the maxilla has an opening called the **infraorbital foramen**. Together with palatine bones, maxillae form the roof of the oral cavity, called the **hard palate**. The part of maxilla that participates in hard palate formation is called the **palatine process of the maxilla** (fig. 6.19). Maxillae also have a hollow air-filled space inside called the **maxillary sinus**.

Nasal bones are scaly, paired triangular bones. They form the roof of the nasal cavity.

Lacrimal bones are located in the anterior upper corner of the orbits. Every lacrimal bone has an opening called a **lacrimal canal**, which leads in a lacrimal sac. It is a part of the lacrimal drainage system. Lacrimal glands in the superio-lateral corner of the eyes secrete tears that moisturize and clean the cornea of the eye. The used tear fluids gather in the inferio-median eye corners and drain into the nasal cavity through the lacrimal canals and lacrimal sac.

The **zygomatic** or **malar bone** forms part of the orbit. Posteriorly, zygomatic bones have long temporal process of zygomatic bone, which fuses with the zygomatic process of the temporal bone, and together they form the zygomatic arch. Inferiorly, the zygomatic bone has alveoli for molar teeth.

The **mandible** in primates is a single bone. In most mammals there are two mandible bones bound at the midsagittal line by a cartilaginous joint called the **symphysis mandibularis** or **mandibular symphysis**. The part of the mandible that carries denture is called the **body** or **shaft of mandible**. The massive flat posterior region is called the **ramus**. The ramus has three prominent projections: a large, flat superior projection called the **coronoid process**; a medial plane transverse to the ramus rounded bar-shaped **condyloid process**; and the inferior **angular process** (fig. 6.20). In life the

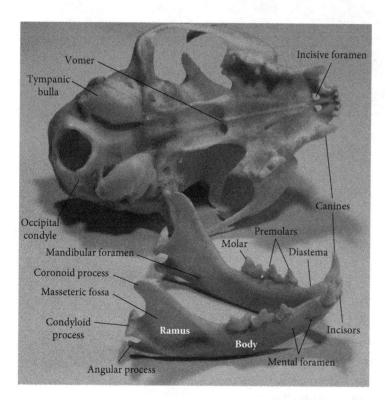

FIGURE 6.20 Cat Skull; Mandible.

condyloid process rests inside the mandibular fossa of the temporal bone and form TMJ. The superior ridge of the mandible is called the **alveolar arch**. It contains sockets (alveoli) for teeth. One, two, or sometimes more tiny holes on the anterio-lateral surface of the body are called **mental foramina**. Mental foramina are passage for blood vessels and nerves to the chin and lower lip. From inside (median side) of the ramus, there is a hole called the **mandibular foramen**. The mandibular foramen permits sensory fibers of the trigeminal nerve and blood vessels to reach the lower denture. The opening of the mandibular foramen is a landmark for local anesthesia when work with mandibular-located teeth is needed.

Palatine bones have the shape of the letter *L*. They form the posterior part of the hard palate and the lateral walls of the nasal cavity. Anteriorly, palatine bones bind with palatine processes of maxillae.

Pterygoid bones are located inside the skull and are not visible outside. They are small, and their function is to support the lateral walls of the pharynx.

The **vomer** is a single bone in the nasal cavity. It is perpendicular to the nasal roof and floor. Together with the perpendicular plate of the ethmoid bone, it forms the **nasal septum**.

VETERINARY APPLICATION

Dogs often have different diseases involving intervertebral discs. Medical examination with spinal radiograph is often required. It is not easy to identify the affected by the lesion area. The vertebra shape is the major landmark, especially the so-called **anticlinal vertebra**. The 11th thoracic vertebra (T11) is called anticlinal because its spinous process, unlike those of the surrounding vertebra, projects straight up. The spinous processes of the thoracic vertebra 1 to 10 are inclined caudally, whereas vertebra T12 and T13 have their spinous processes inclined cranially. This makes the thoracic vertebra T11 easily identifiable. The anticlinal vertebra in cats is also T11. In horses it is T16, in cattle and sheep it is T13, and in swine it is T10.

Turbinate bones or **nasal conchae** are very tiny bones with a complex structure that form the lateral walls of the nasal cavity. There are **dorsal** and **ventral conchae**, the dorsal concha originating from the ethmoid bone and attaching to the maxilla, and the ventral conchae originating from the maxilla and extending further into the nasal cavity. The conchae divide the nasal cavity into nasal ducts or **meatuses**, which branch out from a common nasal meatus, which is adjacent to the nasal septum. There are three nasal meatuses, which branch from the common nasal meatus: **dorsal**, **middle**, and **ventral**. The turbinate bones are covered by mucous membrane, which warms, humidifies, and cleans inhaled air. The dorsal meatus houses olfactory epithelium (tab. 6.3).

The **hyoid apparatus** is composed of several small bones bound by cartilage (fig. 6.21). It is hanged on the temporal bones by two small rods of cartilage. It is located high in the neck above the larynx. It functions as a support bone to help the tongue, pharynx, and larynx swallow food and water.

TABLE 6.3 Facial Bones

Bone	Number
Incisive bone	2
Lacrimal bone	2
Maxilla	2
Nasal bone	2
Zygomatic bone	2
Palatine bone	2
Pterygoid bone	2
Turbinate bone	4
Mandible	1–2
Vomer	1

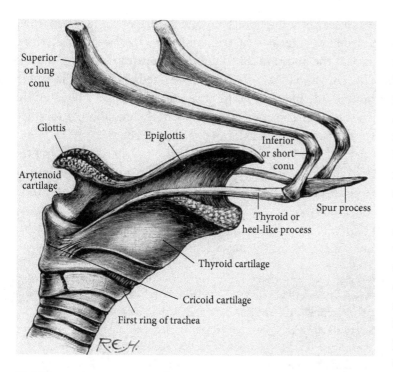

Superior or long conu

Glottis

Epiglottis

Inferior or short conu

Arytenoid cartilage

Spur process

Thyroid or heel-like process

Thyroid cartilage

Cricoid cartilage

First ring of trachea

R.E.H.

FIGURE 6.21   Horse Hyoid Apparatus and Larynx.

The **vertebral** or **spinal column** consists of vertebra (tab. 6.4). It extends from the skull to the tip of the tail. The vertebral column is divided in five regions: cervical, thoracic, lumbar, sacral, and coccygeal. Vertebrae vary in size and shape, especially vertebrae from different vertebral column regions. However, every vertebra has a **body**, which consists of a large ventral middle portion called the **centrum** and a dorsal portion called the **vertebral** or **neural arch**. The body is composed of spongy bone. The cancellous bone is covered by a thin coat of compact bone. The vertebral arch is formed by pedicles and laminae. The pedicles are short thick processes that extend from each dorsal side of the centrum. Each pedicle continues into a dorsally projected **lamina**. Dorsally laminae fuse and complete the arch.

At the place of the laminae fusion arises a **spinous** or **dorsal process**. Above and below the pedicles are shallow depressions called **vertebral notches**. Vertebral notches of two adjacent vertebrae form intervertebral foramina—a passage for vertebral nerves and blood vessels. The two **transverse processes**, one on each side of the vertebral body, project from either side at the point where the lamina joins the pedicle. On the cranial and caudal ends of each vertebra, there are pairs of **articular processes** that form joints between adjacent vertebrae. All vertebrae are joint by **intervertebral discs**, which bind centrums of adjacent vertebra, and synovial joints between their articular processes (fig. 6.22).

TABLE 6.4   Vertebral Formulas of Some Domestic Animals

	Cervical	Thoracic	Lumbar	Sacral	Coccygeal
Cat	7	13	7	3	5–23
Dog	7	13	7	3	20–23
Horse	7	18	6	5	15–21
Cattle	7	13	6	5	18–20
Goat	7	13	7	5	16–18
Pig	7	14–15	6–7	4	20–23
Sheep	7	13	6–7	4	16–18

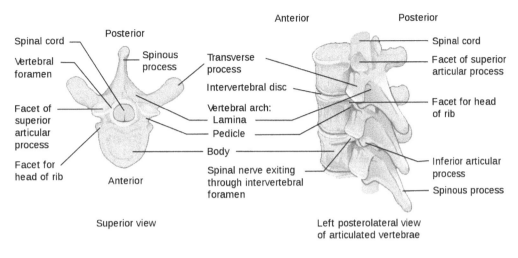

FIGURE 6.22   Anatomy of Vertebra.

Ribs are flat bones (fig. 6.23). They form the lateral walls of the thoracic cage and bind together the vertebral column and sternum. Their dorsal ends carry a small nub called the **capitulum** or **head** separated from the rib shaft or **body** by a narrow **neck**. At the base of the neck there is a short projection called the **tubercle**. Ribs attach to a vertebra at two points: the capitulum attaches to the demifacet on the vertebra's centrum, and the tubercle joints with the transverse costal facet on the transverse process. On the ventral side, the rib is attached to the sternum by costal cartilage. Ribs that are directly attached to the sternum called **true** or **sternal ribs**. The ribs that bind to costal cartilage of other ribs are called **false** or **asternal ribs**. A few pairs of ribs unattached to the sternum are called **floating ribs**.

The **sternum** forms a ventral part of the thoracic cage. It is a structure made of small bones called **sternebra** (pleural sternebrae) (fig. 6.24). The first sternebra at the cranial side is called the **manubrium**. The last caudal sternebra is called the **xiphoid process** or **xiphisternum**. The top of the xiphoid process ends at the **xiphoid cartilage**.

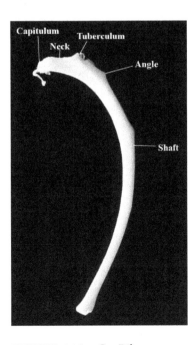

FIGURE 6.23   Cat Rib.

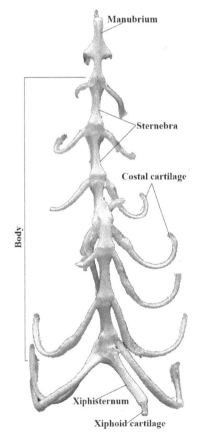

FIGURE 6.24   Cat Sternum.

The Appendicular Skeleton

All terrestrial vertebrates have two pairs of appendages: **thoracic** and **pelvic limbs**.

Thoracic limbs hang on the axial skeleton by the thoracic girdle. In primates the thoracic girdle consists of two pairs of scapula and clavicles. This organization of thoracic limbs is connected with bipedal movement of these mammals and erect position of the upper body parts. Cats and dogs retain remnants of clavicles significantly reduced in size. But they do not form a thoracic girdle. Other mammals may have no clavicle at all. Thus, thoracic limbs have no direct attachment to the axial skeleton. Bones that constitute thoracic limbs are next: scapula, humerus, ulna, radius, and sets of small carpal bones, metacarpal bones, and phalanges.

The **scapula** is flat triangular bone (fig. 6.25). Its lateral side has a longitudinal ridge called a **spine**. Two shallow broad grooves, one above and another beneath the spine, are called **supraspinous** and **infraspinous fossae** correspondingly. From the cranial side the scapula has a shallow, round **glenoid cavity** or **glenoid fossa**. The glenoid fossa functions as an articulation surface for shoulder joint. On the cranial side of the spine there are two projections: the **metacromion** and **acromion**. A small, sharply curved projection above the glenoid fossa is called the **coracoid process**. A concaved ventro-medial side of the scapula is known as the **subscapular fossa**.

The **humerus** constitutes the part of the limb called the **brachium**. Proximally, the humerus is connected with the scapula through the shoulder joint, and distally it is connected with the ulna and radius. The proximal knob-shaped end of the humerus is called the **head**. The head is separated from the rest of the bone by a broad constriction called the **neck**. On two sides, the head is flanked by **greater** and **lesser tuberosities**. The groove between tubercles is known as the **bicipital groove**. It accommodates the tendons of the biceps brachii. On the distal side, the humerus has a hole called the **supracondyloid foramen**. Beneath the supracondyloid foramen there is a wheel-shaped terminal projection called the **trochlea**. From the lateral side, the distal end of the humerus carries nub-shaped projections called **capitulum** (fig. 6.26).

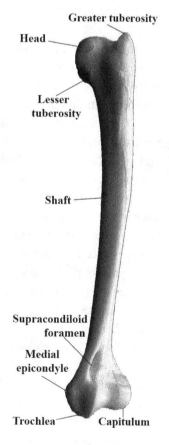

FIGURE 6.26 Cat Right Humerus.

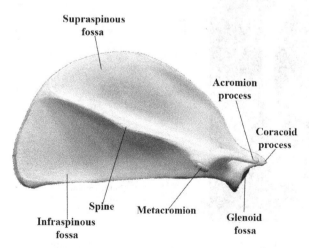

FIGURE 6.25 Cat Right Scapula.

The posterior surface of the distal end of the humerus has a broad, comparatively deep cave known as the **olecranon fossa**. On the anterior surface, there are two small and shallow depressions: **coronoid fossa** between the supracondyloid foramen and trochlea, and **radial fossa** above the capitulum. **Lateral** and **medial epicondyles** are short, robust projections on distal lateral and medial surfaces of the bone.

The **ulna** is a long bone. Together with the radius, it forms part of the forelimb known as the **antebrachium**. The ulna forms a major part of the elbow joint. Proximally, it has a -shaped projection called the **olecranon process**. It provides a surface for attachment of the tendon of the triceps brachii. Beneath the olecranon process is a narrow bowl-shaped notch called the **trochlear notch**. A projection called the **coronal process** follows the trochlear notch from the distal side. On one side the coronal process has an indentation called the **radial notch**. The radial notch accommodates the tablet-shaped radial head. The distal part of the ulna ends in the **styloid process** (fig. 6.27).

The **radius** is shorter and more robust than the ulna (fig. 6.27). Proximally, it has a head that is separated from the radius shaft by a restriction called the **neck**. Imme-

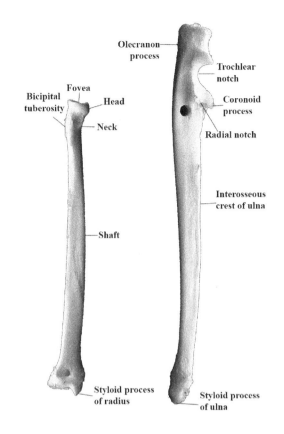

FIGURE 6.27   Cat Right Ulna and Radius.

diately beneath the neck there is a short but strong **bicipital tuberosity**, a point for attachment of the biceps brachii muscle. The distal medial surface of the radius ends in the **styloid process of the radius**.

The **carpal bones** form the **carpus**, or wrist (fig. 6.28). There are eight carpal bones, which are organized in two rows with four bones in a row. The carpus of a horse is referred to as a knee!

The **metacarpal bones** extend from the distal carpal bones. There are five metacarpal bones, which are named by number. They are counted in a medio-lateral direction: the metacarpal bone from the midline is **metacarpal 1**, the next is **metacarpal 2**, and so on. The lateral bone is called **metacarpal 5**. In some mammals (horses, pigs, cattle) metacarpal bones are very reduced and may be absent.

Phalanges constitutes **digits** (fingers or toes) (fig. 6.28). Every digit, except the first one, has three phalanges. The first digit has only two phalanges. Thus, originally a mammalian forelimb has 14 phalanges. Phalanges are named according their position in the digit: **proximal phalanx**, **median phalanx**, and **distal phalanx**.

A horse has only one digit on each limb. It is composed of three phalanges and three sesamoid bones. Their proximal phalanx often is called a long pastern bone; the middle phalanx a short pastern bone; and the distal phalanx a coffin bone. The sesamoid bones in horse forelimbs are two proximal sesamoid bones and one distal sesamoid bone. Two proximal sesamoid bones form a fetlock joint (fig. 6.29).

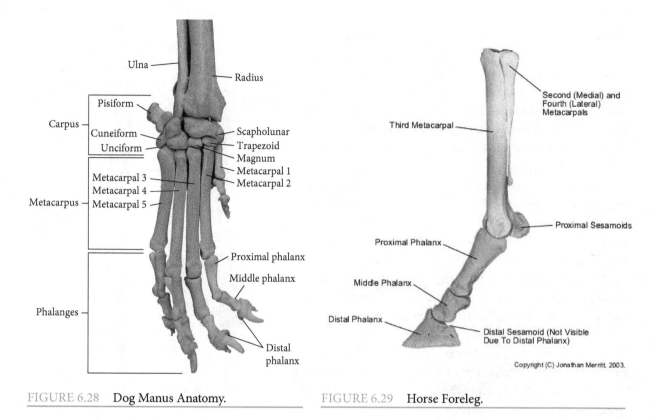

FIGURE 6.28   **Dog Manus Anatomy.**   FIGURE 6.29   **Horse Foreleg.**

Cattle have four digits on each limb. The third and fourth digits support body weight. The second and fifth digits are vestigial and are called dewclaws. Each dewclaw has two small vestigial bones, which do not bind with other bones of the limbs.

In the manus of dogs and cats, a dewclaw is a first digit. Each distal phalanx of these animals has a pointed **ungual process** that is surrounded by the claw.

Pelvic limbs constitute hind legs. They are attached to the axial skeleton through the **pelvic girdle**. The pelvic girdle or pelvis binds with sacrum of the axial skeleton by the **sacroiliac joint**. The pelvis consists of two bone groups that include the **ilium**, **ischium**, and **pubis**. These three bones are firmly fused and form one half of the pelvis or **coxa** (fig. 6.30). These halves are bound along the midline by a cartilage joint known as the **symphysis pubis** or **pubic symphysis**.

The **ilium** is a biggest bone of the pelvis. It occupies the cranial-most position among other pelvic bones. Dorsally, the ilium has a big flat projection called the **wing of ilium** or **ala** (pleural ali). The ridge of the ala is called the **iliac crest**. Anteriorly, the iliac crest may have a sharp angle called the **anterior iliac spine**. The medial side of the ala has a large area with a rough surface. This rough surface is a part of a sacroiliac joint called the **articular surface**. The **body** of the ilium is fused to the pubis and ischium bones. Three bones are fused completely and there are no visible landmarks of the joint between these bones. At the place where the three bones fuse, there is only a deep rounded cave called the **acetabulum**. The acetabulum is a cavity for the femur attachment. Together they form a hip joint.

The **ischium** occupies a caudal position in the pelvis. It is the bone on which cats, dogs, and humans sit. It has a massive projection with rough surface for attachment of strong gluteal and muscles of the upper part of the hind legs called the **ischial tuberosity**. Two indentations on the lateral sides of the bone are called the **lesser** and **greater ischial notches**. These notches are passages for blood vessels and sciatic nerve roots.

The **pubis** is a smallest pelvic bone. It has the shape of the letter *L*. Anterio-ventrally, pubic bones are bound by the symphysis pubis. The pubis and ischium form a bone ring with the biggest hole in the body between them. This hole is known as the **obturator foramen**. The only role of the obturator foramen is to make the pelvis lighter.

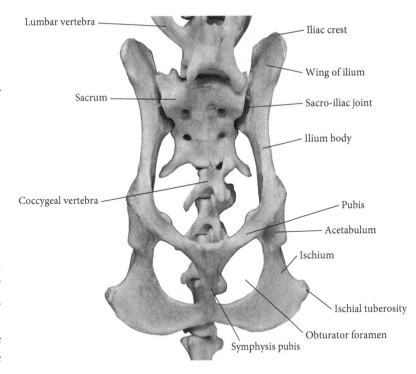

Lumbar vertebra
Sacrum
Coccygeal vertebra
Iliac crest
Wing of ilium
Sacro-iliac joint
Ilium body
Pubis
Acetabulum
Ischium
Ischial tuberosity
Obturator foramen
Symphysis pubis

FIGURE 6.30   Dog Pelvis; Ventral View.

The **femur** is the first proximal bone of the hind leg. It is the biggest long bone in the body in most mammals (fig. 6.31). Proximally, the femur has a ball-shaped projection that perfectly fits the pelvic acetabulum. This projection forms a well moveable ball-and-socket synovial joint and is called the **head of femur**. The head of the femur is separated from the rest of the bone body by a narrow construction called the **anatomic neck**. From both sides, the anatomic neck is flanked by projections known as the **greater** and **lesser trochanter**. At the base of the greater trochanter there is a deep groove called the **trochanteric fossa**. The anterior surface of the femur diaphysis has a pronounced ridge called the **linea aspera**. Distally, there are two wheel-shaped projections called the **lateral** and **medial condyles**. A posterior deep groove between condyles is called the **intercondyloid fossa**. The anterior shallow groove with a smooth surface is known as the **patellar trochlea**. It provides the patella's smooth movement during walking.

The **patella** is a sesamoid bone. Previously, it was believed that it develops as a compression of tendon and ligament tissues. Recent studies show that it develops as a femoral bone projection, which later detaches and becomes independent bone. It is a comparatively small bone with a droplet shape and smooth walls.

The **fabellae** are two small sesamoid bones in dogs and cats. They are located just beneath the femur condyles on the dorsal (posterior) side of the hind leg.

The **tibia** is the main weight-bearing bone of the hind leg. It forms the **stifle joint** with the femur and the **hock joint** with the tarsus below. Two shallow proximal grooves called **tibial condyles** provide a

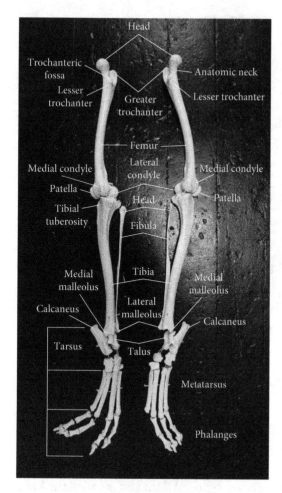

FIGURE 6.31   Dog Hind Leg.

surface for the stifle joint. The anterior proximal surface of the tibia has a visible projection with a rough surface for attachment of the strong quadriceps muscles of the thigh called the **tibial tuberosity**. The ridge on the anterior surface is known as a **tibial crest**. Distally, the tibia bears a finger-like bone projection called the **medial malleolus**.

The **fibula** is a slender weak bone. It does not bear body weight, and its major function is attachment of some tendons and ligaments of the leg and stabilization of the ankle joint. Proximally, the fibula has a small nub called the **head** or **proximal extremity**. Distally, it has a projection called the **lateral malleolus**. The lateral malleolus together with the medial malleolus forms the hock joint.

The **tarsus** forms the ankle or hock. It consists of two rows of eight bones: four bones in a row called the **tarsal bones**. The two largest bones of the proximal row are of special interest. A heel bone called **calcanium** forms the heel. The distal surface of this bone has a rough surface called the **calcaneal tuberosity** for attachment of the **calcaneal** or **Achilles tendon**. A tibial tarsal bone, also called the **talus**, forms the joint between the tibia and tarsus.

The **metatarsus** is made of four **metatarsal bones**. In dogs and cats there are only four metatarsal bone. In these animals, **metatarsus 1** is absent and only **metatarsus 2-5** remain. Horses, of course, have only one fully developed metatarsal bone, called the **cannon bone**, and two small vestigial bones on the both sides of the cannon bone called **splint bones**.

The **phalanges** of the pelvic limb are very similar to those of the thoracic limb. Dogs and cats are different, because they have four digits in their paw on each hind leg.

VETERINARY APPLICATION

The anconeal process of the ulna develops from a secondary growth center that is separate from the primary growth center in the ulnar shaft. In dogs it normally fuses to the rest of the ulna by about six months of age. Sometimes, particularly in large and giant dog breeds, mechanical forces in the elbow break down the fusing tissues and prevent the anconeal process from uniting with the rest of the bone. This results in elbow joint instability that damages the joint surface and causes a secondary osteoarthritis. The diagnostic includes lateral elbow radiography, in fixed position, which will show the unattached process. Treatment usually includes surgical removal of the ununited anconeal process.

The **visceral skeleton** consists of bones that develop within the soft tissues of the body or viscera. The visceral skeleton is highly variable among vertebrates. Not all animals have visceral bones. Three examples of these bones are **os cordis**, **os penis**, and **os rostri**. The os cordis is a bone inside the heart of sheep and cattle. It forms a set of four rings to support heart valves and prevent them from possible closing. Os penis is a bone in the penis of dogs, beavers, raccoons, and walruses. Ventrally, the bone has a groove that partially surrounds the penile urethra (fig. 6.32). Os rostri is a bone in the nose of swine. The function of this bone is obvious: it strengthens the swine's snout for rooting and digging.

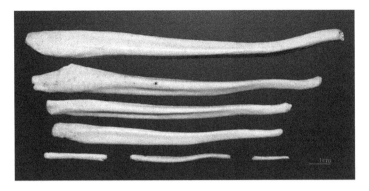

FIGURE 6.32   Os Penis of Brown Bear.

CHECK YOUR UNDERSTANDING

- What bones form the axial skeleton?
- Name all bones of the cranium.
- What is the name of the heel bone?
- What structures constitute the sternum?

CHAPTER SUMMARY

- The skeleton forms the body's shape, holds the body's weight, and together with muscles creates a system of levers for body movement and protects soft organs. Bones have six main functions: 1) **protection**, 2) **support**, 3) **movement**, 4) **mineral storage and acid-base homeostasis**, 5) **blood cell formation**, and 6) **fat storage**. The skeletal system includes bones, cartilage, and joints.

- By origin, bones are classified in three groups: 1) bones that develop by intramembranous ossification are called **intramembranous bones**; 2) bones that develop via cartilage ossification are called **endochondral bones**; and 3) **sesamoid bones**, whose origin is still not clear.

- By shape, bones are divided in five groups: 1) **long**, 2) **short**, 3) **flat**, 4) **irregular**, and 5) **round bones**.

- The long bone has a long shaft or **diaphysis**. On both ends it carries a nub-shaped **epiphysis**. The epiphysis forms a joint with adjacent bones. They are covered by an **articular cartilage** that guarantees smooth frictionless movement. Inside the diaphysis there is a longitudinal hollow space called the **medullary cavity** filled by **yellow bone marrow** that consists of blood vessels and adipose tissue. Compact bone forms the wall of the diaphysis and the outer wall of the epiphysis. Inside, the epiphysis contains spongy or **cancellous bone**. The space between the trabecula is filled by **red bone marrow** that consists of blood vessels and hematopoietic stem cells.

- Bone is covered by a connective tissue membrane called the **periosteum**. The ECM of the periosteum has collagen type 1. Its fibers intertwine with the collagen of tendons and bone ECM and firmly hold skeletal muscle attached to bone. The medullary cavity is lined by the **endosteum**: a thin, vascularized membrane. Both membranes harbor osteogenic cells and osteoblasts.

- Short, flat, irregular, and sesamoid bones have no diaphysis, epiphysis, or medullary cavity. They have a capsule made of compact bone tissue and an internal core of spongy bone tissue.

- Four cell types form bone: **osteogenic cells**, **osteoblasts**, **osteocytes**, and **osteoclasts**. Besides these, bone also has blood cells, chondrocytes, and fibroblasts. ECM contains collagen and solid ground matter made of inorganic compounds of calcium (bones contain 80 to 85 percent of all body calcium) and phosphate. Collagen fibers in ECM form a mesh network that holds salt crystals together and does not let them crumble. The organic component of the ECM is called **osteoid**. In healthy bone, 35 percent of total weight consists of osteoid and 65 percent of inorganic component.

- Osteoblasts originate from **osteogenic cells** located in the periosteum, endosteum, and walls of osteon central canals. Osteogenic cells communicate via paracrine signaling molecules, such as prostaglandins, with osteoblasts, osteocytes, and osteoclasts and also with the cells of nervous tissue, tissues of the gut, muscles, adipocytes, and testis. These signals control osteogenic cells division and development into osteoblasts. Osteoblasts form bone ECM. They are concentrated in the periosteum and endosteum. Trapped inside a small, fluid-filled space surrounded by solid ECM, osteoblasts transform into osteocytes. Osteocyte is a permanent bone cell. Its survival in solid, hard ECM is guaranteed by a fluid-filled **lacuna**. Osteocytes monitor the state of ECM and via paracrine signaling molecules control osteoblasts and osteogenic cells.

- Osteoclasts are large multinucleated cells that originated from monocytes. They are sedentary cells whose cytoplasm contains vesicles with strong hydrolytic enzymes and acids. Release of both components destroys bone tissue. The process of bone destruction is called **bone resorption**.

- Compact bone is strong and heavy. Eighty-five percent of this bone is ECM, 65 percent of which is inorganic calcium salts. The structural unit of compact bone is the **osteon** or **Haversian system**. It is a long tube with thick walls. At the center, osteons have a central canal with blood vessels and nerve fibers. Tissue is organized around the central canal in concentric rings called **lamellae**. Lacunae with osteocytes are located in these lamellae. Every lacuna is connected with other lacunae and a central canal by a network of tiny canals called **canaliculi**. Canaliculi supply osteocytes with oxygen and nutrients. **Perforating** or **Volkmann's canals** bind central canals of adjacent osteons. The old osteons called **interstitial lamellae** remain between new osteons.

- Spongy or cancellous bone forms the interior of long bones and most of the epiphysis. The ECM of spongy bone is organized in spicules called **trabeculae**. Trabeculae form a network with a space for red bone marrow. Trabeculae are covered by the periosteum and on cross section contain lamellae with osteocytes in lacunae.

- Flat bones of the cranium on section look like a sandwich. From both sides they are covered by compact bone with a core made of spongy bone, which is called **diploë**. Some bones have air sacs or **pneumatic diverticula** (frontal, ethmoid, and maxilla bones). Pneumatic diverticula reduce body mass—an adaptation that allows pterosaurs and birds to fly.

- The process of bone formation is called **ossification** or **osteogenesis**. There are two major methods of bone formation: **intramembranous** and **endochondral**.

- Flat bones are formed between two membranous sheets. Bones that develop from this tissue are called **primary bones**. They are temporal and are replaced by permanent **secondary bones**. During intramembranous ossification, the internal spongy bone forms first. Superficial compact bone that covers spongy bone from both sides is formed later. The events of intramembranous ossification are as follows: 1) Mesenchymal cells divide and form dense clusters called the **nidus**. 2) Nidus cells transform into osteogenic cells. 3) Osteogenic cells multiply by mitosis. Some of them develop into osteoblasts, and the nidus becomes a primary ossification center. 4) Osteoblasts of the primary ossification center manufacture and release collagen type 1 fibers. Collagen fibers form a mesh network. 5) Osteoblasts accumulate calcium and deposit calcium salts inside the network of collagen fibers: this process is called **calcification**. 6) Osteoblasts enclose themselves in lacunae and become osteocytes. 7) Osteoblasts on the periphery of the primary ossification center continue to produce ECM and form trabeculae. 8) The spongy bone is growing in all directions from the primary ossification center. It invades the periosteum, where cancellous bone reorganizes into osteons of compact bone. 9) Vascular tissue between trabeculae form bone marrow. 10) There are multiple primary ossification centers, and flat bones grow around these centers, until they fuse and form a single bone. Ossification continues after birth, and a newborn has soft membranous areas called **fontanels**.

- Endochondral ossification takes place inside an embryonic cartilaginous model. The embryonic model consists of hyaline cartilage covered by the **perichondrium**. The perichondrium contains fibroblasts and cartilage stem cells, called **chondrogenic cells**. The cartilage model grows in length by a process called **interstitial growth**. The chondrogenic cells divide and become **chondroblasts**, which form cartilage ECM and, finally, transform in chondrocyte inside lacuna. The first site of ossification is called the **primary ossification center**. It is located in the middle of cartilage model diaphysis. The following events take place: 1) **The periosteum is formed.** Blood vessels grow inside the perichondrium, and chemical signals from blood trigger conversion of chondroblasts into osteogenic cells. Osteogenic cells develop in osteoblasts, and the perichondrium transforms into the periosteum. 2) **The bone collar is formed.** Osteoblasts in the periosteum secrete osteoid at the primary ossification center called bone collar. 3) **The matrix calcifies.** Chondrocytes in the cartilage inside the primary ossification center grow in size (hypertrophy). They secrete alkaline phosphate, an enzyme essential for mineral deposition. Production of alkaline phosphate causes calcification of the cartilage matrix. Calcification of the cartilage matrix and development of the bone collar cut off chondrocytes' blood supply, and they die. 4) **Blood vessels grow inside the emptied space, and osteoblasts replace chondrocytes.** Osteoclasts clean dead chondrocytes from the space and create pathways for blood vessels. Osteoblasts enter the cavity using the calcified matrix as a scaffold. Osteoid deposition forms the early bone trabecula. Osteoclasts continue their activity, break down spongy bone, and form the medullary cavity. The process spreads from the primary ossification center toward both ends of the cartilage model. 5) **A secondary ossification center develops on both epiphyses.** As ossification progresses, the calcified cartilage is replaced by bone. Osteoclasts degrade most of the early spongy bone and clean the space for the medullary cavity. The medullary cavity fills with bone marrow. About the time of birth, cartilage remains in only two locations: deep inside the epiphysis called the **epiphyseal plate** and on the apical surface of the epiphysis called **articular cartilage**. A secondary ossification center appears in each epiphysis. The epiphyseal plate includes all cartilage between the primary and secondary ossification centers. Chondrocytes of the epiphyseal plate continue to form new cartilage. This cartilage is replaced by bone in the same way as in the primary ossification center. The growth of new cartilage and its replacement by bone results in a bone growing in length. Growth continues until the complete ossification of cartilage in the epiphyseal plate. The point of union of the primary and secondary ossification centers is called the **epiphyseal line**.

- Bone growth in length is called **longitudinal growth**. It occurs in the epiphyseal plate by mitotic divisions of chondrocytes. The epiphyseal plate has five zones: 1) **reserve cartilage zone.** The chondrocytes in this zone do not participate in bone growth. Their role is to maintain hyaline cartilage of the epiphyseal plate and provide reserve cells for cellular division; 2) the following zone is called the **proliferation zone**. This zone is responsible for major longitudinal bone growth; 3) next zone is called the **hypertrophy and maturation zone**. Chondrocytes of this zone grow above regular size (hypertrophy); 4) in the **calcification zone** chondrocytes do not grow, but deposit calcium salts in ECM. When ECM is completely calcified, chondrocytes die, suffocated by the absence of oxygen and nutrients; 5) most remote from the epiphysis is the **ossification zone**, which is invaded by osteoclasts that degrade dead chondrocytes and clean space for the following osteoblasts that deposit bone tissue.

- Bone growth in width is called **appositional growth**. It is usually associated with physical stress experienced by the bone. New bone layers are organized in concentric rings called **circumferential lamellae**. With formation of new circumferential lamellae, the old circumferential lamellae reorganize into osteons. Osteoclasts in the endosteum resorb compact bone in the medullary cavity, and the diameter of the medullary cavity also grows.

- Growth hormone, also known as somatotropin, promotes active cell division. Insufficient growth hormone production or lack of sensitivity of target cells to it results in slow bone and cartilage growth, and dwarfism. An excess of this hormone causes gigantism or acromegaly. Calcitonin stimulates activity of osteoblasts, which increase synthesis of osteoid and promote bone growth. Parathyroid hormone stimulates osteoclast activity in bone resorption and the release of calcium in blood flow.

- The sex hormones estrogen and androgen have a strong influence on the postnatal growth of bones and are responsible for characteristic skeletal sexual dimorphism among male and female mammals. These hormones are important for homeostasis of bone tissue during adulthood. A decline in the circulating levels of sex steroids leads to loss of bone mass and their functional integrity. Estrogen is more potent than testosterone. It promotes chondrocyte mitosis and causes fast growth of females in puberty. Because estrogen has a higher impact on bone growth, at the period of sexual maturation females grow faster than males. The fast growth also causes early closing of the epiphyseal plate, and females stop growing earlier than males. Testosterone effects not only longitudinal but also appositional growth. That is why male bones are not only longer but also bigger in diameter.

- Fat-soluble (steroid) vitamins, **vitamin D**, **A**, and **K**, have a strong impact on the state of bones. The main effect vitamin D exerts is on absorption of food calcium in the small intestine. The vitamin also promotes calcium retention in kidneys. Vitamin A is needed for production of retinoic acid, which is an important hormone-like growth factor. It facilitates bone growth, and deficiency in vitamin A causes slow bone growth and ossification. Vitamin K plays an essential role as a cofactor for synthesis of osteocalcin, a calcium ion–binding glycoprotein secreted by the osteoblasts, and plays an essential role in the formation of mineral in bone. Water-soluble **vitamin C** is required for collagen synthesis. Inadequate intake of vitamin C results in a decrease in collagen synthesis and in fragile bones.

- Bones may be fractured in many ways. When tissues and organs around a fractured bone are unaffected, the fracture is called **simple**. **Compound fractures** involve nearby tissues and organs. If the broken bone does not penetrate the skin and is not exposed outside the body, the fracture is called **closed**. An **open fracture** is characterized by exposure of the broken bone and profound bleeding. The bone may be broken only on one side, whereas the opposite side remains unbroken. This type of fracture is called a **greenstick fracture**. It is the easiest to repair and heal. The most difficult fracture types are **oblique**, **spiral**, and **comminuted fractures**.

- The process of a fracture healing proceeds in four steps: 1. **Hematoma development.** Blood from the ruptured blood vessels fills the fracture and forms a blood clot, or **hematoma**. The Hemathma seals broken blood vessels and ends bleeding. Fibrous proteins in the blood clot seal the space between the bone's broken pieces. 2. **Formation of soft callus.** Fibroblasts from the periosteum invade the hematoma. Blood vessels also grow inside the hematoma. They deliver oxygen and nutrients to migrating fibroblasts. Fibroblasts form irregular dense connective tissue in the fracture. Osteogenic cells from the endosteum become chondroblasts that secrete hyaline cartilage. The complex of hyaline cartilage and irregular dense connective tissue is called **soft callus**. 3. **Bone callus development.** Osteoblasts from the periosteum secrete a collar of bone tissue around the soft callus. Osteoblasts migrate inside the soft callus and form bone tissue. 4. **Remodeling**. A bone callus is not a strong structure; osteoclasts and osteoblasts replace it with a secondary bone.

- There are three groups of cartilage tissues: **hyaline**, **elastic**, and **fibrocartilage**. The principal cells are **chondrocytes** that originate from **chondroblasts**. Chondroblasts secrete ECM and transform in chondrocytes. Chondrocytes reside in the fluid-filled lacunae.

- Hyaline cartilage has less fibrous proteins in ECM than other cartilages. It is glossy, transparent, resilient, and slippery. It forms the fetal skeleton model. In an adult, it is present in joints as an articular cartilage.

- Elastic cartilage constructs earlobes (pinna), eustachian (auditory) tube, and epiglottis of the larynx. Its matrix contains elastin fibers that have a yellow color. It is also called yellow cartilage.

- Fibrocartilage is a strong shock-absorbing tissue. This cartilage forms strong shock-absorbing joints, such as symphysis, vertebrate discs, and menisci in knee joints.

- Cartilage is avascular. It is supplied with oxygen and nutrients by diffusion. Diffusion through the cartilage ECM is a very slow process, and cartilage is slow to grow and repair after injury. There are two means of cartilage growth: **interstitial** and **appositional**.

- Growth hormone stimulates chondrocytes to proliferate and grow. Estrogen and testosterone also affect cartilage growth and ossification. Cortisol reduces the rate of bone formation and prolongs cartilage life in the epiphyseal plate.

- The skeleton consists of three functional units: **axial**, **appendicular**, and **visceral skeletons**. The principal differences among them are: 1) The axial skeleton forms a main body axis. It provides attachment for other bones and viscera. 2) The appendicular skeleton forms limbs. The girdle is the part of the appendicular skeleton that fixes limb position on the axial skeleton. 3) The visceral skeleton consists of bones and cartilage that form and support structural organization of viscera, such as fibrocartilage rings around heart valves.

CHECK YOUR KNOWLEDGE

LEVEL 1. CHECK YOUR RECALL

1. Which of the following is **not** a step in the formation of endochondral bone?
   A. Hyaline cartilage develops into the shape of the future bone.
   B. The periosteum develops from connective tissue on the outside of the developing bone.
   C. Hyaline cartilage is replaced by the adipose tissue.
   D. Osteoblasts deposit osseous tissue in the area of disintegrated cartilage.
   E. Osteoclasts dissolve and digest dead cells and cellular debris.

2. Red bone marrow functions to _____, whereas yellow bone marrow functions to _____.
   A. accumulate fat; produce red cells, white cells, and other blood former elements
   B. produce red cells, white cells, and other blood former elements; store fat
   C. create strong frame of bone; produce red cells, white cells, and former elements
   D. produce osteocytes; produce osteoblasts
   E. produce red blood cells; produce white blood cells and blood former elements

3. Bone cells that resorb bone tissue are:
   A. Fibroblasts
   B. Chondrocytes
   C. Osteoblasts
   D. Osteoclasts
   E. Osteocytes

4. The connective tissue membrane that covers bone from the outside is called:
   A. Pleural
   B. Parietal
   C. Visceral
   D. Periosteum
   E. Endosteum

5. Osteoclasts are _____, whereas osteoblasts are _____.
   A. bone-destroying (degrading) cells; bone-building (growing) cells
   B. bone-building (growing) cells; bone-destroying (degrading) cells
   C. red bone marrow cells that produce blood; yellow bone marrow cells that store fat
   D. yellow bone marrow cells that store fat; red bone marrow cells that produce blood
   E. major cell type of cartilage; major cell type of bone

6. Which bones form via intramembranous ossification?
    A.   Irregular bones
    B.   Flat bones
    C.   Sesamoid bones
    D.   Long bones
    E.   Short bones

7. Long bones grow in length from the:
    A.   Diaphysis line
    B.   Epiphyseal line
    C.   Epiphyseal plate
    D.   Medullary cavity
    E.   Articular cartilage

8. A hole in the bone is called:
    A.   Condyle
    B.   Foramen
    C.   Fossa
    D.   Process
    E.   Tuberosity

9. The anatomical name of the hip joint is:
    A.   Sacro-iliac joint
    B.   Symphysis pubis
    C.   Symphysis mandibularis
    D.   Acetabulofemoral joint
    E.   Temporo-mandibular joint

10. The part of the long bone that never ossifies during the entire life span is:
    A.   Epiphyseal plate
    B.   Epiphyseal line
    C.   Secondary ossification center
    D.   Primary ossification center
    E.   Articular cartilage

11. Skeletal cells that are mitotic active are called:
    A.   Osteocytes
    B.   Osteoclasts
    C.   Osteoblasts
    D.   Chondrocytes
    E.   Adipocytes

12. The structural unit of compact bone is _____, whereas of spongy bone it is _____ .
     A. lacunae; canaliculi
     B. canaliculi; lacunae
     C. interstitial lamellae; circumferential lamellae
     D. circumferential lamellae; interstitial lamellae
     E. osteon; trabeculae

13. A big hole in the occipital bone is called _____, and in the pelvis is called _____ .
     A. mental foramen; supracondyloid foramen
     B. supracondyloid foramen; mentyal foramen
     C. foramen magnum; obturator foramen
     D. obturator foramen; foramen magnum
     E. foramen magnum; mental foramen

14. Lacunae in cartilage contain _____, whereas in bone there are _____ .
     A. chondroblasts; osteoblasts
     B. chondrocytes; osteocytes
     C. osteoclasts; osteogenic cells
     D. osteoblasts; osteoclasts
     E. osteocytes; chondrocytes

15. The region of the epiphyseal plate where chondrocytes divides is known as _____, and the region where osteoblasts secrete osteoid is known as _____ .
     A. calcification; reserving zone
     B. reserving zone; proliferation zone
     C. proliferation zone; ossification zone
     D. ossification zone; hypertrophy zone
     E. hypertrophy zone; reserve zone

16. True or false: Blood vessels in the central canal receive blood flow input through perforating canals.
17. True or false: The distal projection of the ulna is called the lateral malleolus.
18. True or false: Posteriorly, frontal bones are bordered by parietal bones.
19. True or false: Proximally, the humerus joins with the scapula through the acetabulum.
20. Match the term with its description:

     _____ Osteocyte   a. Occipital bone
     _____ Osteoblast   b. Mandibular bone
     _____ Osteoclast   c. Maxilla
     _____ Chondrocyte   d. Humerus
     _____ Mental foramen   e. Principal cartilage cell
     _____ Supracondyloid foramen f. Principal bone cell
     _____ Foramen magnum   g. Bone resorbing cell
     _____ Infraorbital foramen   h. Bone-building cell

LEVEL 2. CHECK YOUR UNDERSTANDING

1. In your own words, explain why vitamin D is important for healthy bone growth.
2. Explain the effects of calcitonin and parathyroid hormone (PTH) on bones.
3. What would happen if osteoclasts did not function properly?
4. Explain why a disease of the primary cartilage affects bone development.
5. Explain why female bone mass lowers during pregnancy.

LEVEL 3. APPLY YOUR KNOWLEDGE TO REAL LIFE

1. Explain why a fracture of the lower jaw in a dog usually happens through the jaw's midline.
2. Why does the cat declawing procedure require removing the distal phalanx?
3. Explain why long-lasting stress associated with profound secretion of cortisol causes slow body growth.
4. In fig. 6.33, there is a horse bone fracture. What kind of fracture do you see in this image? Do you recognize the bone?

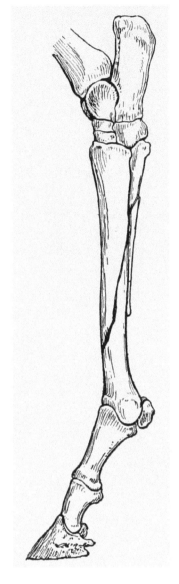

FIGURE 6.33   Horse Bone Fracture.

Chapter 7

Joints

LEARNING OBJECTIVES

Joints are the junctions between bones. They are indispensable elements of the skeletal system. Some joints firmly attach bones to each other, whereas others permit some freedom of movement. Their structural organization is a perfect example of correspondence between form and function. In this chapter you will find information on body joints and possible movement. It is expected that when you finish reading this chapter, you will be able to:

1. Understand the structure and function of different joints.

2. Explain what movement is possible in this or that joint.

3. Understand the basic principles of maintaining healthy joints.

INTRODUCTION

Joints are indispensable structures of the animal skeleton. There are hundreds of joints in the mammalian body. Altogether, they serve three principal functions:

1. Joints bind bones together and guarantee stability of skeleton organization. There are many joints that do not allow movement between bones. These joints organize bones in a strong structure that provide effective protection of internal organs.

2. Joints enable body movement. The freedom and type of movement depends on the structural organization of the joint. These movements are part of the daily animal activity. Thus, joints guarantee animals success for survival and a healthy life.

3. Joints allow bones to grow. Long bones grow from the epiphyseal plates. The epiphyseal plate, as a matter of fact, is a joint made of hyaline cartilage. This cartilage provides major longitudinal bone growth. In an adult organism healthy joints guarantee healthy bones. The compromise of joint stability as a rule causes compensatory modification of bone shape, as happens in osteoarthritis.

In this chapter we will examine joints' structural organization and function. We also will discuss different types of body movements and how these movements correspond with joint structure.

7.1   Classification of Joints

There are two principal ways of joint classification: by joint function or by joint structure. Functionally, joints fall in three groups:

1. **Synarthrosis** are joints which do not allow any bones' movement. Synarthrosis guarantees a high stability of the joint.
2. **Amphiarthrosis** are joints which permit very little movement between bones. Amphiarthrosis provides less stability of the junction between bones.
3. **Diarthrosis** are joints which allow different degree movement. Diarthrosis gives significant freedom of movement but compromises stability of the joint.

There are two classifications of joints according to constructive organization and materials that constitute the joint. Clinical classification takes into account the number of connections between bones that together form the joint. This numerical classification identifies three classes of joints:

1. **Monoarticular**—when the joint has one single junction between bones
2. **Oligoarticular** or **pauciarticular**—when there are two to four junctions between bones in the joint
3. **Polyarticular**—when there are five or more junctions between bones in the joint

Joints are divided in three classes according the tissues that constitute the joint:

1. **Fibrous joints.** Fibrous joints are made of regular dense connective tissue. Collagen fibers of the tissue fasten adjacent bones. Most of these joints are very strong and completely immoveable; that is, they are synarthrosis.
2. **Cartilaginous joints.** These joints are made of cartilage: a resilient pressure-resistant material. These joints also are strong, but some of them allow a light movement in response to external pressure; that is, they are amphiarthrotic.
3. **Synovial joints.** Synovial joints have the most complex organization. These joints are characterized by presence of a synovial cavity between bones. Absence of direct connection between bones permits them to move more or less freely. These joints belong to a diarthrosis type.

CHECK YOUR UNDERSTANDING

- To what type of functional group do synovial joints belong?

- What is the difference between diarthroses and amphiarthroses joints?

7.2   Fibrous Joints

Fibrous joints are made of regular dense connective tissue (see chapter 4, page 117). The tissue contains collagen type 1 fibers. These fibers are very strong and stretch resistant. Collagen fibers of the joint are intertwined with collagen in matrix of both bones, which makes these joints very strong. There are three groups of fibrous joints: **suture**, **syndesmosis**, and **gomphosis**.

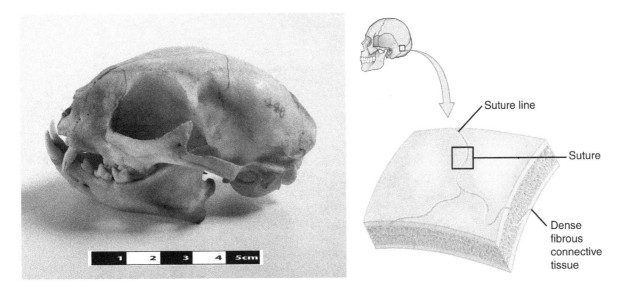

FIGURE 7.1A AND 7.1B Suture.

Sutures

Sutures are joints between the flat bones of the skull. Suture binds bones' edges along their length. As a rule, in the area of contact the edge of the bone is wavy with projections and notches. Two edges of adjacent bones fit each other like a zipper. Collagen fibers of the suture firmly sew both bones (fig. 7.1). During flat bone development, when primary mesenchyme membrane is still not completely ossified and there are remain membranous regions, suture allows some restricted movement, like bending. When a flat bone finally ossified, this movement is completely stopped. With aging, some of the sutures can also be ossified and become a so-called **synostosis**. A synostosis fuses two bones into one single bone. Suture is a synarthrosis.

Depending on the shape of the bones' edges, sutures are divided in three groups (fig. 7.2):

1. **Serrate** suture has interlocking wavy lines. To this group belong the coronal, sagittal, and lambdoid sutures in the skull.
2. **Lap (squamous)** suture has overlapping beveled edges, like the joint between the temporal and parietal bones.
3. **Plane (butt)** suture has straight, nonoverlapping edges. Palatine bones and palatine processes of the maxillae are bound by this type of suture.

Gomphosis

A **gomphosis** is an immovable or synarthrosis joint. This joint also is called **dentoalveolar syndesmosis** to emphasize the fact that these joints bind teeth to the bony teeth sockets, or alveoli, of the maxilla or mandible. Regular dense connective tissue that constitutes the joint forms a **periodontal ligament**. The periodontal ligament makes a connection between the maxilla or mandible and the cementum of the tooth. The gomphosis is the only joint in which a bone does not join another bone, because teeth are not

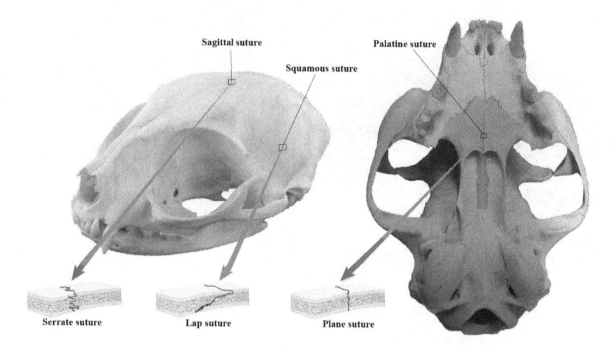

FIGURE 7.2   Three Types of Sutures.

bones. A gomphosis is a specialized fibrous joint in which a conical process or peg of tooth fits into a hole or socket of the bone (*gomphos* is a Greek word that means "bolt"). A small quantity of fibrous tissue holds bones and tooth together. No movement is possible at such peg-and-socket joints (fig. 7.3).

Syndesmosis

A **syndesmosis** is a fibrous joint at which two bones are bound by collagen fibers that are longer than in the suture or gomphosis. This gives bones some mobility. Thus, a syndesmosis is an amphiarthrosis. Regular dense connective tissue which constitutes syndesmosis is organized in a membrane called the **interosseus membrane**. The most movable syndesmosis is the interosseus membrane between the radius and ulna. The long collagen fibers of this membrane allow partial rotation of these two bones around each other (fig. 7.4). This mutual rotation of the radius and ulna allows a special movement of the forelimbs called **supination** and **pronation**. The less movable syndesmosis is between the tibia and fibula. Movement of the tibia and fibular around each other permit some animals to move the tarsus sole medially or laterally in movements called **inversion** and **eversion** correspondingly.

7.3   Cartilaginous Joints

Cartilaginous joints are made of different type of cartilage. You are already familiar with the epiphyseal plate—a cartilaginous joint made of hyaline cartilage. This joint allows little if any movement of bone's epiphysis. There are two types of cartilaginous joints: **synchondrosis** and **symphisis**.

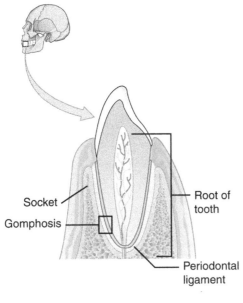

FIGURE 7.3   Gomphosis.

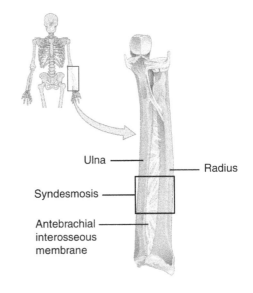

FIGURE 7.4   Syndesmosis between Radius and Ulna.

Synchondrosis

A synchondrosis is a joint made of hyaline cartilage. Hyaline cartilage is a resilient shock-absorbing tissue, which actually almost does not permit bones' movement. These joints functionally are synarthroses. The epiphyseal plate is an example of a synchondrosis (see chapter 6, page 168). Two synchondroses that bind the first rib to the manubrium of the sternum are called **sternocostal** and **costochondrtal joints** (note that all other ribs are attached to the sternum through the synovial joints). These joints persist into adulthood.

Symphysis

A symphysis is a permanent fibrocartilage joint. Fibrocartilage is a strong shock-absorbing tissue that allows slight movement between bones. This joint is an amphiarthrosis. In symphysis mandibularis and symphysis pubis, two adjacent bones are joined by **intermanbidular** and **interpubic discs**, correspondingly. Discs are made of a fibrocartilage and may contain a fluid-filled cavity. The ends of both pubic bones are covered by a thin layer of hyaline cartilage attached to the fibrocartilage. The disc is reinforced by a series of ligaments. These ligaments stabilize the joint and make it stronger.

   Intervertebral discs are another type of symphysis joint. Intervertebral discs have the shape of a tablet. They consist of an outer fibrous coverage called the **anulus fibrosus** and an inner gel-like pulp center called the **nucleus pulposus**. The anulus fibrosus consists of several layers (laminae) of fibrocartilage. The stiff laminae can withstand outside compressive forces. The nucleus pulposus consists of hyaline cartilage. It prevents the development of stress concentration in the vertebral column and acts as a shock-absorbing pad. There is one disc between each pair of vertebrae, except for the two first cervical vertebra (fig. 7.5). The first cervical vertebra called the **atlas** and the second cervical vertebra called the **axis** are designed as a ring around the rod. This joint allows the atlas to rotate around the axis projection called the **dense** or **odontoid process**, which allows the neck to swivel.

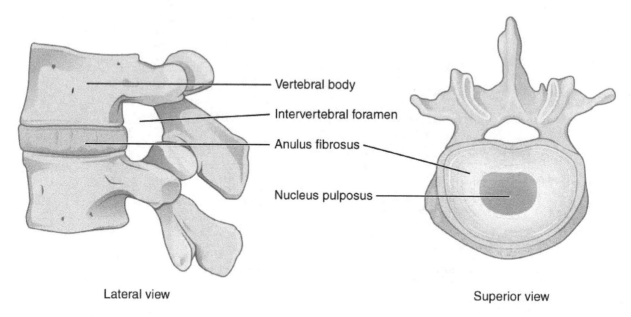

Vertebral body
Intervertebral foramen
Anulus fibrosus
Nucleus pulposus

Lateral view

Superior view

FIGURE 7.5   Intervertebral Disc, an Example of a Symphysis Joint.

CHECK YOUR UNDERSTANDING

- Why are suture and gomphosis counted as synarthroses, whereas a syndesmosis is an amphiarthrosis?

- Why are synchondroses counted as synarthroses, whereas a symphysis is an amphiarthrosis?

- What is the structural difference between a synchondrosis and a symphysis?

7.4   Synovial Joints

Synovial joints have a complex structure. These joints permit different degrees of free movement and, thus, are classified as diarthroses. Because movement compromises structural stability, synovial joints are usually accompanied by additional supporting structures outside of the joint, such as ligaments.

Structure of Synovial Joint

Synovial joints are very diverse in their design, but there are some components common to all synovial joints (fig. 7.6):

1. In all synovial joints, adjacent bones do not physically touch each other. There is a space between bones called the **synovial cavity** filled with slippery fluid called **synovial fluid.** Synovial fluid contains protein lubricin, a lubricating component, secreted by synovial fibroblasts. It is responsible for lubrication, which reduces friction between opposing bone surfaces. Synovial fluid has a nonconstant viscosity coefficient. The fluid viscosity increases and the fluid thickens over a period of continued stress. It also contains phagocytes that remove microbes and the debris that results from normal wear and tear in the joint.

2. The apical ends of both bones in the joint are covered by the **articular cartilage** (see chapter 6, page 160). Articular cartilage is hyaline cartilage: a slippery glossy tissue with some ability to repair, if it is damaged. The function of the articular cartilage is, together with the synovial fluid, to provide a smooth frictionless movement. The ability of hyaline cartilage to have slow growth and repair gives it some guarantee to maintain the joint in a healthy state.

3. From the outside the joint is covered by the connective tissue membrane that forms the **synovial capsule**. The synovial capsule encloses ends of adjacent bones and completely covers their surfaces, except the areas covered by the articular cartilage. The internal surface of the synovial capsule is lined by a **synovial membrane** (fig. 7.6). Synovial membrane is made of a special type of connective tissue called **synovial tissue**. Synovial tissue is composed of vascularized connective tissue that lacks a basement membrane. It has two types of cells, known as a type A and type B cells. Type A cells are derived from white blood cells known as monocytes. As you remember (see chapter 5, page 139, and chapter 6, page 162), monocytes are progenitors of all phagocytes in the body. The function of these cells is to remove the bacteria and wear-and-tear debris from the synovial fluid. Type B cells produce the hyaluronic acid, lubricin, proteinases, and collagenases of the synovial fluid.

Other components of the synovial joint include adipose tissue, nerve fibers, and blood vessels. Adipose tissue is packed into fat pads that fill every available space. Adipose tissue easily changes shape and may be squeezed when joint is in motion. Pads cushion a joint and prevent its injury. Blood delivers oxygen and nutrients and removes waste products. Nerves monitor the state of the joint and control body position and movement.

Some synovial joints have a fibrocartilage that grows inward from the joint capsule.

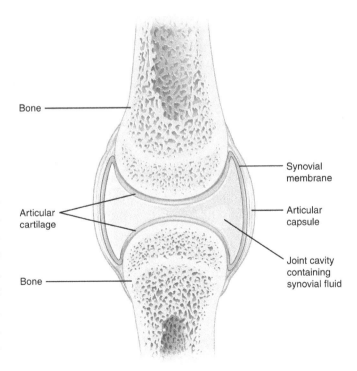

FIGURE 7.6   Principal Organization of the Synovial Joint.

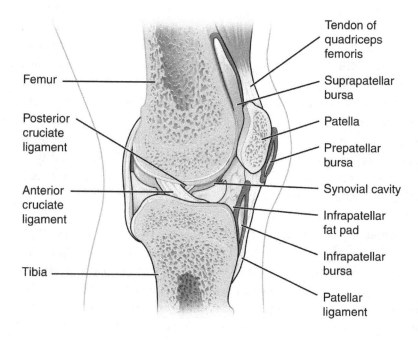

Labels (left side, top to bottom): Femur; Posterior cruciate ligament; Anterior cruciate ligament; Tibia

Labels (right side, top to bottom): Tendon of quadriceps femoris; Suprapatellar bursa; Patella; Prepatellar bursa; Synovial cavity; Infrapatellar fat pad; Infrapatellar bursa; Patellar ligament

FIGURE 7.7   Human Knee Joint, an Example of a Synovial Joint.

Sometimes this fibrocartilage completely crosses the entire joint capsule between articulating bones. These fibrocartilage plates are called an **articular disc.** Articular discs are found inside the temporomandibular joint (TMJ), distal radioulnar joints, sternoclavicular, and acromioclavicular joints. **Menisci** (singular *meniscus*) are fibrocartilage pads that have the shape of a flat donut, with a thick border and thin central region. They do not divide the synovial cavity completely. In the knee, menisci extend inward from the left and right but do not entirely cross the joint. These cartilages absorb shock and pressure, guide bones across each other, improve the fit between bones, stabilize the joint, and reduce the chance of dislocation (fig. 7.7).

Some synovial joints are enforced by so-called **intracapsular ligaments**. For example, in the hip joint the **ligamentum teres** fastens a rounded depression on the virtue of the femur's head called the **fovea** and the depression on the bottom of the acetabulum called the **acetabular notch**. The ligamentum teres does not let the head of the femur fall out of the socket of the acetabulum and prevents hip joint dislocation. The knee joint is stabilized by a set of intracapsular ligaments. A pair of **cruciate ligaments**—anterior (ACL), also known as a cranial (CCL), and posterior (PCL)—bind the lateral condyle of the femur with the anterior intercondylar area of the tibia and the medial condyle of the femur with the posterior intercondylar area of the tibia correspondingly. The ACL prevents the tibia from being pushed too far anterior relative to the femur. It is often torn during twisting or bending of the knee. The PCL prevents posterior displacement of the tibia relative to the femur. The **transverse ligament** connects lateral and medial menisci (fig. 7.7).

VETERINARY APPLICATION

Anterior (cranial) cruciate ligament rupture is an injury that may happen in sport dogs. A wrong step of the dog can result in a rupture or tearing of the anterior cruciate ligament (ACL). The injury may occur when the dog is running and turning. The damage of the ACL causes stifle joint instability. Instead of hinging on each other like they normally do, the femur and tibia slide forward and backward relative to each other. This can damage other joint structures, such as the menisci, and can lead to development of osteoarthritis in the joint.

Rupture of the ACL is diagnosed by palpating the stifle joint and producing what is called anterior drawer movement. Therapy for the anterior cruciate ligament rupture includes restriction in exercises, weight reduction, some physical therapy, and surgical intervention.

Stabilizing and Supporting Structures of Synovial Joints

Additional accessory structures associated with synovial joints include:

1. A **bursa** is a sac lined by synovial membrane and filled with synovial fluid. It resembles a balloon filled with water. A bursa may be attached to the synovial capsule or completely separated. It occupies a position at the heaviest pressure from tendons, ligaments, and muscles. Thus, it is usually found between adjacent muscles, where tendon passes over bone, or between bone and skin. The bursa cushions muscles, helps tendons slide more easily over joints, and corrects direction of tendon pull.

2. A **tendon** is a rope or sheet of tough collagenous regular connective tissue that attaches muscle to bone. It is the most important structure in stabilizing a joint. Tendons pull bones when muscle contracts and press on them holding bones together. For example, the tendon of the long head of the biceps brachii presses on the head of the humerus and holds it inside the glenoid cavity.

3. A **ligament** is a strip or sheet of irregular dense connective tissue. It connects bone to bone or bone to viscera other than skeletal muscle.

4. A **tendon sheath** is an elongated cylindrical bursa wrapped around a tendon. A tendon sheath protects the tendon and directs its course. Tendon sheaths provides friction-free tendon movement and facilitate pressure on the bones of the joint.

5. A **retinaculum** is a broad ring band around limbs. A retinaculum is made of irregular dense connective tissue. It forms a protected pathway for tendons and hold small bones of the limb's extremities in the right position.

VETERINARY APPLICATION

Patellar luxation in dogs is caused by a tendon of the quadriceps off the midline of the joint. Normally, the tendon rides secure inside the trochlea on the distal end of the femur. The quadriceps tendon presses on the patellar from the top along the midline and does not let it to off the trochlea. The physical abnormalities in knee development can cause a shift of the tendon from the midline, and its pressure securing the joint becomes compromised. If this happens, the patellar may pop out of the trochlea, usually toward the body midsagittal plane. This most common type of patellar luxation occurs in small and miniature dog breeds. The patellar luxation causes a periodic, skipping-type gait characteristic for this disorder. The condition is easily diagnosed by extending the stifle joint and palpating the easily displaced patellar. The treatment usually includes different types of surgery.

CHECK YOUR UNDERSTANDING

- Name the three major elements of a synovial joint.

- What is the difference between an articular disc and meniscus?

- What is the role of the intracapsular ligaments?

- What is a bursa? How does it relate to the tendon sheath?

- What role do tendons and ligaments play in synovial joints?

Different Types of Synovial Joints

Synovial joints are very diverse by their construction and the motion they allow. The correspondence between synovial joint organization and allowed movement is one more perfect illustration of the principle of correspondence between form and function. Structurally, synovial joints fall in six groups: **plane** or **gliding, hinge, pivot, condylar, saddle,** and **ball-and-socket joints.**

A **plane** or **gliding joint** is the simplest synovial joint. Bones in this joint have flat articulate surfaces, which gives this joint its first name. The only possible movement in a plane joint is sliding or gliding one bone over the flat surface of the other, which gives this joint its second name. Joints between carpal and tarsal bones are of this type. Sliding or gliding joints have no axis around which bones move. That is why plane joints are classified as **nonaxial joints**, or joints that have no axis.

A **hinge joint** really looks like a hinge: one bone of the joint has a convex groove (fossa) perpendicular to the bone's main axis, whereas another bone has a bar-shaped projection (condyle). The condyle exactly fits the fossa. The only movement possible in this joint is rotation condyle inside the fossa at a right angle to the longitudinal axis of both bones. Because bones move in one plane around one single axis created by the fossa, these joints are also called **uniaxial**. The elbow joint is a classic example of a hinge joint.

A **pivot joint** also allows rotation around one single axis and is classified as a uniaxial joint. The joint is formed by a finger-like rounded projection in one bone and a groove in the other bone. The joint integrity is guarded by a ring ligament that presses on the finger-like projection and holds it inside the groove. It allows the second bone to rotate or pivot around the finger-like projection of the first bone. The **atlantoaxial joint** between the first (atlas) and second (axis) cervical vertebra is of this type. The **dense** or **odontoid process** of the axis (C2) functions as the axis around which the atlas rotates (fig. 7.8).

A **condylar joint** is also often called an **ellipsoid joint**. In this joint one bone forms rounded fossa and the other bone has a nub-shaped condyle. The condyle is located inside the fossa. This joint allows movement in two perpendicular planes. A joint that can move in two directions is called **biaxial**. Joints between metacarpal and phalangeal bones are condylar.

A **saddle joint** is also biaxial, because it allows movement in two planes. It forms by two bones with saddle-shaped articular surfaces. The saddle-shaped surfaces of both bones are stacked one over the other in such a way that their concave surfaces are inserted inside each other. Carpal trapezium bone and metacarpal 1 bones form this joint in primates and human.

A **ball-and-socket joint** is the most moveable joint. It permits movement in all directions. A joint which allows free movement in all directions is called **multiaxial**. The name of the joint exactly describes its construction: one bone has a rounded or ball-shaped projection (head), and the other bone has a round cave (fossa). The ability of free movement compromises joint stability. That is why ball-and-socket joints, as a rule, have strong external support structures such as cartilaginous cuffs, ligaments, or muscles with tendons (fig. 7.8).

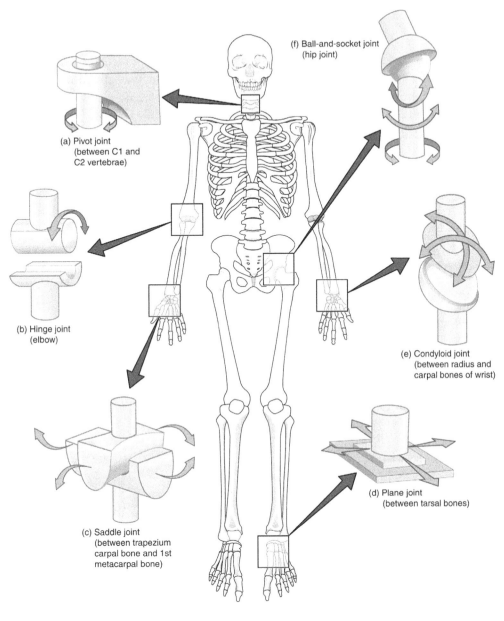

FIGURE 7.8   Six Types of Synovial Joints.

CHECK YOUR UNDERSTANDING

- Why are plane joints called nonaxial?

- Why is a hinge joint classified as a uniaxial joint?

- Name two biaxial joints.

7.5   Different Types of Movement

Synovial joints allow many different types of movement. The movement that bends limbs or a body is called **flexion**. Muscles that flex body are called **flexor muscles**. The opposite movement of stretching a limb or the body is called **extension**. Muscles that extend limbs or the body are known as **extensor muscles**. Movement of the limb away from the body or body's main axis is called **abduction**, and movement of the limb toward the body or body's main axis is called **adduction**. Movement of a limb around its longitudinal axis is called **rotation**. When a limb draws a ring by its distal end, this movement is called **circumduction**. Movement of the head forward is called **protraction**, and movement back toward the body is called **retraction**. The process of moving a body part up is an **elevation**, and moving it down is a **depression** (fig. 7.9). **Pronation** is moving the plantar or palmar surface ventrally, or toward the ground. **Supination** is moving the plantar or palmar surface dorsally, or away from the ground. In general, supination of the paw is only possible in carnivores and pigs. All movements are organized in pairs, where for every movement in one direction, there is a countermovement in the opposite direction. Thus, major animal body movements may be presented by pairs:

> **flexion ↔ extension**
>
> **abduction ↔ adduction**
>
> **protraction ↔ retraction**
>
> **elevation ↔ depression**
>
> **pronation ↔ supination**

and a not complete fit to this scheme pair:

> **rotation ↔ circumduction**

CHECK YOUR UNDERSTANDING

- What is movement of the leg away from the body called?

- When your dog sniffs the air, what movement does it make?

- When your cat scratches the scratching post, what two movements do its digits perform?

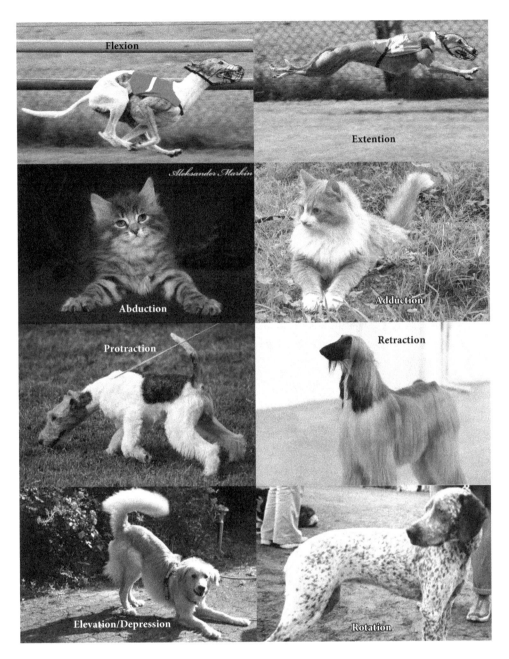

FIGURE 7.9   Animal Movements.

CHAPTER SUMMARY

- Joints are indispensable structures of the animal skeleton. They have three principal functions: 1) bind bones together and guarantee stability of skeleton organization; 2) enable body movement; and 3) allow bones to grow.

- Functionally joints fall in three groups: 1) **Synarthroses** are joints that do not allow any motion. Synarthroses guarantee high stability of the joint. 2) **Amphiarthroses** are joints that permit very little movement. 3) **Diarthroses** are joints that allow a different degree of free movement.

- Numerical classification identifies three classes of joints: 1) **monoarticular**—when there is one single connection between bones; 2) **oligoarticular** or **pauciarticular**—when there are two to four connections between bones in the joint; and 3) **polyarticular**—when there are five or more connections between bones in the joint.

- Joints are divided in three classes according the tissues that constitute the joint: 1) **fibrous joints** are made of regular dense connective tissue; 2) **cartilaginous joints** are made of cartilage; and 3) **synovial joints** are joints with a complex organization and characterized by the presence of a synovial cavity.

- Fibrous joints are made of dense connective tissue. The tissue contains collagen type 1 fibers. It is very strong and stretch resistant. Collagen fibers are intertwined with collagen fibers in the matrix of both bones. There are three groups of fibrous joints: **suture**, **syndesmosis**, and **gomphosis**.

- Sutures are joints between the flat bones of the skull. Suture binds bones' edges along their length. The area of contact between bones is wavy, and the edges of both bones fit each other like a zipper. Collagen fibers of the suture firmly sew both bones. Suture is a synarthrosis. Sutures are divided in three groups: 1) **serrate** suture has interlocking wavy lines; 2) **lap (squamous)** suture has overlapping beveled edges; and 3) **plane (butt)** suture has more or less straight, flat, nonoverlapping edges.

- A **gomphosis** is an immovable or synarthrosis joint. This joint also is called **dentoalveolar syndesmosis** to emphasize the fact that it binds the teeth to the walls of alveoli in the maxilla, zygomatic bone, or mandible. Regular connective tissue of the joint forms a **periodontal ligament**. The periodontal ligament makes connection between bone and cementum of the tooth. The gomphosis is only joint where bone does not join another bone (teeth are not bone).

- A **syndesmosis** is a fibrous joint at which two bones are bound by collagenous fibers that are longer than in a suture or gomphosis. This gives bones a little mobility. A syndesmosis is an amphiarthrosis. Dense connective tissue of the joint is organized in a membrane called **interosseus membrane**.

- Cartilaginous joints are made of different type of cartilage. These joints allow very little if any movement. There are two types of cartilaginous joints: **synchondroses** and **symphises**.

- A synchondrosis is a joint made of hyaline cartilage. Hyaline cartilage is a resilient shock-absorbing tissue, which actually almost does not permit any motion. Functionally, these joints are synarthroses.

- A symphysis is a permanent fibrocartilage joint. The joint is an amphiarthrosis. In symphysis mandibularis and symphysis pubis, two adjacent bones are joined by an **interpubic**, in symphysis pubis, **or intermanbidular**, in the symphysis mandibularis, **discs**. The discs are made of a fibrocartilage and may contain a fluid-filled cavity. The ends of both pubic bones are covered by a thin layer of hyaline cartilage attached to the fibrocartilage. The disc is reinforced by a series of ligaments. These ligaments stabilize the joint. Intervertebral discs have the shape of a tablet. They consist of an outer fibrous capsule called the **anulus fibrosus** and an inner gel-like center called the **nucleus pulposus**. The anulus fibrosus consists of several layers (laminae) of fibrocartilage. The nucleus pulposus consists of hyaline cartilage.

- Synovial joints permit different degrees of free movement and are diarthroses. Synovial joints are the most complex organized joints. Every synovial joint has a space between the bones called a **synovial cavity** filled with **synovial fluid.** Synovial fluid lubricates and reduces friction between bones. Synovial fluid also contains phagocytes that remove microbes and the debris that results from normal wear and tear in the joint. The apical ends of bones are covered by **articular cartilage**. Articular cartilage is hyaline cartilage. The articular cartilage together with synovial fluid provides a smooth frictionless movement. From outside joint is covered by the connective tissue membrane that forms a **synovial capsule** which encloses the synovial cavity. The internal layer of the membrane is known as a **synovial membrane**.

- Synovial joints include adipose tissue, nerve fibers, and blood vessels. Adipose tissue is packed into fat pads that fill all available space. Adipose tissue easily changes shape and may be squeezed when the joint is in motion. Pads cushion the joint and prevent its injury. Blood delivers oxygen and nutrients and removes waste products. Nerves monitor the state of the joint and control body position and movement.

- Some synovial joints have a fibrocartilage that grows inward from the joint capsule. When this fibrocartilage completely crosses the entire joint capsule between articulating bones, it forms an **articular disc. Menisci** are fibrocartilage pads that have shape of a flat donuts, with a thick border and thin central region. They do not divide the synovial cavity completely. In the knee, menisci extend inward from the left and right but do not entirely cross the joint. These cartilages absorb shock and pressure, guide bones across each other, improve the fit between bones, stabilize the joint, and reduce the chance of dislocation.

- Synovial joints are enforced by **intracapsular ligaments**. In the hip joint the **ligamentum teres** fastens a rounded depression on the virtue of the femur head called the fovea and a depression on the bottom of the acetabulum called the acetabular notch. The ligamentum teres does not let the head of the femur pop out of the acetabulum and prevents hip joint dislocation. The knee joint is stabilized by a set of intracapsular ligaments. A pair of **cruciate ligaments**—anterior (ACL) and posterior (PCL)—bind the lateral condyle of the femur with the anterior intercondylar area of the tibia and the medial condyle of the femur with the posterior intercondylar area of the tibia correspondingly. The **transverse ligament** connects the lateral and medial menisci.

- A **bursa** is a sac lined by synovial membrane and filled with synovial fluid. It resembles a balloon filled with water. A bursa may be attached to the synovial capsule or completely separated. It occupies a position at areas of high stress. It is found between adjacent muscles, where tendon passes over bone, or between bone and skin. A bursa cushions muscles, helps tendons slide more easily over joints, and corrects direction of tendon pull.

- A **tendon** is a rope or sheet of tough collagenous regular connective tissue that attaches muscle to bone. It is the most important structure that stabilizes a joint. Tendons pull bones when muscle contracts and hold bones together during motion.

- A **ligament** is a strip or sheet of irregular dense connective tissue. It connects bone to bone or bone to viscera other than skeletal muscle.

- A **tendon sheath** is an elongated cylindrical bursa wrapped around a tendon. A tendon sheath protects a tendon and directs its course. Tendon sheaths provides a friction-free tendon movement and facilitate a tendon's pressure on bones in the joint.

- A **retinaculum** is a broad ring band around limbs. A retinaculum is made of irregular dense connective tissue. It forms a protected pathway for tendons and hold small bones of the limb's extremities at their right position.

- Structurally, synovial joints fall in six groups: **plane** or **gliding, hinge, pivot, condylar, saddle,** and **ball-and-socket joints.**

- The bending of limbs or the body is called **flexion**. The opposite movement of stretching a limb or the body is called **extension**. Movement of a limb away from the body or body's main axis is **abduction**. The movement of a limb toward the body or body's main axis is called **adduction**. The movement of a limb around its main axis is called **rotation**. When a limb draws a ring by its distal end, it does a **circumduction** movement. Movement of the head forward is called **protraction**, and movement back toward the body is called **retraction**. The process of moving a body part up is called an **elevation** and moving it down is called a **depression. Pronation** is moving the plantar or palmar surface ventrally or toward the ground. **Supination** is moving the plantar or palmar surface dorsally, or toward the top. In general, supination of the paw is only possible in carnivores and pigs.

CHECK YOUR KNOWLEDGE

LEVEL 1. CHECK YOUR RECALL

1. The movement of a limb around an axis is:
   A. Rotation
   B. Adduction
   C. Supination
   D. Protraction
   E. Flexion

2. The movement of a limb away from the body's midline is called:
   A. Rotation
   B. Adduction
   C. Abduction
   D. Protraction
   E. Flexion

3. Muscles that stretch the leg are called:
   A. Flexors
   B. Extensors
   C. Rotators
   D. Pronators
   E. Retractors

4. The skull bones are tightly joined along lines called:
    A. Fossa
    B. Intercalated disc
    C. Sinus
    D. Symphysis
    E. Suture

5. The joint between two pubic bones is called:
    A. Pubic arch
    B. Obturator foramen
    C. Symphysis pubis
    D. Pubic crest
    E. Ischial tuberosity

6. The sacrum is bound with coxa by fibrocartilage of:
    A. Sacral foramina
    B. Sacral crest
    C. Sacroiliac joint
    D. Sacral hiatus
    E. Sacral promontory

7. Movement of the part of body ventrally, or below the horizontal midplane, is called:
    A. Depression
    B. Elevation
    C. Circumflexion
    D. Pronation
    E. Rotation

8. The movement of a leg toward the midline of the body is called:
    A. Flexion
    B. Extension
    C. Rotation
    D. Adduction
    E. Abduction

9. When a dog smells prey, it moves the head anteriorly. This movement is called _____.

10. Which of the following is fibrous, and which is a cartilaginous joint?
    A. Ball and socket; plane joint
    B. Gomphosis; syndesmosis
    C. Suture; symphysis
    D. Hinge joint; pivot joint
    E. Saddle joint; synarthrosis

11. The radius and ulna are bound by a _____ joint.
    A.   suture
    B.   symphysis
    C.   synovial
    D.   gomphosis
    E.   syndesmosis

12. A nonaxial joint that allows only sliding movement is a:
    A.   Ball-and-socket joint
    B.   Saddle joint
    C.   Plane joint
    D.   Hinge joint
    E.   Pivot joint

13. Which of these joints is freely moveable?
    A.   Synarthrosis
    B.   Amphiarthrosis
    C.   Diarthrosis
    D.   All of the above
    E.   None the above

14. Which type of fibrous joint connects the tibia and fibula?
    A.   Syndesmosis
    B.   Symphysis
    C.   Suture
    D.   Gomphosis

15. An example of a wide fibrous joint is:
    A.   The interosseous membrane of the forearm
    B.   A gomphosis
    C.   A suture joint
    D.   A synostosis

16. A gomphosis:
    A.   Is formed by an interosseous membrane
    B.   Connects the tibia and fibula bones of the leg
    C.   Contains a joint cavity
    D.   Anchors a tooth to the jaw
    E.   Is made of the hyaline cartilage

17. A syndesmosis is:
    A. A narrow fibrous joint
    B. The type of joint that unites bones of the skull
    C. A fibrous joint that unites parallel bones
    D. The type of joint that anchors the teeth in the jaws

18. A synovial joint is_____, whereas a suture is _____.
    A. diarthrotic; synarthrotic
    B. synarthrotic; amphiarthrotic
    C. amphiarthrotic; diarthrotic
    D. diarthrotic; amphiarthrotic
    E. synarthrotic; diarthrotic

19. Moving a body part up is called _____, and moving it down is called _____.
    A. protraction; retraction
    B. elevation; depression
    C. abduction; adduction
    D. pronation; supination
    E. flexion; extension

20. True or false: A bursa is a sack made of synovial membrane and filled with synovial fluid.
21. True or false: An intervertebral disc is an example of a symphysis joint.
22. True or false: A meniscus is a pad of adipose tissue inside the synovial capsule.
23. True or false: The periodontal ligament is part of a synchondrosis joint.
24. Match the term with its description:

    _____ Symphysis   a. A movement of body part down.
    _____ Synarthrosis   b. A stretch of legs
    _____ Plane joint   c. A freely moveable joint
    _____ Syndesmosis   d. A movement of body part up
    _____ Synovial cavity   e. An amphiarthrosis cartilage joint between bones
    _____ Depression   f. A completely immoveable joint
    _____ Diarthrosis   g. A fluid-filled cavity inside a free moveable joint
    _____ Elevation   h. An amphiarthrosis dense connective tissue joint
    _____ Extension   i. An uniaxial synovial joint

LEVEL 2. CHECK YOUR UNDERSTANDING

1. What is the difference between a tendon and a ligament?
2. Labrum is a cartilage cuff around some ball-and-socket joints, like shoulder and hip joints. Explain why undeveloped labrum makes the shoulder joint unstable?
3. Make the following joint movements with your own body: 1) abduction, 2) adduction, 3) rotation, 4) circumduction, 5) extension, 6) flexion, 7) elevation, and 8) depression.

LEVEL 3. APPLY YOUR KNOWLEDGE TO REAL LIFE

1. Vitamin A is a precursor for synthesis of the hormone-like growth factor that promotes the hyaline cartilage ossification process. Why does an overdose of vitamin A cause stiffness in the neck or limpness in the legs of your pet?

2. Explain why weak or nonfunctioning muscles, for example biceps brachii, may cause synovial joint dislocations.

Chapter 8

Muscles and Muscular System

LEARNING OBJECTIVES

In this chapter you will learn basic principles of muscular system organization. When you have read the chapter, you will be able to:

1. Understand the role of the muscular system in body functioning and the major characteristics of muscle cells.

2. Describe three muscle types and explain the differences among them.

3. Describe the gross anatomy of muscle organs and the role of tendons and aponeuroses.

4. Give definitions and identify the origin and insertion of a muscle.

5. Explain why muscles are organized into groups and give definitions for agonist, synergist, and antagonist muscles.

INTRODUCTION

The first and most obvious role of muscles is body movement. Together with the skeletal system, muscles create a system of movers and levers. Contractile muscle cells move the body with the use of the motor protein molecules **myosin** and **actin**. Myosin converts energy of chemical bonds of ATP molecules into mechanical energy of movement. Muscles maintain body posture. Muscles act on viscera—lungs, blood vessels, gall bladder, and so on—and regulate activity of these internal organs. Cardiac muscle contractions facilitate the heart's ability to pump blood. Sphincters in the urethra control urination. The diaphragm, together with intercostal muscles, expands the thoracic cavity for ventilation of the lungs. Muscles make moveable joints strong and stable by holding bones together. Muscles create the walls of the body and help keep the body's shape.

Not all energy released from ATP molecules is converted into mechanical energy of movement. Part of this energy is released in heat. In a cold air, we often shiver—this is a reaction that helps us maintain body temperature. Skeletal muscles have a glycogen storage that may be used as a source of glucose to maintain a glucose level in the blood. Muscle contraction is accompanied by noise and a body's electromagnetic field. Some predator fishes, like sharks, have very sharp receptors that may detect these tiny noises and electromagnetic signals, even when the prey is hidden or buried in the sand. Specialized muscle organs of some fishes are able to generate voltage electricity, and they have electric organs. These electric organs are used as much for defense as for attack.

8.1 Properties of Muscle Cells

The cumulative efforts of muscle cells include moving the body, propelling food along the digestive tract, and moving secretions along the ducts of multiple exocrine glands. These abilities are the result of five common properties of all muscle cells:

1. **Contractility.** Contractility is ability of muscle cell to shorten. However, there are a number of special muscle cells that may contract without change of their length. Different muscle cells have a different ability to contract. For example, a skeletal muscle cell may contract up to 40 percent of its original length, whereas a smooth muscle cells may contract up to 80 percent.
2. **Excitability.** The ability of a cell to react to different stimuli is called excitability. Muscle cells may respond to many different stimuli, such as chemical signals from motor neurons or hormones of the endocrine system, concentration of chemicals in body fluids, mechanical stretching, or electrical signals. For example, smooth muscles in the skin associated with the hair root—*Arrector pili* muscles—contract in the presence of the hormone epinephrine. That is why the hairs of a scared cat or dog stand up.
3. **Conductivity.** When a muscle cell is excited, its plasma membrane (sarcolemma) becomes leaky for positively charged sodium and potassium ions. That leads to a change of the electrical charge on the walls of the sarcolemma. This change of electrical charge is like a wave that propagates along the entire cellular wall—the property called conductivity.
4. **Extensibility.** Extensibility is an ability of the cell to be stretched without damage. Muscle cell is extensible, because it can be stretched to three times its original length without any visible damage. Most cells of the body cannot do that and if stretched will just rupture.
5. **Elasticity.** When a stretched muscle cell is released, it immediately, like a stretched rubber bend or spring, returns to its original shape. This property is called elasticity. Elasticity results from the special organization of muscle cells' contractile units, such as sarcomeres in skeletal and cardiac muscle cells.

CHECK YOUR UNDERSTANDING

- Name the major functions of muscles.
- Name the five common properties of muscle cells.
- Explain the difference between extensibility and elasticity.

8.2 Classification of Muscles

In correlation with location, muscles may be divided in two groups: **somatic**—muscles that move bones and cartilage; and **visceral**—muscles that control activity of internal organs, such as stomach or blood vessels. Muscles also may be classified into **voluntary**—those that are under the immediate conscious control and cannot contract without signals from the central nervous system (CNS); and **involuntary**—muscles that are not controlled consciously and are able generate autonomic contraction without CNS stimulation.

For example, the heart continues its rhythmic contraction even when an animal is in an unconscious state or coma. A group of specialized cardiac muscle cells called the **pacemaker** have the ability to generate waves of muscle contraction autonomously. Histological studies show that skeletal and cardiac muscles have a sequence of dark and light stripes along their length, whereas smooth muscles have a monotonous coloration. This striation is a result of special organization of contractile units inside the cell body called sarcomeres. The presence or absence of striation, thus, indicates the presence or absence of sarcomeres in the cell body. According to this characteristic, skeletal and cardiac muscles are classified as **striated** and smooth muscles as **not striated** muscle fibers. A natural classification of muscle cells has to take into account all these properties and create one unitary system of simple and precise muscle cell identification.

The most widely used classification divides all muscle tissues in three groups: **skeletal**, **cardiac**, and **smooth** muscles (fig. 8.1). It is based on the combination of different characteristic of muscle cells. Skeletal muscle, as follows from the name, is associated with bones and has a striated appearance on the microscopic slide. Cardiac muscle also has dark and light stripes, when you look at it with a microscope, but is found only in the heart. The last property gives the name to this muscle. Both skeletal and cardiac muscles have striation and are

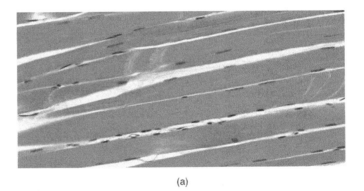

(a)

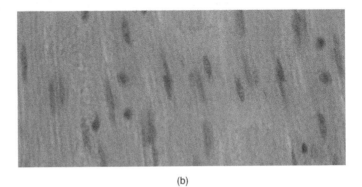

(b)

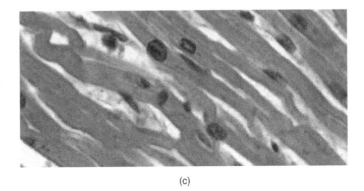

(c)

FIGURE 8.1 Muscular Tissue. A. Skeletal Muscle; B. Smooth Muscle; C. Cardiac Muscle.

also called **striated muscles**, as opposed to **smooth muscle**. Smooth muscle cells have no visible signs of striation (see fig. 8.1.B). Skeletal muscle is under the immediate conscious control, and it belong to the voluntary type, whereas cardiac and smooth muscles are not controlled consciously and belong to the involuntary type of muscles. Because skeletal muscle is associated with bones and cartilage, it also belongs to the somatic type. At the same time, cardiac and smooth muscles are associated with internal organs and may be classified as visceral. Muscle classification is presented in table 8.1.

TABLE 8.1 Classification of Muscle Cells

Muscle type	Skeletal	Cardiac	Smooth
Striation	Striated	Striated	Not striated
Location	Somatic	Visceral	Visceral
Nervous control	Voluntary	Involuntary	Involuntary
Associated with	Bones and cartilage	Heart	Skin, internal organs

CHECK YOUR UNDERSTANDING

- Name the two types of striated muscles.

- What is the difference between striated and smooth muscles?

- What is the difference between voluntary and involuntary muscles?

- Explain what type of muscle is in the heart wall and what type is in the aorta wall.

8.3   Skeletal Muscle

Structure of Skeletal Muscle

When we talk about skeletal muscle, we have to be clear about what we mean. As a matter of fact, skeletal muscle has at least two different meanings: muscle organ and muscle cell. *Biceps femoris*, for example, has all the necessary characteristics to call it an organ. First of all, it is made, like all organs, of different tissues. Of course, the major part of *Biceps femoris* is made of skeletal muscle cells, but there are also a number of membranes that are made of different types of connective tissues, such as loose connective tissue, regular dense connective tissue. There is also blood in blood vessels and nervous tissue. Every skeletal muscle occupies a particular position. Every skeletal muscle has a specific role in the body, and has a very special relationship with other body organs. Thus, *Biceps femoris* has all necessary characteristics to call it an organ.

Looking at a skeletal muscle cell with a microscope shows it has sequence of dark and light cross stripes. These stripes are a result of a structurally highly organized cytoplasmic content (fig. 8.1.A). The name of the skeletal muscle also declares the intrinsic association of these muscles with bones and cartilage. It is a skeletal muscle that moves body parts, but muscle contraction is under the complete control of the CNS. Without stimulation from motor neurons, skeletal muscle cell does not contract and, because of that, it is also called voluntary. Each skeletal muscle is a long (about 5 cm), multinucleated cell. Individual cells can be attached to each other end to end to form a long composite fiber. Every muscle fiber is coated by a connective tissue membrane called the **endomysium**.

Individual muscle fibers together with their endomysium are organized into a group of muscle fibers called **fascicle**. Every fascicle is surrounded by a strong connective tissue membrane called the

perimysium. The number of muscle fibers in fascicle varies from 10 to 100 muscle fibers per fascicle. The entire muscle organ—for example, *Biceps femoris*—is made of a number of such fascicles with their perimysiums. From the outside, muscles such as *Biceps femoris* are wrapped by a strong connective tissue membrane, the **epimysium** (fig. 8.2). At the ends, where muscles attached to bones, the epimysium creates an extension made of regular dense connective tissue that binds muscle to bone, cartilage, or other muscle. When this attachment has a shape of cord or rope, it is called a **tendon**. Tendon is made of a regular dense connective tissue rich with strong type 1 collagen fibers in matrix (see chapter 4, page 117). Collagen fibers of the tendon interlace with collagen fibers of the periosteum and firmly bind muscle with bone. Often muscle is attached to bone or other muscle by a broad, flat connective tissue sheet, called an **aponeurosis**. *Linea alba* is an example of such an aponeurosis that binds together left and right parts of the *Rectus abdominis* muscle (fig. 8.6).

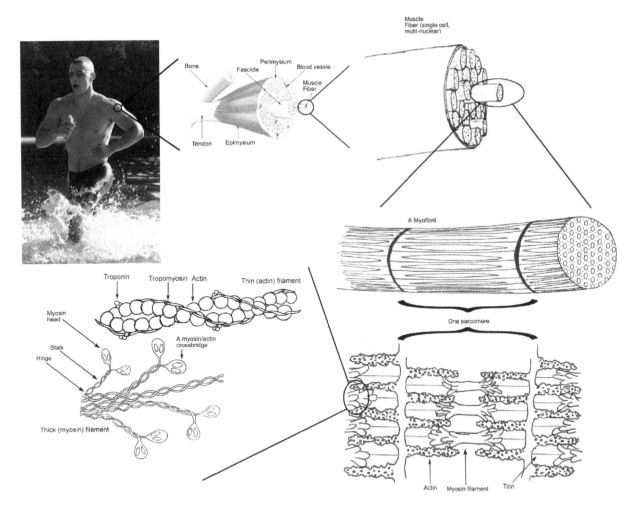

FIGURE 8.2   Structure of Skeletal Muscle Organ.

CHECK YOUR UNDERSTANDING

- Name the three connective tissue structures that cover muscle, fascicle, and muscle fiber.

- Which connective tissue membrane covers fascicles?

- What is the difference between tendons and aponeuroses?

- Explain what relationship exists between epimysium and perimysium.

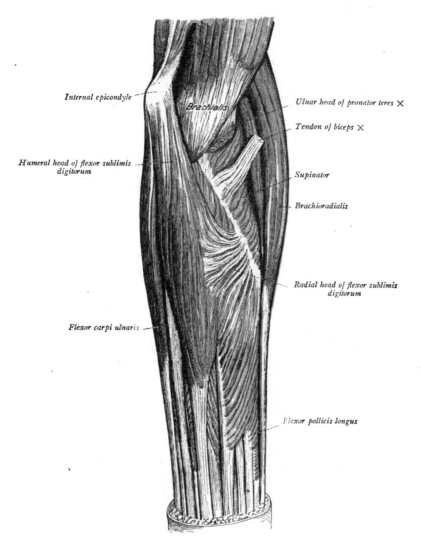

Internal epicondyle

Brachialis

Humeral head of flexor sublimis digitorum

Flexor carpi ulnaris

Ulnar head of pronator teres ✕

Tendon of biceps ✕

Supinator

Brachioradialis

Radial head of flexor sublimis digitorum

Flexor pollicis longus

FIGURE 8.3   Human Arm with Muscles and Tendons.

Muscle Attachment

Tendons transmit muscle force to a distant point. For example, the limb muscles of cursorial animals are usually located close to the animal's body, and tendons transmit the force of these muscles' contraction to the distal bones of the legs. Tendons also permit precise control by distributing forces among digits of the fingers in raccoon or primate hands (fig. 8.3). Regular dense connective tissue of tendons is an avascular tissue, which makes tendon very economic metabolically. They require little maintenance and consume little energy compared with an active and metabolically expensive muscle fibers. Tendons allow the metabolically expensive muscle fibers to be just long enough to produce the required amount of force to move bones. On the other hand, avascular tissues, as a rule, are slow to grow and to heal the damage that may result from a number of special diseases.

VETERINARY APPLICATION

When a horse jumps, it presses on the hind legs with all its weight. Extension of these legs releases a huge amount of energy that launches a half-ton body into the air. When the horse lands on the protracted forelimbs, they work as shock absorbers. This movement requires precise coordinated work of muscles and their associated tendons and ligaments. There are four main tendons and ligaments at the posterior side of a horse leg, organized in two functional groups: 1) **suspensory** and **inferior check ligaments** and 2) **deep digital** and **superficial digital flexor tendons**. The injuries of these structures are called a "bow" and, according to the severity of the injury, are classified in four types:

1. **Type 1 lesion** is a result of a light stretch of tendons and ligaments. It is characterized by local swelling. The swollen area may be warm and painful. Lameness may or may not be present. It is difficult to observe and may not be visible

2. **Type 2 lesion** results from tearing of collagen fibers. Type 2 lesion is a mild tearing characterized by the appearance of swelling, pain, and lameness that is visible from time to time.

3. **Type 3 lesion** is a more severe tearing that causes increased signs of heat, swelling, and pain. The horse often is lame, which is especially apparent at the trot.

4. **Type 4 lesion** is a severe damage of tendons and/or ligaments. It results in severe lameness, with heat, pain, and swelling.

In general, strains are better than tears, small tears are better than large ones, and damage that occurs away from a bone is better than damage right at the bone. These injuries are most common in the forelimbs since they bear 60 percent of the horse's weight. The least severe is an injury of the suspensory check ligament. This ligament serves to stabilize the leg when it takes the body's weight load. An injury of the inferior check ligament injury may cause a large amount of swelling, but usually only a little pain or lameness. The superficial digital flexor tendon is responsible for stability and flexion of the leg. An injury to the superficial digital flexor tendon also causes lameness, but even severe damage may not be the end of horse's career. The deep digital flexor tendon stabilizes the leg when it adapts the maximum load of a full horse's weight and flexes all of the lower leg joints during hoof flight. Serious damage to this tendon is always accompanied by lameness, heat, pain, and swelling. Often, this lesion causes the end of a horse's career.[1]

---

1   J. Posniakoff, "Help for Tendon and Ligament Injuries," *Horse Illustrated Magazine*, June 2006.

To be able to move the body, muscle has to be attached to different bones to pull them toward each other. When a particular muscle contracts, one attached bone moves and changes its position, whereas the other bone does not. The immovable bone that plays the role of a muscle anchor is called the **origin**. The moveable bone at the other end of the muscle is called the **insertion** (fig. 8.4).

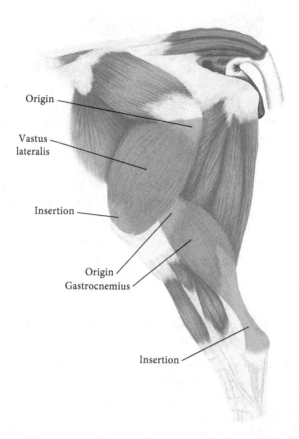

Origin

Vastus
lateralis

Insertion

Origin
Gastrocnemius

Insertion

FIGURE 8.4   Muscles *Vastus Lateralis* and
Gastrocnemius and Their Origins and Insertions in
a Cow.

CHECK YOUR UNDERSTANDING

- *Biceps brachii* is a flexor muscle. On one end it is attached to the scapula, and on the other to the radius. Where is the origin, and where is the insertion of this muscle?

- *Sternomastoid* is a head rotator. It is attached to the mastoid process of the temporal bone and the manubrium of the sternum. Explain where the insertion and where the origin of this muscle are.

- *Rectus femoris* is a hind leg extensor. It is attached to the iliac spine and tibial tuberosity. Where is the insertion, and where is the origin of this muscle?

Muscle Shape

Shape and muscle function depend on the orientation and organization of fascicles. Patterns of fascicles orientation include **parallel**, **fusiform**, **convergent**, **pennate**, and **circular** (fig. 8.5).

Fascicles in **parallel** muscle are lined parallel with each other, and the muscle has more or less the same diameter along all its length. The parallel muscle usually has a stripe everywhere with the same width, like *Atlantoscapularis* and *Pectoantebrachialis* muscles (fig. 8.6).

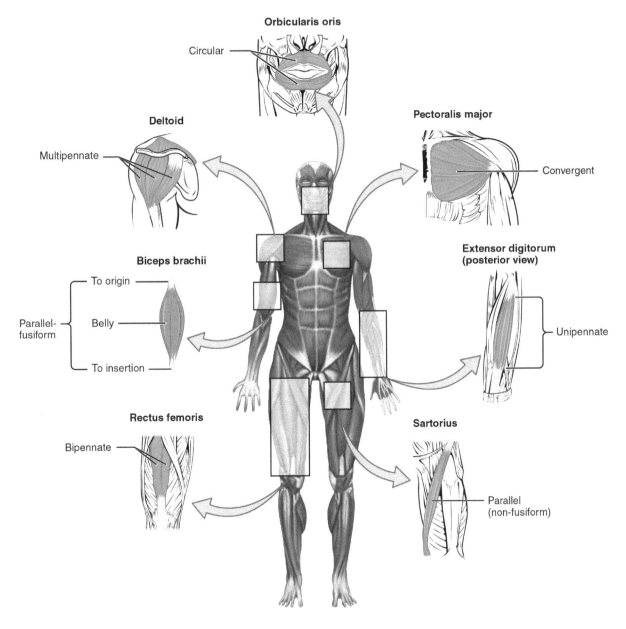

FIGURE 8.5 Arrangement of Fascicles Results in a Different Skeletal Muscle Shape.

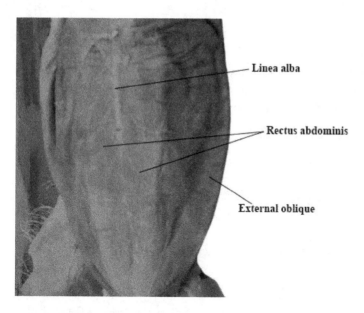

FIGURE 8.6   Cat **Rectus Abdominis** Muscle is an Example of Parallel Muscle.

A **fusiform** muscle has bigger diameter in the middle and is narrow at both ends. The thicker middle region is called the muscle's **belly** or **gaster**. An example of this type of muscle is the *Biceps brachii*.

A **convergent** muscle is broad on one side and narrow on the other. As a rule, this muscle has a triangular shape and has a fan-like arrangement of fascicles, as in the *Serratus ventralis* and *Subscapularis* muscles (fig. 8.7).

A **pinnate** muscle has fascicles that are attached to the tendon at an angle that makes it looks like a feather. The *Rectus femoris* is an example of a bipennate muscle.

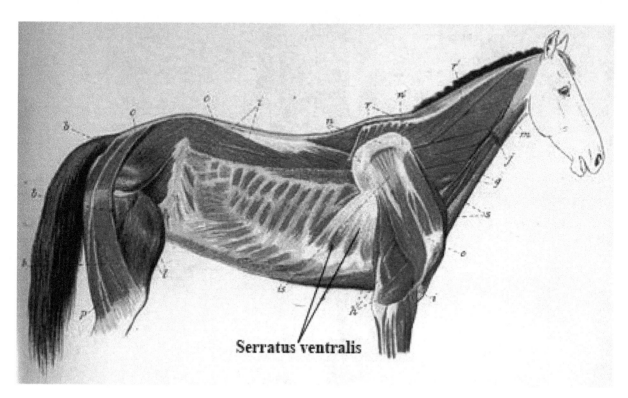

FIGURE 8.7   *Serratus Ventralis* Muscle: An Example of a Convergent Muscle.

Fascicles in a **circular** muscle are organized into concentric rings. The *Orbicularis oculi* and *Orbicularis oris* are examples of this type of muscle. Often circular muscles also called **sphincters** (fig. 8.8).

CHECK YOUR UNDERSTANDING

- Explain how the terms *pinnate* and *convergent* relate to fascicles orientation.

- Why are circular muscles often called sphincters?

- What is the difference between parallel and fusiform muscles?

Functional Muscle Groups

The muscle responsible for bone movement is called a **prime mover** or **agonist**. The agonist moves a particular bone and usually is the biggest or strongest muscle responsible for this movement. However, it is a rare situation when only one muscle generates some movement. As a rule, the agonist moves bone in cooperation with other muscles. Those muscles that help the agonist move the bone are called **synergists**. For example, the *Rectus femoris* is a muscle that extends the hind legs, and it is an agonist extensor muscle of a pelvic limbs. However, the *Rectus femoris* extends the leg in company with three *Vastus* muscles: the *Vastus lateralis*, *Vastus medialis*, and *Vastus intermideus*. These three muscles are synergists, and their role is to help the *Rectus femoris* extend the hind leg (fig. 8.9). In contrast to these four leg extensor muscles (that have a common name *Quadriceps* muscles),

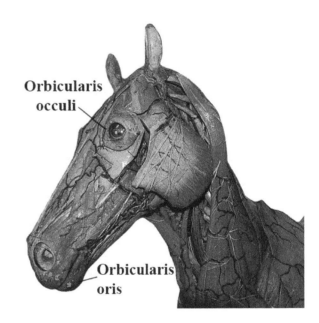

FIGURE 8.8   Circular Muscles ***Orbicularis Occuli*** and ***Orbicularis Oris*** of a Horse.

there is a group of muscles that oppose extension of the hind leg and bend (flex) it. Those muscles that work in opposition to the prime mover (agonist) are called **antagonists**. In the hind leg the antagonists that are responsible for leg flexion (flexor muscles) are the *Biceps femoris*, *Semitendinosus*, and *Semimembranosus* muscles (fig. 8.9).

The definitions of agonist, synergist, and antagonist are relative. In relation to one movement the muscle may be an agonist, whereas in relation to another movement it may be identified as an antagonist. Thus, if we are interested in hind leg flexion, then we have to call the *Biceps femoris* an agonist. In this case, the *Semitendinosus* and *Semimembranosus* would be synergists, whereas *Quadriceps* muscles work against flexion and are antagonists (fig. 8.10).

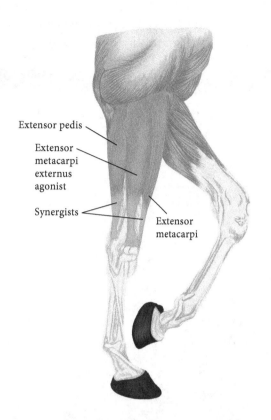

Extensor pedis

Extensor metacarpi externus agonist

Synergists

Extensor metacarpi

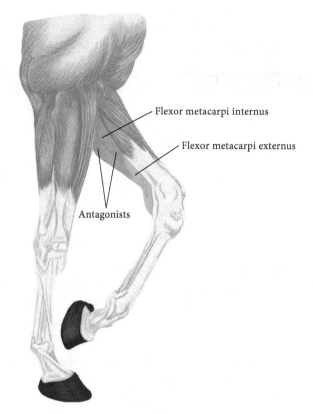

Flexor metacarpi internus

Flexor metacarpi externus

Antagonists

FIGURE 8.9   Horse Thoracic Limb Extensor Muscles.

FIGURE 8.10   Horse Thoracic Limb Flexor Muscles.

CHECK YOUR UNDERSTANDING

- The *Rectus femoris* is the major knee extensor muscle. Three *Vastus* muscles—*V. medialis*, *V. lateralis*, and *V. intermedius*—help the *Rectus femoris*. What relationship exists among these muscles and the *Rectus femoris*?

- The muscles *Biceps femoris* and *Semitendinosus* are knee flexors. What is the relation of these muscles to the *Rectus femoris*?

- If you analyze flexion of the knee, which muscles are the prime mover, synergist, and antagonists?

CHAPTER SUMMARY

- All muscle cells have five properties that allow them to function as movers: **contractility**—the ability of muscle cells to shorten; **excitability**—the ability to react to different stimuli; **conductivity**—the ability of muscle fiber to conduct action potential along its whole length; **extensibility**—the ability of the cell to be stretched without damage; and **elasticity**—the ability of muscle fiber always to restore the original shape of the cell.

- There are three main muscle groups: **skeletal**, **cardiac**, and **smooth** muscles. Skeletal muscle is associated with bones and cartilage. Cardiac muscle is found only in the heart. Both skeletal and cardiac muscles have striation and are called **striated muscles**. Smooth muscle cell has no striation. Skeletal muscle is under control of the cerebral cortex and is called voluntary. Cardiac and smooth muscles are independent or controlled only by autonomous division of the nervous system and are called involuntary.

- Skeletal muscle is a long, multinucleated cell. Muscle are attached to each other end to end and form a long composite muscle fiber. Every muscle fiber is coated with a connective tissue membrane called the **endomysium**. Individual muscle fibers together with their endomysium are organized into groups of muscle fibers called **fascicle**. Every fascicle is surrounded by a strong connective tissue membrane called the **perimysium**. The number of muscle fibers in fascicle varies from 10 to 100 muscle fibers per fascicle. The entire muscle organ is made of many fascicles with their perimysiums. On the outside, the muscle organ is coated by a strong connective tissue membrane called the **epimysium**. At the ends, where muscle is attached to bones, the epimysium extends into a cord-like structure called a **tendon**. Tendon is made of a regular dense connective tissue rich with strong collagen fibers. Collagen fibers of the tendon interlace with collagen fibers of periosteum and firmly fasten muscle with bone. Often muscle is attached to bone or other muscle by a flat sheet, called an **aponeurosis**.

- The immovable bone that plays the role of a muscle anchor is called the **origin**. The moveable bone at the other end of the muscle is called the **insertion**.

- Muscles have a different shape depending on the orientation of fascicles: **parallel**, **fusiform**, **convergent**, **pennate**, and **circular.**

- The strongest muscle that is responsible for movement is called the **prime mover** or **agonist**. Muscles that help or assist agonist are called **synergists**. Muscles that resist the prime mover (agonist) are called **antagonists**.

CHECK YOUR KNOWLEDGE

LEVEL 1. CHECK YOUR RECALL

1. The type of muscle cell that lacks striation and has a single central nucleus is:
   A. Skeletal muscle
   B. Cardiac muscle
   C. Voluntary muscle
   D. Smooth muscle
   E. Somatic muscle

2. A rope-shaped regular dense connective tissue that binds skeletal muscle to the bone is called:
    A. Endomysium
    B. Tendon
    C. Perimysium
    D. Ligament
    E. Fascia

3. A group of skeletal muscle fibers together with the surrounding perimysium form a(n):
    A. Ligament
    B. Endomysium
    C. Perimysium
    D. Fascicle
    E. Myofibril

4. The muscle end attached to a relatively immovable bone or part of the body is called:
    A. Fascia
    B. Origin
    C. Insertion
    D. Fossa
    E. Aponeurosis

5. The muscle that assists the prime mover is termed:
    A. Agonist
    B. Antagonist
    C. Protagonist
    D. Retractor
    E. Synergist

6. The muscle that resists the prime mover's action is called:
    A. Synergist
    B. Symbiont
    C. Agonist
    D. Antagonist
    E. Protagonist

7. Which muscle type has a ring-like fascicle pattern?
    A. Fusiform
    B. Circular
    C. Parallel
    D. Pennate
    E. Convergent

8. Walls of the heart are made of _____ , whereas walls of blood vessels are made of _____ .
   A. smooth muscles; skeletal muscles
   B. smooth muscles; cardiac muscles
   C. cardiac muscles; smooth muscles
   D. cardiac muscles; skeletal muscles
   E. skeletal muscles; smooth muscles

9. In pennate muscle, fascicles have a _____ pattern, whereas in convergent muscle, they are organized in a _____ pattern.
   A. feather-shaped; fan-shaped
   B. parallel; ring
   C. fan-shaped; ring
   D. parallel; feather-shaped
   E. ring; fan-shaped

10. Extensibility is the ability of a muscle cell to _____ , whereas elasticity is the ability to _____ .
    A. conduct electrical impulse; shorten
    B. shorten; respond to stimulus
    C. be stretched; shorten
    D. be stretched; restore original shape
    E. restore original shape; be stretched

11. True or false: The aorta has cardiac muscles in its walls.
12. True or false: Smooth muscles have no striation.
13. True or false: A synergist is a muscle that resists an agonist muscle.
14. Match the term with its description:

    _____ Parallel muscle   a. Moveable end of muscle attachment
    _____ Origin   b. Muscle's ability to return to original state
    _____ Agonist   c. Immovable end of muscle attachment
    _____ Elasticity   d. Muscle most responsible for particular movement
    _____ Insertion   e. Muscle with parallel fascicle organization
    _____ Antagonist   f. Muscle that supports the prime mover muscle
    _____ Synergist   g. Muscle that resists the prime mover muscle

LEVEL 2. CHECK YOUR UNDERSTANDING

1. Why is cardiac muscle involuntary? Why is this muscle type not under complete CNS control?
2. If a skeletal muscle cell loses its elasticity, how will that affect its function?
3. Can skeletal muscle be attached to the same bone, or must it be attached to at least two bones?

4. Why are skeletal muscles organized in functional groups? (Hint: In legs there are extensor muscles [one group] and also flexor muscles [another group].)

5. The masseter is a muscle of mastication (chewing). Superiorly, it is attached by a thick aponeurosis to the maxillary process of the zygomatic bone and the anterior border of the zygomatic arch, and inferiorly, it is attached to the lateral surface of the ramus of the mandible. Which bone(s) serve(s) as the origin, and which bone(s) is/are the insertion? Explain your answer.

LEVEL 3. APPLY YOUR KNOWLEDGE TO REAL LIFE

1. As you learned in chapter 4, skeletal muscle cells, when they become mature cells, do not undergo mitosis. From this chapter, you also learned that skeletal muscle cells are organized into fascicles that create a pattern of a particular shape for every muscle.

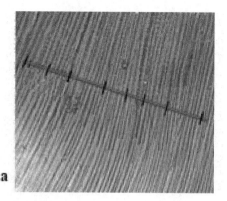 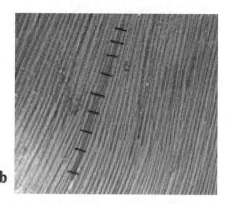

On the presented diagrams you see surgical incisions through muscles. According your educated opinion, which one is done right and which one is done wrong, if the lines demonstrate fascicles orientation? Explain your answer.

Chapter 9

Muscle Cells and Physiology

LEARNING OBJECTIVES

In this chapter you will learn basic principles of muscle cell organization and physiology. When you have completed reading the chapter, you will be able to understand the following:

1. Structural organization of skeletal, cardiac, and smooth muscle cells.

2. Sarcomere organization and the sliding-filament theory of skeletal muscle contraction.

3. Organization and function of the neuromuscular junction.

4. The three phases of the muscle contraction process (excitation, excitation-contraction coupling, and contraction) and the mechanism of muscle cell relaxation.

5. Energy sources and classification of skeletal muscles.

6. Phases of muscle twitch and the effect of frequency of stimulation.

7. Motor unit, recruitment, and muscle tone.

8. The excess post-exercise oxygen consumption and recovery process.

9. Special characteristics of the physiology of cardiac and smooth muscles.

INTRODUCTION

Muscle cell is a very highly specialized type of cell. Its major specialization is moving the body, generating heartbeats, and moving food and fluids in body tubes. As a result of this specialization, muscle cell construction and physiology are designed to successfully performing these functions. As other highly specialized cells, like for example neurons, muscle cells have lost the ability to reproduce—that is, undergo mitosis—they are not able to do what other cells can. On the other hand, their role is unique and all their organization is adapted to it.

As you already know, there are three major types of muscle cells: skeletal, which binds with bones and cartilage and moves the body; cardiac, which generates the heartbeat and pumps blood in blood vessels; and smooth, which is widely distributed inside body viscera. In our review of the microanatomy and physiology of muscular tissues, we will begin with skeletal muscles, and then will provide a short comparison with cardiac and smooth muscles.

9.1 Structure of Skeletal Muscle Cells

Skeletal muscle fiber is a long cell with many nuclei on the inner surface of the cellular membrane. These multinucleated cells originate from embryonic mesoderm. Embryonic cells, called **myoblasts**, fused into a single skeletal fiber with multiple nuclei. Some fibers are about 100 μm in diameter and 30 cm long (fig. 9.1).

Skeletal muscle cell has the same structures as other body cells, but many structures have very special characteristic. Scientists who study skeletal muscle cells give these structures special names. Thus, skeletal muscle cell plasma membrane is known as **sarcolemma**, smooth endoplasmic reticulum is called **sarcoplasmic reticulum**, and cytoplasm is known as **sarcoplasm**. Most special organelles of the sarcoplasm are oriented along a major axis of muscle cell cylindrical structures called **myofibrils**. These myofibrils are made of the contractile proteins **actin** and **myosin** and organized into special structures called **sarcomeres**.

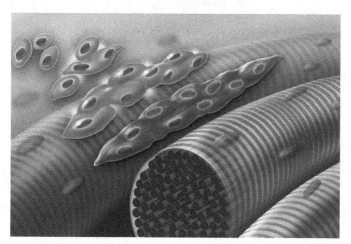

FIGURE 9.1   Skeletal Muscle Cell Development.

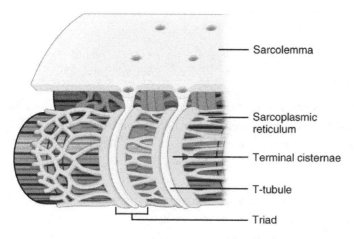

Sarcolemma

Sarcoplasmic reticulum

Terminal cisternae

T-tubule

Triad

FIGURE 9.2   Structure of the Skeletal Muscle Cell.

Another unique organelle of the sarcoplasm is the **sarcoplasmic reticulum (SR)**, a modified smooth endoplasmic reticulum. The sarcoplasmic reticulum at some regions is enlarged and developed into **terminal cisternae**—special calcium storage chambers. The sarcolemma has long **transverse tubules (T-tubules)**. T-tubule expands deep inside the cell interior. It opens outside of the cell on one side and blindly ends on the other. T-tubules create a network of tunnels inside the cell. Extracellular fluid freely flows through the T-tubules' openings and may reach the center of a muscle cell. Every T-tubule from both sides is flanked by a terminal cisterna. The membranes of T-tubule and terminal cisternae walls are bound together by two membrane proteins: the **dihydropyridine receptor** in the wall of the T-tubule, and the **ryanodine** receptor in the wall of sarcoplasmic reticulum. These proteins are linked directly with each other in a one-to-one fashion. The dihydropyridine is a receptor protein sensitive to membrane potential. Ryanodine is a Ca^{2+} channel protein. When an action potential reach T-tubule, the dihydropyridine changes shape and opens a gate in the ryanodine channel. Thus, the T-tubule together with two terminal cisternae from both sides creates a unitary structure known as a **triad** (fig. 9.2).

Sarcomere Organization

As you can see in fig. 9.3, a skeletal muscle cell (muscle fiber) contains hundreds of **myofibrils** made of two types of **myofilaments**. Every myofibril is a structure made of special protein molecules. Myofibril is subdivided into units following each other along its length, like cars in a train. Every myofibril contains hundreds or thousands of such units, called a **sarcomere**. From both sides every sarcomere is bordered by Z discs that play a role as anchors for contractile proteins (fig. 9.3). There are three types of protein molecules that make sarcomere:

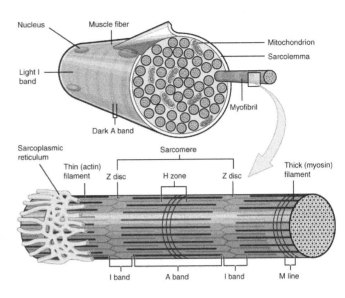

FIGURE 9.3   Myofibril Organization.

1. **Structural proteins.** Structural proteins create the frame of the sarcomere, make its shape, and anchor other proteins.
2. **Contractile proteins.** Two proteins—actin and myosin—produce tension and decrease the length of the sarcomere.
3. **Regulatory proteins.** A group of proteins that control ability of actin and myosin molecules to interact and to generate tension in muscle cell.

The structural protein **desmin** creates a scaffold around Z discs of adjacent myofibrils to hold them together. This scaffold extends to the cytoplasm and interlaces with a cytoskeleton of the cell. Altogether it creates a robust structural organization of the muscle cell and helps it withstand contraction and extension. **Titin** forms a core axis of thick filaments. One side this giant molecule is elastic and attached to the Z disc; the other side is rigid and attached to the M line. Titin holds thick filaments at the center of the sarcomere and its elastic region like a spring returning sarcomere to its original position when myofilament relaxes after contraction. The protein **nebulin** creates the frame of thin filaments. **Obscurin** is associated with the M line and binds it with the sarcoplasmic reticulum. **Dystrophin** is a structural protein that anchors the sarcolemma to the surrounding connective tissue and to the myofibrils. Dystrophin supports muscle fiber strength and is responsible for its mechanical stability.

The contractile proteins **actin** and **myosin** are organized into thin and thick filaments. **Thick filaments** are composed of **myosin** molecules. From 200 to 400 myosin molecules are organized around a rigid titin region. Myosin is a large ATP-dependent motor protein. A myosin molecule has two distinct regions. Two long heavy polypeptide chains coil around each other and create a "tail." At the end of both heavy tail, the chains have short globular structures called a "head." The head has two special sites: one for binding to an active site of actin molecule, and the other for binding and hydrolyzing ATP molecules. The head and tail regions are connected by a flexible hinge region called the "neck" that may bend. Myosin tails interlace and are found only in the middle region of thick filament. Myosin heads are on both ends of thick filament: half of myosin heads are on one end and the other half are on the other end (fig. 9.4).

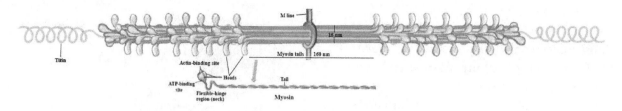

FIGURE 9.4   Myosin Molecule and Thick Filament.

A thin filament is made of a contractile protein **actin** and two regulatory proteins—**tropomyosin** and **troponin**. A globular bead-shaped actin molecule has a special region called an **active site** that may create a reversible chemical bond with the head of a myosin molecule called a **cross bridge**. Many actin molecules are held together by a nebulin and tropomyosin molecules like beads in a necklace. Two strings of such necklaces are intertwined into a single thin filament. Troponin molecules stabilize this structure by holding together tropomyosin and actin molecules (fig. 9.5).

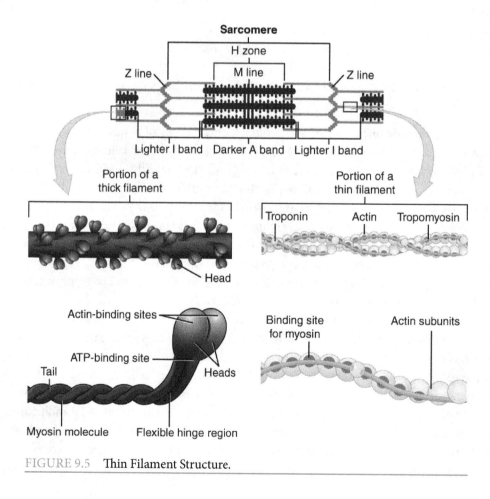

FIGURE 9.5   Thin Filament Structure.

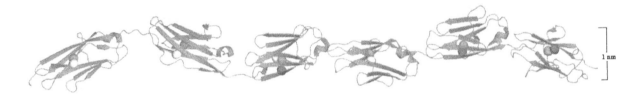

FIGURE 9.6   Elastic Filament.

In addition to thick and thin filaments, there are also **elastic filaments**. Elastic filaments are made of giant titin molecules. Elastic filaments hold thick filaments in the center of the sarcomere, resist overstretching of myofibril, and, like a spring, return the sarcomere to its original length when muscle fiber is relaxed (fig. 9.6).

In a sarcomere cross section, thick and thin filaments alternate each other like sandwich: thick filament always occupies a position between thin filaments, and every thin filament is surrounded by thick filaments. In longitudinal section thin and thick filaments are arranged in sequence where there are only thin filaments, following the region with thin and thick filaments altogether, and the region with thick filaments is only at the center of the sarcomere (fig. 9.7). Now, looking at this structure, you understand why skeletal muscle cell has striations. The regions with thin filaments only (I band) are more transparent to light and, thus, look like light stripes. The regions where thin and thick filaments overlap (A bend) are less transparent and under a microscope look like dark stripes.

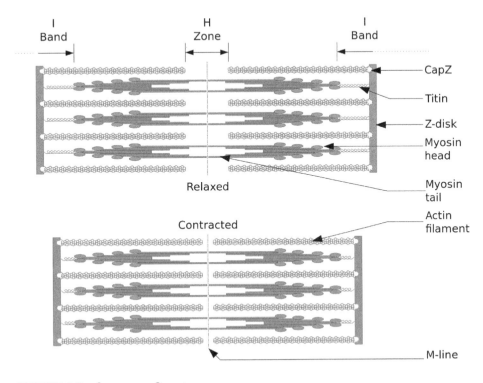

FIGURE 9.7   Sarcomere Structure.

CHECK YOUR UNDERSTANDING

- What molecule(s) form elastic filaments? What is the role of elastic filaments?

- What is a triad?

- Why does skeletal muscle have striation?

- Name contractile proteins and describe how they are organized in myofilament.

9.2 Mechanism of Muscle Contraction: Sliding-Filament Theory

As you can see, a contractile unit of skeletal muscle cell is a sarcomere. The modern theory of muscle contraction was independently proposed in 1954 by two groups of scientists and is called the **sliding-filament theory**. This theory states that muscle cell contraction is based on movement of thick and thin filaments toward each other (sliding). Previously scientists believed that during contraction, thick and thin filaments become shorter and this creates tension inside muscle cell. The sliding-filament theory states that it is not true. Muscle fiber becomes shorter because thin filaments of the sarcomere slide over thick filament toward the center of the sarcomere. As a result, the sarcomere becomes shorter. Every muscle cell has hundreds of parallel, cylindrical myofibrils, each of which contains a sequence of hundreds to thousands of sarcomeres arranged end to end. When all these sarcomeres become shorter, a strong force of their mutual pulling constricts the muscle fiber. The movement of filaments toward each other is generated by chemical interactions between thick and thin filaments. For that, the myosin heads of the thick filament have to create a chemical bond with the active site of an actin molecule—create **cross bridges**. When the cross bridges develop, thick myofilaments "grab" the thin filament and pull it toward the M line. This pulling force moves thin filaments toward the M line and forces Z discs on both ends of the sarcomere move close to each other. As a result, the total length of the sarcomere decreases (fig. 9.8).

However, sarcomere contraction does not happen by itself. Cross bridges between thick and thin filaments do not develop because tropomyosin molecules block active sites of actin molecules and prevent myosin heads from binding them. Troponin molecules guard positions of actin and tropomyosin molecules firmly. A stimulation of a motor neuron is needed to open active sites of actin molecules. Otherwise, muscle fiber remains relaxed. Thus, to understand muscle cell contraction in depth, we have to examine the mechanism of stimulation of the skeletal muscle fiber by a motor neuron.

CHECK YOUR UNDERSTANDING

- What is a cross bridge, and how do cross bridges relate to muscle contraction?

- What prevents the formation of cross bridges?

- Which structure in myofilament contracts?

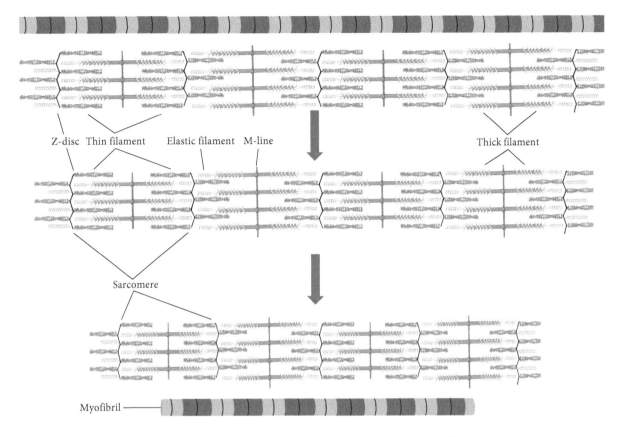

Z-disc Thin filament   Elastic filament M-line   Thick filament

Sarcomere

Myofibril

FIGURE 9.8   The Mechanism of Sarcomere Contraction According the Sliding-Filament Theory.

Sodium-Potassium Pump and Resting Membrane Potential

When we studied transport through a plasma membrane, we learned about the sodium-potassium pump that creates an electrochemical gradient across the membrane (see chapter 3, page 72). Recall that the phospholipid bilayer of the plasma membrane is impermeable for electrically charged particles such as Na^+, K^+, Ca^{2+}, and others. To help these ions cross the plasma membrane, there are special transport proteins. Some of these proteins provide passive movement of ions and electrically charged molecules from an area where their concentration is high to an area where their concentration is low. This type of movement across the plasma membrane is called facilitated diffusion. Proteins that provide facilitated diffusion are called **leak channels**. Thus, aquaporin is an example of a leak channel protein. There are other transport proteins that actively push substances from one side of the plasma membrane to the other in one direction, even when the gradient of concentration is against this movement. This movement of substance from a place of low concentration to an area where its concentration is high is similar to moving a heavy load up a hill, and because of that, these proteins need an energy influx from ATP molecules. This type of transport is called active transport, and the proteins are called **ATP-dependent pumps**. The sodium-potassium pump transports sodium and potassium ions across the membrane. This pump moves sodium ions out of the cell and moves potassium ions from outside to inside the cell. Every cycle this pump moves three sodium ions out of the cell and two potassium ions inside the cell (fig. 9.9).

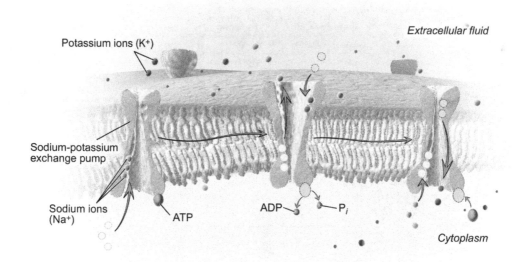

FIGURE 9.9   Sodium-Potassium Exchange Pump.

As a result of sodium-potassium pump activity, concentration of sodium outside of the cell is about ten times higher than inside. At the same time, concentration of potassium ions inside the cell is seven times higher than outside. This inequality of distribution of chemical elements is also accompanied by an inequality in the electrical charge inside and outside of the cell membrane. A region of cytoplasm close to the plasma membrane inside the cell becomes negatively charged but outside the cell is positively charged. The difference between the inner membrane surface and interstitial fluid on outer surface varies from −60 to −95 μV. The minus demonstrates the fact that electrical charge inside the cell is negative and outside is positive. Electrochemical potential generated by sodium-potassium pump cannot exist for a long time. According to the principles of thermodynamics, substances tend to move in direction from a high concentration to lower concentration, until their concentration (and electrical charge) will be equalized. Maintaining the electrochemical gradient at a particular level requires a continuing energy influx. This energy comes from ATP molecules that energize the sodium-potassium pump. The electrochemical potential created by the sodium-potassium pump is characteristic of cells at rest and is called the **resting membrane potential**.

CHECK YOUR UNDERSTANDING

- Why is the sodium-potassium pump called ATP-dependent?

- Describe the mechanism of development of resting membrane potential.

- How will membrane potential change if the level of sodium ions in the blood is elevated, for example, by salty food?

Action Potential

The sodium-potassium pump is not the only channel protein for Na^+ and K^+. There is a number of different channel proteins in cellular membranes that facilitate movement of these ions. Leak channels permit constant flow of Na^+ and K^+ following the gradient of their concentration. There are so called **gated channels** that may be "closed" or "open," like a door or a gate. When this channel is open, substances may move through it in both directions. When it is closed, the movement stops. A gated channel opens when it receives a special signal or stimulus. The signal may be of different kind and origin. Some channels open when they bind with special signaling molecules from the interstitial fluid. These channels are called **ligand-gated channels**. Other channels open when the electrical charge of a plasma membrane—membrane potential—is changed. These channels are called **voltage-gated channels**.

A quick temporary change of electrical charge in a region of plasma membrane is called **action potential**. Action potential is a voltage-dependent change in membrane permeability to ions. Ion channels that produce action potential are voltage-gated channels. During an action potential, the membrane potential changes from the negative resting value to a positive value and then returns to its original negative value. All these changes happen very rapidly in a few milliseconds. When the changing membrane potential reaches some critical value, the voltage gated Na^+ channels open. This critical value of the membrane potential is called **voltage threshold** (step 2 on fig. 9.10). The opening of the voltage-gated Na^+ channels causes a rapid rise of the membrane potential (remember that resting membrane potential is negative: -60 to -95 μV) (step 3 in fig. 9.10). The positive charged sodium ions rush inside the cell (Na^+ concentration outside of the cell is about 10 times higher than inside). This influx of Na^+ neutralizes the negative charge of cytoplasm—the process called **depolarization**. The rapid increase of membrane potential value may reach 0 and even becomes positive (overshoot). At this point, Na^+ channels close and K^+ voltage-gated channels open. Na^+ movement stops, but K^+, because their concentration inside the cell is high, rushes out of the cell. Potassium ions are also carrying positive electric charge, and electric charge inside the cell again returns back to a negative value. This process is called **repolarization**. The membrane potential for a few milliseconds may even drop below the resting membrane potential value. This state is called **hyperpolarization** (step 5 on fig. 9.10).

Once initiated, an action potential propagates along the sarcolemma without a decrease in amplitude and at a constant velocity. It does not develop until the threshold level is reached, and as far as this level is reached, it propagates with the same strength all over the muscle fiber. That is why we characterize action potential as an **all-or-nothing** process.

CHECK YOUR UNDERSTANDING

- What is the difference between voltage-gated and ligand-gated channels?
- What is the role of voltage-gated channels in the development of action potential?
- Which channels are responsible for membrane depolarization?
- Describe the role of potassium channels in membrane repolarization.

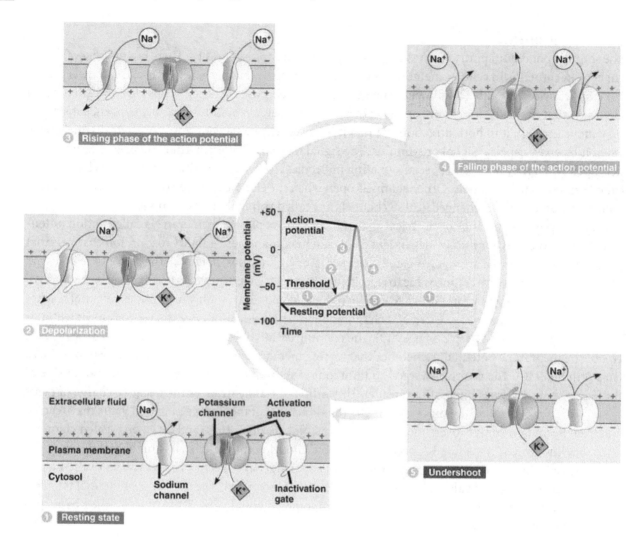

FIGURE 9.10   Mechanism of action potential: *1. Resting state.* In a resting state the plasma membrane maintains its resting membrane potential. At this state the activation gates on the Na^+ and K^+ channels are closed. *2. Depolarization.* A stimulus opens the activation gates on some Na^+ channels. Na^+ moves inside cell through these channels and depolarizes the membrane. *3. Rising phase* of the action potential. If the depolarization reaches the threshold level, it opens the activation gates on most Na^+ channels. Massive opening of most Na^+ channels triggers an action potential. At this phase K^+ channels activation gates remain closed. The Na^+ influx changes the inside surface of the membrane positively charged. *4. Falling phase* of the action potential. During this phase the inactivation gates on most Na^+ channels close and stop Na^+ influx. At the same time, the activation gates on most K^+ channels open and K^+ moves out of the cell, which restores the inner side of the cell membrane to negative again. *5. Undershoot or hyperpolarization.* Both gates of the Na^+ channels are closed, but activation gates on some K^+ channels are still open. When these gates close and inactivation gates open on Na^+ channels, the cell membrane returns to the resting membrane potential.

Neuromuscular Junction

A skeletal muscle cell at rest has a resting membrane potential. For development of action potential, voltage-gated channels have to be open. What triggers alteration of resting membrane potential and opening of voltage-gated channels? The skeletal muscle fiber has to be stimulated by a nerve cell—a **motor neuron**—to contract. Motor neuron is located somewhere in the CNS—in the brain or spinal cord. A long tubular outgrowth—an **axon**—connects motor neurons with muscle fiber. Nerve impulse is a signal that nerve send to the muscle fiber. This signal is generated at the base region of axon, called an **axon hillock**. The motor nerve impulse propagates to the end of the axon, called the **axon terminal** (fig. 9.11).

The area where the motor neuron communicates with muscle fiber is called the **synapse**. The synapse, together with skeletal muscle cell, creates the **neuromuscular junction (NMJ)**. There is no direct physical contact between the axon terminal and the sarcolemma, called the **motor end plate**. Between the axon terminal and the motor end plate there is a narrow gap called the **synaptic cleft**, and nerve impulse cannot jump from the axon terminal to the motor end plate. Thus, a synapse has three components (fig. 9.12):

1. **axon terminal**—the enlarged end of the axon
2. **synaptic cleft**—a narrow space between the axon terminal and muscle cell sarcolemma
3. **motor end plate**—a specialized folded region of the muscle cell membrane (sarcolemma) designed to receive signals from the motor neuron

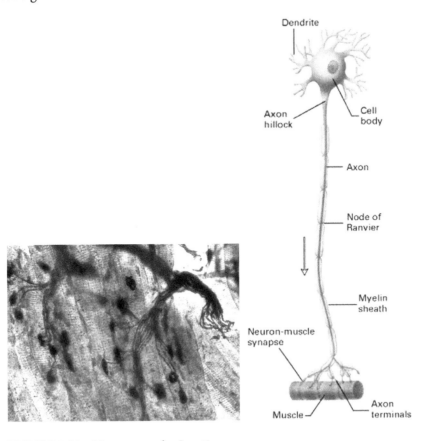

FIGURE 9.11   Neuromuscular Junction.

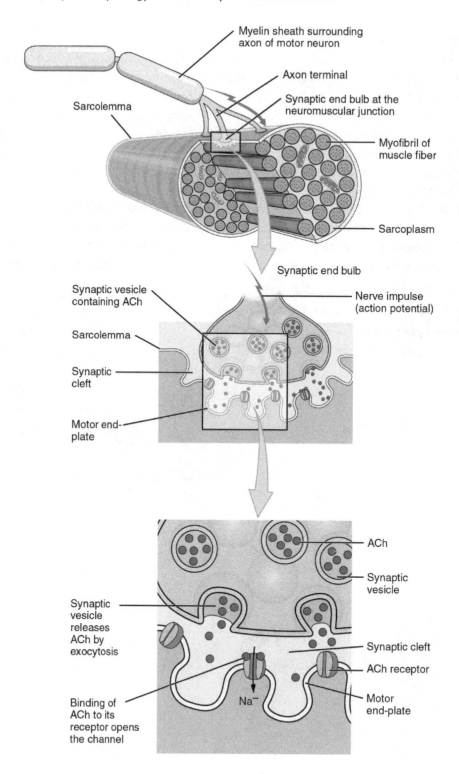

FIGURE 9.12   Neuromuscular Junction.

The agent that transmits nerve impulse from the axon terminal to the motor-end plate is called a **neurotransmitter**. There are many different neurotransmitters that play different roles in communication among nerve cells, and neurons and effector organs. A neurotransmitter that transmits nerve impulse to the motor end plate is known as **acetylcholine (ACh)**. Acetylcholine is stored in special **synaptic vesicles** inside the axon terminal. When the nerve impulse reaches the end of the axon, ACh is released into the synaptic cleft. ACh very fast diffuses across the synaptic cleft and reach motor end plate. Sarcolemma in a motor end plate contains a special receptor protein for ACh that are ion ligand-gated channel proteins. When ACh binds with this protein, it changes its confirmation (3-D shape—see chapter 3, page 72) and opens for sodium ions (fig. 9.12).

There is a very interesting story about discovery of neurotransmitters. For this discovery, Otto Loewi received a Nobel Prize in 1936. At the beginning of the 20th century, physiologists were split between those who thought that nerve cells communicate with each other through electrical impulses and those who thought there are special messenger molecules that transmit nerve impulse. One night, Loewi woke up very agitated: he had a dream about how to make a simple definitive experiment that may solve this dilemma. A happy and relieved Loewi went back to sleep looking forward to the next day, when he would go to his laboratory and do this experiment.

When he woke up the next morning, he suddenly realized with horror that he forgot the design of the experiment. He remembered only that he definitely had the solution, but he did not remember what it was. For several very frustrating weeks, he tried to restore his memory. Happily, one night in a deep sleep Loewi again saw how the experiment had to be organized. Having had the frustrating experience with the previous dream, he did not go back to bed. He got dressed and in the middle of the night went to his laboratory.

The experiment was simple and beautiful. He prepared two beakers with saline. In one beaker he put the heart of a frog with an associated vagus nerve. In another beaker he placed a frog heart only (the vagus nerve was removed). When all preparations were finished, he stimulated the free vagus nerve in the first beaker. The nerve stimulation caused the heart rate to slow down. After that, he took a sample of saline from the first beaker and poured it over the frog heart in the second beaker and observed that this heart rate slowed down too. The evidence was obvious: there is a chemical substance in the solution produced by the vagus nerve in the first beaker that controls heart rate. The conclusion you may make by yourself: **the vagus nerve controls heart rate through the chemical agent, not by electrical impulses.**

CHECK YOUR UNDERSTANDING

- Name three elements of a neuromuscular junction.

- Describe the major characteristics of the motor end plate.

- How can you identify what is a neurotransmitter, and which neurotransmitter can be found in the synaptic cleft of a neuromuscular junction?

Skeletal Muscle Contraction

To contract, skeletal muscle fiber has to be excited—stimulated by a motor neuron. The wave of excitation has to spread over the whole muscle fiber and reach structures that are responsible for the fiber contraction—sarcomeres with their thick and thin filaments. Inside the sarcomere, myosin and actin molecules create cross bridges that cause thin filaments slide over thick filaments and force the sarcomere to contract. Contraction of sarcomeres result in shortening of myofilaments inside muscle fiber. The total length of muscle fiber decrease. The process of skeletal muscle contraction is divided into three steps or phases:

I. Excitation phase
II. Excitation-contraction coupling phase
III. Contraction phase

Now, let's look at these three phases in details.

I. Excitation phase. During excitation phase, an action potential of nerve impulse is converted into an action potential of muscle fiber. It begins with arrival of a nerve impulse to the axon terminal and release of ACh into the synaptic cleft. ACh binds with Na+ ligand-gated channels and generates alteration of motor-end plate membrane potential that leads to development of action potential in sarcolemma. The whole process proceeds in five steps (fig. 9.13):

Step 1: An action potential (nerve impulse) from the CNS (brain or spinal cord) reaches the axon terminal of the motor neuron and triggers release of the ACh from the synaptic vesicles into the synaptic cleft through exocytosis.

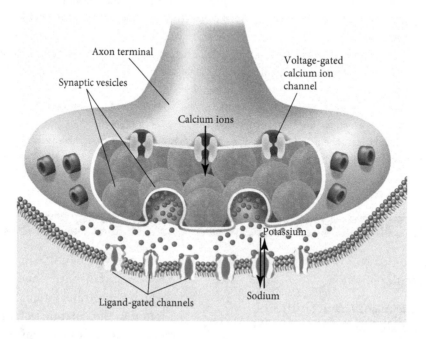

FIGURE 9.13   Excitation-Contraction Coupling, Step 1—Action Membrane Potential Development.

Step 2: ACh diffuses across the synaptic cleft—a fluid-filled space between axon terminal and motor end plate.

Step 3: ACh binds to ligand-gated ion channel proteins in the walls of the motor end plate.

Step 4: Ligand-gated sodium ion channels open and positive charged sodium ions enter the cytoplasm of muscle fiber.

Step 5: Entry of sodium ions depolarizes sarcolemma locally. Local depolarization of sarcolemma of the motor end plate is called the **end-plate potential** (tab. 9.1).

Stimulation of the muscle fiber by a motor neuron is terminated by a special enzyme called **acetylcholinesterase (AChE)** that degrades ACh. After ACh is removed from the synaptic cleft, motor neuron stimulation of the muscle fiber stops.

TABLE 9.1   Sequence of Events in Excitation Phase

Nerve impulse (action potential) arrives at axon terminal of the motor neuron
↓
Voltage-gated calcium channels open and calcium enters the axon terminal
↓
Calcium entry causes synaptic vesicles to release acetylcholine (neurotransmitter) by exocytosis into the synaptic cleft
↓
Aceylcholine diffuses across the synaptic cleft and binds to Acetylcholine-receptors in the sarcolemma
↓
Acetylcholine binds to receptors and opens sodium and potassium channels. Sodium and potassium move across the sarcolemma and membrane potential changes (depolarization). Wave of depolarization propagates along the cell membrane

VETERINARY APPLICATION

Myasthenia Gravis. Myasthenia gravis is an autoimmune disease. Serum analysis shows the presence of antibodies to acetylcholine receptor proteins. It means that an animal's immune system attacks and destroys ACh receptors in the motor-end plate. Destruction of ACh receptors results in disruption of nerve impulses to muscle fibers. The most common symptom in dogs is muscle weakness, which becomes worse with exercise and improves with rest. Another common symptom affects the esophagus, and dogs have trouble swallowing and drinking. They may also regurgitate food. In some situations, affected dogs aspirate food and water inside respiratory organs, which can cause pneumonia.

Some breeds are at risk for the myasthenia gravis. Among these breeds are Jack Russell terriers, springer spaniels, and smooth fox terriers.

CHECK YOUR UNDERSTANDING

- Describe the sequence of events of the excitation phase.

- Where is acetylcholine stored?

- Describe the role of acetylcholinesterase.

- What would happen if acetylcholinesterase becomes blocked (inhibited)?

II. Excitation-contraction coupling phase. This phase connects muscle fiber excitation by a motor neuron and muscle fiber contraction, "coupled" these two phases. The series of events that happen during this phase consists of three steps (tab. 9.2).

Step 1: The end-plate potential generates an action potential. The end-plate potential is a local minute change of membrane potential that may spread some distance and die without causing further changes. However, when the end-plate potential is strong enough and reaches some particular value called the **threshold level**, it may reach nearby voltage-gated sodium ion channels and open them. The opening of the voltage-gated sodium channels causes development of action potential (fig. 9.14).

Step 2: The action potential propagates along the sarcolemma like falling dominos. The depolarization of the sarcolemma in one area causes opening of voltage-gated channels in a nearby territory and the whole process spreads along the sarcolemma. Its strength does not change, and when it reaches the entrance of a T-tubule, it moves along the walls of the T-tubule deep inside the muscle fiber interior (fig. 9.14).

TABLE 9.2   Sequence of Events During the Excitation-Contraction Coupling Phase

The end-plate potential generates development of action potential
↓
The action potential propagates along sarcolemma and enters T-tubules
↓
Depolarization of walls of T-tubules opens calcium voltage-gated channels in terminal cisternae and calcium ions enter cytosol

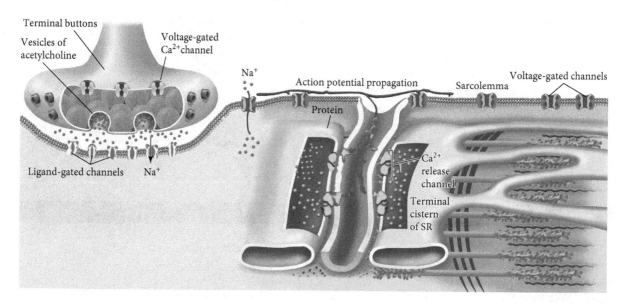

FIGURE 9.14   Excitation-Contraction Coupling. Step 2.

Step 3: Walls of T-tubules depolarize. Ca^{2+} voltage-gated channel proteins of the terminal cisternae from both sides of the T-tubule are linked with special proteins in the walls of T-tubules and open when the T-tubule walls are depolarized (see page 240). Opening of Ca^+ channels in terminal cisternae releases Ca^+ and it rush into the cytosol. The Ca^+ flood triggers the beginning of contraction phase (fig. 9.15).

VETERINARY APPLICATION

Botulinum Toxin. Botulinum toxin is most lethal biological poison. One gram of crystalline toxin can kill about 1 million adult people. The toxin is produced by anaerobic bacterium *Clostridium botulinum*. The toxin binds to motor neurons in the neuromuscular junction and blocks the release of ACh from synaptic vesicles. This toxin activity blocks muscle contraction. The blockage of neuromuscular junctions of respiratory muscles causes death from respiratory failure.

Diluted to miniscule concentration, the toxin is widely used in medicine for relief from painful muscle spasms and migraine headaches. In veterinary practice, botulinum toxin drugs are used in treatment of distemper, arthritis, masticatory myositis, and essential blepharospasm.

CHECK YOUR UNDERSTANDING

- What is a threshold level?

- What happens when ACh binds with ACh receptors?

- Describe the role of T-tubules in excitation-contraction coupling.

III. Contraction phase. According to the sliding-filament theory, muscle contraction is a result of shortening of sarcomeres. Sarcomeres are shortening because cross bridges between actin and myosin molecules pull thin filaments toward the center of the sarcomere. In a relaxed skeletal muscle cell regulatory protein tropomyosin holds actin molecules together and blocks actin to create chemical bonds with myosin molecules. As long as actin-binding sites are closed by tropomyosin molecules, the development of cross bridges is not possible. Another regulatory protein troponin guards the

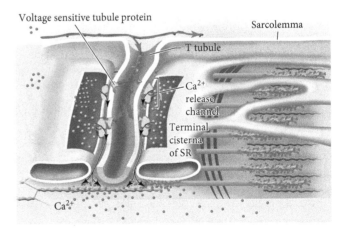

FIGURE 9.15   Excitation-Contraction Coupling. Step 3—Release of Ca^{2+} from Terminal Cisternae.

position of tropomyosin molecules and does not let it to open actin active sites. Ca2+ play a role of trigger in this process. The phase is divided into six steps:

Step 1: After release of calcium ions from terminal cisternae, Ca^{2+} floods into cytosol and binds with regulatory protein troponin that has three subunits. One subunit binds with calcium ion, the next one binds with actin molecule, and the third subunit binds with tropomyosin molecule. When Ca^{2+} binds with the calcium subunit, the troponin molecule changes its shape and ease the hold over the tropomyosin molecule.

Step 2: As far as troponin eases its grip, the tropomyosin slides from its original position and opens active sites of actin molecules. This step creates an opportunity for cross bridges development.

Step 3: Before myosin head binds with the active site of an actin molecule, it has to take a high-energy position—to be "cocked." This requires energy provided by an ATP. Recall that myosin head has an ATPase site. When ATP molecule binds with this site, ATPase hydrolyzes (breaks down) ATP molecule on ADP and phosphate group (P_i). The released energy "cocks" the myosin head in a "ready to create cross bridge" high-energy position.

Step 4: The cocked myosin head immediately binds with an actin active site and creates a cross bridge.

Step 5: This step is called the **power stroke**. As far as the myosin head creates a cross bridge with an actin molecule, the neck of the myosin molecule bends and moves from the high-energy position to its relaxed low-energy position. This bending of the neck pulls the thin filament toward the center of the sarcomere. The change of the position of myosin molecule head frees ADP and P_i, and leaves a vacant ATPase site.

Step 6: Now, being in a relaxed low-energy position, ATPase of the myosin head is open for a new ATP molecule. Attachment of new molecule of ATP breaks down the cross bridge and returns head to a high-energy cocked position. The ATP molecule splits on ADP and P_i (tab. 9.3).

Until Ca^{2+} binds with troponin molecules, the cycle may repeat again and again, from step 3 to step 6. In average muscle contraction, this cycle repeats 20 to 40 times for each myosin head in all sarcomeres of a myofibril (fig. 9.16).

TABLE 9.3 Sequence of Events during the Contraction Phase L

Calcium binds to troponin molecules and changes its shape (confirmation)
↓
Tropomyosin molecules slide and open active sites of actin molecules
↓
ATPase in the head of myosin molecules hydrolyses ATP into ADP and phosphate group and released energy put myosin head in a high energy position
↓
The myosin heads bind to the active sites of actin molecules and create cross-bridges
↓
The necks of myosin molecules bend and pull thin filaments towards the center of the sarcomere. ADP and phosphate group moves away and free ATPase site of myosin head
↓
Another ATP molecule binds to the ATPase site of the myosin molecule and breaks the cross-bridge between actin and myosin. The myosin head returns back to high energy position and the whole process may repeat again and again

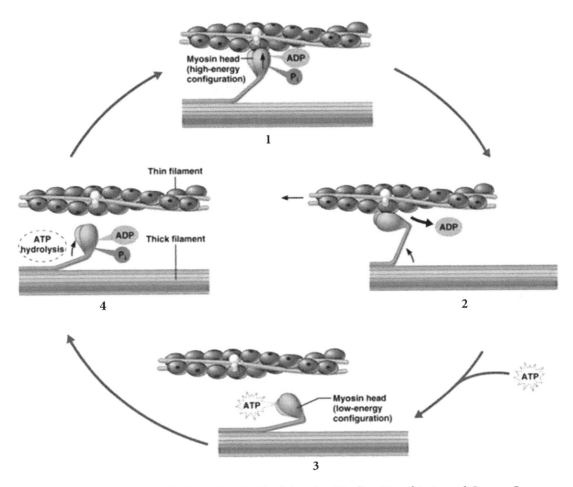

FIGURE 9.16   Contraction Cycle: 1. Myosin Head Attaches Binding Site of Actin and Creates Cross Bridge; 2. Phosphate Group (P$_i$) is Released Initiating Power Stroke. Myosin Neck Bends and Pull Thin Filament toward the Center of the Sarcomere (M Line). Finally, ADP Is Released; 3. A New ATP Attaches to Myosin Head. The Link between Actin and Myosin Weakens and Cross Bridge Detaches; 4. ATP Splits to ADP and P$_i$. Myosin Head Returns to High-Energy Position (Cocks).

CHECK YOUR UNDERSTANDING

- Describe the role of Ca^{2+} in muscle contraction.

- Describe the sequence of a power stroke.

- Describe the role of regulatory proteins in cross bridges development.

- Describe the role of ATP in muscle contraction.

Muscle Relaxation

The cycles of power strokes in muscle fiber will continue until calcium ions are present in the cytosol and there are some available ATP molecules. However, even when ATP molecules are completely spent, muscle fiber cannot relax. Calcium bonded to troponin molecules leaves active sites of actin molecules open for cross-bridge formation, and the muscle cell remains in a contracted position. It will not be able to contract more, but it also will not be able to relax. In order to relax, Ca^{2+} has to be removed out of the cytosol back into the terminal cisternae. The motor neuron stimulation also has to be stopped. Thus, muscle fiber relaxation is an active process and it may be described in four steps:

Step 1: Acetylcholinesterase degrades ACh in synaptic cleft and stop muscle stimulation. Without ACh ligand-gated channels in the motor end plate close and new action potentials do not generated.

Step 2: Sarcolemma restores its resting membrane potential. The voltage-gated calcium channels in walls of terminal cisternae close and calcium is trapped in sarcoplasmic reticulum.

Step 3: Active transport calcium channels in terminal cisternae pump calcium back into sarcoplasmic reticulum from cytosol. As all active transport proteins, this pump needs ATP for its activity. If ATP in the cell is absent, the muscle relaxation is not possible.

Step 4: The concentration of Ca^{2+} in cytosol decreases. Troponin is freed of Ca^{2+}. It restores the resting shape and binds with tropomyosin. Tropomyosin returns back and blocks the active sites of actin molecules. This prevents formation of cross bridges and the elastic fibers of titin molecules return the sarcomere to its original relaxed position.

Overview: From Motor Nerve Impulse to Muscle Contraction

In conclusion, let us put together all the preceding knowledge into one picture (table 9.4).

CHECK YOUR UNDERSTANDING

- Why does ACh have to be removed from the synaptic cleft to allow muscle fiber to relax?

- Explain why skeletal muscle fiber cannot relax until Ca^{2+} concentration in cytosol remains high.

- Why can muscle cell not relax if it runs out of ATP?

TABLE 9.4   Sequence of Events in Skeletal Muscle Fiber Contraction

Excitation	Excitation-Contraction Coupling	Contraction	Relaxation
1. Action potential arrives axon terminal and opens voltage-gated calcium channels ↓	1. The end-plate potential generates development of action potential ↓	1. Calcium binds to troponin. Troponin changes its shape (confirmation) ↓	1. Acctylcholinesterase degrades ACh in synaptic cleft. Muscle stimulation stops. Without ACh ligand-gated channels close ↓
2. Synaptic vesicles release ACh into syanptic cleft ↓	2. The action potential propagates along the sarcolemma and enters T-tubules ↓	2. Tropomyosin slides and open active site of actin ↓	2. Sarcolemma restores resting membrane potential. Voltage-gated calcium channels in terminal cisternae close and calcium trapped in sarcoplasmic reticulum ↓
3. ACh binds with ligand-gated ion channel in motor-end plate ↓	3. Depolariztion of T-tubules opens calcium voltage-gated channels in the walls of terminal cisternae and calcium enters the cytosol	3. ATPase hydrolyses ATP and released energy put myosin head in a high energy position ↓	3. Calcium pump in terminal cisternae moves calcium back to sarcoplasmic reticulum ↓
4. Ion channels open and sodium ions enter the cell ↓		4. The myosin heads bind to the active sites of actin ↓	4. Troponin restores its original shape; myosin covers actin binding sites ↓
5. Sodium entry depolarizes local region of sarcolemma, generating an end-plate membrane potential		5. Necks of myosin bend and pull thin filaments towards the center of sarcomere ↓	5. Elastic filaments return thin and thick filaments to their resting position
		6. ATP breaks cross-bridges. Myosin heads return back to high energy position. All may repeat again	

9.3   Energy Sources for Skeletal Muscle and Skeletal Muscle Classification

Thus, muscle fiber contraction and relaxation both need energy. The energy is needed to energize the sodium-potassium and calcium pumps, provide power strokes, and cock the myosin heads. This energy comes from ATP molecules stored in muscle cell. Surprisingly, the storage of ATP in muscle cell is limited to a few seconds of muscle fiber contraction. This means that for more or less prolonged muscle activity, new molecules of ATP must be produced.

The ATP molecules are synthetized in process of cellular respiration which may be subdivided into two major steps: 1) **glycolysis**—the splitting of a glucose molecule into two pyruvate molecules that takes place in cytosol and does not requires oxygen; 2) **citric acid cycle** and **oxidation-phosphorylation reactions** that take place in mitochondria and require oxygen; 3) there is also an immediate way to get ATP—just restore ATP molecules from ADP molecules available in the cytosol by adding a phosphate group (P_i). Thus, we have three recourses of ATP in muscle cell.

Immediate Sources of Energy

The first and immediate recourse of energy for muscle contraction is ATP storage that, as we already found, is consumed in a few seconds. At the same time a regeneration of ATP begins. The most important donor of P_i for ATP resynthesis is **creatine phosphate**. Creatine phosphate is a temporal storage of high-energy phosphate group. The creatine phosphate donates P_i to ADP to produce ATP (fig. 9.17).

Creatine phosphate is produced from creatine and ATP molecules when muscle cell is at rest. The regeneration of ATP from creatine phosphate is driven by a simple mass action: as most chemical reactions, ATP molecule formation from ADP and creatine phosphate may go in both directions **ADP + Creatine Phosphate ↔ ATP + Creatine** and when total mass of ADP overweight the total mass of ATP, the reaction is driven to the right side. This simple relation is very important, because ATP synthesis can be accelerated instantaneously and rapidly. As a result, the rate of ATP supply to muscle contraction thanks to creatine phosphate increases. Until creatine phosphate present in the cell, the rate of ATP regeneration is remarkably high. However, the storage of the creatine phosphate is also limited and its supply is consumed in a short time. When the muscle runs out of creatine phosphate, a long-term mechanisms of ATP synthesis takes over.

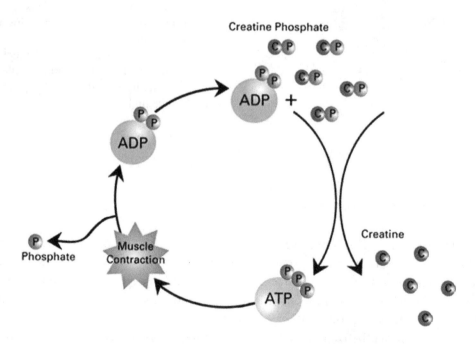

FIGURE 9.17   Creatine Phosphate as an Immediate Source of Energy for ATP Regeneration.

Glycolytic Sources of Energy

A mechanism of ATP formation in organism is a cellular respiration. It is a very complex process based on breaking down a glucose molecule ($C_6H_{12}O_6$) and harvesting the energy released from glucose chemical bonds in ATP molecules. This process may be subdivided in two phases. The first phase takes place in cytosol and does not requires oxygen. The second phase occurs in mitochondria and requires oxygen. The first phase is called **glycolysis** and, because it goes without oxygen, it also called **anaerobic phase**. The second phase depends on oxygen and is called **oxidative** or **aerobic**. When muscle cell runs out of creatine phosphate, the major resource of ATP production becomes anaerobic glycolysis.

In most general form, glycolysis may be described as a split down of glucose molecule into two pyruvic acid molecules and generation of 2 ATP molecules: $C_6H_{12}O_6 \rightarrow 2C_3H_6O_3 + 2ATP$. The rate of ATP synthesis through anaerobic glycolysis is lower than that from creatine phosphate. As a result, the rate of ATP supply decreases, although it remains comparatively high. Muscle cell uses this recourse as long as the glucose remains available. Thus, its length depends on the storage of glucose. Usually, glucose is stored in glycogen.

If oxygen supply in muscle cell is absent or very low, the breakdown of glucose is finished and products of glycolysis accumulate in organism. Unfortunately, pyruvic acid is converted into a lactic acid. Accumulation of the lactic acid leads to lowering of pH, acidosis, misbalance of electrolytes, and, as a result, to muscle fatigue.

Oxidative Sources of Energy

Oxidative catabolism cumulatively may be expressed as oxidation of pyruvic acids produced during a glycolytic phase: $C_3H_6O_3 + O_2 \rightarrow H_2O + \uparrow CO_2 + 15–17ATP$. You can see that it harvests much more ATP molecules per one molecule of glucose (30–34 ATP molecules) than glycolysis (only two ATP molecules). It demonstrates the effectiveness of oxidative catabolism. Oxidative or aerobic reactions are not accompanied by accumulation of lactic acid and acidosis. So, a muscle that uses an oxidative ATP synthesis can work for a long time without fatigue. After one minute of skeletal muscle activity, 100 percent of ATP supply is produced by oxidative aerobic catabolism. For that muscle cell needs a constant and sufficient supply of oxygen. Thus, the availability of oxygen is a main restrictive factor for this type of ATP production.

Rigor Mortis

Three to four hours after death, the entire body begins to progressively stiffen. Muscle spasms over the entire body that develop after death is called rigor mortis. Rigor mortis is caused by leakage of Ca^{2+} from terminal cisternae into cytosol and a lack of ATP fuel to pump Ca^{2+} back into the sarcoplasmic reticulum. As a result, Ca^{2+} remains in the cytosol, where it binds with troponin and initiates muscle contraction. Contracted muscle fiber also cannot relax without ATP. Thus, muscle spasms persist and the body remains stiff, until the proteins of myofilaments begin to degrade. The degradation of muscle fiber proteins begins about 42–72 hours after death, depending on the temperature.

There are two major ways to provide sufficient and continuing supply of oxygen: 1) create an oxygen storage inside the cell, and 2) create an efficient system of oxygen delivery. A special protein **myoglobin** creates oxygen storage. This protein (**Mb** or **MB**) is similar to hemoglobin. Both proteins have a special

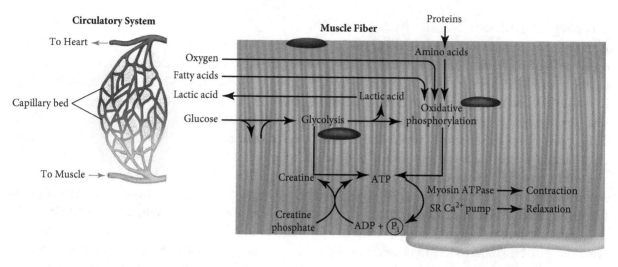

FIGURE 9.18   Major Sources of Energy for Skeletal Muscle.

iron-containing structure (group) that binds oxygen molecule. Hemoglobin is an oxygen transporting molecule in the blood. The myoglobin is an oxygen-binding protein in skeletal muscles of most vertebrates and almost all mammals. Like a hemoglobin, a myoglobin molecule has an intensive red-to-brown color, when it binds with oxygen. The oxygen molecule is loosely bond to myoglobin and oxygen donation for ATP production is an easy process. Another important resource of oxygen is an oxygen delivered by blood from lungs (fig. 9.18). To provide a sufficient oxygen supply, its delivery has to match the rate of oxygen consumption. Oxygen transport by blood takes time, and its usage has to be comparatively slow so that oxygen consumption does not overrun the delivery. The muscle cell that relies on oxidative energy source has to have a well-developed system of blood vessels.

CHECK YOUR UNDERSTANDING

- What immediate resources of ATP production do you know?

- Why does glycolytic production of ATP cause muscle fatigue?

- Why does oxidative production of ATP not cause muscle fatigue?

Classes of Skeletal Muscle Fibers

Every muscle fiber can use all sources of ATP formation. However, there are muscle fibers that mostly use an immediate and fast glycolytic source of energy, whereas other fibers rely on oxidative catabolic reactions. In relation to these energy resources skeletal muscle cells may be divided into two groups: **type 1 slow-twitch fibers** and **type 2 fast-twitch fibers**.

Type 1 slow-twitch fibers, as the name suggests, contract slowly. The rate of these muscle fibers contraction equalizes the rate of oxygen consumption with its delivery by blood. A sufficient oxygen supply allows slow-twitch fibers to receive energy from oxidative catabolism. That is why they are also called **oxidative muscle fibers**. These fibers have substantial amount of myoglobin in their cytoplasm that hold a significant amount of oxygen. An extensive number of blood vessels guarantees continuous oxygen delivery. The cytoplasm of type 1 fibers is reach of mitochondria, where oxidative reactions take place. Type 1 fibers have an intensive dark red color and are called **red/dark muscles**. Because oxidative catabolism does not accumulate lactic acid by-product, these muscles virtually never tire, no matter how long they work. This property suggests a name **fatigue-resistant**. In short, type 1 slow twitch fibers are oxidative, red, and fatigue-resistant. They are very good for long-lasting endurance muscle activity, such as running a marathon or a fly long distance like a migrating bird.

Type 2 fast-twitch fibers, as their name reflects, contract very fast and have no time to wait a new fresh oxygen delivery by blood. They receive their energy from immediate sources of ATP and glycolysis. They do not have as much myoglobin in their cytoplasm as type 1 fibers, and their vascularization is also comparatively low. Because of that, these fibers have white color and are called **white fibers**. They are also called **glycolytic fibers**, because most energy they take from anaerobic glycolysis. Final product of glycolysis is pyruvic acid that decreases pH of body fluids and disturbs electrolyte homeostasis. The loss of homeostasis leads to fatigue. That is why the type 2 fibers are known as **fatigue fibers**. This type of fiber is very fast in contraction and also fast to fatigue. They are very good for a short-term maximum activity, such as a 100 m sprint or a running cheetah.

VETERINARY APPLICATION

Carnitine. Race horses demonstrate an amazing speed and endurance. However, these two qualities contradict each other. Horses with fast-twitch type 2 muscles demonstrate the best results in a short distance, but they are quick to fatigue and cannot run for long distances. On the other hand, horses with a high ratio of slow-twitch type 1 can run for a long distance, but their speed is far from sprinter horses.

In sport there are many food supplements that are designed to improve horse performance. Carnitine is needed for optimal mitochondrial oxidation. A long-term dietary supplementation with carnitine in conjunction with exercises demonstrates an increased endurance of sprinter horses. The research demonstrates an increase of percentage of type 2 fibers. It was observed an increase of capillary-to-muscle ratio, which results in an increase in muscles' blood perfusion. Carnitine supplementation also increases a spare muscle glycogen.

Visual difference between type 1 and type 2 fibers can be seen if you look at the white meat of chicken and dark meat of duck breasts. While ducks fly great distances, all a chicken can do is jump to the roof of a two-story house. As a matter of fact, most muscle fibers have an intermedium between these two type's characteristics. The real muscle organ is a combination of these different types of fibers. The ratio between type 1 and type 2 fibers in muscle organs is determined genetically (fig. 9.19).

CHECK YOUR UNDERSTANDING

- How long does oxidative catabolism fuel muscle activity?

- Explain why oxidative catabolism is referred to as "aerobic"?

- Would creatine phosphate supplementation improve muscle performance?

- What type of muscle fibers of whales and dolphins allows them to take deep dives that last a long time?

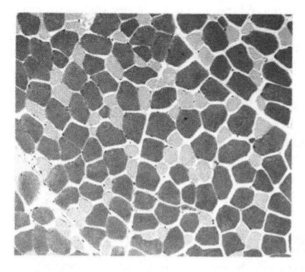

FIGURE 9.19 Type 1 Slow-Twitch Red Fatigue-Resistant Muscle Fibers and Type 2 Fast-Twitch White Fatigue Muscle Fibers in Muscle Organs.

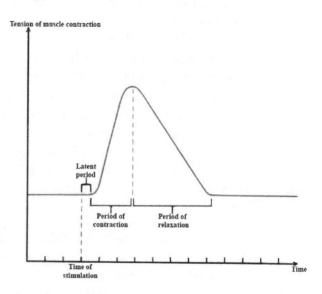

FIGURE 9.20 Record of Muscle Twitch.

Twitch Contraction

Contraction of isolated single muscle fiber is called **muscle twitch**. A recorded contraction, triggered by a direct electrical stimulation, is called a **myogram**.

On the myogram in fig. 9.20, one can see that muscle fiber twitch consists of three consecutive periods:

1. **Latent period.** It is a very short period, about 1–2 ms. At the beginning of this period muscle fiber receives a signal from a motor neuron and becomes excited, but contraction is still not observed. This phase includes a period when action potential spreads over the sarcolemma, reach transverse tubules, moves inside them, opens Ca2+ voltage-gated channels in the terminal cisternae of sarcoplasmic reticulum, and Ca2+ enter cytosol. This phase ends by binding of Ca2+ to troponin molecules which now let tropomyosin molecules open binding sites on actin molecules.

2. **Contraction.** When active sites of actin are open, myosin heads create cross bridges. Cross bridges create a tension. They pull thin filaments toward the center of a sarcomere and muscle fiber contracts.

3. **Relaxation.** The relaxation phase begins only when acetylcholinesterase decomposes ACh in synaptic cleft and Ca2+ pump in sarcoplasmic reticulum removes Ca2+ back to terminal cisternae. Troponin molecules freed of Ca^{2+} restore their hold on tropomyosin and actin molecules. Tropomyosin returns to initial position and closes actin binding sites. Cross bridges now cannot be formed and thanks to elastic forces from titin molecules, sarcomeres return to their original length.

From the start of the latent period to some point in muscle contraction, the fiber remains unresponsive to new stimuli from motor neurons. This period of inability to react on to new stimuli is called the **refractory period**. Different muscle cells have different refractory periods. Most of the skeletal fibers have refractory period that continues from the moment when fiber becomes excited and up to beginning of contraction phase.

Relation between Muscle Tension and the Timing and Frequency of Stimulation

Muscle fiber responses on motor neuron stimulus by all-or-nothing way. It contracts completely, or does not contract at all. A **refractory period** is a time period when muscle fiber cannot response to new stimulation. Until the end of this period muscle fiber cannot start new contraction. However, at the end of a refractory period muscle fiber may start a new contraction, even if it is not relaxed completely. Laboratory studies of effect of stimulation frequency on skeletal muscle fiber show that with increase of frequency individual twitches overlap and may fuse in one continuous powerful muscle contraction.

When the rate of stimulation is comparatively low—less than 10 stimuli per second—muscle fiber has enough time to relax. A new contraction begins after complete relaxation of muscle fiber and muscle twitches are separated from each other. The tension of muscle fiber of all twitches also remains the same (fig. 9.21.A).

If the frequency of stimulation is increased and varies from 10 to 20 stimulations per second, the muscle fiber has no time to remove all Ca^{2+} back to sarcoplasmic reticulum and some amount of these ions remain in cytosol. The following stimulation releases more Ca^{2+} from cisternae. That leads to forming more cross bridges. As a result, next contraction is stronger. On the myogram it looks like a stepwise increase in strength of contraction and is called **treppe** (fig. 9.21.B).

Stimulation of muscle fiber with frequency 20 to 50 stimuli per second demonstrates further increase in strength of fiber tension. The next contraction begins when fiber is not relaxed. Consecutive twitches fuse in continuous **sustained contraction** (fig. 9.21.C). The fusion of individual twitches is called **summation**. Summation leads to development of **wave summation** or sustained contraction.

When stimulations follow with frequency higher than 50 stimuli per second, individual twitches fuse completely and form a continuous prolonged contraction called a **tetanus** (fig. 9.21.D).

CHECK YOUR UNDERSTANDING

- Why does increase of frequency of muscle fiber stimulation above 20 stimuli per second lead to wave summation?

- Can cardiac muscle have a tetanus contraction, if its refractory period ends when the muscle relaxes completely?

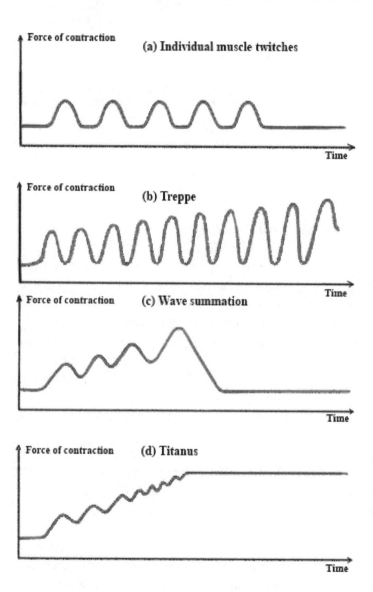

FIGURE 9.21   Skeletal Muscle Fiber Response to Stimulus Frequency.

Motor Unit, Recruitment, and Muscle Tone

You know that skeletal muscle fiber contracts only if it is stimulated by a motor neuron. In vertebrates every muscle fiber is associated only with one motor neuron. On the other hand, a single motor neuron is always associated with a group of muscle fibers. In this way, an impulse from one motor neuron leads to contraction of many fibers together. This organization—a motor neuron and a group of associated skeletal muscle fibers—is called a **motor unit**. On average a single motor unit has about 150 muscle fibers, but their number varies significantly, from small motor units with 10 fibers to big motor units with 2,000 to 3,000 muscle fibers. Different muscle organs have different size of motor units. Usually, a comparatively weak muscle that requires a very precise control of movement, such as *Levator palpebrae* muscle, has small motor units. A big strong muscle whose movement does not need to be precise but powerful, such as *Latissimus dorsi*, has big motor units where a single motor neuron innervates a thousand muscle fibers. In most cases we have a combination of small and big motor units in one organ.

Every motor unit have only one type of muscle fibers. Those motor units that have type 1 slow-twitch muscle fibers are termed **slow motor units**; and those are made of type 2 fast-twitch muscle fibers are called **fast motor units**.

Subdivision of muscle organ into fascicles and motor units allows muscle precisely control force and energy for body movement. It is obvious that when you take a pen from your desk, you spend much less energy than when you move an armchair. Every time when we do something, our brain evaluate the force we have to use to accomplish the task and activate as much motor units as needed, but does not more. However, very often life makes a correction. For example, you want to take a box you expected is empty. Your brain activates some number of motor units expecting that it is enough for the task. But when you take the box, you feel that it is very heavy. Your brain immediately does correction and activates additional motor units. This increase of number active motor units in muscle contraction is called **recruitment**. In muscle contraction, usually slow motor units are activated first. The fast motor units come to play later.

Normally, even when we are at rest, our muscles remain in state of partial tension. Even when most of motor units are at rest, there always are some activated motor units that keep some minimal tension in muscle. Motor units alter each other. When one active motor unit relaxes, the other motor unit becomes active. This maintains some minimal level of tension in muscle known as **muscle tone**. Muscle tone is very important for normal body functioning. The abnormally low muscle tone is called **hypotonia**. The chronic hypotonia may result in development of some pathogenic processes. Hypotonic muscle is soft and flattened. It does not create a tension needed, for example, for stabilizing associated with this muscle joint. As a result, joint may be enlarged and can be easily dislocated. The opposite is a state of abnormally high tone called **hypertonia**. Hypertonic muscle feels like a rock. Its contraction may be painful. **Spastic hypertonia** involves uncontrollable muscle spasms, stiffening or straightening out of muscles, or shock-like contractions. It may be a result of a spinal cord injury.

CHECK YOUR UNDERSTANDING

- Explain what a motor unit is. What is motor unit recruitment?

- Explain a mechanism of muscle tone.

- Why does hypotonia of muscle associated with a particular joint lead to the joint's instability?

Excess Post-Exercise Oxygen Consumption and Recovery Period

Physical activity is always accompanied by an increased rate and depth of breathing. Working muscles need more oxygen. Often the breath rate remains increased even when activity is over. It demonstrates the fact that body needs a time to restore preactivity state. This time is known as **recovery period**. The increased breath rate is called **excess post-exercise oxygen consumption (EPOC)**. Back in time it also was known as an **oxygen debt**, means that during physical activity organism spends more oxygen than receives.

EPOC develops because physical activity causes depletion of ATP, creatine phosphate, and oxygen storages. At the same time, metabolic by-products, such as lactic acid, are accumulated. Altogether, these disturbs body homeostasis. To return body homeostasis, organism needs energy of ATP molecules that mostly are produced by cellular respiration. The process of disturbed homeostasis restoration includes:

1. Return to normal body temperature. During physical activity the rate of catabolic reactions increased. This generates additional amount of heat and body temperature, as a rule, increases. To return to normal body temperature additional body heat has to be dissipated, which requires increased activity of some organs, for example, sweat glands.
2. Production of lactic acid during glycolysis leads to change of body fluids pH and electrolytes' imbalance. To restore pH and electrolytes homeostasis, organism has to 1) restore normal concentration of electrolytes, first of all—sodium, potassium, and calcium; 2) oxidize lactic acid to get ATP; 3) convert excess lactic acid back into glucose; 4) remove accumulated excess of carbon dioxide from blood flow.

All these processes require oxygen. Oxygen is a terminal receptor of electrons in an oxidative-phosphorylation reaction in mitochondria that generates major amount of ATP needed to restore homeostasis. Thus, EPOC is measured by the amount of oxygen an organism needs to restore homeostasis.

CHECK YOUR UNDERSTANDING

- What is EPOC?

- What does an organism have to do to restore body homeostasis after intensive physical activity?

- Why are beverages rich in electrolytes, such as Gatorade, are recommended to athletes after vigorous exercises?

9.4 Cardiac Muscle

Cardiac muscles have some characteristics similar to those of skeletal muscle fibers. They have striations, which shows that cardiac muscles, like skeletal muscles, have myofibrils that are made of sarcomeres. They also have T-tubules and terminal cisternae. However, cardiac muscle cell has fewer triads than skeletal fibers. Cardiac muscles are short, branched, and have only one nucleus. They have a lot of mitochondria and a lot of myoglobin. All these shows that cardiac muscle cells are slow-twitch oxidative fatigue-resistant muscles. Another important feature of cardiac muscles are **intercalated discs**—a special type of gap and desmosome junction between cells. The intercalated discs link cardiac muscle cells physically and electrically. Thanks to that, cardiac muscles can conduct action potential from one cell to another and transmit a wave of contraction through a myocardium. As a result, cardiac muscle contract as one single unit (fig. 9.22). Muscles that contract as one single unit also are called **syncytium**.

As we learned previously, cardiac muscle for contraction does not need stimulation from nervous system. Myocardium generates its own action potential. This property is called **self-exciting**. A group of cells in the region known as **sinoatrial node (SAN)** or **pacemaker** rhythmically generates action potentials. The intercalated discs help these action potentials propagate along the myocardium.

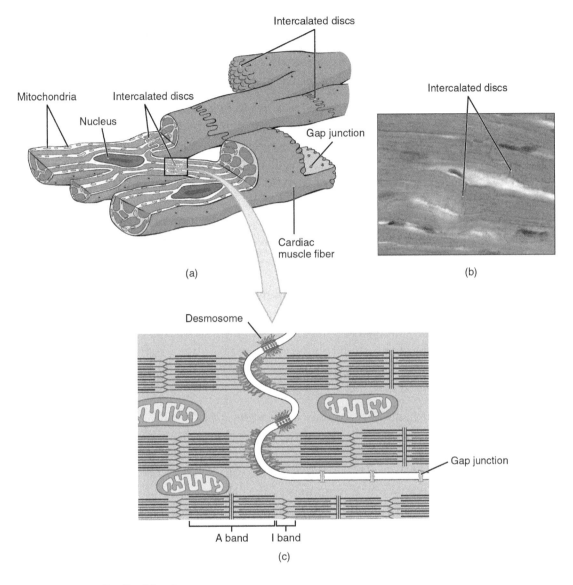

FIGURE 9.22   Cardiac Muscle.

CHECK YOUR UNDERSTANDING

- Describe the major characteristics of cardiac muscle cell.

- What is an intercalated disc?

9.5   Smooth Muscle

Smooth muscles are everywhere in walls of all internal organs. *Arrector pili* muscles in the dermis raise the hairs of the body when it is cold or when an animal is frightened. Smooth muscles of the iris regulate the amount of light that enters an eyeball. Among the major functions of smooth muscles are:

1. **Smooth muscles make sphincters.** Sphincters are circular muscles along tubular parts of hollow organs that control movement of substances. A sphincter may be open or closed, depending the state of the organ. A closed sphincter stops movement of substances through the tube. The activity of these muscles is regulated by a negative feedback. For example, the *internal urethral sphincter* opens when the urinary bladder is stretched by urine accumulated inside and closes when the bladder is empty.

2. **Regulation of flow in hollow tubular structures.** Constriction of smooth muscles in walls of tubular organs decreases diameter of the organ and, by that, decreases flow of substances through these organs. Thus, smooth muscles contraction in walls of blood vessels may decrease blood flow and redirect blood flow to another body region.

3. **Wavelike contraction of sheets of smooth muscles in walls of ducts and tubes facilitates movement of substances in these organs.** In the walls of many organs, such as the digestive tract, ureters, urethra, vagina, and so on, smooth muscles are organized in two layers: circular and longitudinal. Rhythmic contraction and relaxation of these layers results in waves of contraction that rhythmically propagates along the tubular organs. These kind of rhythmic waves of contractions are known as **peristalsis**.

Smooth muscles get their name from microscopic studies, which showed that these muscles have no striation like skeletal and cardiac muscles. Absence of striation means these cells have no myofilaments and sarcomeres. However, their contractile proteins are the same: myosin and actin. However, the arrangement of these proteins is different from that of skeletal and cardiac muscles. Actin filaments are organized into group oblique to the main axis of the cell. The position of thin filaments is fixed by structural proteins that form **dense bodies**. Some of these dense bodies anchored thin filaments to sarcolemma and other dense bodies bind them to nearby cell. Thus, through dense bodies tension transmits from one cell to another. A group of thin filaments spreads from dense body and is arranged around thick filament (fig. 9.23). Compared with skeletal muscle, in smooth muscle one thick filament

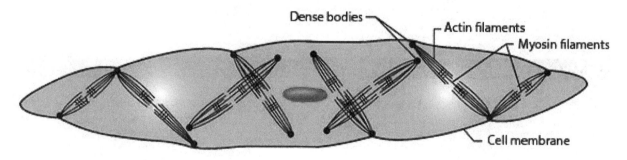

FIGURE 9.23   Smooth Muscle.

associated with more thin filaments. Smooth muscle cell has no troponin. The place of this regulatory protein occupies **calmodulin**.

Contraction of smooth muscle is not controlled by motor neurons. Smooth muscles may be excited by many different sources: neurons of autonomic nervous system, endocrine system, stretch and chemical receptors, and so on. Some cells are able to generate their own action potential and play role of a **pacemaker**. These cells with some rhythmicity generate waves of contraction.

The mechanism of contraction in smooth muscle is very similar to that of skeletal muscle. Because smooth muscle has no terminal cisternae with Ca^{2+}, contraction depends of an influx of Ca^{2+} from outside of the cell. Ca^{2+} binds to calmodulin. The rest of the events are more or less similar. Thanks to the oblique position of thick and thin filaments smooth muscle can contract up to 80 percent of its resting length. For comparison, a skeletal cell can contract no more than 40 percent of its resting length. Smooth muscle cell consumes only 1/100 of ATP molecules that normally are consumed a skeletal muscle fiber. The position and ratio of thin and thick filaments allows only a slow development of cross bridges. As a result, smooth muscles contract slowly, but their contraction is very strong (fig. 9.24). Besides that, smooth muscle can hold a contraction state for a long time with very low consumption of energy.

There are two types of smooth muscle: **multi-unit** and **single-unit smooth muscle**. Single-unit smooth muscles get their name from the fact that these muscles are organized into big groups, usually sheets. They are linked electrically by gap junctions which facilitate propagation of excitation wave among cells. This organization creates muscular structure that contracts as a one unit. Very often single-unit smooth muscles demonstrate peristalsis, as do single-unit smooth muscles in the walls of digestive tract or ureters (fig. 9.25).

Multi-unit smooth muscles are comparatively rare. Their name reflects the fact that they are not organized into groups by gap junctions and every cell contract independently. This type of smooth muscle is found where there is a need in precise graded regulation of force of contraction. They constitute such organs as the *iris* of eye and the *Arrector pili* muscle.

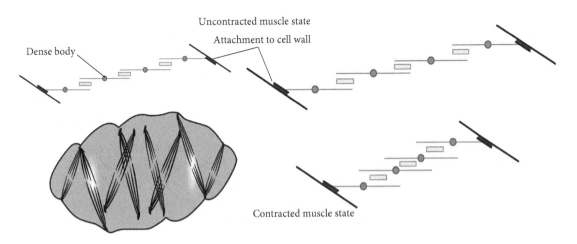

FIGURE 9.24   Mechanism of Smooth Muscle Contraction.

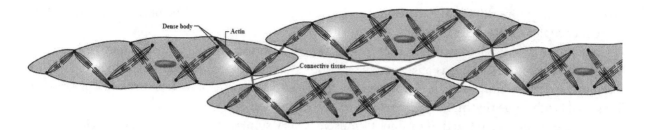

FIGURE 9.25   Single-Unit Smooth Muscle.

CHECK YOUR UNDERSTANDING

- What roles do smooth muscles play in an organism?

- What is the difference between single-unit and multiple-unit smooth muscles?

- What is the difference in organization of the contractile structures of smooth muscles and the sarcomeres of skeletal fibers?

CHAPTER SUMMARY

- A **sarcoplasmic reticulum (SR)** is a modified smooth endoplasmic reticulum of skeletal muscle cell. Sarcoplasmic reticulum at some regions forms **terminal cisternae**—special calcium storage spaces. Plasma membrane of the skeletal muscle is called sarcolemma. It has long, open outside and expanded inside the cellular interior blindly ended tubes called **transverse tubules (T-tubules)**. T-tubules create a network of tunnels inside the cell. From T-tubule both sides are flanked by terminal cisternae. The structures formed by t-tubule and two terminal cisternae are known as triad.

- A sarcomere is made of three type of proteins: 1) structural proteins create the frame of the sarcomere, make its shape, and anchor other proteins; 2) two contractile proteins: actin and myosin produce tension and decrease length of the sarcomere; 3) regulatory proteins control ability of actin and myosin molecules to generate tension in muscle cell.

- **Actin** and **myosin** are organized into thin and thick filaments. **Thick filaments** are composed of 200 to 400 myosin molecules. A myosin molecule has two distinct regions: two long heavy polypeptide chains create a "tail," and short globular structures called "head." The head has two sites: one for attachment to actin molecule, and the other for hydrolysis of ATP. The head and tail regions are connected by a flexible hinge region called "neck" that may band. Myosin tails interlace and are found only in the middle region of thick filament. Myosin heads are on both ends of thick filament. A thin filament is made of a contractile protein **actin** and regulatory proteins **tropomyosin** and **troponin**. Actin molecules are hold together by tropomyosin like beads in a necklace. Troponin holds together tropomyosin and actin molecules. There are elastic filaments made of titin. Elastic filaments hold thick filaments in the center of the sarcomere, resist overstretching of myofibril, and, like a spring, return the sarcomere to its original length when the muscle fiber is relaxed.

- The area where the motor neuron communicates with muscle fiber is called **synapse**. The synapse together with skeletal muscle cell creates **neuromuscular junction (NMJ)**. The synapse has three components: **axon terminal**—the enlarged end of the axon; **synaptic cleft**—a narrow space between axon terminal and muscle cell sarcolemma; and **motor end plate**—a specialized folded region of sarcolemma. The agent that transmits nerve impulse from the axon terminal to the motor-end plate is called **neurotransmitter**. Neurotransmitter of NMJ is known as **acetylcholine (ACh)**. Acetylcholine is stored in **synaptic vesicles** inside the axon terminal.

- The process of skeletal muscle contraction proceeds in three steps or phases: **excitation phase**; **excitation-contraction coupling phase**; and **contraction phase**. In the excitation phase nerve impulses reach the axon terminal and trigger a release of ACh into synaptic cleft. ACh binds with ACh receptors and opens Na^+ channels. The influx of Na^+ inside muscle fiber depolarizes motor end plate membrane and, if it reaches threshold level, generates action potential. During excitation-contraction coupling action potential propagates along the muscle fiber towards T-tubules. Depolarization of the membrane of T-tubules opens voltage-gated Ca^{2+} in terminal cisternae and Ca^{2+} flood cytosol. During contraction Ca^{2+} binds with troponin molecules and initiates power stroke cycles.

- Muscle fiber can relax only when the enzyme acetylcholinesterase degrades ACh in synaptic cleft and stops muscle stimulation; sarcolemma restores resting membrane potential; voltage-gated calcium channels close and trap Ca^{2+} in sarcoplasmic reticulum; Ca^{2+} pumps return Ca^{2+} into terminal cisternae; concentration of Ca^{2+} in cytosol decreases and formation of new cross bridges ends; finally, of titin returns the sarcomere to its original relaxed position.

- For contraction and relaxation muscle fiber needs ATP energy. The first and immediate recourse of energy for muscle contraction is an ATP. The next resource of energy is **creatine phosphate** which donates P_i to ADP and regenerates ATP. When ATP and creatine phosphate storage end, glycolytic synthesis of ATP begins to play a leading role. Glycolysis is a chemical process: $\textbf{C}_6\textbf{H}_{12}\textbf{O}_6 \rightarrow \textbf{2C}_3\textbf{H}_6\textbf{O}_3 + \textbf{2ATP}$. In absence of oxygen the products of glycolysis accumulate and pyruvic acid is converted into a lactic acid. Accumulation of lactic acid leads to lowering of pH, acidosis, misbalance of electrolytes, and, as a result, muscle fatigue. If there is enough oxygen, pyruvic acid is decomposed to water and carbon dioxide. This harvests a maximum of 34 ATP molecules per 1 molecule of glucose. Oxidative or aerobic reactions are not accompanied by accumulation of lactic acid and acidosis. The muscle that uses an oxidative ATP synthesis can work for a long time without fatigue. After one minute of skeletal muscle activity, all ATP is produced by oxidative aerobic catabolism. The oxygen for these reactions is provided from 1) oxygen stored in myoglobin, and 2) oxygen delivered by blood.

- In relation to energy resources, skeletal muscle cells are divided in two groups: **type 1 slow-twitch fibers** and **type 2 fast-twitch fibers**. Type 1 slow-twitch fibers receive energy from oxidative catabolism. These fibers have substantial amount of myoglobin and extensive vascular system to guarantee sufficient supply of oxygen. The type 1 fibers are reach of mitochondria, where oxidative reactions take place. The type 2 fast-twitch fibers receive energy from immediate sources of ATP and glycolysis. They do not have much myoglobin and their vascularization is comparatively low. These fibers are very fast in contraction and also fast in fatigue. They are very good for a short-term maximum activity.

- The contraction of individual muscle fibers is called muscle twitch. Muscle twitch has three periods: 1) a very short, about 1–2 ms, latent period; 2) a contraction period, when Ca^{2+} influx initiates development of cross bridges that pull thin filaments towards the center of a sarcomere; 3) a relaxation phase that begins with decomposition of ACh by acetylcholinesterase, Ca^{2+} pump in sarcoplasmic reticulum removes Ca^{2+} back to terminal cisternae, troponin molecules freed of Ca^{2+} grabs tropomyosin and actin molecules together, and elastic forces of titin return sarcomeres to their original length.

- When the rate of stimulation is less than 10 stimuli per second, muscle fiber has enough time to relax. A new muscle twitch is separated from previous. The tension of muscle fibers of all twitches also remains the same. When frequency of stimulation increases (10 to 20 stimulations per second) the muscle fiber has no time to remove all Ca^{2+} back to SR. The following stimulation releases more Ca^{2+}. As a result, next contraction is stronger. A stepwise increase in strength of contraction is called **treppe**. Stimulation of muscle fiber with frequency 20 to 50 stimuli per second, causes further increase in strength of fiber tension: the next contraction begins when fiber is not relaxed, consecutive twitches fuse in continuous **sustained contraction**. The fusion of individual twitches is called **summation**. When frequency of stimulation is higher than 50 stimuli per second, individual twitches fuse and form a continuous prolonged contraction without relaxation called **tetanus**.

- In vertebrates every muscle fiber is associated with only one motor neuron, but a single motor neuron is always associated with a group of muscle cells. In this way, an impulse from one motor neuron leads to contraction of many fibers together. This organization—a motor neuron and a group of associated skeletal muscle fibers—is called a **motor unit**. On average, a single motor unit has about 150 muscle fibers, but their number varies, from small motor units with 10 fibers to big motor units with 2,000 to 3,000 muscle fibers. Different muscle organs have different size of motor units. In most cases we have a combination of small and big motor units in one organ. Every motor unit have only one type of muscle fibers. The motor units that have type 1 slow-twitch muscle fibers are termed **slow motor units**; and those are made of type 2 fast-twitch muscle fibers are called **fast motor units**. The increase of number active motor units is called **recruitment**. In muscle contraction, usually slow motor units are activated first. The fast motor units come to play later. Even, when most of motor units are at rest, there always are some activated motor units that keep some minimal tension in muscle. They maintain some minimal level of tension in muscle known as **muscle tone**.

- Working muscles need oxygen. Physical activity depletes ATP, creatine phosphate, and glucose storage and body needs a time to restore preactivity state. This time is known as **recovery period**. The increased breath rate is called **excess post-exercise oxygen consumption (EPOC)**. To return body homeostasis, organism needs to 1) return to normal body temperature. For that, additional body heat has to be dissipated, which requires increased activity of some organs, for example, sweat glands; 2) restore pH and electrolytes homeostasis: sodium, potassium, and calcium, oxidize lactic acid to get ATP, conversion of lactic acid excess back into glucose, remove accumulated carbon dioxide from the blood flow. All these require oxygen. Thus, EPOC is measured by an amount of oxygen needed to restore homeostasis.

- Cardiac muscles are short, branched, and have only one nucleus. They are slow-twitch oxidative fatigue-resistant muscles. Another important feature of cardiac muscles are **intercalated discs**—a special type of gap and desmosome junction between cells. The intercalated discs link cardiac muscle cells physically and electrically. Cardiac muscles can conduct action potential from one cell to another and transmit a wave of contraction through a myocardium. As a result, cardiac muscles contract as one single unit.

• Smooth muscles have no striation. Their contractile protein actin is organized into a group oblique to the main axis of the cell. The position of thin filaments is fixed by structural proteins that form **dense bodies**. Some of these dense bodies anchored thin filaments to sarcolemma and others bind them to nearby cell. Thus, through dense bodies tension transmits from one cell to another. A group of thin filaments are arranged around a thick filament. The troponin in smooth muscle is replaced by **calmodulin**. Smooth muscles become excited by many different sources: neurons of autonomic nervous system, endocrine system, stretch and chemical receptors, and so forth. Some cells are able to generate their own action potential and play the role of a **pacemaker**. These cells with some rhythmicity generate waves of contraction. The mechanism of contraction in smooth muscle is similar to that of skeletal muscle. Because smooth muscle has no terminal cisternae with Ca^{2+}, contraction depends of an influx of Ca^{2+} from outside of the cell. Smooth muscle can contract up to 80 percent of its resting length, whereas a skeletal cell contracts no more than 40 percent of its resting length. Smooth muscle cell consumes only 1/100 of ATP molecules that normally are consumed a skeletal muscle fiber. There are two types of smooth muscle: **multi-unit** and **single-unit smooth muscle**. Single-unit smooth muscles get their name from the fact that these muscles are organized into big groups, usually sheets. They are linked electrically by gap junctions which facilitate propagation of excitation wave among cells. This organization creates muscular structure that contracts as a one unit. Often single-unit smooth muscles demonstrate peristalsis. Multi-unit smooth muscles are comparatively rare. They are not organized into groups and every cell contracts independently.

CHECK YOUR KNOWLEDGE

LEVEL 1. CHECK YOUR RECALL

1. Which of the following statements about myofilaments is true?
   A. Elastic filaments are made of myosin molecules.
   B. Thin filaments contain regulatory proteins troponin and tropomyosin.
   C. Both thick and thin filaments are made of actin molecules.
   D. Thick filaments have actin molecules organized around titin.
   E. Both thick and thin filaments during muscle contraction become shorter.

2. Myofibrils are composed primarily of:
   A. Acetylcholine
   B. ATP and ADP molecules
   C. Actin and myosin molecules
   D. Troponin and tropomyosin molecules
   E. Titin and dystrophin molecules

3. What is the function of the transverse tubules?
   A. They store sodium ions for the generation of action potential at the cell surface.
   B. They transmit action membrane potential impulses into the muscle cell interior.
   C. They connect actin and myosin fiber during contraction.
   D. They store neurotransmitters, such as acetylcholine.
   E. They have acetylcholine receptors and receive nerve signals.

4. The striated appearance of skeletal muscle cell results from the:
   A. Pattern of the transverse tubules in the cell
   B. Organization of the sarcoplasmic reticulum
   C. Sarcomere arrangement inside the cell
   D. Pattern of cisternae distribution inside the cell
   E. Pattern of deposition of some substances, such as creatine

5. Which structure of the skeletal muscle cell stores calcium?
   A. Cisternae of the sarcoplasmic reticulum
   B. Sarcolemma
   C. Transverse tubules
   D. A bands
   E. Myofilaments

6. The stiffness of skeletal muscles after death (rigor mortis) results from:
   A. ACh release and excess of ATP in muscle cells
   B. Ca^{2+} release in the muscle and lack of ATP to remove it back to cisternae
   C. Accumulation of lactic acid in the muscle cell after glucose breakdown
   D. Excess glucose in the muscle cell
   E. Na^+ leaking into the muscle cells through the broken plasma membrane

7. Which of the following is **not true** when comparing red and white muscle type cells?
   A. Red muscles contract more slowly than white.
   B. Red muscles contain more myoglobin than white.
   C. Red muscles have fewer mitochondria than white.
   D. Red muscles fatigue slower than white.
   E. Red muscles have better blood supply than white.

8. What is the role of enzyme acetylcholinesterase?
   A. It helps create cross bridges between actin and myosin microfilaments.
   B. It activates generation of action potential.
   C. It decomposes acetylcholine molecules in the synaptic cleft.
   D. It binds tropomyosin molecules to actin.
   E. It opens sodium channels in the motor end plate.

9. In recording muscle twitch, the delay between the time a stimulus is applied and the time when the muscle responds to this stimulus is called:
    A. Refractory period
    B. Relaxation period
    C. Latent period
    D. Contraction period
    E. Stress period

10. The very brief moment following stimulation when a muscle remains unresponsive to new stimulus is called:
    A. Refractory period
    B. Relaxation period
    C. Latent period
    D. Contraction period
    E. Stress period

11. The threshold stimulus is defined as the:
    A. Maximum stimulus required to cause muscle contraction
    B. Amount of acetylcholine required to cause muscle contraction
    C. Minimal motor neuron stimulus needed to cause muscle contraction
    D. Minimal membrane potential required to cause muscle contraction
    E. Amount of Ca^{2+} needed to cause muscle contraction

12. The rhythmic, wavelike movements made by smooth muscles in tubular organs is called:
    A. Summation
    B. Sustained contraction
    C. Eccentric contractions
    D. Concentric contractions
    E. Peristalsis

13. By the term *muscle tone*, we mean:
    A. Completely relaxed muscle at rest
    B. Muscle contracted for a long time without any relaxation
    C. Muscle that contracts and relaxes rhythmically
    D. Muscle sensitivity to a new stimulus
    E. Muscle in a continuous state of partial contraction

14. Recruitment of motor units is:
    A. A process of gradual contraction of muscle fibers
    B. An increase in the strength of nerve impulses that leads to stronger muscle cell contraction
    C. The minimal strength of nerve impulses needed for muscle contraction
    D. The increase in a number of active motor units
    E. The moment when a motor neuron impulse reaches the axon terminal

15. Summation is a(n):
    A. Force of maximum twitch
    B. Series of separated muscle contractions
    C. Process that combines forces of individual twitches into one sustained contraction
    D. Increase in the strength of a muscle contraction without changing its length
    E. Slow muscle contraction without changing its tonus

16. What event causes a troponin-tropomyosin complex to regain its original relaxed shape?
    A. Return of Ca^{2+} into the sarcoplasmic reticulum
    B. ACh receptors bind with ACh
    C. Diffusion of Na^+ back into transverse tubules
    D. Complete depletion of ATP and creatine phosphate
    E. Breakdown of glucose

17. Thick filaments are made of _____, whereas thin filaments are made of _____.
    A. titin; nebulin
    B. nebulin; titin
    C. myosin; actin
    D. actin; myosin
    E. troponin; tropomyosin

18. The sodium-potassium pump generates _____, whereas voltage-gated channels generate _____.
    A. cross bridges formation; cross bridges degradation
    B. action potential; cross bridges formation
    C. motor end plate potential; resting membrane potential
    D. action potential; motor end plate potential
    E. resting membrane potential; action potential

19. ACh is stored in _____, whereas ACh receptors are in _____.
    A. synaptic cleft; motor end plate membrane
    B. axon terminal vesicles; motor end plate membrane
    C. motor end plate membrane; synaptic cleft
    D. synaptic cleft; axon terminal vesicles
    E. axon terminal vesicles; synaptic cleft

20. Cross bridges are chemical bonds between _____ and _____.
    A. titin; actin
    B. actin; troponin
    C. troponin; tropomyosin
    D. myosin; actin
    E. tropomyosin; myosin

21. True or false: Muscle fiber becomes short because its contractile proteins actin and myosin shorten.
22. True or false: Muscle fiber does not need ATP energy for relaxation.
23. True or false: Oxidative muscle fibers are faster than glycolytic.
24. True or false: Glycolytic muscle fibers tend to fatigue quickly.
25. True or false: Oxidative muscle fibers are rich in myoglobin to bind oxygen in cytosol.
26. Match the term with its description:

_____ Troponin	a. Gap and desmosome junction between cells
_____ Myosin	b. A contractile protein that makes thick filaments
_____ Sarcomere	c. Another name for muscle cell
_____ Muscle fiber	d. A contractile structure of muscle cell
_____ Thin filament	e. A regulatory protein of the thin filaments
_____ Lactic acid	f. A structure in a sarcomere made of actin
_____ Intercalated disc	g. A final by-product of glycolysis

LEVEL 2. CHECK YOUR UNDERSTANDING

1. Skeletal muscle response to a motor neuron stimulus is called "all-or-nothing." Why?
2. Name the functional contractile unit of the myofibril.
3. Why can skeletal muscle not relax without ATP?
4. Why do whale muscles have a very dark brown color?
5. In your own words, explain why smooth muscles can contract up to 80 percent of their initial length, whereas skeletal only 40 percent?

LEVEL 3. APPLY YOUR KNOWLEDGE TO REAL LIFE

1. When running a comparatively long distance, there usually is a moment when you feel that you get a new strength in your muscles. Athletes call it a "second wind." Can you explain what happens at this moment?
2. Back in time, Indians of Central America hunted with arrows soaked in a liquid from the skin of small tropical frogs. The skin glands of these frogs release the poison curare. Curare binds to ACh receptors in the neuro-muscular junction. What will happen when the arrow soaked in curare poison wounds an animal? Is this poison used in veterinary medicine?
3. **Parturient paresis** (milk fever) is a disease caused by low blood calcium. The first milk produced by dairy cattle (called **colostrum**) contains high concentration of Ca^{2+}. A cow needs to produce 3 g of Ca^{2+} per hour for colostrum. When a cow does not have a sufficient calcium supply, it can develop milk fever within 72 hours following parturition. Symptoms include muscle weakness, labored breathing, and paralysis of the hind legs. If left untreated, the cow can collapse into coma and die. Can you explain why a Ca^{2+} imbalance causes these symptoms?
4. Predict the effect of an overdose of salt in the diet on skeletal muscles. What effect can a high level of Na^+ in the blood have on skeletal muscles?

Chapter 10

Introduction to the Nervous System

LEARNING OBJECTIVES

In this chapter you will learn about the histology of the nervous system and the nature of nerve impulses. When you finish reading the chapter, you will have knowledge about the following:

1. The major role of the nervous system and its principal organs.

2. The cells that create nervous tissue and their role in the normal functioning of the nervous system.

3. The nature and mechanism of nerve impulses.

INTRODUCTION

The nervous system unites the organs in an organism by control of their activity. Cells that create nervous tissue are highly specialized cells. Among these cells, neurons play a principal role. These cells are characterized by the ability to generate an action potential and conduct it along significant distances thanks to long cytoplasmic projections. In this chapter you will learn about the nature of nerve impulses—how a nerve impulse is generated and transmitted. You will also learn what role numerous neuroglia cells play in the functioning of the nervous system.

10.1 Overview of the Nervous System

Anatomically, the nervous system is divided into the **central nervous system (CNS)** and **peripheral nervous system (PNS)**. The CNS consists of the **brain** and **spinal cord**. The PNS is made of **nerves** and **ganglia**. The PNS gathers information from receptors, conducts this information for processing to the brain or spinal cord, and conveys commands to effector organs. The CNS is a processing center, where all collected information is analyzed and decisions are made. According to this distribution of functions, the PNS carries **sensory** and **motor functions**, whereas the CNS is responsible for **integrative function**. Depending the nature of the incoming and outgoing information, anatomists divide **sensory** and **motor divisions** of the PNS into **somatic**, where receptors and effector organs are associated with skin, skeletal muscles, and tendons; and **visceral**, which is associated with viscera or internal organs such as the heart, lungs, liver, and so on. As a result, the sensory division of the

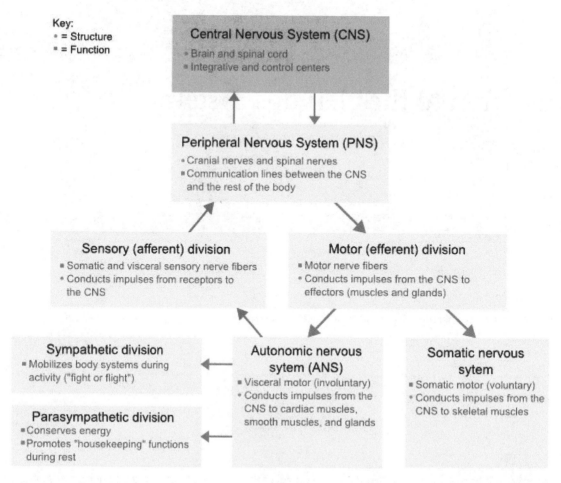

FIGURE 10.1   Divisions of the Nervous System. Arrows Demonstrate the Direction of Nerve Impulses.

PNS is subdivided into somatic and visceral divisions; and the motor division is subdivided into somatic and visceral (usually called the **autonomic nervous system**, or **ANS**) divisions (fig. 10.1).

Organs of the nervous system are composed of different tissues, but the principal is a nervous tissue made of **neurons** and **neuroglia** or just **glia** cells. Nervous tissue is highly cellular. The ground mater constitutes only 20 percent or less of the tissue volume.

CHECK YOUR UNDERSTANDING

- To what division of the nervous system does the facial cranial nerve belong?

- What division of the nervous system innervates the heart?

- To what division of the nervous system does the neuron that serves skeletal muscle belong?

10.2   Neurons

Neurons are major cells of nervous tissue responsible for receiving and sending nerve signals. Their principal characteristic is excitability—an ability to generate action potential (see chapter 9, page 247). Neurons create a network through which essential information is conducted and processed. Neurons are among the most specialized cell types in organism. They have no centrioles and, as a result, they do not have the ability to divide. That is why neurons have a very long life span and can survive the entire life of the organism.

Neurons vary in size, shape, and function. A neuron's body is also called a **neurosoma**. **Dendrites** are cellular projections that receive and carry signals toward the cell body. A single projection called an **axon** takes signals away from the neuron body (fig. 10.2).

The neuron cell body is much bigger in comparison to other cell bodies. It has a very high metabolic activity that is necessary to maintain a huge cytoplasmic volume of the cell and manufacture proteins that facilitate major neuron functions. Metabolically active neurons consume 4.93 to 7.05 $*10^{-9}$ µmol of glucose per minute. This high metabolic activity is maintained by 1) a large number of free ribosomes and great total volume of the rough endoplasmic reticulum, reflecting a high rate of proteins' synthesis. Clumps of a just synthesized protein molecules are known as **Nissl bodies**; 2) a remarkably enlarged Golgi apparatus that accumulates and processes new proteins; 3) a very large number of mitochondria responsible for oxidation of glucose molecules and generation of energy (fig. 10.3).

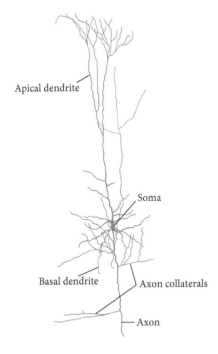

FIGURE 10.2   Pyramidal Neuron. Soma and Dendrites Are in Red; Axon Is Blue.

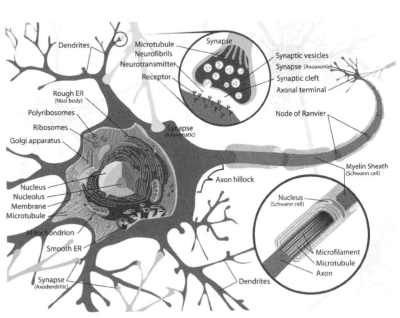

FIGURE 10.3   A Neuron Diagram.

A cytoskeleton is made of intermediate filaments combined into **neurofibrils**. Neurofibrils provide structural support of the cell body and extend into dendrites and axon. Beside structural function, the cytoskeleton plays the role of a "railroad." It participates in the transport of chemicals on a long distance towards the tips of dendrites and axon. Some animals have axons about meters long. Supply of axon terminals with necessary substances on such long distances through diffusion is not effective. It may take days or even weeks to reach the tip of a long axon. Microtubules run along the axon and provide "tracks" for fast transportation. The motor proteins kinesin and dynein bind to microtubules and move cargoes. Vesicular cargoes move relatively fast (50–400 mm/day), whereas diffusion takes much more time (about 8 mm/day).

VETERINARY APPLICATION

Retrograde transport moves substances and particles from axon terminals toward the cell body. Retrograde axonal transport is mediated by the motor protein dynein and is used to send chemical messages and some products back to the cell body. The retrograde transport can cover 10–20 centimeters per day.

Some pathogens exploit this process to invade the nervous system. They enter the distal tips on an axon and travel to the soma by retrograde transport. Examples include tetanus toxin, the herpes simplex, rabies, and polio viruses. In these infections, the delay (latent period) between infection and the onset of symptoms corresponds to the time needed for the pathogens to reach the cell body.

Dendrites are "receiving" extensions of neuron. Typically, they are short, highly branched, and look like a tree, which suggested the name for these projections. They receive input and transmit it to the cell body. The cytoplasm of dendrites contains the same organelles as the cytoplasm of the cell body. Plasma membrane of dendrites bears numerous receptor proteins with sodium and potassium gated channels and sensitive to different neurotransmitters. Dendrites can grow and branch throughout entire neuron life. Recent studies demonstrate that growth and "pruning" of dendrites is increased during learning. It is now accepted that branching and creation of new connections between neurons is a major way of development of new skills and long-term memory.

A neuron may have only one axon, also called a **nerve fiber**. An axon is an extension of the cell body that can generate and conduct action potential. Usually, the axon conducts this action potential from the cell body to the distal end of axon. However, there are some neurons whose axon may conduct action potential in both directions. The area of the cell where axon arises is called **axon hillock** (fig. 10.3). It is an enlarged part of the axon. The plasma membrane or **axolemma** of the axon hillock carries a huge number of voltage-gated sodium and potassium channels, which is necessary for generation of action potential (see chapter 9, page 247). The slender axon fiber greatly varies in length. Thus, a motor neuron that innervates muscles of the foot in elephants or giraffes is located in the lumbar region of spinal cord, whereas effector muscles are a meter away. Close to the distal part, the axon may have branches that arise at a right angle to the main axis of the axon. These branches are called **axon collaterals**. At the ends, the axon and its collaterals split into tiny fine branches known as **telodendria**. On the tip of the telodendria there is an **axon terminal** or **synaptic knob** that communicates with another neuron or effector organ. Usually, an axon has 1,000 or more axon terminals.

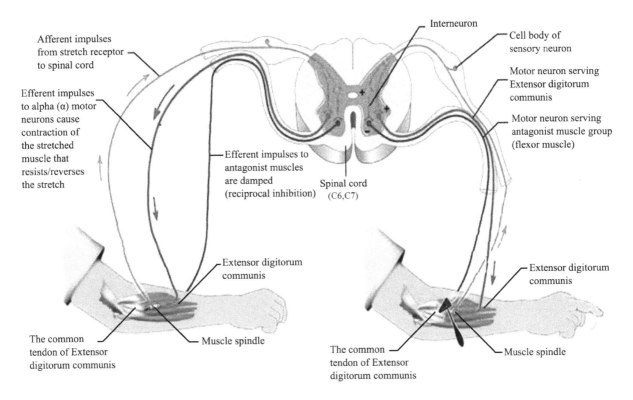

FIGURE 10.4   Simple Spinal Reflex Arc Made of a Sensory Neuron, Interneuron, and Motor Neuron.

Neurons are classified in three functional groups: sensory, motor, and interneurons. Neurons that collect sensory information from receptors and conduct this information to the CNS are called **sensory** or **afferent neurons**. Neurons that conduct nerve impulse from CNS to the effector organ on the periphery of the body are called **motor** or **efferent neurons**. Neurons of the CNS that connect sensory and motor neuron are called **interneurons** or **association neurons** (fig. 10.4).

Neurons are divided in three groups, according their shape or structural organization:

1. **Multipolar neurons** have many branched dendrites. Most of the interneurons in the brain and spinal cord belong to this group. Altogether, 99 percent of body neurons are of this type.
2. **Bipolar neurons** have only two processes: one dendrite and one axon. Bipolar neurons are a rare type of neurons. They are found in the retina of the eye and the olfactory epithelium in the nasal cavity.
3. **Pseudounipolar neurons** formerly were called unipolar neurons. However, recent studies show that these neurons begin their development as a bipolar neuron and later dendrite and axon fuse and create a one single process that later splits in two branches. These two branches are called peripheral process and central process. The majority of sensory neurons belong to this type (fig. 10.5).

Different kinds of neurons

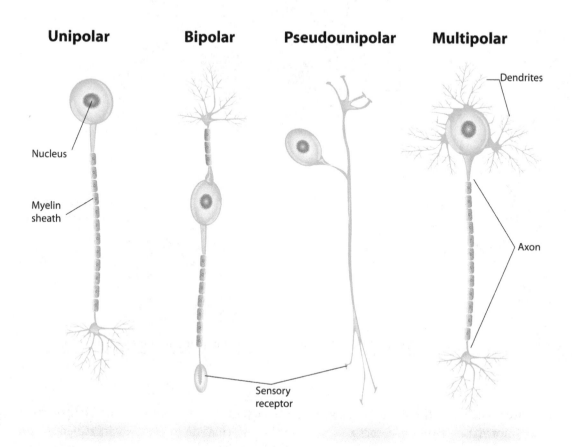

FIGURE 10.5   Three Morpho-Functional Types of Neurons.

CHECK YOUR UNDERSTANDING

- What is the function of a dendrite?

- What is the difference between multi-polar and pseudounipolar neurons?

- Describe the functional differences between motor and sensory neurons.

10.3   Electrophysiology of Neuron

Neurons have two principal properties: **excitability** and **conductivity**. Excitability is an ability to respond to different stimuli, such as chemical, electrical, and mechanical, by changing the resting membrane potential of the cell membrane. Conductivity is an ability to conduct electrical changes across the plasma membrane. At rest neuron has a resting membrane potential. The resting membrane potential is generated by the sodium-potassium pump (Na^+/K^+ pump; see chapter 9, page 245). Na^+/K^+ pump transports Na^+ ions out of the cell and K^+ ions inside the cell. As a result of this activity, the external extracellular fluid becomes positively charged compare to internal cytosol (fig. 10.6).

The electrical changes that may happen with the resting membrane potential are of two types: 1) **local potential** is a change of the membrane potential that travels a short distance and disappears with increased distance; 2) **action potential** that, once generated, propagates along the axon with the same strength until it reaches the axon terminal.

Often the stimulus is weak and cannot create an action potential, but it still generates a small local change in the membrane potential. Such small local changes in the resting membrane potential are called **graded potential**. They vary in strength and in degree of change in resting membrane potential. However, they do not have enough strength to generate an action potential, and the membrane soon returns to the resting membrane potential.

There are three principal differences between the local potential changes and action potential:

1.   The local potential is graded; that is, it generates changes in the membrane potential of different degree. Action potential always has the same strength that equal to maximum depolarization the neuron can generate. In other words, action potential develops as an **all-or-none** event: if action potential

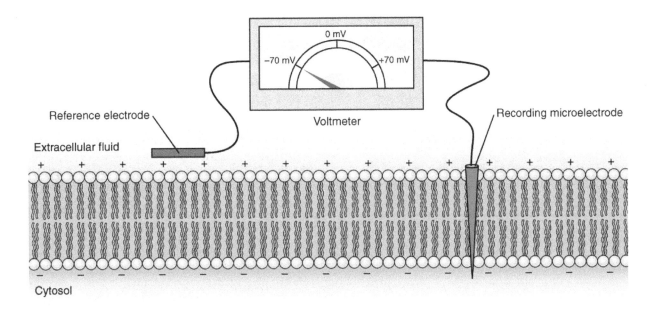

FIGURE 10.6   The Resting Membrane Potential.

happens, it develops in complete strength or does not happen at all. The local potential is a change of membrane potential of any strength and does not follow the all-or none principle. The action potential may happen only when the stimulus reaches a **threshold level** and, when the threshold level of depolarization is reached, the action potential develops in the full strength. The local potential depends on the strength, size, or frequency of stimuli. Strength of the local potential depends on the strength of the stimulus. The action potential does not depend of the stimulus. It always has the same strength of depolarization, and it does not matter how strong, long, or frequent the stimuli are.

2. The local potential is reversible. Once the stimulation of the neuron stops, ion channels immediately close, local potential disappears, and resting membrane potential restores. On the other hand, the action potential is irreversible: once develops it cannot be stopped and has to proceed completely.

3. The local potential never proceeds for a long distance. Local potential decreases and disappears in a short distance. The action potential does not decrease its strength with distance and proceeds until it reaches the axon terminal. This property makes the action potential a physical foundation of the nerve impulse, which is simply a wave of action potential propagated on a long distance (fig. 10.7).

When a neuron fires an action potential, it sequentially opens its voltage-gated ion channels, and to restore the resting membrane potential, first of all, these channels have to be closed. The closing of voltage-gated channels takes a time. Any new incoming signal cannot generate a new action potential until voltage-gated channels, at least partially, will not be closed. During the period of closing voltage gated channels, the neuron is not sensitive to new incoming signals. A brief period, when the neuron is not responsive and cannot fire a new action potential, is called the **refractory period**. The refractory period has two phases: the **absolute refractory period** and **relative refractory period**. Absolute refractory period is characterized by the complete absence of ability to fire new action potential, no matter how strong the new stimuli are. This period continues until at least some sodium voltage-gated channels return to the rest state. The relative refractory period follows the absolute refractory period. It is characterized by increased ability to fire an action potential in response to high intensity stimuli. Relative refractory period begins when the sodium voltage gated channels already are close, but potassium voltage channels are still open.

The nerve impulse is a wave of an action potential propagated along the axon. Action potential propagates mostly in one direction, from the trigger zone on the axon hillock toward the axon terminal. Opening of the voltage gated channels in the trigger zone, where these ion channel proteins are most dense, causes nearby voltage-gated ion channels to open. Their opening generates depolarization of the membrane around and, when the depolarization reaches the threshold level, all nearby voltage-gated channels open. This leads to the further depolarization and further opening of voltage-gated channels,

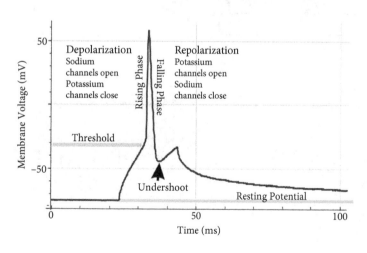

FIGURE 10.7   Action Membrane Potential.

and so on, until the wave reaches the end of the axon. You may compare it with a line of dominoes. When the first domino falls, it hits the next one, and it falls. The fall of the second triggers the fall of the next, and so on, until the last domino in the line falls. To initiate this process, you only have to push the first domino and the process continues by itself. Propagation of the action potential proceeds in one direction, because the membrane in the previous section—that is, behind the action potential—at that time is still in a refractory period.

At the end, axon terminal creates a junction with other neuron or effector organ, for example a skeletal muscle, called **synapse**. It is very rare that membranes of both neurons have direct physical contact. This kind synapse is called **electrical synapse**. An electrical synapse is created by a gap junction between plasma membranes of two neurons. Electrical synapse creates a link that conducts an action potential from one neuron to the other. However, in most cases, neurons are separated by a gap called **synaptic cleft**. Thus, synapse has three elements: 1) plasma membrane of the axon terminal, called **presynaptic membrane**; 2) synaptic cleft; and 3) plasma membrane of receiving signal neuron, called **postsynaptic membrane**. Special molecules called **neurotransmitters** carry signals between neurons. This type of synapse is called **chemical synapse**. You are already familiar with one neurotransmitter—acetylcholine (ACh). Scientists have discovered more than 60 different neurotransmitters. These molecules belong to different chemical compound types, such as amino acids (glutamate, aspartate, D-serine, γ-aminobutyric acid, and glycine),

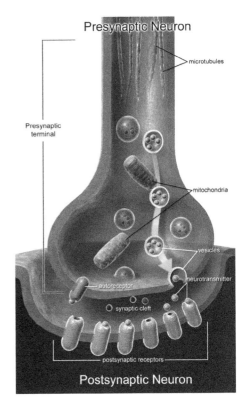

gases (nitric oxide and carbon monoxide), monoamines (dopamine, norepinephrine, epinephrine, histamine, and serotonin), and many others. Neurotransmitters are stored in **synaptic vesicles** in axon terminal of the presynaptic neuron. Plasma membrane of the postsynaptic neuron has **receptors**: proteins that create chemical bonds with neurotransmitters. Receptors are linked with ion channels, so when neurotransmitter binds with receptor, it causes opening of ion channels and leads to a local potential change in the postsynaptic membrane.

In general, the process of nerve impulse transition from one neuron to the other can be described in four steps:

1. An action potential of the presynaptic neuron reaches axon terminal, where it triggers opening of Ca^{2+} voltage-gated channels.
2. Ca^{2+} enters the cytoplasm of axon terminal and cause synaptic vesicles to release a neurotransmitter into the synaptic cleft by exocytosis.
3. Molecules of neurotransmitter diffuse across the synaptic cleft and bind with receptors in the postsynaptic membrane.
4. The binding of neurotransmitters to the receptors opens ion channels and causes local membrane potential changes (fig. 10.8).

FIGURE 10.8 Nerve Impulse Transition in Synapse.

VETERINARY APPLICATION

In mammals, carbon monoxide is naturally produced by the action of heme oxygenase 1 and 2 in the process of he-moglobin breakdown. In 1993 it was found that together with nitric oxide and hydrogen sulfide, carbon monoxide is a normal neurotransmitter. In many tissues, all three gases are known to act as anti-inflammatories and vasodilators.

There is a hypothesis that in some synapses that participate in development of a long-term memory, the receiving cells make carbon monoxide. In response to a new signal, the receiving neuron releases carbon monoxide and back-transmits it to the presynaptic neuron. This back transmitting of carbon monoxide plays role of a message that tells to transmit signals more readily in future. It was shown that some such neurons contain guanylate cyclase, an enzyme that is activated by carbon monoxide.

The local membrane potential may or may not lead to development of the action potential in the post-synaptic neuron. An action potential develops only when the local membrane potential in the postsynaptic neuron (called **postsynaptic potential**) reaches a threshold level. Any postsynaptic membrane potential change that brings the membrane potential closer to the threshold level is called **excitatory postsynaptic potential (EPSP)**. The local membrane potential changes in the postsynaptic neuron, which leads to hyperpolarization and decreases chance to reach the threshold level, is called **inhibitory postsynaptic potential (IPSP)**. When postsynaptic potential hits the threshold level, postsynaptic neurons generate their own action potential. The summation of local postsynaptic potential may result from two events: spatial and temporal summations. Under spatial summation specialists designate a situation when some number of presynaptic neurons simultaneously send their signals to the postsynaptic cell. Temporal summation results from frequent stimulation of the postsynaptic neuron by the same presynaptic cell when stimuli overlap and finally reach threshold level.

The synaptic transmission of nerve impulse is terminated when the neurotransmitters are removed from the synaptic cleft. It may happen in three ways:

1. Diffusion: some neurotransmitters simply diffuse away from the synaptic cleft into the interstitial fluid.
2. Degradation: some neurotransmitters are degraded in the synaptic cleft by enzyme. For example, ACh is degraded by acetylcholinesterase.
3. Reuptake: some neurotransmitters are removed from the synaptic cleft by transporting them back into the synaptic vesicles of presynaptic neuron.

Neurons are organized into functional groups. They create networks called **neuronal pools** and **neuronal circuits**. Neuronal pool is an anatomic or structural characteristic. It includes all neurons connected through their dendrites and axons, even when the cell bodies may be located in the different parts of the nervous system (in the brain and spinal cord, for example). The neuronal circuit is a functional characteristic of the neuronal network. It characterizes the pathway of nerve signals along the network.

- What is resting membrane potential?

- What do the terms *depolarization*, *repolarization*, and *hyperpolarization* mean?

- What is local potential, and why it is also called graded potential?

- Give the definition of action potential.

- Explain the difference between absolute and relative refractory periods.

10.4   Neuroglia

Neuroglia cells have many functions that may be characterized as maintenance of stable environment around neurons, protection, and assistance in functioning. Neuroglia cells are able to undergo mitosis and may fill the vacant space when neuron dies. There are six major types of neuroglia cells: two types are found in the PNS and four in CNS.

The four glial cells of the CNS are **astrocytes**, **oligodendrocytes**, **microglia**, and **ependymal cells**. Astrocytes get their name from their star-shaped cell body (fig. 10.9.A). The cell has cytoplasmic extensions ended with end-feet. The membrane of the end-foot contacts with wall of the blood vessel or plasma membrane of the neuron. Transport proteins in the membrane of the end-feet move oxygen, carbon dioxide, nutrients, and waste products between blood flow and neuron. This transport activity creates neuron-blood barrier. The astrocyte holds neuron at some distance from blood vessels. Astrocytes regulate ion balance and absorb neurotransmitters from the extracellular fluid. Astrocytes are mitotically active cells. When the damaged neurons die, astrocytes fill freed space and create a scar. The overactive astrocytes may cause development of pathological processes such as astrocytoma.

Aged and old dogs may develop a brain tumor. The tumor may be a meningioma or glioma. The gliomas are the most frequent in dogs. Astrocytoma is the most common glioma tumor that may develop everywhere in the brain or spinal cord. There are five forms of astrocytoma:

- Grade I: **Pilocytic astrocytoma**
- Grade II: **Diffuse astrocytoma/low-grade astrocytoma**
- Grade III: **Anaplastic astrocytoma**
- Grade IV: **Glioblastomas** (also called glioblastoma multiforme, GBM, or grade IV astrocytoma). Anaplastic astrocytoma is malignant and accounts for more than 50 percent of all astrocytomas. This tumor grows and spreads very aggressively.

Brain stem gliomas arise in the brain stem. A tumor in this area is difficult to treat. The most common brain stem gliomas are high-grade astrocytomas. Symptoms of brain tumor (astrocytoma) in dogs include 1) abnormal pupil reflex to light, 2) seizures from mild to severe, 3) anorexia, 4) loss of appetite, 5) collapse, 6) nystagmus, 7) circling, 8) disorientation, 9) blindness, 10) head pressing, and 11) dyspnea.

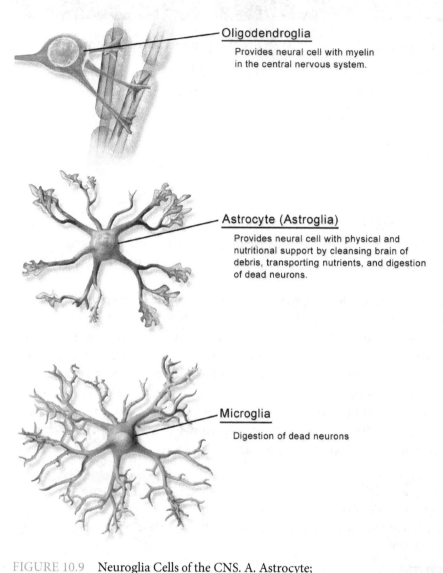

Oligodendroglia
Provides neural cell with myelin in the central nervous system.

Astrocyte (Astroglia)
Provides neural cell with physical and nutritional support by cleansing brain of debris, transporting nutrients, and digestion of dead neurons.

Microglia
Digestion of dead neurons

FIGURE 10.9   Neuroglia Cells of the CNS. A. Astrocyte; B. Oligodendrocyte; C. Microglia.

Oligodendrocytes also have cytoplasmic extensions (fig. 10.9.B). Some of these extensions are flattened at the end. These flattened ends wrap around the axon and create a concentric layer known as **myelin**. A sequence of myelin segments covering the axon is called a **myelin sheath**. Each oligodendrocyte has several projections and creates myelin around axons of many neurons (figs. 10.11; 10.12.C).

Microglia originates from white blood cells monocytes. They are phagocytes—wandering cells that clean and digest pathogenic agents, disease-causing organisms, dead cells, and cellular debris (fig. 10.9.C).

Ependymal cells line cavities filled with **cerebrospinal fluid (CSF)** inside the CNS. They have cilia, whose wavy movements create a slow flow of the CSF within the brain **ventricles** and **central canal** of the spinal cord. These cells participate in formation of the CSF and monitor its composition (fig. 10.11).

In the PNS there are two types of glial cells: **Schwann** and **satellite cells**. Schwann cells create myelin sheath around axons in the PNS. They also play principal role in repairing of damaged axons in the PNS.

Satellite cells are flat cells like shingles that cover bodies of neurons in the PNS. Their role in the PNS remains unknown. However, it is known that these cells create isolation and protection of neurons in the PNS (figs. 10.10; 10.11).

Oligodendrocytes and Schwann cells create myelin sheath around axons: oligodendrocytes in the CNS and Schwann cells in the PNS (fig. 10.12). Myelin is composed of plasma membranes of these cells many times wrapped around axon. Like plasma membranes of other cells, the plasma membrane of oligodendrocytes and

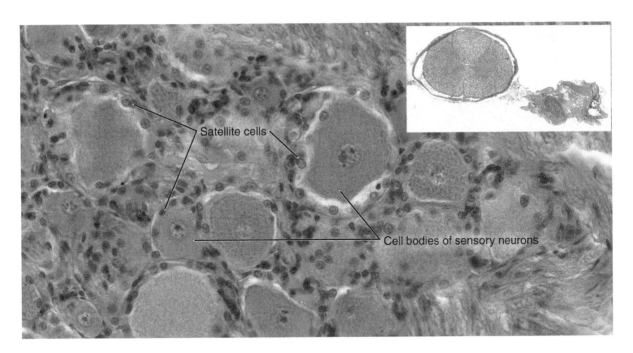

FIGURE 10.10   Satellite Cells in Dorsal Root Ganglion Covered Bodies of Sensory Neurons.

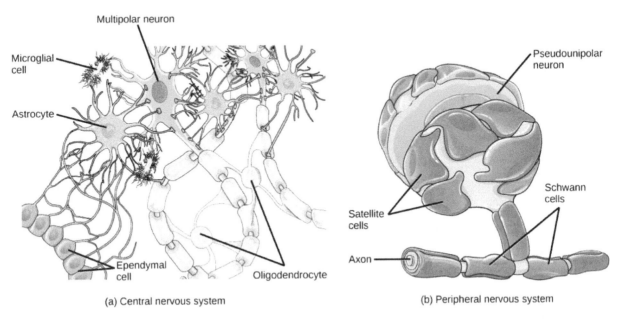

FIGURE 10.11   Neuroglia Cells.

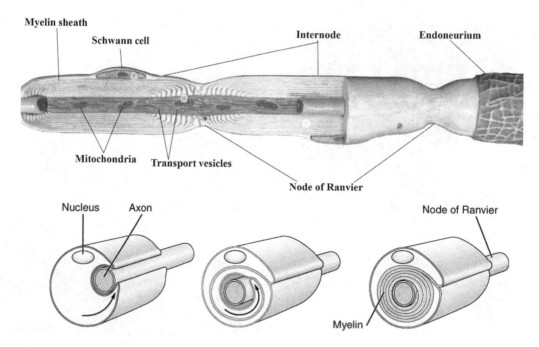

FIGURE 10.12   Myelin Sheath in the CNS Made by: A. Oligodendrocytes, and the PNS Made by B. Schwann Cells. Difference between C. Oligodendrocyte and D. Schwann Cell Myelination Process.

Schwann cells is made of a phospholipid bilayer with inclusions of cholesterol and glycoprotein called myelin. Plasma membrane of oligodendrocytes and Schwann cells is also different from other cells by the total amount of fat in their membranes that constitutes 70 to 80 percent. Fat molecules of the myelin sheath prevent movement of electrically charged ions that makes myelin a perfect insulator. Thus, the **internodes**—a portion of axon covered by myelin—are completely isolated from the interstitial fluid. The movement of sodium and potassium ions across the plasma membrane in this region is not possible. As a matter of fact, internodes have no Na^+, K^+ and other ion channels. As a result, the myelinated axon regions cannot generate an action potential. All voltage-gated channels of the myelinated axons are concentrated in the **nodes of Ranvier**—unmyelinated portions of the axon between two myelinated internodes. Myelination and patched distribution of voltage-gated channels on the nodes of Ranvier cause action potentials are generated only in nodes of Ranvier and skip internodes. You may compare the propagation of the nerve impulse in myelinated axons with jumps of the action potential from one node of Ranvier to the next. This type of nerve impulse conduction is called **saltatory conduction** (fig. 10.13). Saltatory conduction increases the speed of the nerve impulse propagation 15 to 150 times. Because fat molecules in general have a white waxy color, myelinated nerve fibers also have a white color, whereas the neuron's body and dendrites are gray. Thus, **white matter** of the nervous tissue is made of myelinated axons, whereas **gray matter** consists of dendrites and neuron bodies.

Among other factors that influence the speed of the nerve impulse is the diameter of an axon. The general rule states that axons with a larger diameter have a higher speed of nerve impulse conduction than axons with a smaller diameter. When small unmyelinated fibers conduct impulses 0.5 to 2.0 m/s, small, myelinated fibers conduct nerve impulse 3 to 15.0 m/s, and large myelinated

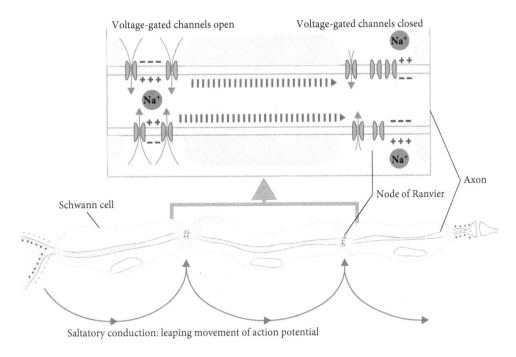

Voltage-gated channels open

Voltage-gated channels closed

Na⁺

Schwann cell

Node of Ranvier

Axon

Saltatory conduction: leaping movement of action potential

FIGURE 10.13   Saltatory Conduction of Nerve Impulse.

fibers—up to 120 m/s. Different organs are innervated by different nerve fibers. Thus, slow signals supply the stomach and dilate pupil where speed is less of an issue. At the same time, reflexes associated with body balance, for example knee jerk reflex, are supplied by thick myelinated fibers with the highest velocity of nerve impulses. According the speed of the nerve impulse conduction, axons are classified in three groups:

1. **Type A fibers** are the largest and myelinated fibers. They conduct the fastest nerve impulses. They serve where the high speed of nerve impulse is vital: sensory neurons and some skeletal muscles.
2. **Type B fibers** are intermediate by diameter and usually myelinated. In most found in the autonomic nervous system associated with glands.
3. **Type C fibers** are smallest and unmyelinated. They have low conduction speed and are associated with autonomic nervous system and some sensory axons that transmit pain, temperature, and pressure sensations.

CHECK YOUR UNDERSTANDING

- What functions do astrocytes have?

- What is the function of microglia?

- What is the difference between myelin made by oligodendrocyte and by Schwann cell?

- Why is the speed of nerve impulse conduction higher in myelinated axons than in unmyelinated?

CHAPTER SUMMARY

- The principal function of the nervous system is to create a harmonious functioning of the organism. The nervous system monitors the status of every organ, collects and analyze changes in internal and external environment, and sends instructions to organs. The nervous system is a key system responsible for successful maintaining of homeostasis.

- The nervous system has two parts: the **central nervous system (CNS)** and **peripheral nervous system (PNS)**. The CNS consists of **brain** and **spinal cord**. The PNS includes **nerves** and **ganglia**. PNS carries **sensory** and **motor functions**. The CNS has **integrative function**. The PNS has **sensory** and **motor divisions**. The sensory division is subdivided in somatic and visceral divisions; and the motor division is subdivided in somatic and visceral (**autonomic nervous system**, or **ANS**) divisions.

- Nervous tissue consists of **neurons** and **neuroglia (glia)** cells. A neuron has a cell body—**neurosoma, dendrites**— cellular projections that receive and deliver signals to the neurosoma; and an **axon**—a single projection that takes signal away from the neurosoma. The plasma membrane of dendrites bears receptor proteins with ion gated channels.

- An axon is an extension of the cell body that generates and conducts action potential. Axons arise from an **axon hillock**. The **axolemma** of an axon hillock carries a huge number of voltage-gated sodium and potassium channels, which is necessary for generation of action potential. The distal part of the axon may have branches called **axon collaterals**. At the ends, the axon and its collaterals splits into fine branches called **telodendria**. The tip of every telodendria has axon terminals, or **synaptic knobs.**

- Neurons are classified in three functional groups: sensory, motor, and interneurons. Sensory (afferent) neurons collect sensory information from receptors and conduct this information to the CNS. Motor (efferent) neurons conduct motor commands from the CNS to the effector organs. Interneurons connect sensory and motor neurons. By shape neurons are divided in three groups: multipolar neurons have many dendrites; bipolar neurons have only two processes: one dendrite and one axon; and pseudounipolar neurons have only one single projection that has two ends: axon and dendrite.

- Neurons have two properties: **excitability** and **conductivity**. Excitability is ability to response on stimuli. Conductivity is ability to conduct electrical changes across the plasma membrane. At rest neuron has a resting membrane potential generated by the sodium-potassium pump (Na^+/K^+ pump). The electrical changes that happen with the resting membrane potential are of two types: 1) **local potential** and 2) **action potential**.

- Action potential always has the same strength that equal to maximum depolarization. Action potential develops as an **all-or-none** event: if action potential happens, it develops in complete strength or does not develops at all. The action potential may happen only when the stimulus reaches a **threshold level**. Local potential is graded. It generates changes in the membrane potential of different degree. The local potential is reversible. Once the stimulation of the neuron stops, ion channels close and local potential disappears. Local potential never proceeds for a long distance.

- A brief period, when a neuron is not responsive and cannot fire a new action potential, is called **refractory period**. The refractory period has two phases: **absolute refractory period** and **relative refractory period**.

- The nerve impulse is a wave of an action potential moving along the axon. Action potential propagates in one direction from the trigger zone on the axon hillock toward the axon terminal. At the end, the axon terminal has a junction with other neurons or an effector organ called a **synapse**. There are two types of synapses: **electrical** and **chemical synapse**. An electrical synapse has a gap junction between membranes of two neurons. Electrical synapse creates a link that conducts an action potential from one neuron to the other. In chemical synapses neurons are separated by a gap called **synaptic cleft**. This synapse has three elements: 1) the plasma membrane of the axon terminal, called the **presynaptic membrane**; 2) a synaptic cleft; and 3) the plasma membrane of the neuron that receives the signal, called the **postsynaptic membrane**. Special molecules of **neurotransmitters** carry signals between neurons. Neurotransmitters are stored in **synaptic vesicles** in axon terminal of the presynaptic neuron. Plasma membrane of the postsynaptic neuron has **receptor** proteins that bind with neurotransmitters. Receptors are linked with ion channels, and when a neurotransmitter binds with a receptor, the ion channels open and the postsynaptic membrane depolarizes.

- Action potential develops only when the local membrane potential in the postsynaptic neuron (called **postsynaptic potential**) reaches threshold level. A postsynaptic potential that brings the membrane potential closer to the threshold level is called **excitatory postsynaptic potential (EPSP)**. The local membrane potential changes in the postsynaptic neuron, which leads to hyperpolarization and decreases chance to reach the threshold level, is called **inhibitory postsynaptic potential (IPSP)**.

- Neurons are organized in functional groups: **neuronal pools** and **neuronal circuits**. Neuronal pool is an anatomic or structural characteristic. It includes all neurons connected through their dendrites and axons. The neuronal circuit is a functional characteristic of the neuronal network. It characterizes the pathway of nerve signals.

- There are four glial cells in the CNS: **astrocytes**, **oligodendrocytes**, **microglia**, and **ependymal cells**. Astrocytes create a neuron-blood barrier. They regulate ion balance and absorb neurotransmitters from the extracellular fluid. Astrocytes are mitotically active cells and create a scar after neurons' death. Oligodendrocytes create concentric layers of **myelin** around axons in the CNS. Microglia are phagocytes. They clean and digest pathogenic agents, disease-causing organisms, dead cells, and cellular debris. Ependymal cells line cavities filled with the **cerebrospinal fluid (CSF)** inside the CNS. They have cilia, which biting creates a slow movement of the CSF within the **ventricles** of the brain and **central canal** of the spinal cord. They form and control composition of the CSF.

- There are two types of glia cells in the PNS: **Schwann cells** and **satellite cells**. Schwann cells create myelin sheath around axons in the PNS. They also play principal role in repairing of damaged axons. Satellite cells are flat cells that like a shingles covers bodies of neurons in the PNS. These cells create isolation and protection of neurons in the PNS.

- Myelin is composed of plasma membranes of oligodendrocytes and Schwann cells wrapped around axon. About 70 to 80 percent of plasma membrane of these cells is phospholipids, cholesterol, and glycoprotein myelin. The **internodes**—a portion of axon covered by myelin—are completely isolated from the interstitial fluid. The movement of sodium and potassium ions across the plasma membrane in this region is not possible. As a result, the internodes cannot generate an action potential. All voltage-gated channels of myelinated axons are concentrated in **nodes of Ranvier**—unmyelinated parts of axon between internodes and action potentials are generated only in nodes of Ranvier. The result: nerve impulse in myelinated fibers jumps from one node of Ranvier to the next. This type of nerve impulse conduction is called **saltatory conduction**. Saltatory conduction increases the speed of the nerve impulse propagation 15 to 150 times. Fat molecules in general have white waxy color and myelinated axons also have white color. The neuron's body and dendrites have gray color. Thus, **white matter** of the nervous tissue is myelinated axons, whereas **gray matter** is dendrites and neurosomas.

- The diameter of the axon also effects speed of nerve impulse conduction. Axons with bigger diameter have higher speed of nerve impulse than axons with smaller diameter. Small unmyelinated fibers conduct impulses with speed 0.5 to 2.0 m/s; small myelinated fibers conduct impulses with a speed 3 to 15.0 m/s; large myelinated fibers conduct impulses with speed up to 120 m/s.

CHECK YOUR KNOWLEDGE

LEVEL I. CHECK YOUR RECALL

1. The neuron's extensions that form a major surface for reception of external signals are:
   A. Myelin sheath
   B. Collaterals
   C. Axon terminals
   D. Nissl bodies
   E. Dendrites

2. Neurons are connected each other through:
   A. Synapse
   B. Node of Ranvier
   C. Myelin sheath
   D. Terminal button
   E. Soma

3. Which of the following is a neuroglia cell of the PNS?
   A. Astrocyte
   B. Oligodendrocyte
   C. Schwann cell
   D. Microglia
   E. Ependymal cell

4. Brain and spinal cord together form:
   A. Autonomic nervous system
   B. Peripheral nervous system
   C. Sensory division of the nervous system
   D. Motor division of the nervous system
   E. Central nervous system

5. How does myelination affect the propagation of an action potential?
   A. It speeds propagation by increasing the density of voltage-gated channels at nodes of Ranvier.
   B. It speeds propagation by increasing electrochemical gradients favoring Na⁺ entry.
   C. It slows down propagation because Na⁺ channels exist only at nodes of Ranvier.
   D. It slows down propagation because myelin sheath isolates axon and prevents ion movement across axon membrane.

6. In a neuron, what creates the electrochemical gradient, a resting membrane potential?
   A. Voltage-gated K^+ channels
   B. Na^+/K^+ ATPase (pump)
   C. Voltage-gated Na^+ channels
   D. Ligand-gated Na^+/K^+ channels
   E. Leaking channels for Ca^{2+}

7. Neurons completely located within the CNS are termed:
   A. Afferent neurons
   B. Efferent neurons
   C. Motor neurons
   D. Interneurons
   E. Sensory neurons

8. The areas of the neuron most densely impregnated with voltage-gated ion channels are:
   A. Dendrites
   B. Neurosoma plasma membrane
   C. Nodes of Ranvier
   D. Internodes
   E. Synaptic knobs

9. The glial cells responsible for immune defense within the CNS are:
   A. Microglia
   B. Satellite cells
   C. Ependymal cells
   D. Oligodendrocytes
   E. Astrocytes

10. Saltatory conduction is characteristic of:
    A. Chemical synapses only
    B. Electrical synapses only
    C. Axon hillock only
    D. Myelinated axons only
    E. Unmyelinated axons only

11. Nerve cells that collect information from receptors are called:
    A. Sensory neurons
    B. Motor neurons
    C. Interneurons
    D. Efferent neurons
    E. Multipolar neurons

12. The nerve cell that conduct nerve impulse away from the CNS is called:
    A. Afferent
    B. Efferent
    C. Sensory
    D. Interneuron
    E. Unipolar neuron

13. The area on the neuron cell membrane where the action potentials are generated is:
    A. Dendrite terminal
    B. Axon terminal
    C. Membrane of the soma
    D. Axon hillock

14. Why do biologists say that positive feedback occurs during action potential?
    A. The action potential is an all-or-none event, meaning that once starts, it goes to end.
    B. The opening of K^+ channels repolarizes the membrane, making it less likely that Na^+ channels will open and depolarize the membrane.
    C. Once sodium channels open and membrane starts to depolarize, it is more likely that more channels will open and the wave of depolarization runs along the axon.

15. True or false: Cranial nerves are part of the central nervous system.
16. True or false: In the CNS, the myelin sheath is created by oligodendrocytes, whereas in the PNC it is created by Schwann cells.
17. True or false: As a rule, motor neurons are multipolar, whereas sensory neurons are pseudounipolar.
18. True or false: During the refractory period, the voltage-gated sodium channels are not in their resting state.
19. Fill in the blanks: The _____ is the period of time when the neuron completely unable generate a new action potential, whereas the _____ is the period when a larger-than-normal stimulus is required to elicit a new action potential.
    A. action potential; graded potential
    B. absolute refractory period; relative refractory period
    C. postsynaptic potential; presynaptic potential
    D. excitatory potential; inhibitory potential
    E. threshold level; subthreshold level

20. The segment of an axon covered by myelin is called _____, whereas the segment of an axon between two myelinated regions is called _____.
    A. postsynaptic membrane; presynaptic membrane
    B. presynaptic membrane; postsynaptic membrane
    C. internode; node of Ranvier
    D. node of Ranvier; internode
    E. telodendria; axon hillock

21. Match each neuroglia cell with its function:

    _____ Schwann cell   a. Phagocytes of the CNS.
    _____ Ependymal cell   b. Cells that cover neuron bodies in the PNS
    _____ Astrocyte   c. Cells that create myelin sheath in the PNS
    _____ Oligodendrocyte   d. Create nerve-blood barrier and maintain extracellular environment
    _____ Microglia   e. Cells that create a myelin sheath in the CNS
    _____ Satellite cell   f. Ciliated cells that line ventricles and central canal of the CNS

LEVEL 2. CHECK YOUR UNDERSTANDING

1. What would happen if a drug blocked sodium channels in the axon and dendrites?
2. Explain why salutatory conduction is much faster than continuous conduction.
3. Describe the main characteristics of an electrical synapse.

LEVEL 3. APPLY YOUR KNOWLEDGE TO REAL LIFE

1. During a surgery, an anesthesiologist administers an inhalation anesthetic agent that opens Cl⁻ channels in the postsynaptic membranes of the brain neurons. Explain why this will result in a deep sleep during the whole surgical procedure.
2. The drug **lidocaine** blocks sodium channels. Explain the mechanism of the numbing effect created by this drug.

Chapter 11

Overview of Anatomy and Physiology of the Nervous System

LEARNING OBJECTIVES

In this chapter you will learn about the anatomic organization of the nervous system. When you have finished reading it, you will have knowledge about:

1. Principal organs of the nervous system.

2. Structure and basic roles of organs of the central and peripheral nervous systems.

3. Organization of nervous system structures in functional groups.

4. Difference between somatic and autonomic nervous systems.

INTRODUCTION

The principal function of the nervous system is to unite organs into an organism through the control of their activity. The nervous system monitors the status of every organ, collects and analyzes information about vital changes in internal and external environment, and sends instructions to organs. In this chapter you will learn about the structure and functions of organs of the nervous system and how nervous system controls critical life functions. Effector organs include mechanical effectors, such as muscles, and chemical effectors, such as glands. Thus, the response of nervous system results in muscle contraction and glandular secretion.

11.1 Overview of CNS

The basic role of the CNS is processing sensory input information, making decision, and send commands through motor neurons to muscles or glands. That what is called integrative function. Interneurons responsible for this integrative function are multipolar neurons organized in two organs: brain and spinal cord. The border between brain and spinal cord is a line made by the edges of the foramen magnum. Groups of neurons create gray matter of the brain and spinal cord. The white matter is made of myelinated axons. In some areas of the brain, there are regions of white matter with inclusions of more or less big islands of gray matter. Such inclusions of gray matter inside the white matter are called **nuclei** (single nucleus). From the outside the CNS is covered by three

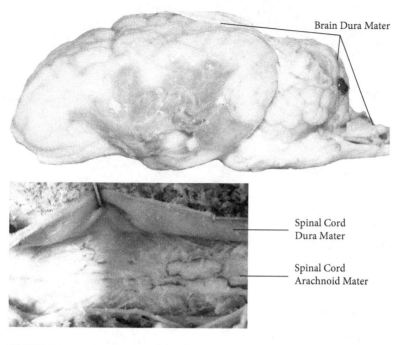

Brain Dura Mater

Spinal Cord
Dura Mater

Spinal Cord
Arachnoid Mater

FIGURE 11.1   Meninges of the Brain and Spinal Cord.

connective tissue membranes collectively known as meninges. The matrix of the outermost membrane contains collagen fibers that make it strong and tough. This membrane is called the **dura mater**. Beneath the dura mater is a web-like **arachnoid mater**. This membrane is carrying blood vessels that feed underlying tissues. The delicate **pia mater** covers the brain and spinal cord. Both the brain and spinal cord are hollow inside. Chambers of the brain are called **ventricles** and a single continuous hollow tube in the spinal cord is called **the central canal**. They are connected by one continuous pathway and filled with cerebrospinal fluid (CSF). CSF is produced by the **choroid plexus**, a small tufts of blood vessels associated with ependymal cells that project into ventricles (figs. 11.1–11.3).

The organization of the CNS is easy to understand by looking at nervous system development in embryogenesis. The nervous system develops from the ectoderm, a superficial cellular layer that covers a developing embryo. The dorsal part of the ectoderm creates a flattened stripe of cells along the

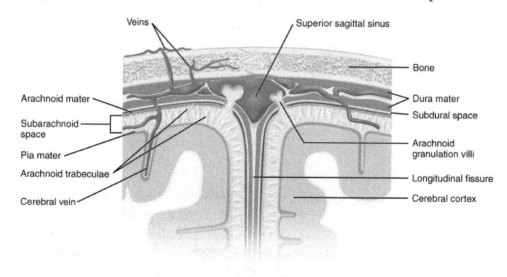

Veins

Superior sagittal sinus

Bone

Arachnoid mater

Dura mater

Subdural space

Subarachnoid space

Pia mater

Arachnoid granulation villi

Arachnoid trabeculae

Longitudinal fissure

Cerebral vein

Cerebral cortex

FIGURE 11.2   Diagram of Meninges.

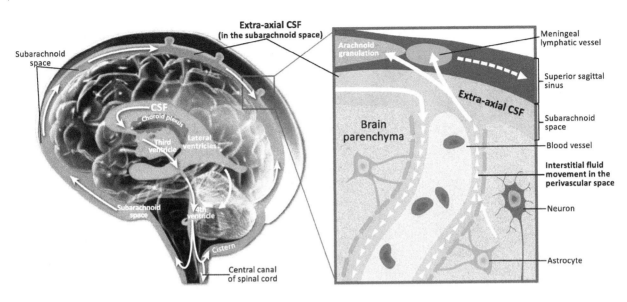

FIGURE 11.3   Ventricles of the Brain and Central Canal of Spinal Cord of Dog.

anterio-posterior axis of the embryo called the **neural plate**. Ectodermal cells move inside the growing embryo and the neural plate folds into groove. This groove continues to move deeper and deeper inside the body and, finally, folds into a tube. The tube closes from the dorsal side by remaining ectodermal cells. This tubular structure close to the dorsal surface is called the **neural tube**. The space inside the tube fills with fluid. The anterior portion of the neural tube later develops into brain, whereas its posterior part remains tubular and becomes the spinal cord. Some ectodermal cells organize into two longitudinal stripes on the both sides of the neural tube. These groups of cells are called **neural crest**. The neural crest gives rise to the ganglia and nerves of the PNS (fig. 11.4).

CHECK YOUR UNDERSTANDING

- What is the neural tube?

- Which structures generate cerebrospinal fluid?

- List and describe four brain ventricles.

- Name three meninges and explain their function, from superficial to deep.

11.2   Brain

In the brain, the central canal enlarges into continuous fluid-filled ventricles. The neural tube in the brain region also enlarges and differentiates into three regions: **forebrain**, **midbrain**, and **hindbrain**. Later, the forebrain develops into two structures: **cerebrum** and **diencephalon**. The midbrain remains, and the hindbrain develops into three regions: **cerebellum**, **pons**, and **medulla oblongata**. The midbrain, pons, and medulla oblongata together form the **brain stem** (fig. 11.8).

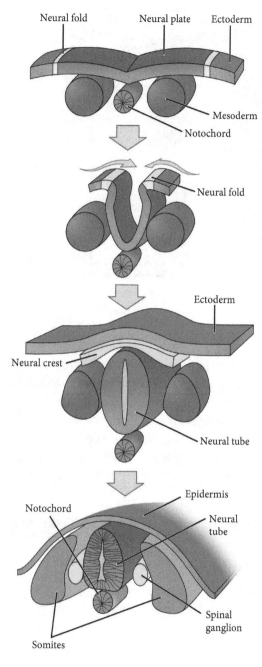

FIGURE 11.4   Nervous System Development (Neurulation).

The cerebrum is an anterior portion of the brain. Its gray matter creates a narrow superficial layer called the **cerebral cortex**. It has a pair of expanded lobes called **cerebral hemispheres** and **olfactory bulbs**. The subcortical region is made of white matter. The surface of the cerebral hemispheres is wavy. These waves are called **convolutions**. Ridges of convolutions are called **gyri** (singular **gyrus**) and shallow grooves between them—**sulci** (singular **sulcus**). However, in the platypus, opossum, and many rodents, the cerebral cortex is smooth. A few deep grooves named **fissure** separate cerebral hemispheres from each other (**longitudinal fissure**) and from cerebellum (**transverse fissure**). Two ventricles are located deep inside the cerebrum and called left and right **lateral ventricles**. Neurons of the left and right cerebral hemispheres communicate via big groups of myelinated axons that create a well visible white colored structures called **commissures**. The biggest commissure is named the **corpus callosum**. The corpus callosum is found only in eutherian mammals and absent among other vertebrates (fig. 11.5). Each hemisphere is divided into five areas or lobes. The anterior lobe, which lays under the frontal bone is known as a **frontal lobe**. It is separated from the other cortex areas by a **central sulcus**. Anterior to the central sulcus lays **precentral gyrus**, which houses motor neurons that control all skeletal muscles of the body. That is why this region has the name **primary motor center**. Posterior to the central sulcus is the **parietal lobe**. The most anterior gyrus of the parietal lobe located along the central sulcus is called the **postcentral gyrus**. It functions as a **primary sensory center** that accumulates a sensory cutaneous input from the whole body. The **temporal lobe** is located above the temporal bone on the lateral side of the hemisphere. It is separated from the frontal lobe by a **lateral fissure**.

Neurons of this lobe process hearing information. The **occipital lobe** occupies the posterior position. It is separated from the parietal lobe by the **parieto-occipital sulcus**. The occipital lobe is a primary center of procession visual information. The **insula** is separated from other lobes. It resides deep inside the cerebrum. Its neurons are associated with taste receptors and internal organs.

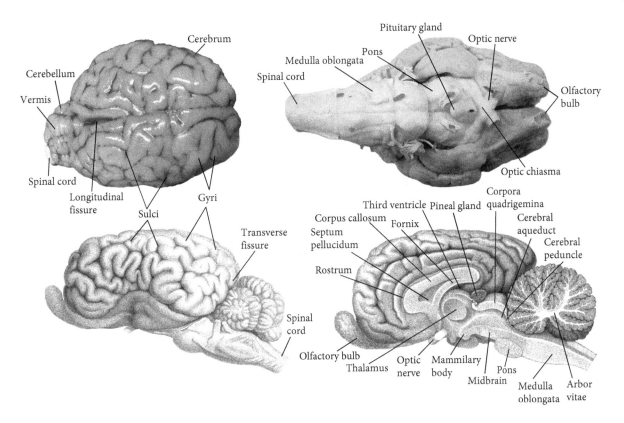

FIGURE 11.5   Sheep Brain in Dorsal, Ventral, and Lateral View, and Midsagittal Section.

Basal nuclei are groups of neurons in the floor of the cerebrum surrounded by white matter. From the diencephalon they are separated by a mass of white matter called internal capsule. The principal basal nuclei are **caudate nucleus, putamen**, and **globus pallidus** (fig. 11.6). These nuclei receive sensory input from **substantia nigra**: a nucleus in the midbrain. The basal nuclei control movement. They integrate information on body position and motivation state, and transforms it in motor activity or inhibition of inappropriate movements. Pathological process in basal nuclei may cause involuntary movements known as dyskinesias (Parkinson's disease is an example of dyskinesias).

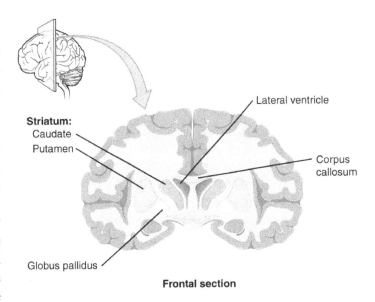

FIGURE 11.6   Basal Nuclei in Cross Section of Human Brain.

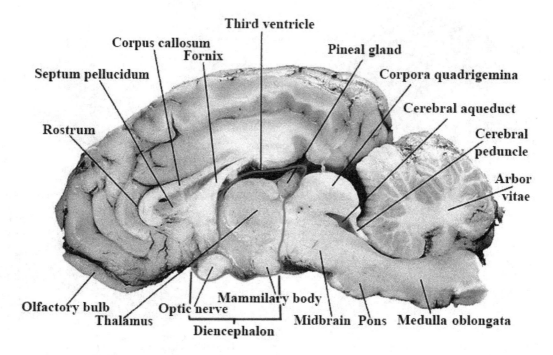

Third ventricle
Corpus callosum
Fornix
Septum pellucidum
Pineal gland
Corpora quadrigemina
Rostrum
Cerebral aqueduct
Cerebral peduncle
Arbor vitae
Olfactory bulb
Optic nerve
Mammilary body
Thalamus
Diencephalon
Midbrain Pons Medulla oblongata

FIGURE 11.7   Sheep Brain: Diencephalon.

The diencephalon includes four regions: the **epithalamus, dorsal thalamus, ventral thalamus,** and **hypothalamus**. The epithalamus consists of two structures: the **pineal gland** and **habenular nucleus**. The role of the habenular nucleus is still unknown. The pineal gland controls production of pigment by melanocytes and regulates diurnal and seasonal cycles of animal activity. The dorsal thalamus is the largest part of the diencephalon often just called thalamus. The dorsal thalamus is the master coordinating center. It receives sensory input from all receptors except olfactory and transmits these stimuli to the corresponding sensory area in the cerebral cortex. The hypothalamus forms the floor of the **diencephalon**. The most prominent parts of the hypothalamus are **mammillary bodies** (11.7). These bodies are a part of so called Papez circuit—a structure involved in reproductive behavior and short-term memory. The hypothalamus consists of set of nuclei that are involved in many homeostatic mechanisms, such as regulation of body temperature, blood pressure, satiety and thirst centers, and so on. Neurosecretory cells of the hypothalamus produce hormones that regulate activity of anterior pituitary gland. Thus, hypothalamus is a center for integration activities of nervous and endocrine systems. Hypothalamus and thalamus are important part of the **limbic system** involved in emotional behavior, spatial (orientation in the space) and short-term memory. The **third ventricle** is narrow and located between two lobes of the diencephalon. The **interventricular foramens** connect the third ventricle with left and right lateral ventricles (fig. 11.7).

The cerebellum monitors and modifies, but does not initiate, motor output. Its signals pursue two goals: maintain body equilibrium and control precise muscle activity. The cerebellum receives detailed sensory input about external space and is involved in motor memory. Destruction of the vermis—a midline region of the cerebellum—causes a loss of coordination of limbs, body, or eye movement called ataxia.

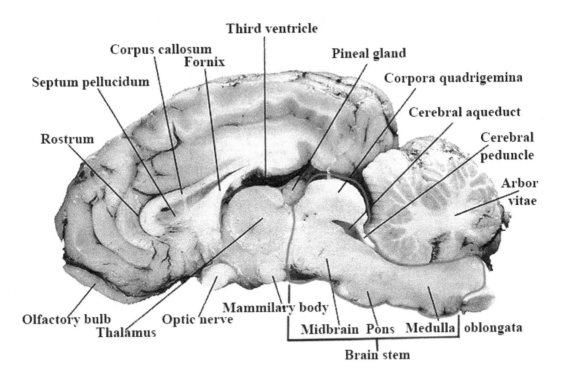

FIGURE 11.8   Sheep Brain: Brain Stem.

Destruction of the cerebellar hemispheres results in under- or overshooting a target called dysmetria. Beneath the cerebellum is the **fourth ventricle**. Anteriorly, the fourth ventricle is connected with the third ventricle via the **cerebral aqueduct**. Posteriorly, the fourth ventricle is connected with the central canal of the spinal cord (figs. 11.5; 11.7).

The brain stem consists of three parts: midbrain, pons, and medulla oblongata. The roof of the midbrain is called the **tectum** or **corpora quadrigemina**. The corpora quadrigemina contains two pairs of nervous masses: **superior** and **inferior colliculi**. The superior colliculi are the centers of visual sensory information and control of eye movement. The inferior colliculi are centers of auditory sensory input and following of sounds by hearing organs.

The pons occupies position between the midbrain and medulla oblongata. It is a prominent part of the brain stem. The anterior part of the pons contains the descending motor tracts (groups of myelinated axons), which through the pons continue to the spinal cord. The posterior portion of the pons contains the **reticular formation nuclei** and **nuclei of cranial nerves**. The reticular formation consists of a neuron's network distributed within midbrain, pons, and medulla oblongata nuclei. The pontine nuclei have many functions such as motor, breathing, sleep, and arousal centers.

The medulla oblongata operates primarily at the reflex level. First of all, it houses primary nuclei of cranial nerves VII to XII. Second, it is a route to main ascending and descending pathways to and from the higher brain centers. Third, the medulla oblongata contains such reflex centers as the respiratory center, heartbeat center, and intestinal motility. Damage to the medulla oblongata is life threatening because these reflex centers control fundamental vital functions.

CHECK YOUR UNDERSTANDING

- What structures constitute the brain stem?

- What is the primary function of the cerebrum?

- Which component of the diencephalon produces the hormone melatonin?

- Explain the difference between functions of the basal nuclei and cerebellum.

11.3   Spinal Cord

The spinal cord has two principal functions: it creates simple spinal reflexes, and it contains ascending tracts for sensory input and descending pathways that transmit motor signals to effector organs. The spinal cord is made of two regions: white and gray matter. In the spinal cord gray matter occupies the center, whereas white matter has a peripheral position. In cross section the mass of the gray matter has the shape of a butterfly. The wings of this butterfly have dorsal, ventral, and, in some regions, lateral extensions of gray matter correspondingly called **dorsal horns**, **ventral horns**, and **lateral horns**. The dorsal horns contain interneurons that receive sensory input from afferent neurons. These neurons process received information and send command impulses to motor neurons, which are located in the ventral and lateral horns. The ventral horns are made of somatic motor neurons associated with skeletal muscles. The lateral horns have motor neurons of the visceral or autonomic division associated with cardiac or smooth muscles and glands (fig. 11.9).

Spinal reflexes are based on closing the circuit between sensory neurons that reach the spinal cord through the dorsal horn and motor neurons that leave the spinal cord through ventral (for somatic) or lateral (for autonomic) horns without involvement of neurons in the brain. For example, if an animal put its leg on a sharp object, the withdraw reflex has to be very fast and has to include as few as three neurons.

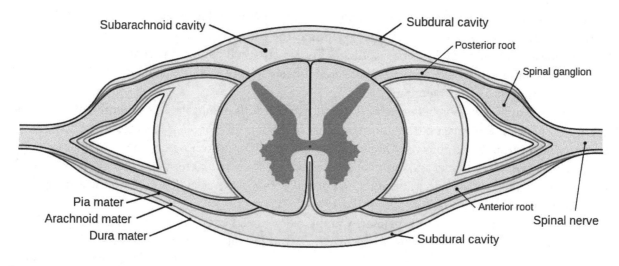

FIGURE 11.9   Spinal Cord.

Spinal tracts connect upper and lower regions of the CNS via myelinated nerve fibers. Nerve tracts may be ascending that conduct sensory impulses from the peripheral sense receptors to centers in the brain. The descending tracts convey command impulses to muscles and glands. There is a tendency for nerve fibers that conduct similar information to travel together and occupy specific regions in the spinal cord. Very often, these tracts are named for the region of their origin and destination. For example, the spinothalamic tract originates in the spinal cord and ends in the thalamus. Somatic motor neurons are organized in two groups: upper motor neurons and lower motor neurons. Upper motor neurons have comparatively large bodies located in the primary motor centers within the cerebral frontal lobe. Dendrites and axons of these neurons also lay inside the CNS, and activity of these neurons is restricted by the brain and spinal cord. Lower motor neurons have small bodies located in the nuclei of the cranial nerves (except cranial nerves I, II, and VIII) or in the ventral horn of the spinal cord. Axons of the lower motor neurons form the peripheral nervous system—cranial or spinal nerves. Thus, the somatic motor nerve impulse generated by the upper motor neuron in the primary motor center travels to the lower motor neuron in the brain stem or the ventral horn of the spinal cord, where it is transmitted to the lower motor neuron. The last neuron sends a motor signal to the effector muscle.

CHECK YOUR UNDERSTANDING

- Describe the functions of the neurons in the three horns of spinal gray matter.

- What is the difference between ascending and descending spinal tracts?

11.4 Peripheral Nervous System

The peripheral nervous system is made of nerves and has two divisions: sensory and motor. The sensory division is formed by nerves that carry sensory or afferent input impulses. The motor division contains nerves carrying motor or efferent output commands to muscles and glands. Motor neurons that control visceral activity constitute the **autonomic nervous system (ANS)**. Anatomically, nerves are divided in **cranial** and **spinal nerves**.

Nerves consist of many axons. On the outside, nerves are covered by a tough connective tissue membrane called **epineurium**. As a rule, nerve fibers that originate in the same region and innervate the same organ tend to be organized in groups called **fascicles**. Every fascicle is separated from the other fascicles by deep connective tissue membrane called **perineurium**. Inside the fascicle, every axon, whether myelinated or not, is also covered by a connective tissue called **endoneurium** (fig. 11.10). Does it remind you of the structural organization of skeletal muscle? Nerve structure may be compared to a cable. Inside, a cable is made of many isolated wires. If axons that create a nerve conduct only sensory input, this nerve is called a **sensory nerve**. **Optic** and **vestibulocochlear nerves** are examples of sensory nerves. Nerve that carry only motor signals to muscles or glands are called **motor nerve**. **Oculomotor** and **abducens nerves** are examples of such motor nerves. But most of nerves carry as sensory as motor fibers. These nerves are called **mixed nerves**. **Trigeminal** and **glossopharyngeal nerves** are mixed nerves and have both types of fibers.

Spinal nerves originate in the spinal cord and have two roots: the **dorsal root of spinal nerve** and **ventral root of spinal nerve**. The dorsal root of spinal nerve contains sensory fibers that enter the spinal cord

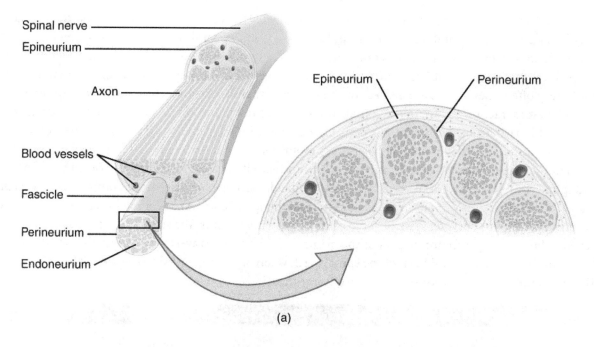

(a)

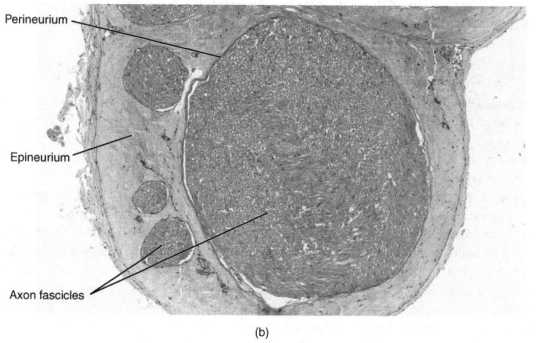

(b)

FIGURE 11.10   Nerve Structure.

via the dorsal horn, where they synapse with interneurons of the spinal cord. The bodies of sensory neurons are outside the CNS. They are organized in groups that are located in the dorsal root and called **dorsal root ganglion**. Bodies of motor neurons reside in the gray matter of spinal cord. The somatic motor neurons are in ventral horns of the gray matter; and visceral (autonomic) motor neurons are in lateral horns. Motor neurons send their axons through the ventral root of spinal nerve. Lateral to the dorsal root ganglion both roots fuse and form spinal nerve. Thus, a spinal nerve is always a mixed nerve. It carries both motor and sensory fibers (fig. 11.11).

The spinal nerve is short. It splits into two branches called the **ventral** and **dorsal rami** (singular **ramus**) immediately after leaving a vertebral cavity. The rami contain sensory and motor fibers. Both rami are mixed nerves. The dorsal ramus travels to the dorsal side of the body. The ventral ramus travels to the ventral side, but before that it gives a small branch made of visceral or autonomic motor fibers only. This small branch of autonomic nerve fibers is called **ramus communicans** (plural **rami communicantes**). Rami communicantes have exclusively visceral motor nerves. The ventral rami of the spinal nerves in cervical, lumbar, and sacral regions come together and merge to form complex network called **nerve plexuses**. Thus, there are **cervical, brachial, lumbar,** and **sacral plexuses** (the last two are often called **lumbosacral plexus**). An advantage of such organization is that the injury of one or another spinal nerve does not cut off motor and sensory innervation to some part of the body (figs. 11.12–11.15).

The right and left cervical plexuses are found deep in the neck between the first and fourth cervical vertebra. They also receive small contribution of trigeminal and hypoglossal cranial nerves. Nerves of cervical plexus supply the skin of the neck, part of the head, chest, and shoulders. The biggest nerve of this plexus is the **phrenic nerve** that supplies the diaphragm and plays a principal role in breathing (fig. 11.12).

The ventral rami of C5–T1 nerves form the brachial plexus. The five major nerves that sprang from the brachial plexus

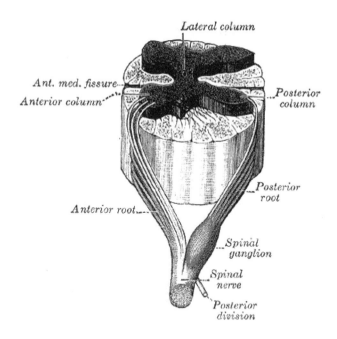

FIGURE 11.11   Spinal Nerve.

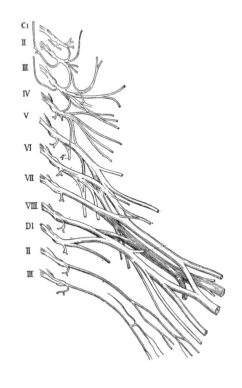

FIGURE 11.12   Cervical Plexus.

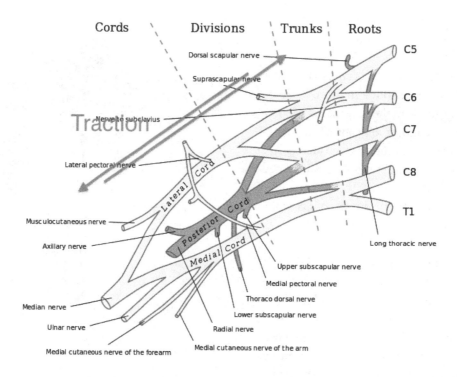

FIGURE 11.13   Brachial Plexus.

are **axillary**, **radial**, **musculocutaneous**, **median**, and **ulnar nerves**. The axillary nerve supplies muscles around the axilla, including deltoid and teres minor muscles. The radial nerve runs along the radial side of the forelimb. It supplies the triceps brachii and extensor muscles of the forelimb. The musculocutaneous nerve innervates most muscles of the dorsal side of the forelimb, including the biceps brachii and brachialis. The median nerve is located between the radial and ulnar nerves. It supplies the digital flexor muscles. For that it passes beneath the **flexor retinaculum**. This position of the median nerve beneath the strong connective tissue of the retinaculum may cause **carpal tunnel syndrome**, when the pressure from the retinaculum on the nerve is increased. The ulnar nerve, as its name suggests, travels along the ulna and innervates flexor muscles (fig. 11.13).

VETERINARY APPLICATION

Swelling of the carpal canal usually means that one of the flexor tendons from the branches of the median nerve that runs through it has been injured or that one of the structures within or associated with the canal have been injured. The carpal canal can also become infected either through the blood, a wound, or an injection. Compression by the flexor retinaculum, a band of connective tissue at the back of the canal, can cause pain and irritation.

The condition can be treated by injections in the area of the median nerve and the top of the canal with a mixture of lidocaine, sarapin, and a low dose of corticosteroid. In some cases, the condition may require surgical dissection of the carpal canal.

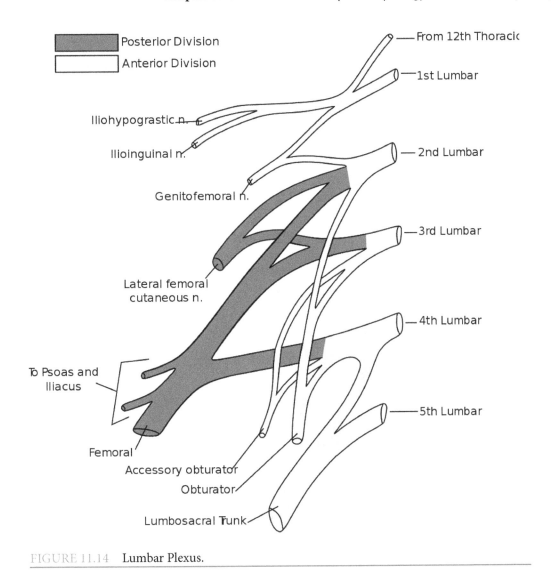

FIGURE 11.14   Lumbar Plexus.

The lumbar plexus is formed by the ventral rami of L1–L4 nerves. Nerves of this plexus supply structures of the pelvis and the hindlimbs. The largest nerves of this plexus are **obturator** and **femoral nerves**. The first nerve serves to adductor muscles, whereas the second serves the quadriceps muscles of the femur (fig. 11.14).

The largest nerve of the sacral plexus is the **sciatic nerve**. It serves the hip joint. In the lower part of the thigh, it splits into the **tibial** and **common fibular nerves** (fig. 11.15).

There are 12 pairs of cranial nerves (fig. 11.16). Cranial nerves that serve special sense organs (sight, hearing, olfaction, taste) are called **special cranial nerves**. Cranial nerves that serve widely distributed viscera are called **general cranial nerves**. Traditionally, cranial nerves in addition to the name are numbered by Roman numerals from I to XII. **Olfactory nerve (I)** is a sensory nerve concerned with the sense of smell. **Optic nerve (II)** is also a sensory nerve that serves to conduct visual information. Actually, both nerves are not real nerves, but projections of the brain and, strictly speaking, are tracts.

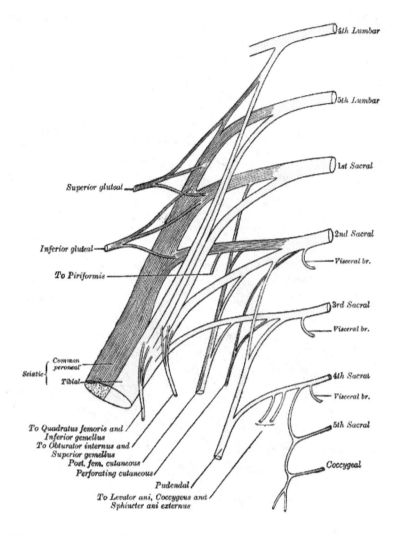

FIGURE 11.15   Sacral Plexus.

Oculomotor nerve (III), as its name indicates, is a motor nerve that supplies the rectus and inferior oblique extrinsic muscles of the eye and also carries autonomic motor fibers to iris and ciliary bodies of the eye. **Trochlear nerve (IV)** is also a motor nerve that serves to extrinsic superior oblique muscle of the eye. **Trigeminal nerve** or **trigeminus (V)** has three branches: **ophthalmic**, **maxillary**, and **mandibular**. Trigeminus is a mixed nerve. It has both sensory and motor fibers. **Abducens nerve (VI)** is a third motor nerve. It innervates the extrinsic lateral rectus muscle of the eyeball. **Facial nerve (VII)** is a mixed nerve. Its sensory fibers conduct sensory impulses from taste buds and skin. Its motor fibers control activities of the facial muscles, tongue, and salivary glands. **Vestibulocochlear, octaval**, or **auditory nerve (VIII)** is a sensory nerve that collect auditory and body balance information from cochlea and vestibular apparatus. **Glossopharyngeal nerve (IX)** is a mixed nerve, whose fibers supply taste buds and the muscles of the tongue and pharynx. **Vagus nerve (X)** is a mixed nerve. Its motor

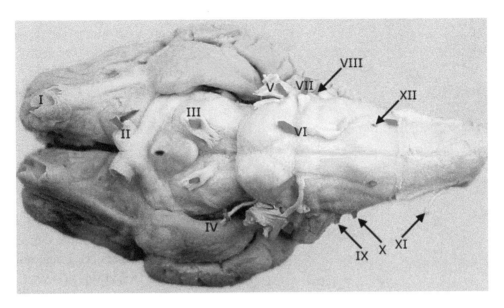

FIGURE 11.16   Cranial Nerves in Sheep's Brain.

fibers present the biggest parasympathetic nerve. Vagus nerve widely branched and serves areas of the mouth, pharynx, and most of the body viscera from heart to intestines and kidney. **Accessory nerve (XI)** is a motor nerve that serves to sternomastoid and trapezius muscles. Some of its fibers join to the vagus nerve to serve the pharynx and larynx. **Hypoglossal nerve (XII)** is a motor nerve that innervates the hyoid and tongue muscles.

CHECK YOUR UNDERSTANDING

- Describe the difference between somatic and visceral motor divisions.

- What is a ganglion?

- Compare the structure of nerve and skeletal muscle.

- Why are spinal nerves always mixed nerves?

11.5   Autonomic Nervous System

As observed from since ancient times, the nerve fibers that supply viscera or internal organs seem unable to be voluntarily controlled and demonstrate their autonomous activity. Nerve fibers that control and regulate activity of visceral organs have a collective name: the **autonomic nervous system**. Autonomic sensory fibers monitor the internal environment of the body: concentration of oxygen and carbon dioxide, body temperature and blood pressure, tension in the urinary bladder, and heart rate. Motor fibers of the autonomic nervous system innervate cardiac muscles, smooth muscles, and glands. Like a somatic sensory neuron, an autonomic sensory neuron resides in a dorsal root ganglion. On the other hand, the motor pathway includes two neurons: the first neuron resides in a lateral horn of the spinal cord and called the **preganglionic neuron**. The second neuron resides in ganglia outside the CNS and is called the **postganglionic neuron**. Thus, the

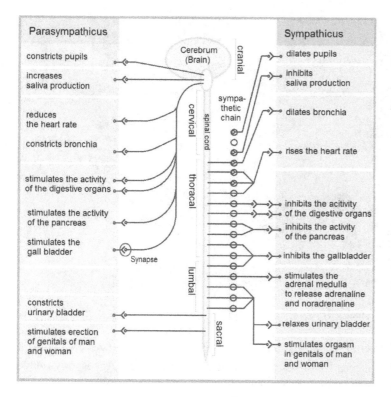

FIGURE 11.17   Autonomic Nervous System (ANS).

motor command to the internal organ has to pass two motor neurons and the synapses between them. In mammals, every internal organ is innervated by two types of autonomous fibers. When one of these fibers stimulates organ activity, the other fiber inhibits. Thus, the autonomic nervous system functionally is divided in two divisions: the **sympathetic** and **parasympathetic** (fig. 11.17).

The parasympathetic nervous system consists of autonomic motor fibers of cranial nerves III (oculomotor), VIII (facial), IX (glossopharyngeal), X (vagus), and sacral nerves S2–S4. In general, the parasympathetic system restores the body's balance by decreasing activity of body organs and establishing of restful vegetative state. Parasympathetic system slows heart rate, decreases blood pressure, constricts coronary blood vessels, and promotes deposition of glycogen. At the same time, it elevates activity of the digestive system. That is why this system often is called "rest and digest."

Parasympathetic preganglionic fibers are long and, as a rule, reach effector organs (for example, heart or liver). Postganglionic fibers are short. The ganglion, where preganglionic and postganglionic fibers synapse, is located nearby or directly on the surface of the effector organ. Both preganglionic and postganglionic neurons release the acetylcholine (ACh) to transmit signal in ganglion synapse between neurons and in synapse between postganglionic neuron and effector organ (fig. 11.18).

VETERINARY APPLICATION

Canine dysautonomia is a degenerative disease of the autonomic nervous system. The cause of the disease is not known. Symptoms include disruption of digestion, clumsy motions, confusion, sleepiness, and inability to stand. Other clues are painful urination, dilation of the eyes, lack of pupil reaction to light, inflammation of the bladder, dry mouth, dry nose, dry eyes, loss of appetite and weight (extreme), vomiting, diarrhea, losing control of bowels and urination, weakness, lack of tear production, photophobia (fear of light), swollen third eye, abdominal tenderness, coughing, depression, loss of motor reflexes, a slow weak heart rate, and breathing difficulty. The lack of pupil contraction and absent reflexes are usually indicative of dysautonomia. An echocardiograph (ECHO) is an important tool in diagnosis and will likely show systolic dysfunction and enlargement of the atrium or aorta. Other tests needed for diagnosis are serum analysis, complete blood count (CBC), liver enzyme panel, urinalysis, and fecal examination. Abdominal and thoracic X-rays and ultrasound usually show bladder distention, enlarged esophagus, and aspiration pneumonia. Treatment of dysautonomia is not usually successful no matter how early it is found. There is no known cure at the moment. Most dogs diagnosed with the disease are usually euthanized within a few weeks or months.

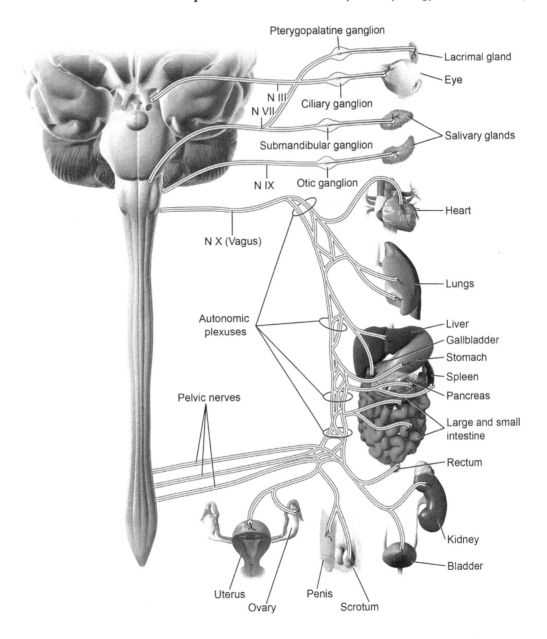

FIGURE 11.18   Parasympathetic Nervous System.

The sympathetic nervous system is constructed from thoracic and lumbar spinal nerves (fig. 11.19). In general, sympathetic nervous system mobilize organisms to emergency or strenuous actions. Signals from this system increase activity of most viscera: increases heart rate, blood pressure, blood flow, and so forth. At the same time, it decreases activity of the digestive system. This effect of the sympathetic system is reflected in name that is often used for this system: "fight or flight."

The preganglionic neuron of the sympathetic system has short preganglionic axons and long postganglionic axons. The sympathetic ganglion is located near the vertebral column. All sympathetic ganglia

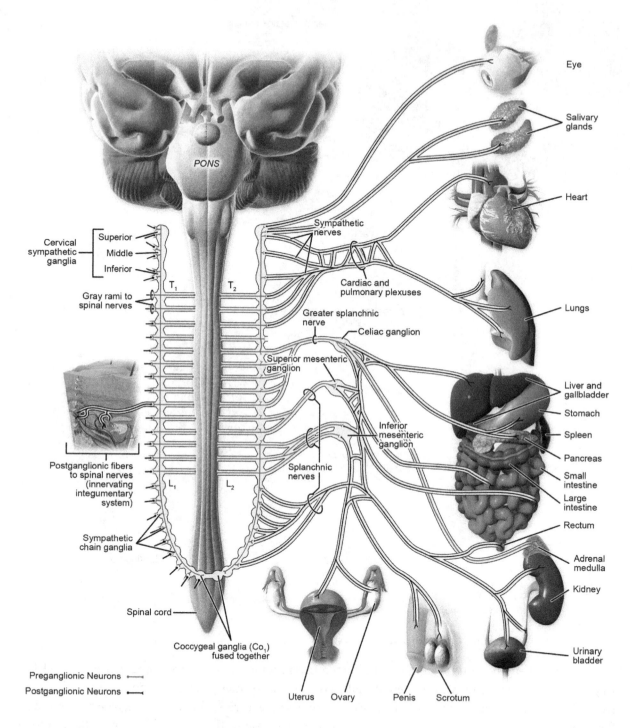

FIGURE 11.19   Sympathetic Nervous System.

longitudinally are connected by **sympathetic trunks**. The resulting structure is called **sympathetic chain ganglia**. The sympathetic chain ganglia extend along the thoracic and lumbar spinal cord from the superior cervical ganglion to the inferior sacral ganglion on both sides of the vertebral column (figs. 11.19–11.20). Bodies of the sympathetic preganglionic neurons are located in the lateral horns of the spinal cord. They send their axons via ventral roots of spinal nerves together with lower somatic motor neurons. The axons of these neurons travel with axons of other motor neurons to spinal nerve and ventral ramus for a short distance, and branch off to form small nerves called **white rami communicantes**. These rami are called white because they are always myelinated. From the rami communicantes axons enter sympathetic ganglion, where they synapse with postganglionic neuron. Some of preganglionic neurons do not synapse with postganglionic neuron of their level, but send their axons through the sympathetic trunk to other ganglia or to the **collateral ganglia** located near the target organ. Finally, there are three ways to synapse:

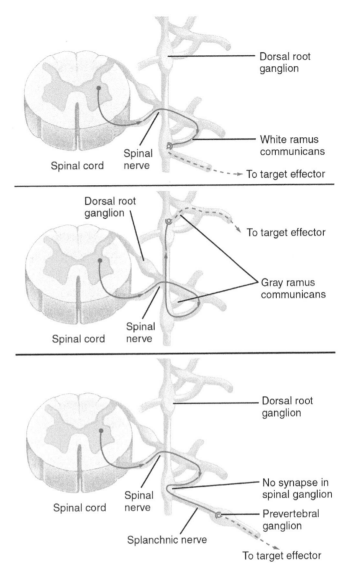

FIGURE 11.20   Sympathetic Chain Ganglion.

1. The axon synapses with the postganglionic neuron of the same level in the sympathetic chain ganglion.
2. The axon passes the same-level ganglion and via the sympathetic trunk makes a synapse to the postganglionic neuron in the nearby (ascending or descending) chain ganglion.
3. The axon may pass the chain ganglion and synapses with a postganglionic neuron in a collateral ganglion.

The postganglionic neuron innervates the target cells. The axons of postganglionic neurons exit the chain ganglia via small **gray rami communicantes**, and again join the spinal nerve. They travel with other spinal nerve fibers until reach the target organ. The postganglionic rami are called gray because they are not myelinated (fig. 11.20).

The preganglionic neuron communicates with postganglionic by ACh like parasympathetic neurons. The postganglionic axons in their turn release one of three neurotransmitters: ACh, **norepinephrine** (also known as **noradrenalin**), or **epinephrine** (also known as **adrenalin**). About 80 percent of postganglionic neurons release norepinephrine. To be able to receive neurotransmitter signal, receiving cell has to have receptor proteins in postsynaptic membrane sensitive to the particular neurotransmitter. The receptors that bind with ACh are called **cholinergic receptors**. Receptors sensitive to norepinephrine and epinephrine are called **adrenergic receptors**.

There are two types of cholinergic receptors: **muscarinic** and **nicotinic**. Muscarinic receptors are G-protein coupled transmembranous protein molecules. On the external surface of the plasma membrane, these proteins have ACh-binding site and on the internal site they are bound with G-protein. ACh forms chemical bonds with receptor ACh-binding site, which cause conformational transformation of the receptor protein resulted in release of G-protein at the inner surface of the membrane. The released active G-protein acts as an enzyme that triggers cascade of chemical reactions in cytoplasm of the postsynaptic neuron. The molecules that participate in these metabolic reactions are termed secondary messengers. These reactions, finally, lead to opening of sodium channels, influx of the sodium into the postsynaptic cell, and local membrane depolarization that produces postsynaptic potential. Thus, muscarinic receptors generate response to the stimulus by changing cellular metabolism via second messenger cascade reactions. It takes a sequence of chemical reactions before a postsynaptic neuron generates its own response. Muscarinic receptors generate a slow response and, as a rule, present in those synapses, where the speed of nerve impulse transmission is not critical. Muscarinic receptors were discovered when scientists studied the effect of water-soluble toxin extracted from poisonous mushrooms *Amanita muscaria* that cause muscle convulsions, which may cause death. Muscarinic receptors are involved in a large number of physiological functions, including heart rate and force, and contraction of smooth muscles. There are five subtypes of muscarinic receptors: M1–M5. All five are found in the CNS. M1 receptors are common in secretory glands; M2 are found in cardiac muscles; M3 are found in smooth muscles and glands.

Nicotinic receptors were discovered in studies of tobacco's nicotine effect on the nervous system. These studies show that neurons have a group of specific cholinergic receptors. These cholinergic receptors are ligand-gated Na^+ channel proteins in the neuron plasma membrane. This channel opens and allows Na^+ to enter the cell when nicotine binds to it. The influx of sodium ions depolarizes the neuron plasma membrane and may cause development of action potential. Nicotinic receptors do not need secondary messengers, and neuron response on nicotinic ligand is straightforward, immediate, and fast. Nicotinic receptors present in a wide range of neuron-neuron and neuromuscular synapses. A wide range of different neurotoxins bind with nicotinic receptors and block the opening of Na^+ channels. According sensitivity to a snake venom toxin, a-bungarotoxin, nicotinic receptors are classified in two principal groups: **a-bungarotoxin-sensitive** and **a-bungarotoxin-insensitive** receptors.

The adrenergic receptors are classified into two major groups: **alpha (α) receptors** and **beta (β) receptors**. There are two main types of **alpha (α) receptors**:

1. **Alpha-1 ($α_1$) receptors** are found in plasma membranes of smooth muscle cells.

2. **Alpha-2 (α_2) receptors** are found in plasma membranes of the preganglionic sympathetic neurons. The binding of the norepinephrine to these receptors causes hyperpolarization of the membrane and, as a result, canceling the action potential.

There are three main types of **beta (β) receptors**:

1. **Beta-1 (β_1) receptors** are found in plasma membranes of cardiac muscle cells, some cells of the kidney, and adipocytes.
2. **Beta-2 (β_2) receptors** are characteristic of plasma membranes of smooth muscles in walls of the trachea, bronchi, urinary system, and blood vessels that serve skeletal muscles, liver, and pancreas. They also were found in cells of salivary glands and some skeletal muscles.
3. **Beta-3 (β_3) receptors** are mostly found on the plasma membranes of adipocytes and smooth muscles in the wall of the digestive tract.

This diversity of receptors on neurotransmitters results in a diversity of responses of target cells. Not only can different neurotransmitters cause different reaction of target cell, but also the same neurotransmitter may generate a different response depending on the type of receptor protein in the plasma membrane of the cell. Thus, the parasympathetic system slows down the heart rate because ACh released by the vagus nerve hyperpolarizes the plasma membrane of cardiac muscle. At the same time, the sympathetic stimulation increases heart rate because the β_1 receptors open and depolarize cardiac muscle membrane when bound to norepinephrine. When β_2 receptors cause relaxation of smooth muscles of the blood vessels that supply skeletal muscles, β_3 receptors in smooth muscles of the digestive tract causes their contraction.

VETERINARY APPLICATION

The existence of different subtypes of sympathetic nervous system receptors allows to design drugs that are specific for particular receptor types. These drugs may be antagonists that block the receptor and prevent norepinephrine binding, or they are agonist that bind the receptor and mimic the effect of norepinephrine. Thus, there were developed next drugs that bind to sympathetic receptors:

Alpha-1 blockers (antagonists) bind to α_1 receptors, particularly those on the smooth muscle cells lining blood vessels. They block the action of norepinephrine and prevent the blood vessels to constrict, an effect that lowers blood pressure and is useful in treating hypertension.

Alpha-2 agonists bind to the presynaptic α_2 receptors and activate them, which decreases the output of both preganglionic and postganglionic sympathetic neurons. The α_2 agonists are the only single class of anesthetic drugs that induce reliable, dose-dependent sedation, analgesia, and muscle relaxation in dogs and cats. Used at low doses in combination with inhalational anesthetics, α_2 agonists reduce the amount of anesthetic drug required to induce and maintain anesthesia.

Beta-blockers are antagonists that bind to β_1 receptors on the heart and decrease its rate and force of contraction.

Beta agonists bind to β_2 receptors on the smooth muscles of airways and cause bronchodilation. Thus, β_2 agonist *isoproterenol* (*ISO*) causes tracheal relaxation in dogs.

11.6 Reflex Arc and Reflexes

Organized programmed or automatic responses to different stimuli are called **reflexes**. Every reflex begins with a sensory stimulus and finishes with a rapid motor response. Thus, each reflex develops as a signal from a receptor, is conducted to the CNS through the sensory (afferent) neuron, and has a motor output through effector organ stimulated by a particular motor neuron. This anatomic organization of automatic response is called **reflex arc**. The simplest reflex arc has three neurons: sensory neuron, interneuron, and motor neuron.

Depending on the location of the reflex arc, there are two types of reflexes: **cranial** and **spinal**. The difference between these two types of reflexes is obvious: cranial reflexes are mediated by the cranial nerves, whereas spinal reflexed are mediated by the spinal nerves. Cranial reflexes include the closure of the eyelids when something touches the cornea, or gagging when the back of the throat is irritated. Depending on the number of neurons that participate in the reflex arc, reflexes are classified as **monosynaptic**, where there are only two neurons: sensory and motor with a single synapse between them; or **polysynaptic**, where there are more than two neurons and many synapses. Depending the type of motor neurons, reflexes are divided into **somatic** and **visceral** or **autonomic**.

Most of the spinal somatic reflexes include three neurons. The body of the somatic sensory neuron is located in the dorsal root ganglion. Its axon travels through the dorsal root to dorsal horn and synapse here with interneuron. The interneuron transmits nerve impulse to the same or the opposite side of the ventral horn of the spinal cord, where it synapses with motor neuron. The motor neuron then sends motor command via the ventral root to a somatic effector (fig. 11.21).

The visceral reflex arc structurally is more complex. Unlike the somatic reflex, motor visceral reflex arc contains two motor neurons. Preganglionic neurons are located in lateral horns of spinal cord. Postganglionic neurons are located in chain or collateral ganglion. Thus, the simplest visceral reflex arc includes four neurons (fig. 11.21).

Somatic reflex arc

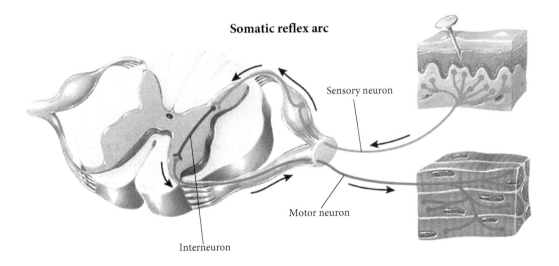

Sensory neuron

Motor neuron

Interneuron

Autonomic reflex arc

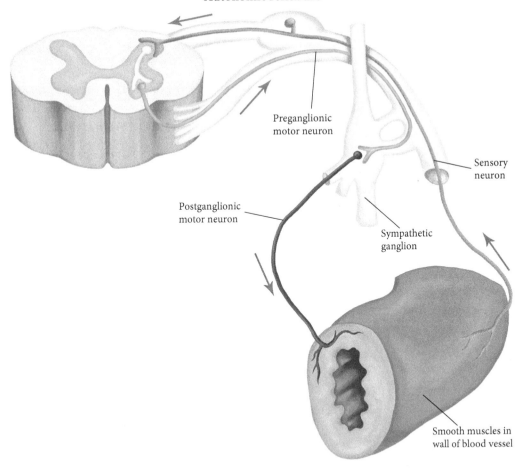

Preganglionic
motor neuron

Sensory
neuron

Postganglionic
motor neuron

Sympathetic
ganglion

Smooth muscles in
wall of blood vessel

FIGURE 11.21   Somatic and Autonomic Reflex Arcs.

CHAPTER SUMMARY

- The principal function of the nervous system is to create harmonious functioning of the organism through the organs' control. The nervous system monitors the status of every organ, collects and analyze information from internal and external environment, and sends instructions to organs. The nervous system is a key system responsible for successful maintaining of homeostasis.

- The nervous system has two parts: the **central nervous system (CNS)** and **peripheral nervous system (PNS)**. The CNS consists of the **brain** and **spinal cord**. The PNS includes **nerves** and **ganglia**. The PNS carries **sensory** and **motor functions**. The CNS has **integrative function**. The PNS has **sensory** and **motor divisions**. The sensory division is subdivided into somatic and visceral divisions; and the motor division is subdivided in somatic and visceral (**autonomic nervous system**, or **ANS**) divisions.

- The brain and spinal cord are covered by three connective tissue membranes known as **meninges**. The outermost strong and tough membrane, the **dura mater**, contains a lot of collagen fibers. Beneath the dura mater is the web-like blood vessel-carrying **arachnoid mater**. The delicate **pia mater** covers the brain and spinal cord.

- The brain and spinal cord are hollow inside. Chambers of the brain are called **ventricles**. A hollow tube in the spinal cord is called the **central canal**. Ventricles and the central canal are connected and filled with cerebrospinal fluid (CSF) produced by the **choroid plexus**, small tufts of blood vessels associated with ependymal cells that project into ventricles.

- The brain is divided in three regions: **forebrain, midbrain,** and **hindbrain**. The forebrain has two structures: **cerebrum** and **diencephalon**. The hindbrain has three regions: **cerebellum, pons,** and **medulla oblongata**. The midbrain, pons, and medulla oblongata create morpho-functional unity called **brain stem**.

- The **cerebral cortex** is a superficial layer of neurosomas. It has a pair of lobes called **cerebral hemispheres** and **olfactory bulbs**. The subcortical region is made of white matter. The surface of the cerebral hemispheres is covered by wavy **convolutions**. Ridges of convolutions are called **gyri** (singular **gyrus**) and shallow grooves between them are **sulci** (singular **sulcus**). Deep grooves or **fissure** separate cerebral hemispheres from each other (**longitudinal fissure**) and from cerebellum (**transverse fissure**). Deep inside the cerebrum are left and right **lateral ventricles**. Neurons on the left and right hemispheres communicate via groups of myelinated axons called **commissures**. The biggest commissure is **corpus callosum**. The hemisphere is divided in five regions or lobes: **frontal, parietal, temporal, occipital,** and **insula**. Posteriorly, the frontal lobe is limited by a **central sulcus**. The **precentral gyrus** houses **primary motor center**. The anterior gyrus of the parietal lobe is called **postcentral gyrus**. It functions as a **primary sensory center**. The **temporal lobe** is separated from the frontal lobe by **lateral fissure**. This lobe process hearing information. The **occipital lobe** occupies posterior position. It is separated from the parietal lobe by the **parieto-occipital sulcus**. Occipital lobe is a center of procession visual information. The **insula** is located deep inside the cerebrum. Its neurons are associated with taste receptors and internal organs.

- **Basal nuclei** are groups of neurons in the cerebral floor. From the diencephalon they are separated by a mass of white matter called internal capsule. The principal basal nuclei are the **caudate nucleus, putamen,** and **globus pallidus**. The nuclei receive sensory input from the midbrain nucleus, the **substantia nigra**. The basal nuclei initiate and control movement.

- The diencephalon includes four regions: the **epithalamus, dorsal thalamus, ventral thalamus**, and **hypo-thalamus**. The epithalamus consists of two structures: the **pineal gland** and **habenular nucleus**. The pineal gland produces melanin and regulates diurnal and seasonal cycles. The dorsal thalamus is a coordinating center. It receives sensory input from all receptors except olfactory and transmits these stimuli to the corresponding sensory areas in the cerebral cortex. The hypothalamus forms the floor of the **diencephalon**. The most prominent parts of the hypothalamus are **mammillary bodies**. These bodies are a part of the Papez circuit—a structure involved in reproductive behavior and short-term memory. The hypothalamus is a center of many homeostatic mechanisms. Hypothalamic neurosecretory cells produce hormones. The **third ventricle** is located between the diencephalon lobes. The **interventricular foramens** connect the third and lateral ventricles.

- The cerebellum maintains body equilibrium and control precision of muscle activity. Beneath the cerebellum is **fourth ventricle**. Anteriorly, the fourth ventricle is connected with the third ventricle via the **cerebral aqueduct**, and posteriorly with the central canal of the spinal cord.

- The **corpora quadrigemina** is a dorsal structure of the midbrain. The corpora quadrigemina has two pairs: the **superior** and **inferior colliculi**. The superior colliculi are the centers of visual sensory information and control of eye movement. The inferior colliculi are centers of auditory sensory input and a center of hearing reflexes.

- The pons occupies a position between the midbrain and medulla oblongata. The anterior part of the pons contains descending motor tracts. The posterior portion of the pons contains the **reticular formation** and **nuclei of cranial nerves**.

- The medulla oblongata operates as a reflex center. It houses the nuclei of cranial nerves VII to XII. It is also a pathway for main ascending and descending tracts.

- Gray matter of the spinal cord concentrates in the center and has projections called **dorsal, ventral**, and **lateral horns**. The dorsal horns contain interneurons that receive sensory input from afferent neurons. The ventral horns are made of somatic motor neurons associated with skeletal muscles. The lateral horns have motor neurons of the visceral or autonomic division associated with cardiac or smooth muscles and glands.

- Nerves consist of many axons. From outside, nerves are covered by a tough **epineurium**. Inside, nerve fibers are organized in groups called **fascicles**. Every fascicle is separated from other fascicles by **perineurium**. Inside the fascicle, every axon is also covered by an **endoneurium**.

- Spinal nerves have two roots: **dorsal** and **ventral**. The dorsal root contains axons of sensory neurons that enter the spinal cord via the dorsal horn, where they synapse with interneurons. The bodies of sensory neurons outside the CNS are organized in groups called **dorsal root ganglion**. Motor neurons from the gray matter of the spinal cord send axons through the ventral root of spinal nerve. Both roots fuse and form spinal nerve. Thus, a spinal nerve is always a mixed nerve and carries both motor and sensory fibers.

- A spinal nerve is short and splits in two branches: **ventral** and **dorsal rami**, both with sensory and motor fibers. The ventral ramus gives a small branch with visceral (autonomic) motor fibers—**ramus communicans**. The ventral rami of the spinal nerves in some regions merge and form **nerve plexuses: cervical, brachial, lumbar**, and **sacral plexuses**.

- There are 12 pairs of cranial nerves: **olfactory nerve (I)** is a sensory nerve concerned with the sense of smell; **optic nerve (II)** is a sensory nerve that conducts visual information; **oculomotor nerve (III)** is a motor nerve that supplies rectus and inferior oblique extrinsic muscles of the eye and carries autonomic motor fibers to iris and ciliary bodies of the eye; **trochlear nerve (IV)** is a motor nerve that serves to extrinsic superior oblique muscle of the eye; **trigeminal nerve** or **trigeminus (V)** has three branches: **ophthalmic**, **maxillary**, and **mandibular**. Trigeminus is a mixed nerve; **abducens nerve (VI)** supplies extrinsic lateral rectus muscle; **facial nerve (VII)** is a mixed nerve. Its sensory fibers serve taste buds and skin. Its motor fibers control the facial muscles, tongue, and salivary glands; **vestibulocochlear nerve (VIII)** is a sensory nerve that collects auditory and body balance information from cochlea and vestibular apparatus; **glossopharyngeal nerve (IX)** is a mixed nerve that supply taste buds, muscles of tongue and pharynx; **vagus nerve (X)** is a mixed nerve. Its motor fibers present the biggest parasympathetic nerve; **accessory nerve (XI)** is a motor nerve that serves to sternomastoid and trapezius muscles; some fibers join vagus to serve pharynx and larynx; **hypoglossal nerve (XII)** is a motor nerve that innervates hyoid and tongue muscles.

- The motor neurons that serve viscera belong to autonomic nervous system. The autonomic motor pathway includes two neurons: the first neuron is in a lateral horn of the spinal cord and is called **preganglionic neuron**. The second neuron resides in ganglia outside the CNS and is called **postganglionic neuron**. Functionally, the ANS is divided in two divisions: **sympathetic** and **parasympathetic**.

- The parasympathetic nervous system consists of motor fibers of cranial nerves III (oculomotor), VIII (facial), IX (glossopharyngeal), X (vagus), and sacral nerves S2–S4. The parasympathetic system restores the body's balance by decreasing organ activity and establishing a restful vegetative state. The parasympathetic system slows heart rate, decreases blood pressure, constricts coronary blood vessels, and promotes deposition of glycogen. At the same time, it elevates activity of the digestive system. Parasympathetic preganglionic fibers are long. Postganglionic fibers are short. The ganglion is near the effector organ. Both preganglionic and postganglionic neurons are cholinergic.

- The sympathetic nervous system consists of thoracic and lumbar spinal nerves. Signals from this system increase activity of most viscera. The preganglionic axons of the system are short and postganglionic are long. The sympathetic ganglion is located near the vertebral column. Sympathetic ganglia longitudinally are connected by **sympathetic trunks**. The resulting structure is called **sympathetic chain ganglia**. The preganglionic neurons of the sympathetic system are located in the lateral horns of the spinal cord. They send axons via ventral roots of spinal nerve together with somatic motor neurons. All axons travel to spinal nerve and ventral ramus. Shortly after leaving the vertebral column, sympathetic preganglionic axons branch off to form **white rami communicantes**. From rami communicantes they enter sympathetic ganglion and synapse with postganglionic neuron. Some axons do not synapse, but continues through the sympathetic trunk to ganglia of another level or to the **collateral ganglia** near the target organ. The axons of postganglionic neurons exit the chain ganglia via small **gray rami communicantes** and join the spinal nerve. They travel with other nerve fibers until the target organ. The preganglionic neurons are cholinergic. The postganglionic axons release one of three neurotransmitters: ACh, **norepinephrine**, or **epinephrine**.

- The effect of the neurotransmitter on the target cell depends of the receptor proteins in the postsynaptic membrane. The **cholinergic receptors** are proteins that bind ACh. Receptors sensitive to norepinephrine and epinephrine are called **adrenergic receptors**. There are two types of acetylcholine receptors: **muscarinic** and **nicotinic**. The muscarinic receptors are coupled with G-protein. They generate slow metabolic response via second messenger cascade reactions. The nicotinic receptors are ligand-gated ion channels that mediate a fast synaptic response. The adrenergic receptors are classified into two major groups: **alpha (α)** and **beta (β) receptors**. Diversity of neurotransmitters and receptors results in diversity of reactions of target cells. Thus, parasympathetic system is slow down the heart rate because ACh released by vagus nerve hyperpolarize plasma membrane of cardiac muscle. At the same time, sympathetic stimulation increases heart rate because the β_1 receptors open and depolarize cardiac muscle membrane.

- A reflex is a programmed automatic response to stimulus. A reflex begins with a sensory stimulus and finishes with a motor response. The anatomic organization of reflex response is called a **reflex arc**. Depending on location, there are two types of reflexes: **cranial** and **spinal**. Cranial reflexes are mediated by cranial nerves, whereas spinal are mediated by spinal nerves. Depending on the number of neurons that participate in the reflex arc, reflexes are classified as **monosynaptic**, when there are only two neurons and one synapse, and **polysynaptic**, when there are more neurons and many synapses. Reflexes may also be **somatic** and **visceral (autonomic)**.

CHECK YOUR KNOWLEDGE

LEVEL I. CHECK YOUR RECALL

1. Central sulcus separates:
   A. Parietal and temporal lobes
   B. Parietal and occipital lobes
   C. Occipital and frontal lobes
   D. Occipital and temporal lobes
   E. Frontal and parietal lobes

2. Which of the follows is not a part of the diencephalon?
   A. Thalamus
   B. Hypothalamus
   C. Basal nuclei
   D. Mammillary bodies
   E. Pineal gland

3. Cerebrospinal fluid (CSF) is produced by:
   A. Choroid plexus
   B. Brachial plexus
   C. Cervical plexus
   D. Lumbar plexus
   E. Sacral plexus

4. The pons is part of the _____, whereas the diencephalon is part of the _____.
    A. midbrain; forebrain
    B. forebrain; midbrain
    C. forebrain; brain stem
    D. brain stem; forebrain
    E. brain stem; midbrain

5. A cluster of nerve cell bodies outside the CNS is called _____, whereas a cluster of nerve cell bodies inside the CNS is called _____.
    A. ganglion; nucleus
    B. nucleus; ganglion
    C. white matter; gray matter
    D. gray matter; white matter

6. Somatic motor neurons innervate _____, whereas autonomic neurons innervate _____.
    A. skeletal muscles; cardiac muscles
    B. cardiac muscles; smooth muscles
    C. cardiac muscles; skeletal muscles
    D. smooth muscles; cardiac muscles
    E. smooth muscles; skeletal muscles

7. Sympathetic preganglionic fibers are _____ and _____.
    A. short; cholinergic
    B. long; cholinergic
    C. short; adrenergic
    D. long; adrenergic

8. Match the term with its description:
    _____ Basal nuclei   a. Cholinergic receptor
    _____ Superior colliculi   b. Putamen and globus pallidus
    _____ Corpus callosum   c. Produces cerebrospinal fluid
    _____ Pons   d. Connects cerebral hemispheres
    _____ Muscarinic receptor   e. Releases norepinephrine
    _____ Adrenergic fiber   f. A middle part of the brain stem
    _____ Choroid plexus   g. Center that controls eye movements

9. True or false: Postganglionic sympathetic neurons as a rule release ACh.
10. True or false: Nicotinic receptors are sensitive to norepinephrine.
11. True or false: Corpus callosum is a white matter.

LEVEL 2. CHECK YOUR UNDERSTANDING

1. Why does brain stem injury usually cause loss of reflex control over autonomic functions?
2. If you run upstairs from the first to the sixth floor, what changes in your body will be initiated by the sympathetic nervous system?
3. How can you identify the difference between an injury of the basal nuclei and the cerebellum?

LEVEL 3. APPLY YOUR KNOWLEDGE TO REAL LIFE

1. What will an injection of a drug that selectively binds to and activates the α_2 adrenergic receptors cause? What veterinary applications might such a drug have?
2. In terms of survival, the injury to which brain part is most dangerous?

Chapter 12

Senses and Sense Organs

LEARNING OBJECTIVES

The principal property of living organisms is an extraordinarily robust organization and ability to adapt to constant changes in the environment. This property is based on multiple homeostatic mechanisms that control and regulate all organism activities, from regulation of blood calcium to foraging and reproductive behavior. This chapter describes sensory receptors: anatomic structures that monitor the external environment and the physiological state of the body. After reading the chapter, you are expected to be able to describe the following:

1. Classification of sensory organs.

2. Structural organization of general sensory organs.

INTRODUCTION

Sensory receptors are organs whose specialty is gathering information about the state of external and internal environments. For that, receptors have to be able to observe changes of specific environmental parameters and convert an energy of these changes into the nerve signals. These nerve impulses are processed in the spinal cord or brain. The sensory impulses processed in spinal cord generate spinal reflexes. The sensory impulses processed in the brain result in cranial reflexes. The sensations processed in the cerebral cortex of the brain are referred to as **perceptions**. In humans, perception is a foundation of high mental processes, such as learning and planning. The perception of the world in many ways depends on the sensory receptors: what parameters of the world they are sensitive to. Parameters of the world detected by sensory receptors are called **receptor modalities**. Modalities include temperature, pressure, chemical content, body damage that causes pain, and so on. Vertebrates are very different in their ability to perceive the world. Bats navigate in the complete darkness of caves through their exceptional hearing. Hawks have amazingly sharp vision that helps them see quickly running rodents from high in the sky. Perception is not a precise result of sensation. Perception is an interpretation of sensation by the brain, and it depends on which receptor is activated. For example, mechanical pressure on the eyeball is interpreted as a sensation of bright light. That is why a strike to the eye causes "seeing of stars."

Sensory receptors are made of different sensory cells, which are sensitive to different stimuli. The ability of the sensory cell to respond to a stimulus of a very low intensity is called **sensitivity**. An ability to distinguish stimuli of different modality, for example pressure from temperature, is known as **sensory specificity**. A **sensory receptor cell** is a cell that specialized to transform energy of the specific stimulus into a nerve impulse. Thus, stimulus is a specific form of energy to which receptor cell is sensitive. This sensitivity can be expressed in opening of ionic channels and, as a result, changing of the resting membrane potential of the plasma membrane; or a change of the metabolic processes inside the cell that may result in release of neurotransmitters into the synapse with the nearby sensory neuron. The forms of energy that cause these changes in the cell are mechanical, thermal, chemical, or electromagnetic. The process of conversion of an energy of a stimulus into nerve impulse is called **sensory transduction**. Sensory transduction needs special molecules in the sensory receptor cell called **receptor molecules**. As a rule, receptor molecule is a transmembrane protein that changes its confirmation (a 3-D molecule shape: see chapter 2, page 48) in response to the stimulus energy. The change of the receptor molecule confirmation opens ion channels or triggers cascade of chemical reactions inside the cell, which leads to change of the membrane potential known as a **receptor potential**. Some sensory cells are, as a matter of fact, sensory neurons. In this case, development of receptor potential may cause depolarization of the plasma membrane and, when depolarization reaches a threshold level, action potential. However, many sensory cells are not neurons and do not generate an action potential. In this case, the sensory cell makes a synapse with a nearby sensory neuron and transmits receptor potential through the neurotransmitters, which it synthesizes.

In most cases, sensory receptor cells do not function alone but as part of a group of cells. Receptor cells organized in groups are known as **sense organs**. Usually, a sense organ has many sensory receptor cells accompanied by different types of supporting cells. For example, the vertebrate eye is a sense organ that contains photoreceptor cells. The supporting tissues of the eye include connective tissue of cornea and blood vessels, together with smooth muscles of iris and secretory epithelial cells of the ciliary bodies. Together with analytical centers of the CNS that process sensory information, sense organs form **sensory systems**. The vertebrate visual system includes the eyes and the brain areas, which process visual information.

CHECK YOUR UNDERSTANDING

- What is a sensory transduction?
- What is a receptor potential?
- What is a receptor modality?

12.1   Classification of Senses

There are four principal sources of energy that may affect sensory receptors: mechanical, thermal, chemical, and electromagnetic. Mechanical sensations include such phenomena as touch, pressure, vibration, tension, stretching. Thermal sensations are of two types: warm and cold. Chemical senses are based on ability of particular molecules; for example, pheromones called **ligands** create chemical bonds with receptor protein molecules. Vision is based on sensitivity of special receptor proteins to electromagnetic fields of different frequency. This includes not only vision but also such phenomenon as bird navigation in electromagnetic field of the earth during migrations.

The source of the stimulus may be located outside or inside the body. In first case, we talk about **external senses**; in the second, **internal senses**. Internal signals may come from skeletal muscles and skin and are called **somatic senses**, or from internal organs, such as the liver, and are called **visceral senses**.

TABLE 12.1   The Senses

Sense	What Is Sensed	Type of Stimulus
General Senses		
Visceral sensations	Hunger, thirst, hollow organ fullness	Chemical, mechanical
Touch	Touch and pressure	Mechanical
Temperature	Heat and cold	Thermal
Pain	Intense stimuli of different type	Mechanical, chemical, or thermal
Proprioception	Body position and movement	Mechanical
Special Senses		
Taste	Tastes	Chemical
Smell	Odors	Chemical
Hearing	Sounds	Mechanical
Equilibrium	Body balance and head position	Mechanical
Vision	Light	Electromagnetic

The sensations that an organism experiences are combinations of these sensory elements and are, for example, external chemical senses, such as smell, and internal chemical senses, such as sensing oxygen concentration in blood. Internal chemoreceptors can sense sore skeletal muscles, resulting from accumulation of lactic acid and electrolyte imbalance in muscular tissue, which is a somatic chemical sense. Sensing oxygen concentration in blood, on the other hand, is a visceral chemical sense. In all, there are ten categories of sensations, which are classified in two groups: five **general senses** and five **special senses** (table 12.1). Every sense category has a specific sensory structure, and the diversity of senses corresponds to the diversity of sense organs.

Sensory receptors respond to stimuli with different speed, intensity, and duration. This observation is expressed by a generalization, which states: *The sensory modality or quality of sensation associated with a particular stimulus depends solely on the type of receptor that was stimulated, but not on how the receptor was stimulated.* That is why electrical stimulation of hearing receptors causes "hearing of sounds." Receptors respond on stimulus with different speed and intensity, and can stop to send signals after some period of time. This receptor response on the stimulus is called **receptor adaptation**. Based on their ability to adapt, receptors are classified in two groups: **rapidly adapting** and **slowly adapting receptors**. As the name implies, rapidly adapting receptors are fast responding. Their response, as a rule, is intense, but its intensity decreases quickly with time. These receptors are important for detecting the beginning of the stimulation and fast response, if the stimulus is life threatening. The slowly adapting receptors, in contrast, react to the stimulus comparatively slow. Their response is not so intense, and signaling continues as long as the stimulus continues without significant decrease of its intensity. Dull and chronic pains are generated by this type of receptor.

CHECK YOUR UNDERSTANDING

- What is the difference between somatic and visceral senses?

- What sense type do you experience when wind blows your hair?

- What is the difference between rapidly and slowly adapting receptors?

- What type of sense is tasting food?

General and Special Senses

Simple considerations divide senses into two major groups: **general** and **special senses**.

1. General senses are external and internal senses that have comparatively simple-constructed receptors distributed all over the body. For example, pain receptors are free ends of sensory neurons located everywhere in the skin (somatic external sense) and in most viscera, such as the stomach (visceral internal sense). The information from general senses is processed in the brain and spinal cord.

2. Special senses require complex-structured receptor organs called sense organs that collect stimuli external to the body and are located in the head. For example, taste is sensed by taste buds: a complex of sensory and accessory cells in the tongue and walls of the oral cavity. Information from the special censes is processed in the cerebral cortex of the brain; that is, it forms perceptions.

12.2 General Senses

General senses include sensations of touch, vibration, pressure, temperature, pain, and **proprioception**. The general sense receptors are simple in organization and widely spread over the body. General senses inform the CNS about the condition inside and outside the body. The CNS processes this information and through the motor neurons send command signals to the skeletal muscles. The motor neurons that directly activate skeletal muscles are multipolar lower motor neurons. Their bodies are located within ventral horns of the spinal cord or a brainstem. Their axons are in the PNS. There are two lower motor neuron types associated with general senses: **alpha motor neurons** and **gamma motor neurons**. Alpha motor neurons are large myelinated neurons that stimulate skeletal muscles to contract. Gamma motor neurons are small and are partially myelinated or not myelinated. Gamma neurons control contraction of the intrafusal muscle cells, which are a part of a muscle spindle organ.

CHECK YOUR UNDERSTANDING

- What is the difference between general and special senses?

- Why is the sense of equilibrium counted as a special sense?

- Why is pain classified as a general sense?

Anatomy of General Sensory Organs

Sensory receptors of the general senses are divided in three anatomical categories: **free, encapsulated**, and **associated nerve endings**. The structure of the nerve ending is designed for the best receiving of the stimulus and increasing of the received signal.

Free nerve endings. A sensory neuron that lacks any special structures on its receptive terminus is called a **free nerve ending** or **free sensory receptor**. Often a free nerve ending is extensively branched to increase the monitored area (fig. 12.1). Free sensory receptors are primarily concerned with pain sensations. The receptors for pain are also called **nociceptors**, and pain sensation is a **nociception**. Nociceptors are slow-adapting, if at all, receptors. The sensory neuron bodies of nociceptors are located in either the **dorsal root ganglia** or the pons. Pain sensory neurons in dorsal root ganglia monitor pain all over the body, except

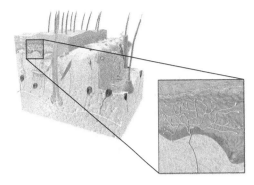

Free Nerve Endings

FIGURE 12.1   Nociceptors—Free Sensory Neurons Endings.

for the head. Pain in the head is monitored through the **trigeminal ganglia** located in the pons. Nociceptors are sensitive only to the high threshold of stimuli. Only when the high threshold of stimulus has been reached does the nociceptor generate a nerve impulse. The nociceptors are classified according to the environmental modalities they respond to. Thus, there are mechanical, thermal, and chemical nociceptors. Some nociceptors respond to more than one modality. These nociceptors are called **polymodal**. Some nociceptors do not respond at all to any stimuli unless some tissue is injured. These receptors are referred to as **silent** or **sleeping nociceptors**. They respond only to damage and inflammation of the surrounding tissues.

There are two different types of axons: **A fibers** and **C fibers**. A fibers are thickly myelinated and conduct an action potential at a rate of about 20 meters per second toward the CNS. C fibers are lightly myelinated or nonmyelinated and can sand a nerve impulse only at speeds of around 2 meters per second (see chapter 10, page 295). As a result, pain comes in two phases. The first phase is mediated by the fast-conducting A fibers, and the second phase is conducted by the C fibers. The pain associated with the A fibers is extremely sharp and feels like an electrical shock. The second phase, generated by the C fibers, is a prolonged dull pain.

There are three major environmental modalities: mechanical, thermal, and chemical that corresponds to three types of nociceptors. **Mechanical nociceptors** respond to excess pressure or mechanical deformation. They also respond to incisions that break the skin surface. **Thermal nociceptors** are activated by noxious heat or cold. There are specific nociceptor sensor protein molecules which respond to the thermal stimulus. One has a threshold temperature of 42°C, when it changes its confirmation and opens sodium ion channels in the plasma membrane. The cool stimuli are sensed by another sensory channel protein molecule at temperatures below 10°C. **Chemical nociceptors** respond to a wide variety of chemical substances, among which are spices. For example, the burn of hot chili peppers is caused by capsaicin molecules. Apart from these external stimulants, chemical nociceptors have the capacity to detect endogenous ligands, and certain fatty acid amines that arise from changes in internal tissues.

Injured tissues release chemicals that stimulate nociceptors. The most potent among all pain stimulating compounds is **bradykinin**. Bradykinin makes organisms aware about the injury and activates cascade of reactions that promote healing. Another powerful pain generating agents are prostaglandins. Histamine and serotonin are also among nociceptors' stimulating agents.

Pain-relieving agents are known as **analgesics**. The analgesic effect of opioids has been known since ancient times. Nowadays many new artificial drugs with a strong analgesic effect have been discovered. It has also been discovered that an organism can produce its own analgesic compounds. These compounds are known as **endogenous opioids**. They are opium-like substances that bind with the same pain receptors as opioids, but are produced internally by organism. Endogenous opioids are secreted by the CNS, pituitary gland, digestive tract, and other organs. Two analgesic oligopeptides called **enkephalins** are 200 times more potent than morphine. Enkephalins are found in high concentration in the brain as well as in the adrenal medulla. Their secretion is triggered by stress reaction as a response to pain. The CNS and anterior pituitary gland secrete **endorphins** and **dynorphins**. Endorphins and dynorphins are large analgesic neuropeptides. Endorphins are naturally produced in response to pain, but their production can also be triggered by various activities such as physical exercises and sports. Laughter may also stimulate endorphin production. A 2011 study showed that attendees at a comedy club showed increased level of endorphins and higher-than-average resistance to pain. These substances are also called **neuromodulators** because they alter neurons' response on neurotransmitters. They can block the transmission of pain signals and produce feelings of pleasure and euphoria.

VETERINARY APPLICATION

Capsaicin is an alkaloid compound produced by hot peppers. This compound causes a feeling of fire in the mouth when you eat a hot pepper. It happens because capsaicin opens ligand gated ion channels in chemical nociceptors. Flow of ions through these channels causes depolarization of the plasma membrane and triggers development of the action potential. As far as the signal is generated in nociceptors, the CNS interprets this signal as pain. The repeated contact of capsaicin with nociceptors leads to their desensitizing. Nociceptors become less sensitive and decrease generation of action potentials in response to pain stimuli. This capsaicin property is used in designing topical applicators and creams for pain relief. These applications are especially effective for local pain relief in disorders of peripheral nerves known as neuropathies and shingles caused by viral infection. Capsaicin does not cure the cause of the pain. It simply makes nociceptors less sensitive to the pain stimuli.

Thermoreceptors are free sense nerve endings. The study of these receptors demonstrates that regularly thermoreceptors are free ends of tiny, unmyelinated, and slow C fibers. According to their location, thermoreceptors are identified as **superficial** and **central thermoreceptors**. Superficial thermoreceptors are located in the skin. They detect changes in skin temperature. Central thermoreceptors are located in the hypothalamus. They monitor temperature of the blood. The transduction of temperature in cold receptors is mediated in part by the TRPM8 channel protein. This channel allows leaking inside the cell Na^+ and Ca^{2+} ions of a magnitude inversely proportional to the temperature. The channel can also be open by the binding with an extracellular ligand. Thus, **menthol** binds with the TRPM8 and opens channel for ions flow. Since the TRPM8 is expressed in neurons which send cold signals, menthol, when it is applied to body surface, creates a sensation of cooling.

Another type of free nerve ending receptors are **hair follicle receptors**. In these receptors free nerve endings wrapped around the base of a hair follicle in the dermis or hypodermis. The network of free endings forms a **hair plexus** or **root hair plexus**. The hair follicle receptor molecules are pressure-sensitive or **stretch-activated channels**. These channels open when the end region of plasma membrane is stretched. The open channels allow sodium ions flow inside the cell and plasma membrane depolarizes. When hair is bended, neuron's plasma membrane depolarizes and, if depolarization reaches a threshold level, an action potential is generated (fig. 12.2).

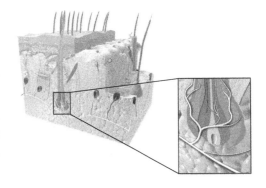

Root Hair Plexus

FIGURE 12.2   Hair Follicle Receptors.

CHECK YOUR UNDERSTANDING

- What is the difference between encapsulated and associated receptors?

- What are sense nociceptors?

- What free nerve ending receptors do you know?

- How do stretch-activated channels function? What is their role in hair follicle receptors?

Encapsulated sensory receptors. Encapsulated sensory receptors have their termini enclosed inside a special structure. This structure is called **encapsulated nerve ending**, or **encapsulated sensory receptor**. The list of these receptors includes **Merkel cell fibers**, **Meissner** or **tactile corpuscles**, **Ruffini endings**, also known as **bulbous corpuscles**, **lamellated** or **Pacinian corpuscles**, and **Krause end-bulbs**.

Merkel cell fibers consist of sensory neuron endings surrounded by a capsule made of Merkel cells. Merkel cell fibers are most important for tactile sensing of form and texture. They are located below the skin epidermis, especially in the most sensitive body regions. These receptors are slow adapting and have the finest spatial resolution among all the skin mechanoreceptors (fig. 12.3).

Meissner corpuscles are formed from two to six sensory neuron endings together surrounded by myelin and collagen. Often, they are intimately associated with Merkel cell fibers. Meissner corpuscles are located in dermal papillae. They are rapidly adapted receptors. They are receptors of touch and form, even are less sensitive than Merkel cell fibers (fig. 12.4).

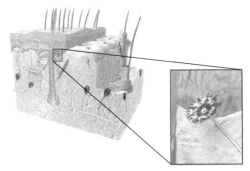

Merkel Cell
(Tactile Disc)

FIGURE 12.3   Merkel Cell.

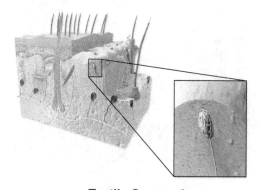

Tactile Corpuscle
(Meissner's Corpuscle)

FIGURE 12.4   Meissner Corpuscle.

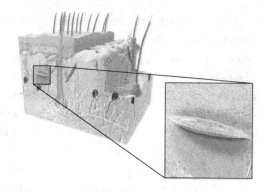

Ruffini Corpuscle

FIGURE 12.5   Ruffini Corpuscle.

Ruffini endings are also known as **bulbous corpuscles**. They are located in the dermis, hypodermis, and ligaments. This spindle-shaped receptor is sensitive to stretch and movement, which causes shifting of body parts. They have the highest density around the fingernails and claws, where they allow control of the grip on an object. Ruffini corpuscles respond to sustained pressure and show very little adaptation. Ruffinian endings are located in the deep layers of the skin and register mechanical deformation within joints, more specifically angle change, with a specificity of up to 2.75 degrees, as well as continuous pressure states. They also act as thermoreceptors (fig. 12.5).

Pacinian corpuscles are located deep in skin, joints, and deep body tissues. For example, Pacinian corpuscles are found in the pancreas. In Pacinian corpuscles, the nerve endings are enclosed in a series of concentric layers called **lamellae** that form an "onion skin" capsule. The capsule acts as a tiny transducer that converts pressure into nerve impulses. The receptor responses on the vibrations. The multiple lamellae absorb the energy of the mechanical stimulus and only rapid and frequent changes in pressure are recorded (fig. 12.6). Pacinian corpuscles adapt rapidly to stimuli.

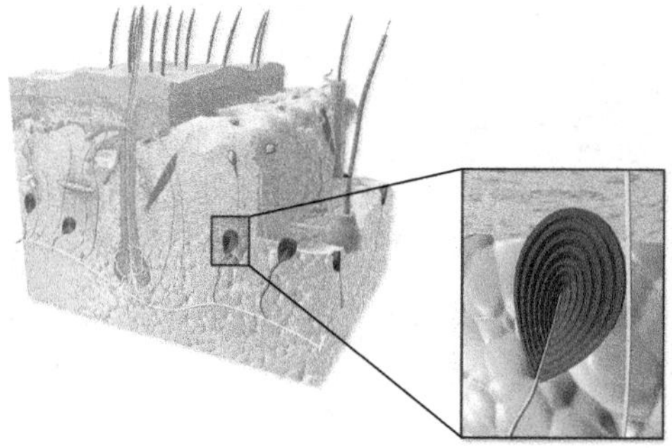

Krause end-bulb receptors are cutaneous thermoreceptors. They have a cylindrical or oval body, consisting of a capsule formed by the expansion of the connective-tissue sheath of a myelinated nerve fiber, and containing a soft semifluid core in which the axis-cylinder terminates either in a bulbous extremity or in a coiled-up plexiform mass (fig. 12.7). End-bulbs are found in the conjunctiva of the eye (in humans they are spheroidal in shape, but cylindrical in most other animals), in the mucous membrane of the lips and tongue, in synovial membranes of some joints, and in the epineurium of nerves. They are also found in the penis and clitoris, where they are called **genital corpuscles**.

Lamellated Corpuscle
(Pacinian Corpuscle)

FIGURE 12.6   Pacinian Corpuscle.

VETERINARY APPLICATION

An abnormally low body temperature is called **hypothermia**. A low temperature slows an organism's metabolic reactions. The heart and respiratory rate slow when an animal's body temperature drops below the norm. The affected animal may lose consciousness and die, if does not warm up in time. Hypothermia can develop not only in animals exposed to low air temperatures, but also in animals under general anesthesia in a veterinary hospital. It happens because most general anesthetic drugs anesthetize the temperature control centers in the brain. This causes a slow fall in body temperature during anesthetic procedures. The situation can worsen if the animal contacts cold surfaces such as a metal surgery table. The low body temperature slows all metabolic processes in the animal's body, including those processes that metabolize and remove anesthetic agent from organism at the end of the procedure. This prolongs the effect of anesthetic drugs and slows the animal's recovery after the procedure. For this reason, veterinarians keep animal warm during the anesthetic procedures by warming the surgery table and cage and holding the animal in warm towels and blankets.

CHECK YOUR UNDERSTANDING

- Which mechanoreceptors are sensitive to a very fine touch?

- What is an encapsulated receptor?

- What is Krause end-bulb receptor function?

Associated sensory receptors. In an associated sensory receptor, a terminus of a sensory neuron wraps around another structure called **associated sensory receptor** or **associated nerve ending**. This receptor monitors state of limb flexion and degree of muscles' contraction. The feeling of limb flexion and tension in constructing muscle is called **proprioception** and its receptors are known as **proprioceptors**. Proprioceptive information is indispensable for determination of body parts' positions and movement. Proprioceptive information is collected by two types of receptors: **muscle spindles** and **Golgi tendon organs**.

A **muscle spindle** organ controls the length of skeletal muscle. These receptors are distributed between the regular skeletal muscle cells, which are called **extrafusal muscle cells** or **fibers**. Extrafusal muscle cells are regular muscle cells in the muscle that surround a capsule of spindle organ. These muscles contract together with all

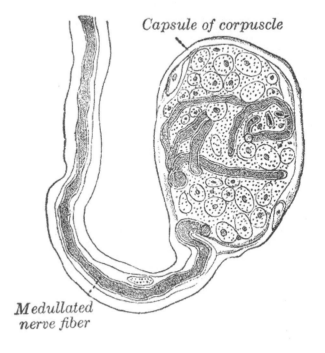

Capsule of corpuscle

Medullated nerve fiber

FIGURE 12.7 Krause End-Bulb.

other muscle cells in muscle and their length is the same as the length of other muscle cells. This contraction together with other muscle fibers allows extrafusal muscle fibers to control a length of skeletal muscle cells in the muscle. The extrafusal muscle cells are innervated by **alpha motor neurons**. The extrafusal muscles surround connective tissue capsule. Inside the capsule, there are packages of fusiform-shaped **muscle spindles** made of modified striated **intrafusal muscle cells**. Each spindle organ contains 2 to 12 intrafusal muscle cells, which are specialized sensory organs. There are two types of intrafusal muscle fibers: the **nuclear bag intrafusal fibers** and **nuclear chain intrafusal fibers**. The nuclear bag intrafusal fibers have nuclei clustered in a swollen region near the middle of the fiber. Their actin and myosin microfilaments are concentrated at the both poles and absent in the middle region. The nuclear bag intrafusal muscle cells are associated with a **primary afferent sensory nerve** or **annulospiral nerve**. The nuclear chain intrafusal fibers has nuclei widely distributed along the cell. It is associated with a **secondary afferent sensory** or **flower spray nerve**. Both primary and secondary afferent sensory neurons contain mechanically (stretch) gated ion channels that open when these muscle cells are stretched. Both types of intrafusal muscles are innervated by the **gamma motor neurons** (fig. 12.8).

Muscle spindle functions to maintain muscle tone. Normal muscle maintains a small amount of tension even when it is relaxed (see chapter 9, page 267). When a muscle relaxes more than normal, the muscle spindle sags. Primary and secondary afferent nerves wound around the intrafusal fibers sense this sag. Through reflex connections in the spinal cord, these afferent neurons synapse with alpha motor neurons to stimulate contraction of extrafusal fibers that stimulate muscle tension and restore muscle tone. The stretching of a muscle lends to its reflex contraction. When postural muscles are stretched or load is added,

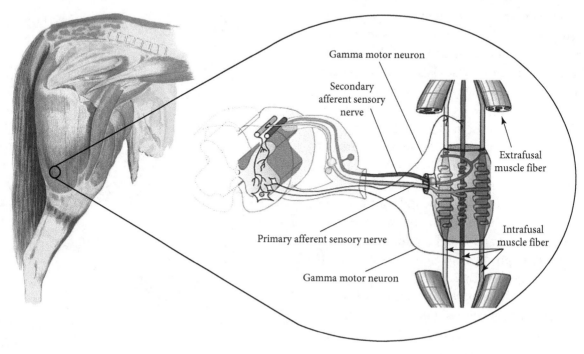

FIGURE 12.8   Spindle Muscle Receptor.

muscle spindles lengthen, initiating the **stretch reflex**. The sensory function of the intrafusal muscle fibers is to inform the nervous system about the rate of change in the length of the extrafusal muscle fibers with which they are associated. This information can initiate a stretch reflex to adjust tonus. It is also relayed to the cerebellum, which modifies muscle activity.

Different body muscle organs have different number of spindle muscle organs. As a rule, the muscles that produce fine muscle contractions, such as the muscles of the eyelids and extraocular muscles, have a large number of muscle spindles. Muscles that generates course powerful contractions, such as dorsal and gluteal muscles like *Latissimus dorsi* or *Gluteus maximus*, have a relatively small number of muscle spindles.

A loss of proprioceptors' sensitivity is called **sensory ataxia**. Sensory ataxia is characterized by the loss of sensitivity to the positions of joint and body parts. Usually, sensory ataxia is associated with damage or dysfunction of dorsal funiculi of spinal cord that carry sensory information from proprioceptors to the CNS.

Golgi tendon organs are sensory receptors in the tendons, located in tendon area close to the junction with muscle. They lie along the line of muscle action and function as tension recorders, supplying the CNS with information about the forces generated by muscles. Golgi tendon organ consists of an encapsulated bundle of collagen fibers attached to about 20 extrafusal muscle fibers. Each Golgi tendon organ contains a single somatic sensory axon whose endings are wrapped around its enclosed collagen fibers. The rate at which these neurons fire depends on the amount of muscle tension generated with each contraction—the greater the tension, the more rapidly they fire (fig. 12.9).

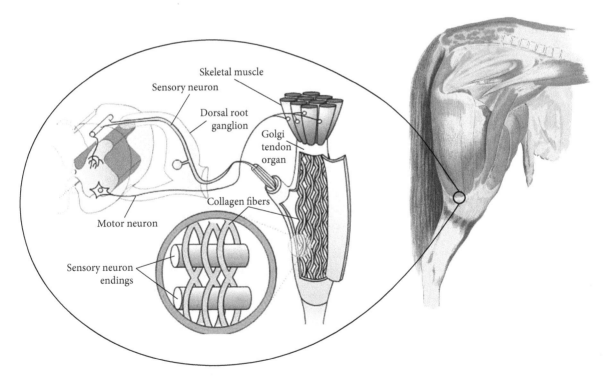

FIGURE 12.9   Golgi Tendon Organ.

CHECK YOUR UNDERSTANDING

- What kind of sense is proprioception?
- What is muscle spindle organ function?

- What kind of information does a Golgi tendon organ generate?

CHAPTER SUMMARY

- Sensory receptors are organs whose specialty is gathering information about the state of external and internal environments. Receptors observe changes and convert an energy of these changes into nerve impulses. These nerve impulses are processed by the CNS. The sensory impulses processes in spinal cord generate spinal reflexes. The sensory impulses processed in the brain generate cranial reflexes. The sensations processed by the brain cerebral cortex are referred to as **perceptions**. The perception in many ways depends on the sensory receptors: what parameters of the world they are detected. Parameters of the world detected by sensory receptors are called **receptor modalities**. Modalities include temperature, pressure, body damage that causes pain, and so on.

- Sensory receptors are made of different sensory cells, which are sensitive to different stimuli. The ability of the sensory cell to respond to a stimulus of a very low intensity is called **sensitivity**. An ability to distinguish stimuli of different modality is known as **sensory specificity**. A **sensory receptor cell** is a cell that specialized to transform energy of the specific stimulus into a nerve impulse. The process of conversion of an energy of stimulus into nerve impulse is called **sensory transduction**. Sensory transduction needs special molecules called **receptor molecules**. Receptor molecule is a transmembrane protein that changes its confirmation in response to the stimulus energy. The change of the receptor molecule confirmation opens ion channels or triggers cascade of chemical reactions inside the cell, which leads to change of the membrane potential known as a **receptor potential**. Some sensory cells are, as a matter of fact, sensory neurons. In this case, development of receptor potential may cause depolarization of the plasma membrane and, when depolarization reaches a threshold level, action potential. However, many sensory cells are not neurons and they do not generate an action potential. In this case, sensory cell makes a synapse with a nearby sensory neuron and transmits receptor potential through the neurotransmitters, which it synthesizes.

- Sensory receptor cells are organized in groups known as **sense organs**. Usually, a sense organ has many sensory receptor cells accompanied by different types of supporting cells. Together with analytical centers in the CNS that process sensory information, sense organs form **sensory systems**.

- There are four principal sources of energy that have an effect on sensory receptors: mechanical, thermal, chemical, and electromagnetic. Mechanical sensations include touch, pressure, vibration, tension, stretching. Thermal sensations are of two types: warm and cold. Chemical senses are based on ability of molecules called **ligands** to create chemical bonds with receptor protein. The electromagnetic senses are based on sensitivity of receptor proteins to electromagnetic fields of different frequency.

- The source of a stimulus may be located outside or inside the body. In the first case, stimuli generate **external senses**; in the second, they generate **internal senses**. Internal signals may come from skeletal muscles and skin and are called **somatic senses**, or from internal organs, such as the liver, and are called **visceral senses**.

- Different types of sensory receptors respond to stimuli with different speed, intensity, and duration. This response on the stimulus is called **receptor adaptation**. Based on their ability to adapt, receptors are classified in two groups: **rapidly adapting** and **slowly adapting receptors**. Rapidly adapting receptors are fast responding. Their response is intense, but its intensity decreases fast with time. These receptors are important for detecting the beginning of the stimulation and fast response to a life-threatening stimulus. The slowly adapting receptors are comparatively slow. Their response is not intense and signaling continues as long as the stimulus continues without significant decrease of intensity.

- Senses are classified in two major groups—**general** and **special senses**—based on a simple definition: 1. General senses are external and internal by origin. They have simple-constructed receptors distributed everywhere in the body. 2. Special senses have complex-structured receptor organs called sense organs. They collect stimuli external to the body and are located in the head.

- General senses include touch, vibration, pressure, temperature, pain, and proprioception. The general sense receptors are simple in organization and widespread over the body. The general senses inform the CNS about the condition inside and outside the body. The CNS processes the information from the general receptors and through the motor neurons send command signals to the skeletal muscles. The motor neurons that execute these commands are multipolar lower motor neurons. Their bodies are located within ventral horns of the spinal cord or in a brainstem. Their axons are in the PNS. There are two major motor neuron types associated with the general senses: **alpha motor neurons** and **gamma motor neurons**. Alpha motor neurons are large myelinated neurons that stimulate skeletal muscles to contract. Gamma motor neurons are small. They control intrafusal muscle cells, which are receptors of a muscle spindle organ.

- Sensory receptors of the general senses are divided in three anatomical categories: **free, encapsulated**, and **associated nerve endings**.

- **Free nerve endings.** Sensory neuron that lacks any special structures on its receptive terminus is called a **free nerve ending** or **free sensory receptor**. Often a free nerve ending is extensively branched to increase the monitored area. Primarily free sensory receptors are concerned with painful sensations. The receptors for pain are called **nociceptors**, and pain sensation is **nociception**. Nociceptors are slowly adapting receptors. The cell bodies of the nociceptor sensory neurons are located in either the **dorsal root ganglia** and observe pain all over the body except head. Pain in the head is monitored through the **trigeminal ganglia**. The nociceptors are sensitive only to a high stimulus threshold. Only when the high threshold has been reached does the nociceptor generate an action potential. The nociceptors are classified according environmental modalities they respond to. Some nociceptors respond to more than one modality and are called **polymodal**. Some nociceptors do not respond at all to any stimuli unless injury has occurred. These receptors are referred to as **silent** or **sleeping nociceptors**.

- Nociceptors have two different types of axons: **A fibers** and **C fibers**. A fibers are thickly myelinated and conduct an action potential at a rate of about 20 meters per second toward the CNS. The C fibers are lightly myelinated or nonmyelinated and can sand a nerve impulse only at a speed of 2 meters per second. As a result, pain comes in two phases. The first phase is mediated by the fast-conducting A fibers, and the second phase is conducted by the C fibers. The pain associated with the A fibers is extremely sharp. The second phase generated by C fibers is a prolonged dull pain.

- Nociceptors are sensitive to three environmental modalities: mechanical, thermal, and chemical. **Mechanical nociceptors** respond to an excess of pressure or mechanical deformation. They also respond to incisions that break the skin surface. **Thermal nociceptors** are activated by noxious heat or cold. There are two receptor protein channels: 1) one has a threshold temperature of 42°C, 2) the other is sensitive to temperatures below 10°C. **Chemical nociceptors** respond to a wide variety of compounds as outside as inside of the body.

- Another type of free nerve ending receptors are **hair follicle receptors**. In these receptors free nerve endings are wrapped around the base of a hair follicle in the dermis or hypodermis. The network of free endings forms a **hair plexus** or **root hair plexus**. The hair follicle receptor molecules are pressure-sensitive or **stretch-activated channels**. The channels open when the end region of plasma membrane is stretched and allow sodium ions flow inside the cell. When hair bends, the neuron's plasma membrane depolarizes and, if depolarization reaches a threshold level, an action potential is generated.

- **Encapsulated sensory receptors.** Encapsulated sensory receptors have their termini enclosed inside a special structure. This structure is called an **encapsulated nerve ending**, or **encapsulated sensory receptor**. These receptors include **Merkel cell fibers**, **Meissner** or **tactile corpuscles**, **Ruffini endings**, also known as **bulbous corpuscles**, **lamellated** or **Pacinian corpuscles**, **Krause end-bulbs**.

- **Merkel cell fibers** consist of sensory neuron endings surrounded by a capsule of Merkel cells. Merkel cell fibers are most important for tactile sensing of form and texture. They are located below the skin epidermis, especially in the most sensitive body regions. These receptors are slow adapting and have the finest spatial resolution of all other skin mechanoreceptors.

- **Meissner corpuscles** are formed from two to six sensory neuron endings together surrounded by myelin and collagen. Often, they are intimately associated with Merkel cell fibers. Meissner corpuscles are located in dermal papillae. They are rapidly adapted receptors. They are receptors of touch and form, even are less sensitive than Merkel cell fibers.

- **Ruffini endings** are also known as **bulbous corpuscles**. They are located in the dermis, hypodermis, and ligaments. This spindle-shaped receptor is sensitive to stretch and movement, which causes shifting of body parts. They have the highest density around the fingernails and claws, where they control the grip on an object. Ruffini corpuscles respond to sustained pressure and show very little adaptation. Ruffinian endings are located in the deep layers of the skin, and register mechanical deformation within joints, more specifically angle change, with a resolution of up to 2.75 degrees, as well as continuous pressure states. They also act as thermoreceptors that respond for a long time, so in case of deep burn there will be pain as these receptors are burned off.

- **Pacinian corpuscles** are located deep in skin, joints, and deep body tissues. In Pacinian corpuscles the nerve endings are enclosed in a series of concentric layers called **lamellae** that form an "onion skin" capsule. The capsule acts as a tiny transducer that converts pressure into nerve impulses. The receptor responses on the phasic motion like a tonic receptor. The multiple lamellae absorb the energy of the stimulus and only rapid and frequent changes of the pressure are recorded. Pacinian corpuscles adapt rapidly.

- **Krause end-bulb** receptors are cutaneous thermoreceptors. They have a cylindrical or oval body, consisting of a capsule formed by the expansion of the connective-tissue sheath of a myelinated fiber, and containing a soft semifluid core in which the axis-cylinder terminates either in a bulbous extremity or in a coiled-up plexiform mass. End-bulbs are found in the conjunctiva of the eye, in the mucous membrane of the lips and tongue, in synovial membranes of some joints, and in the epineurium of nerves. They are also found in the penis and clitoris, where they are called **genital corpuscles**.

- **Associated sensory receptors** have sensory neuron endings wrapped around a receptor structure called an **associated sensory receptor** or **associated nerve ending**. Associated sensory receptors monitor a state of limb flexion and degree of muscles contraction and are called **proprioceptors**. Proprioceptive information is important for determination of a position and movement of body parts. There are two types of proprioceptors: **muscle spindles** and **Golgi tendon organs**.

- **Muscle spindle** organ controls the length of skeletal muscle. Muscle spindles are distributed between the regular skeletal muscle cells, known as an **extrafusal muscle fibers**. The extrafusal muscle fibers control length of skeletal muscle fibers. The extrafusal muscle cells are innervated by **alpha motor neurons**. The space between extrafusal muscle cells is occupied by packages of fusiform-shaped **muscle spindles** that contain **intrafusal muscle cells**. Each spindle organ contains 2 to 12 intrafusal muscle cells. There are two types of intrafusal muscle fibers: the **nuclear bag intrafusal fibers** and **nuclear chain intrafusal fibers**. The nuclear bag intrafusal fibers have nuclei clustered in a swollen region at the middle of the fiber. Their actin and myosin microfilaments are concentrated at cell poles and absent in the middle region. The nuclear bag intrafusal muscle cells are associated with a **primary afferent sensory nerve**. The nuclear chain intrafusal fibers has nuclei evenly distributed along the cell. It is associated with a **secondary afferent sensory nerve**. Both afferent sensory neurons contain stretch-gated ion channels that open when cells are stretched. Intrafusal muscles are innervated by **gamma motor neurons**. Muscle spindle functions to monitor muscle tone. Normal muscle maintains a small amount of tension even when it is relaxed. When a muscle relaxes more than normal, the muscle spindle sags. Primary and secondary afferent nerves wound around the intrafusal fibers sense this sag. Through the spinal reflex arch, afferent neurons synapse with alpha motor neurons and stimulate contraction of extrafusal fibers, which restores muscle tone. When postural muscles are stretched, muscle spindles lengthen, initiating the **stretch reflex**. Muscles have different numbers of spindle muscle organs. Muscles that produce fine muscle contractions have a large number of muscle spindles. Muscles that generate powerful contractions have a relatively small number of muscle spindles.

- **Golgi tendon organs** are proprioceptors in the tendons, located close to the tendon junction with muscle. They lie along the line of muscle action and function as tension recorders, supplying the CNS with information about the muscle pull forces. Golgi tendon organ consists of a group of encapsulated collagen fibers attached to about 20 extrafusal muscle fibers. Each Golgi tendon organ contains a single somatic sensory axon whose endings are wrapped around collagen fibers. The rate at which these neurons fire depends on tension generated by muscle.

CHECK YOUR KNOWLEDGE

LEVEL 1. CHECK YOUR RECALL

1. Nociceptors monitor:
   A. Pain
   B. Change of temperature
   C. Smell of the food
   D. Air movement along the skin surface
   E. Brightness of the sunlight

2. Proprioceptors are located in:
   A. Eyeballs
   B. Olfactory epithelium
   C. Taste buds
   D. Skeletal muscles and tendons
   E. Cochlea and vestibule

3. Receptors that respond to pressure are called:
   A. Nociceptors
   B. Thermoreceptors
   C. Chemoreceptors
   D. Mechanoreceptors
   E. Photoreceptors

4. The sensation of sheets on your skin lessens when you lie still in the bed. This change is due to:
   A. Sensory adaptation of mechanoreceptors
   B. Sensory adaptation of nociceptors
   C. Sensory adaptation because of pH change receptors associated with sleep
   D. Adaptation of the vestibular apparatus
   E. Adaptation of vibration detecting systems

5. Which of the following senses is a general sense?
   A. Equilibrium
   B. Proprioception
   C. Olfaction
   D. Gustation
   E. Vision

6. The branching tips of the dendrites of sensory neurons are called:
   A. Telodendria
   B. Collaterals
   C. Free nerve endings
   D. Terminal buttons
   E. Synapses

7. Which tactile receptors, sensitive to fine touch, pressure, and low-frequency vibration, are abundant in the eyelids, lips, nipples, and external genitalia?
   A. Lamellated (Pacinian) corpuscles
   B. Tactile (Merkel) discs
   C. Tactile (Meissner) corpuscles
   D. Ruffini corpuscles
   E. Krause end-bulb

8. What are receptors that monitor pressure called?
    A. Baroreceptors
    B. Nociceptors
    C. Thermoreceptors
    D. Golgi tendon apparatus
    E. Proprioceptors

9. Receptors that monitor concentration of oxygen, carbon dioxide, and pH in blood are:
    A. Baroreceptors
    B. Nociceptors
    C. Thermoreceptors
    D. Chemoreceptors
    E. Proprioceptors

10. Pain receptors are usually associated with:
    A. Free neuron endings
    B. Tactile (Merkel) discs
    C. Lamellated (Pacinian) corpuscles
    D. Tactile (Meissner) corpuscles
    E. Ruffini corpuscles

11. Spindle muscle and Golgi tendon organ are examples of:
    A. Baroreceptors
    B. Nociceptors
    C. Thermoreceptors
    D. Chemoreceptors
    E. Proprioceptors

12. The most powerful chemical stimulator of pain receptors is:
    A. Histamine
    B. Dopamine
    C. Bradykinin
    D. Prostaglandin
    E. Serotonin

13. Merkel cell fibers are sensors for _____, and Pacinian corpuscles are for _____.
    A. fine touch and surface texture; vibration
    B. vibration; fine touch and surface texture
    C. skeletal muscle tonus; body bending
    D. body bending; skeletal muscle tonus
    E. vibration; skeletal muscle tonus

14. Extrafusal muscles are innervated by _____, and intrafusal muscles by _____.
    A. alpha motor neurons; primary sensory neurons
    B. primary sensory neurons; secondary sensory neurons
    C. gamma motor neurons; alpha motor neurons
    D. secondary sensory neurons; gamma motor neurons
    E. alpha motor neurons; gamma motor neurons

15. The smell of food is a _____, whereas the feeling of an empty stomach is a _____.
    A. chemoreception; nociception
    B. proprioception; chemoreception
    C. special sense; general sense
    D. general sense; mechanoreception
    E. general sense; special sense

16. Thermoreceptors include _____ and _____.
    A. Meisner's corpuscles; Ruffini corpuscles
    B. Pacinian corpuscles; free nerve endings
    C. Merkel cell fibers; Golgi tendon organ
    D. Free nerve endings; Krause end-bulbs
    E. Ruffini corpuscles; Pacinian corpuscles

17. True or false: The function of a receptor cell is to transform the energy of a stimulating factor into a nerve impulse.
18. True or false: A group of sense organs constitute a sensory system.
19. True or false: Sensation depends **only** on the nature of the stimulus.
20. True or false: Nociceptors are general sense receptors presented by free nerve endings.
21. Match the term with its description:

    _____ External senses   a. Lower motor neuron that controls intrafusal muscle
    _____ Intrafusal muscle fiber   b. A proprioceptor that senses muscle tension
    _____ Free nerve ending   c. Pain receptors that respond only to body damage
    _____ Gamma motor neuron   d. Free nerve endings wrapped around a hair follicle
    _____ Golgi tendon   e. Sensation of skeletal muscles and skin
    _____ Hair follicle receptors   f. Senses which monitor external environment
    _____ Sleeping nociceptors   g. Receptor of a spindle muscle organ
    _____ Slowly adapting receptors h. An unspecialized sensory neuron ending
    _____ Somatic senses   i. Conversion of a stimulus' energy in nerve impulse
    _____ Transduction   j. Receptor that does not lose sensitivity for long time

LEVEL 2. CHECK YOUR UNDERSTANDING

1. Why is the proprioceptive sense important to the maintenance of balance and posture?
2. Why are touch mechanoreceptors such as Merkel cell fibers and Meissner's corpuscles rapid adapting, whereas nociceptors and thermoreceptors are slow adapting?

3. What difference does innervation of nociceptors by A and C nerve fibers make? Why is such dual innervation important for animal survival?

4. What are the five types of receptors according to modality of stimulus? Give an example of each type.

LEVEL 3. APPLY YOUR KNOWLEDGE TO REAL LIFE

1. The term *sensory ataxia* designates a loss of proprioception. What symptoms would you expect in a patient with sensory ataxia?

Chapter 13

Special Senses

LEARNING OBJECTIVES

This chapter continues to familiarize you with senses and sensory organs. In it you will learn about special senses that include gustation, or sense of taste; olfaction, or sense of smell; vision; audition, or sense of hearing; and vestibular sensation. The material of this chapter will help you answer questions about:

1. Similarities and differences among general and special senses.

2. The common processes in the foundation of taste and smell senses, and the differences between olfactory and gustatory sense organs.

3. Structure and function of the vertebrate eye.

4. Which common processes create hearing and vestibular sensations, and how the ear and vestibular apparatus are organized.

INTRODUCTION

Special senses are different from general senses by the complexity of sensory organs, location in the head, and exclusive concentration on external stimuli (see chapter 12, page 335). Special senses include taste, smell, vision, hearing, and sensation of body balance and position in space. The modalities that are censored by the special sensory organs include light, chemicals, and sound. The nerve impulses from these organs travel through the cranial nerves to the thalamus and then to the corresponding sensory nuclei. The exception is the olfactory system. Olfactory sensory input travels directly to the olfactory centers in temporal lobes and have no synapses in the thalamus. The receptor cells of the special sense organs are not sensory neurons endings. As a rule, they are specialized epithelial cells that detect specific external stimuli and transform these stimuli into receptor potential. Olfactory receptors again are the only exclusion from this rule: their receptors are neurons that have ligand gated channels to detect odor molecules.

13.1   Anatomy and Physiology of Olfaction

Both olfaction, or sense of smell, and gustation, or sense of taste, are based on chemoreception. Contact of an odorant or food molecules with the appropriate receptors initiates action potentials in sensory neurons.

353

In terrestrial animals, the distinction between taste and olfaction is quite simple. Taste is mediated by specialized chemoreceptive organs in the mouth. Only a few types of chemical compounds generate gustatory sensations. To stimulate sensory receptors, these compounds have to be dissolved in liquid. Olfaction occurs in the nasal cavity. The stimuli are airborne. They must be dissolved in the liquid of the nasal passage before contact with the receptor molecules. For aquatic animals, the distinction between taste and smell is less clear: all chemicals come from the water environment.

All vertebrates have a main **olfactory system**. Besides that, most terrestrial vertebrates also have a system of accessory olfactory organs called the **vomeronasal system**. The receptive surface of the olfactory system is termed the **olfactory epithelium**. The olfactory epithelium contains three types of cells: sensory neuron **receptor cells**, **basal cells**, and **sustentacular cells**. Basal cells are stem cells that produce new and replace old receptor cells. Sustentacular cells are epithelial cells that secrete mucus, support olfactory sensory cells, and produce pigment that gives the olfactory epithelium its color. The olfactory epithelium lines the nasal cavity and constitutes a specific area in the nasal mucosa. This area varies among vertebrates. Its size depends the importance of olfaction in animal life. In humans the olfactory epithelium covers only $2–4 \ cm^2$, whereas in dogs it is $18 \ cm^2$, and in cats it is $21 \ cm^2$. In humans there are around 10^7 olfactory receptor neurons. In dogs there are up to 4×10^9 olfactory receptor neurons.

An olfactory receptor cell is a bipolar neuron. Its cell body is located in the olfactory epithelium among the sustentacular cells. The sensory neuron has a single narrow dendrite that extends from the cell body toward the apical surface of the olfactory epithelium and terminates in a **dendritic knob** embedded into the mucus layer. Apical surface of the dendritic knob carries a tuft of 20–30 projections of plasma membrane termed **olfactory cilia**. The receptor proteins in the plasma membrane of the olfactory cilia are associated with G-protein that opens ion channels. The odorant molecules that are dissolved in mucus interact with receptor protein, the ion channels open, and receptor potential is developed.

The axons of the olfactory sensory neurons are short and unmyelinated. They are among the smallest axons in the nervous system and have a diameter around $0.2 \ \mu m$. It is most correct to apply the term **olfactory nerve** only to these short axons. Through the cribriform plate of the ethmoid bone, axons extend inside the cranium, where they synapse with the **second-order** neurons in the **olfactory bulb**. There are several cell types within the olfactory bulb, the most important of which are **mitral cells**. Axons of the mitral cells form the **olfactory tract**. The olfactory tract conducts nerve impulses to the striatum and limbic system. This is the only sensory pathway that has no synapse in the thalamus.

Olfactory sensory neurons are the only nerve cells exposed to the harsh external environment and, as a result, experience its harmful effect. A regular olfactory sensory neuron has a short life span, about 60 days, before it degenerates. Thus, these neurons have to be regularly replaced throughout animal life. They are the first mammalian neurons discovered to be able to regenerate. New bipolar olfactory neurons develop from **basal cells** in the olfactory epithelium.

The axon of an olfactory receptor neuron terminates within a globular cluster of other axons from many olfactory receptor neurons. Here all of them make a synapse with a mitral cell in the olfactory bulb. Axons of sensory receptor cells and dendrites of mitral cells form a globular network called the **glomerulus**. Every glomerulus carries the olfactory signals from the same particular receptor protein sensitive to the same particular odorant (fig. 13.1). Usually, there are only a few such glomeruli in the olfactory bulb, which are associated with a particular odorant. All axons from the receptor cells that are sensitive

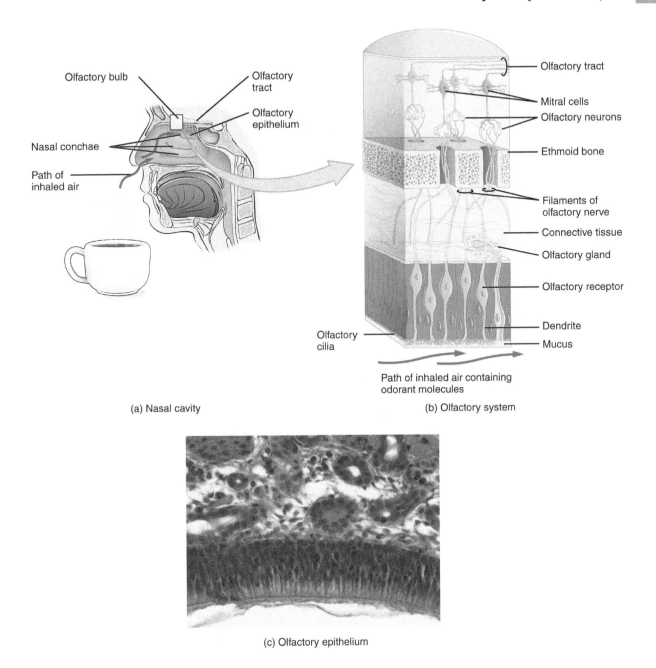

Olfactory bulb

Olfactory tract

Olfactory epithelium

Nasal conchae

Path of inhaled air

Olfactory tract

Mitral cells

Olfactory neurons

Ethmoid bone

Filaments of olfactory nerve

Connective tissue

Olfactory gland

Olfactory receptor

Dendrite

Olfactory cilia

Mucus

Path of inhaled air containing odorant molecules

(a) Nasal cavity

(b) Olfactory system

(c) Olfactory epithelium

FIGURE 13.1 Anatomy of the Olfactory System.

to the same odorant converge and terminate at the same region of the olfactory bulb. In the olfactory cortex, signals from different glomeruli undergo integration. This pathway allows the olfactory bulb and olfactory cortex in the temporal lobes to form an impression about the original smell.

Most mammals (but not humans) also have a second olfactory system called the **vomeronasal organ** (also termed **Jacobson's organ**). It is located below the main olfactory epithelium between the vomer

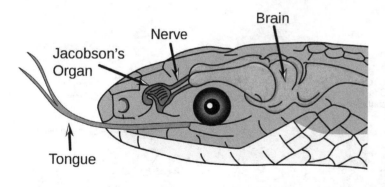

and maxilla bones and forms a self-enclosed pouch usually isolated from the air breathed through the nose. When an animal detects an unusual odor, a pheromone for example, the organ pumps air into the lumen of the vomeronasal organ, where it contacts with the receptor cells. In some reptiles, pheromones are delivered to the organ on the tip of the tongue. A snake or lizard repeatedly sticks out and withdraws its tongue to sample the air and deposits pheromones onto the surface of the vomeronasal organ.

The forked tongue of the snake provides two-point sampling that allows to detect a gradient of pheromone concentration and points on the direction of a pheromone source (fig. 13.2). Histologically, the vomeronasal epithelium is similar to that of the main olfactory epithelium. The vomeronasal receptor cells are very specific and respond only to one or a few compounds. Their sensitivity to these specific odorants is very high.

CHECK YOUR UNDERSTANDING

- What types of cells make up the olfactory epithelium?

- Describe the structure of an olfactory neuron.

- What odors do vomeronasal receptors sense?

13.2   Anatomy and Physiology of Gustation

The sense of food, like the sense of smell, is based on chemoreception. The sense of tasting food is called **gustation**. Gustation begins in a specialized receptor cells in **taste buds**. Taste bud contains a cluster of 20 to 150 cells of three types: **receptor cells**, **basal cells**, and **supporting cells**. Receptor cells constitute only 5 to 15 percent of all cells in the taste buds. The life span of receptor cells is 5 to 15 days. Basal cells on the bottom of the taste bud are stem cells. They produce new receptor cells. Tiny openings on the apex of the taste bud called **taste pore** allow dissolved substances to enter the taste bud and make contact with the sensory receptors. Taste buds are scattered along the tongue and walls of the oral cavity. Every receptor cell synapses with a sensory neuron.

In the tongue, taste buds are located on rounded projections called **papillae**. There are four types of taste buds (fig. 13.3):

1. **Vallate or circumvallate papillae** are dome-shaped round projections. They are the largest papillae with hundreds of taste buds.

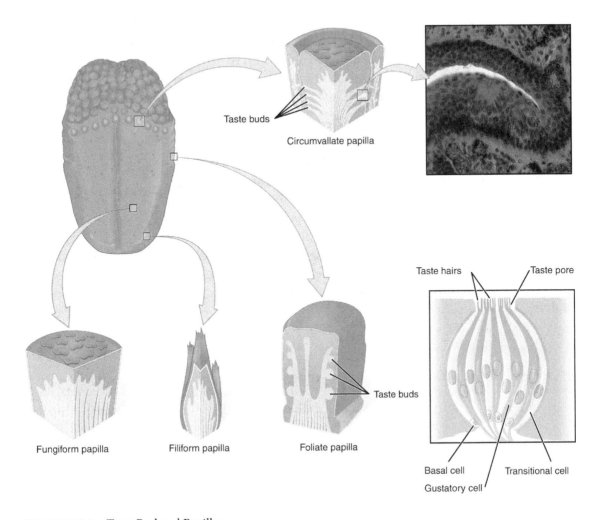

Taste buds

Circumvallate papilla

Taste hairs   Taste pore

Taste buds

Fungiform papilla   Filiform papilla   Foliate papilla

Basal cell   Transitional cell
Gustatory cell

FIGURE 13.3   Taste Bud and Papillae.

2. **Fungiform papillae**, as their name implies, have the shape of a mushroom and possess only a few taste buds.
3. **Foliate papillae** are thick ridges on the lateral sides of the tongue. These papillae have taste buds only in children and puppies. With age they lose their taste buds and do not function in gustation.
4. **Filiform papillae** are long, thin cylinders scattered along the tongue. They have no taste buds, but contain sensory nerve endings to detect food texture and temperature.

There are five principal tastes:

1. **Sweet taste** is a taste of simple sugars, such as glucose, fructose, or galactose.
2. **Sour taste** is based on chemoreceptors that bind hydrogen ion. All acids, such as lemon juice or citric acid, are donors of hydrogen ions and have a sour taste.

3. **Salty taste** is founded on recognition of metal ions in food, such as Na+, K+, or Ca2+.
4. **Bitter taste** is associated with nitrogen-containing compounds. This taste functions to avert appetite and prevent ingestion of toxins and poisons contained in decaying organic matter.
5. **Umami taste** is associated with the taste of meat or broth. This taste is due to monosodium glutamate and aspartate present in food.

The taste stimulus is detected when food molecules bind with the corresponding receptor protein in the plasma membrane of the taste cell. The final food taste sensation is a combination of many signals from different receptors. The smell of the food is also a very important element of taste. Blocking olfactory receptors by nasal congestion makes food tasteless. The real taste of the food is an interpretation of sensations generated by taste and olfactory receptors processed in gustatory centers. Three cranial nerves: facial, glossopharyngeal, and vagus conduct gustatory impulses from receptor cells in the taste buds to the brain. Axons of these nerves terminate in the **solitary nucleus** in the medulla oblongata, where they synapse with central sensory neurons in the thalamus. The vagus nerve in a solitary nucleus also synapses with motor neurons that control saliva production. From the thalamus signals travel to the **primary gustatory cortex** in the parietal lobes.

It is very difficult to judge the gustatory sensation of an animal, but it is obvious that animals are very different in their food preferences. Thus, for a long time it was believed that cats do not taste sweet because normally they do not demonstrate an interest in sweet foods. Recent studies show that cats do have sweet receptors.

VETERINARY APPLICATION

An infection of the upper respiratory tract is usually accompanied by coughing, sneezing, sore throat, and nasal and eye discharges. An upper respiratory tract infection may create a serious danger to domestic animal because of loss of the sense of smell. A sick, sneezing animal can completely lose its sense of smell, which drastically changes its behavior. Animals that lose the sense of smell can completely stop eating and drinking. If this continues for a long time, the animal may become severely dehydrated. In these situations, veterinarians often administer fluids, either orally or through injections, to animals with an upper respiratory tract infection. This allows them to keep the animal properly hydrated and gives them time to take care of the infection.

CHECK YOUR UNDERSTANDING

- Name five basic types of taste.
- What types of papillae do you know?
- Which nerve carries taste sensations to the brain?

13.3   Anatomy of the Eye and Physiology of Vision

Vertebrates develop a variety of organs sensitive to electromagnetic radiation. The photoreceptors in the eye are characteristic to all vertebrates. The vertebrate eye focuses light on photosensitive cells to form a picture of the environment. A group of accessary organs protects the eye and facilitates its function. These accessory structures are **eyelids**, **nictitating membrane**, **eyebrows**, **eyelashes**, **conjunctiva**, **lacrimal apparatus**, and **extrinsic muscles**.

The **eyelids** or **palpebrae** are two skin folds. They cover the anterior part of the orbit. A **levator palpebrae superioris muscle** moves the eyelid up. Contraction of this muscles is controlled by trigeminal (sensory fibers of cranial nerve V) and facial (motor fibers of cranial nerve VII). Together with the brain visual centers, these nerves constitute a circuit, responsible for a **blinking reflex** that protects the eye and facilitates its lubrication with tears. The **orbicularis oculi muscle** is an antagonist to the levator palpebrae superioris. Contraction of this muscle closes the eye. Inside, the eyelid contains a plate of a regular dense connective tissue called the **tarsal plate** that gives a shape to the eyelid. Inside the tarsal plate there are modified sebaceous glands called **tarsal** or **Meibomian glands**. They are holocrine glands, which secrete **meibum**. In fig. 13.4 one can see two rows of tarsal glands. Their secretion is released in a common duct, which opens

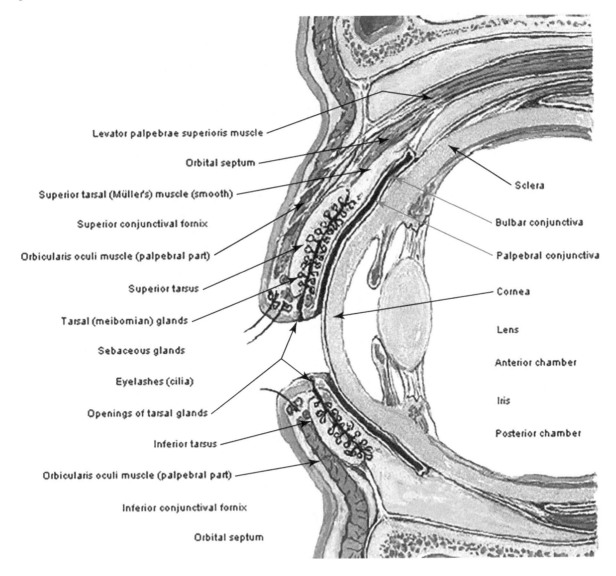

FIGURE 13.4   Eyelid Anatomy.

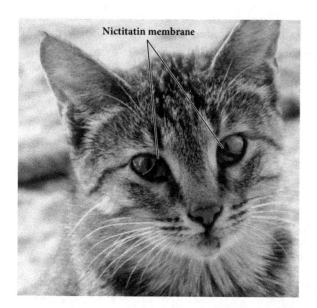

Nictitatin membrane

FIGURE 13.5   Nictitating Membrane.

at the top of the eyelid. Meibum creates an oily film that covers watery tears and prevents evaporation of the tears from the eye surface. Meibum prevents tear spillage onto the cheek, trapping tears between the oiled edge and the eyeball, and makes the closed lids airtight. In human eyes there are approximately 50 glands on the upper eyelids and 25 glands on the lower eyelids. Dysfunctional meibomian glands often cause dry eyes. Tarsal glands open on the top of the eyelids through the tiny ducts. Both eyelids meet at the edges of the orbit at the medial and lateral **commissures** or **canthi**.

The **nictitating membrane** is a transparent third eyelid present in some animals (fig. 13.5). It moves across the eye from the medial canthus. It protects and moisturizes the eye. Often called a **third eyelid** or **haw**, it may be referred as the **plica semilunaris**, **membrane nictitans**, or **palpebra tertia**. Fully developed nictitating membranes are found in fish, amphibians, reptiles, birds and mammals such as camels, polar bears, and seals, but are rare among primates. A gland of the third eyelid is called **Harder's gland**. In some animals it produces up to 50 percent of the tear film. Usually, the nictitating membrane is translucent. In crocodiles, it protects the eye and also helps focus the eye under water. Birds can actively control their nictitating membrane. In birds of prey, the membrane also protects the parents' eyes from their chicks while they are feeding them. Woodpeckers tighten their nictitating membrane a millisecond prior to their beak impacting the trunk of a tree to prevent shaking-induced retinal injury. The membrane also is used to protect the eye while attacking prey, as in sharks. Nictitating membranes can protect eyes from UV radiation, as they do in polar bears to prevent snow blindness.

Eyebrows and **eyelashes** reduce risk of eye injury, by trigger blink reflex. They also prevent eyes from fluids and perspiration running into the eyes and reduce bright light to desensitize receptor cells.

The **conjunctiva** is a thin epithelial membrane. The membrane is folded in two. One fold of this membrane lines the posterior surface of the eyelids, and the other fold covers the anterior portion of the sclera. The fold of the conjunctiva that lines the eyelids is known as the **palpebral conjunctiva**. The conjunctiva that covers the eyeball is called the **bulbar** or **ocular conjunctiva**. A space between the palpebral and ocular conjunctivae is termed the **conjunctival sac**. The conjunctiva is translucent and difficult to see. The conjunctiva protects the eye and provides smooth frictionless movement of the eyeball in orbit. The inflammation of the conjunctiva is called **conjunctivitis**. Viral conjunctivitis can be very contagious.

The **lacrimal apparatus** is made of **lacrimal glands** and ducts that release and remove tears. Lacrimal glands are located at the superior lateral corners of both eyes behind the conjunctiva. Stimulated by autonomic neurons, lacrimal glands release lacrimal fluids and mucus via the tiny ducts into the conjunctival sac. Together with secretion of tarsal glands and nictitating membrane, they create tears. Tears cover the anterior surface of the eye, and moisturize and protect the cornea. Tears have three layers, like a sandwich.

The watery lacrimal fluids form the bottom layer of this sandwich. It moisturizes epithelial cells that cover the eye, protect them from drying and development of pathogenic microflora. Lacrimal fluids contain lysozyme—an enzyme that protects eye from bacteria and fungi. The next tear layer consists of mucus, and on top of it there is an oily secretion of the tarsal glands. This last secretion forms an oily film that prevent tears from evaporating. Altogether tears lubricate eyes and wash away dust particles and pathogenic organisms. Moving down by the gravity, tears finally collected in the medial canthi of the eye, where there are two tiny holes called **lacrimal puncta**. Lacrimal puncta open into the tiny canals known as **lacrimal canaliculi**. Through the lacrimal puncta and canaliculi,

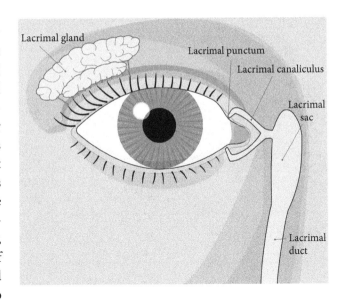

FIGURE 13.6   Lacrimal System.

tears are collected in lacrimal sac that empties into the nasal cavity via the **nasolacrimal duct** (fig. 13.6).

There are six **extrinsic eye muscles** that rotate the eyeball in orbit: four of them are known as **rectus** and two as **oblique muscles**. Muscles help to focus on a particular object and gaze it movement. Extrinsic muscles are skeletal muscles controlled by oculomotor (III), trochlear (IV), and abducens (VI) cranial nerves. The rectus muscles extend from a common tendon ring on the posterior wall of the orbit to insertion on the eyeball. Four rectus muscles are **superior, inferior, medial**, and **lateral rectus muscles**. These muscles rotate the eyeball consequently up, down, medially, and laterally. Two oblique muscles are attached to the superior and inferior surface of the eyeball and are called **superior** and **inferior oblique muscles**. Before to insert to the corresponding site on the eyeball, these muscles make a turn through the fibrous loop called **trochlea**. The superior oblique muscle turns the eye down and laterally. The inferior oblique rotates eye up and laterally (fig. 13.7). Extrinsic eye muscles produce very small, precise movements and are among the most highly innervated skeletal muscles in the body. Their motor units consist only of two or three muscle fibers.

You may compare the construction of the vertebrate eye to that of camera. It has the shape of a sphere located at the anterior side of the orbit. Its walls are made of three layers or **tunics**. The outermost tunic is called **fibrous tunic**. Fibrous tunic is made of a tough dense connective tissue. It protects eye from injuries, and forms the eyeball shape. The middle layer is called **vascular tunic** or **uvea**, because it carries blood vessels and provide oxygen and nutrients to all internal eye structures. The innermost layer is known as a **neural tunic** or **retina** (fig. 13.8). The name of this tunic points on the fact that it is a part of the brain. During the embryogenesis anterior portion of the brain grows and come in contact with epithelial cells of the forehead. The nervous tissue of the brain in place of the contact forms cup-shaped retina and epithelium creates the lens.

Fibrous tunic forms the outer layer of the eye. It makes a tough, dense connective tissue capsule of the eye. The major portion of the tunic is white colored and termed **sclera**. Collagen fibers in sclera allow it to resist

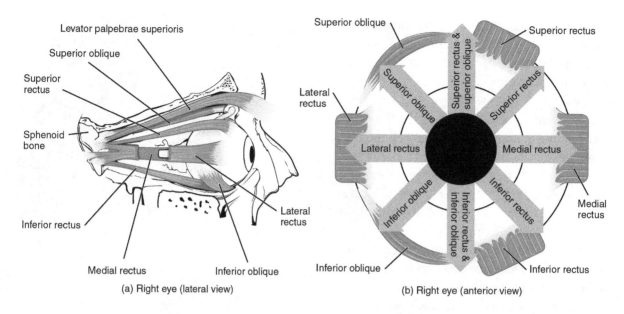

FIGURE 13.7   Extrinsic Eye Muscles.

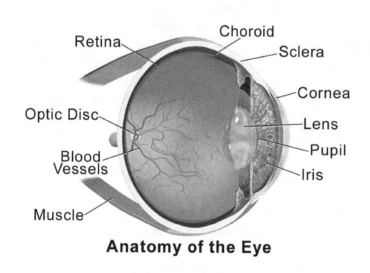

FIGURE 13.8   Eye Anatomy.

deformations and maintain the eye shape. Collagen fibers in sclera are arranged irregularly, which makes it opaque. Collagen fibers in sclera intertwines with collagen fibers of attached to the eyeball extrinsic ocular muscles that rotate the eyeball in the orbit. The sclera forms the shape of the eyeball. In birds, reptiles, and fishes, tiny flat bones called **scleral ossicles** are embedded inside sclera and help it to hold the shape. Anteriorly sclera is replaced by the **cornea**. The border between the cornea and the sclera is called the **limbus**. Collagen fibers in the cornea are organized in regular parallel lines. Regular organization of collagen, very low water in tissue, and absence of blood vessels make the cornea translucent to the light. At the same time, as far as the cornea is avascular, it receives oxygen and nutrients from the aqueous humor in the anterior chamber. The absence of blood vessels in the cornea and the lens makes transplantation of these structures an easy procedure that does not create concern about tissue rejection.

The vascular tunic or uvea constitutes the middle layer of the eye. It is composed of three distinct regions: the **choroid, ciliary body**, and **iris**. The choroid is the largest part of the vascular tunic and occupies all middle and posterior regions. An extensive network of blood vessels of this layer provides oxygen and nutrients to all eyeball structures. The choroid is pigmented. The pigment reduces a light scattering. In most domestic animals, except swine, choroid forms a special reflective surface known as the **tapetum lucidum**. In nocturnal animals the tapetum lucidum reflects a dim night light, amplifies it, and stimulates the light-sensitive receptor cells in the retina. The tapetum lucidum makes animal eyes shine at night in car headlights (fig. 13.9).

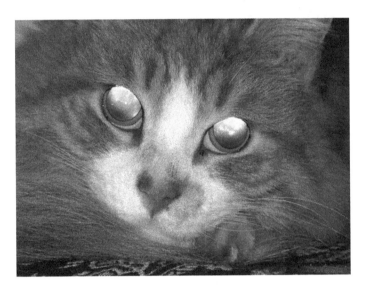

FIGURE 13.9   Shining Tapetum Lucidum in Cat Eyes.

The **ciliary body** is an anterior continuation of choroid. It consists of a tiny circle of smooth muscle called **ciliary muscle**. Tiny threads of **suspensory ligaments** bind ciliary muscles with the lens. Together with the cornea, the lens is responsible for focusing of the light beam on the receptor cells in the retina. The process of adjusting curvature of the lens and focus on object is called **accommodation**. Reptiles, birds, and mammals use the ciliary body to vary the shape of the elastic lens. Fish and amphibians accommodate eye by changing the distance between a rigid lens and the retina with muscles. Ciliary muscles control lens curvature via suspensory ligaments and controls visual accommodation. Contraction of ciliary muscles moves ciliary body closer to the lens. As a result, tension on ciliary ligaments decreases and allows the elastic lens to round up. The relaxation of the ciliary muscles moves ciliary body away from the lens and the tension on the ciliary ligaments increases. Ciliary ligaments pull on the lens and flatten it (fig. 13.10). Besides that, ciliary body secrets **aqueous humor**. Aqueous humor is a watery fluid similar to blood plasma. It delivers oxygen and nutrients to internal tissues of the lens and sclera, as far as there are no blood vessels in this part of the eye.

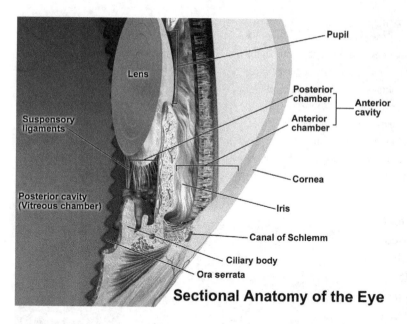

Sectional Anatomy of the Eye

FIGURE 13.10   Sectional Anatomy of the Eye.

The iris is a thin anterior part of the uvea. It consists of tiny pigmented smooth muscles. At the center the iris has an opening called the **pupil**. The iris functions as a diaphragm in a camera. Relaxation and contraction of iris muscles reduce or enlarge the diameter of the pupil and regulate the amount of light that enters the eye interior. Muscles of the iris are organized in two distinctive layers. A group of central smooth muscles are organized in concentric rings and called **pupillary sphincter muscles**. Contraction of these muscles constricts the pupil and reduces amount of light that enters the eye. These muscles are under the control of the parasympathetic nervous system known as the "rest and digest autonomic nervous system." The outer iris muscles layer has a radial orientation and termed **pupillary dilator muscles**. Contraction of these muscles is controlled by sympathetic ("fight or flight") nervous system and causes increase of the pupil for incoming light.

Retina is the innermost layer responsible for eye photosensitivity. It has three layers. The outermost layer, close to the choroid, from which it receives blood supply, contains receptor **rod** and **cone cells**. The next two layers of the retina contain sensory neuron cells. The medial layer known as an **outer plexiform layer** is made of bipolar and horizontal sensory neurons, and the innermost layer called the **inner plexiform layer** is made of amacrine and ganglion neurons. Light enters the eye and falls on the retina. That light has to pass through ganglion, amacrine, bipolar, and horizontal cells sequentially (fig. 13.11). The boundary between anterior retina and posterior edge of the ciliary body is a visible serrated line called the **ora serrata**. Oxygen supply and nutrition retina receives from the capillary network in choroid. The deepest retinal structures are supplied by branches of the central retinal artery that enters the eye together with the optic nerve.

The **lens** is an oval (biconcave) sphere separates anterior and posterior cavities of the eye. Together with the cornea, the lens is responsible for light refraction and focusing it on the receptor cells of the retina. The lens is suspended on the suspensory ligaments. Posterior to the lens is the vitreous body, which, along with the aqueous humor bathes the lens. The anterior surface of the lens is less curved than the posterior. The shape of the lens can change due to accommodation. The lens has three main parts: the **lens capsule**, the **lens epithelium**, and the **lens fibers**. The lens capsule forms the outermost layer of the lens and the lens fibers form its core. The epithelial cells are located only on the anterior side of the lens between the lens capsule and the lens fibers. There are no nerves, blood vessels, or connective tissue in a lens. The lens

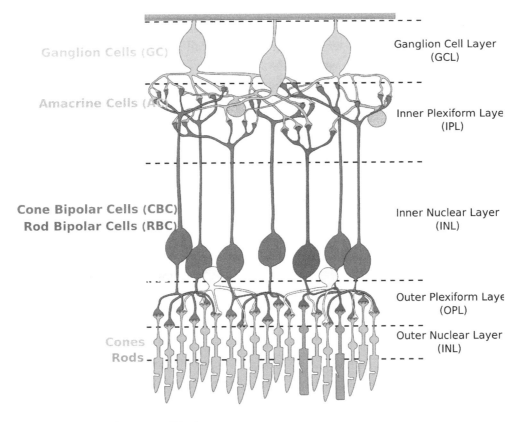

FIGURE 13.11   Anatomy of Retina.

capsule is a smooth, transparent basement membrane that surrounds the lens completely. The capsule is elastic and contains elastic collagen type IV produced by the lens epithelium. The elastic capsule has a globular shape when is not under the tension. The lens epithelium is a simple cuboidal epithelium. The epithelial cells of the lens serve as the progenitors for new lens fibers. The lens fibers are long, thin, transparent cells two-three times longer that wide. The lens fibers are arranged in concentric layers like the layers of an onion. These tightly packed layers of lens fibers are referred to as laminae. New lens fibers are generated from the lens epithelium and are added to the outer cortex. The mature lens fibers are dead cells without organelles and nuclei. They are completely filled with transparent fibrous protein molecules known as **crystalline**.

Within the eye there are three chambers. Two chambers lie anteriorly to the lens. They constitute an anterior eye cavity. The **anterior chamber** is located between posterior wall of the cornea and the iris. The **posterior chamber** creates a space between the iris and the lens. Both chambers are connected through the pupil and filled with an **aqueous humor**—a watery secretion of ciliary bodies in the posterior chamber. To prevent buildup, the fluid is drained at the same rate as it is secreted. It is drained inside the anterior chamber into a blood vessel that circles the anterior edge of the iris, called the **scleral venous sinus** or **canal of Schlemm**. Abstraction of aqueous humor drainage results in accumulation of the fluid and increase of hydraulic pressure inside the eyeball. When this continues for some time, it may cause pathologic changes.

The third and largest chamber occupies posterior eye cavity. It is called the **vitreal chamber**. The vitreal chamber occupies space between the lens and the posterior wall of the eyeball lined by the retina. This chamber is filled by **vitreous humor**, which also often is called a **vitreous body**, because it consists of thick transparent viscous gelatinous material. The vitreous humor gently presses the retina against the choroid. It maintains a normal shape of the eyeball and guarantees regular oxygen and nutrients supply of the retina from blood vessels in choroid. The loss of the vitreous body volume with aging may cause the decrease in pressure and compromise blood supply to the retina. The decrease in retina blood supply may cause diseases such as **macular degeneration**.

VETERINARY APPLICATION

Glaucoma is a group of diseases characterized by increased intraocular pressure that causes pain and can lead to blindness. In domestic animals, glaucoma is most often diagnosed in dogs. An intraocular pressure is measured by tonometer. Glaucoma may have many causes, but the basic mechanism is that aqueous humor is produced faster than drained out of the anterior chamber. Accumulation of aqueous humor causes the rise of intraocular pressure. Therapy for glaucoma usually involves medical or surgical treatments designed to increase the rate at which aqueous humor is drained out of the anterior chamber.

The visual system is a most complex special sense system based on photoreception and processing of visual information. The process is triggered by the solar energy. About half of the solar radiation reaching the earth is within the wavelength of 400 to 700 nm and the wavelength of this range constitute "visible light." All living organisms detect light in the same way: they use a pigment that absorbs the light. A photopigment is a complex composition of a protein called **opsin** and nonpeptide organic molecule called **chromophore**. The chromophore presents in all living organisms from bacteria to mammals and birds. It is known as **retinal**. Retinal is one of the many forms of vitamin A. A combination of retinal and opsin forms pigment known as **rhodopsin**. There are many mammalian rhodopsins with different light-absorption spectra. Because they all use the same chromophore, the difference among rhodopsins is mostly in protein opsin. The absorption of the energy of light causes changes in opsin molecule confirmation (3-D shape), known as a **photochemical reaction**. Change in rhodopsin activates a G-protein signal-transduction cascade that results in release of neurotransmitter in synaptic cleft by receptor cell.

The retina of the vertebrate eye is an outgrowth of the brain. It contains **rod** and **cone photoreceptor cells** (fig. 13.12) and a complex network of neurons: **bipolar cells**, **horizontal cells**, **amacrine cells**, and **ganglion cells**, which perform the first steps of visual integration. A pigmented epithelium lies at the back of the retina. It absorbs light not absorbed by the photoreceptors and has other important tasks, including the control of the ionic balance around the rod and cone cells. All retinal layers are transparent and light easily reaches rod and cone cells. Many retinas have central high-acuity region called **fovea centralis**. The fovea centralis has the highest density of photoreceptors compare with the rest of the retina. It is a region about 1.5–2 mm in diameter clear of blood vessels and other intervening pathway of light tissues. The center of the fovea has highly dense packed cones. Rod receptors are absent in this area. Primates and some birds have well-developed fovea. Other vertebrates have a less well-developed fovea, but most of them have a region called **macula lutea**, which also contains a large number of photoreceptors.

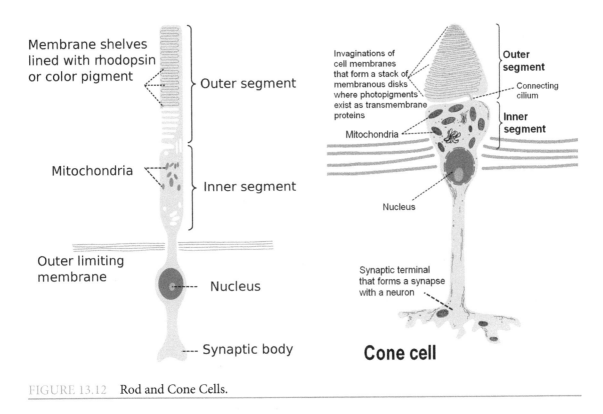

Membrane shelves lined with rhodopsin or color pigment

Outer segment

Mitochondria

Inner segment

Outer limiting membrane

Nucleus

Synaptic body

Invaginations of cell membranes that form a stack of membranous disks where photopigments exist as transmembrane proteins

Outer segment

Connecting cilium

Inner segment

Mitochondria

Nucleus

Synaptic terminal that forms a synapse with a neuron

Cone cell

FIGURE 13.12   Rod and Cone Cells.

The axons of retinal ganglion cells that form optic nerve, come off the inner side of the retina, which facing the lens. These axons exit through the retina at area called **optic disc** (fig. 13.13). Because optic disc contains axons only and has no receptor cells, it creates a **blind spot** in visual field. Rod and cone receptors have different sensitivity to the visual light. Rod cells are more sensitive and used in dim light. Cones are less sensitive, but in a bright light they can be used for color and high-acuity vision. That is why, nocturnal animals tend to have rod cells, whereas cones are characteristic of daytime animals. Both cell types have two distinct regions: an **outer segment** containing the photosensitive membranous structures, and

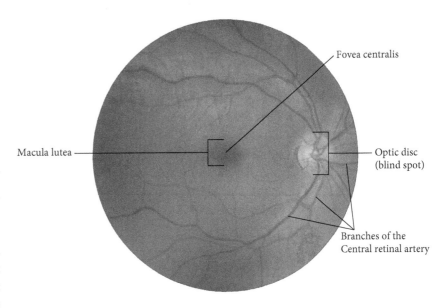

Fovea centralis

Macula lutea

Optic disc (blind spot)

Branches of the Central retinal artery

FIGURE 13.13   Macula Lutea and Optic Disc.

an **inner segment** containing most of regular cell structures, such as nucleus, mitochondria, lysosomes, and so on. The distal end of the inner segment has a synaptic terminal associated with retina neurons. The inner and outer segments are connected by a narrow cytoplasmic bridge. The outer segment contains flattened lamellae of membranes that originates from cell plasma membrane. In the cones, lamellae are just a continuation of plasma membrane and the lumen of each lamellae is connected with the extracellular space. In rods, lamellae are separated from the plasma membrane and form flattened **discs** inside the cell. Discs are paled like pancakes and fill all the space inside the outer segment. Both lamellae contain rhodopsin and are the areas of photochemical reactions.

The transduction of the light into an electrical signal has three steps: 1) light strikes rhodopsin and causes a change in its confirmation; 2) the change in rhodopsin conformation causes decrease concentration of messenger molecules (cyclic guanine-monophosphate or cGMP); and 3) the decrease of cGMP causes closing of ion channels that results in hyperpolarization of plasma membrane. In dark, the cGMP concentration increases and membrane potential returns back to its resting state. This mechanism is designed to turn the response off when the light stimulation is removed. Turnoff in rod cells is slower than in cones. It means that rods are less sensitive to illumination changes than cones. The rods stimulated by a very bright light recover slowly.

Photoreceptors respond to light, but the visual system, which includes photoreceptors, retina, and brain visual centers, responds to **contrast**: changes in level of light and color. In diurnal species, single cone tends to synapse with single bipolar cell in outer plexiform layer of retina. This signal projects to the CNS. The direct one-to-one transfer of impulses between cone and bipolar neuron increases the resolution of the retina and an acuity of the color vision. **Bipolar neurons** receive sensory input from receptor cells and conduct it to amacrine and ganglion cells in the inner plexiform layer. **Horizontal neurons** in outer plexiform layer integrate different areas of retina making synapses with many receptor cells. They organize groups of rod cells in batteries, by making synapses with them. This organization of receptor cells in groups affects the intensity of the signal received by the bipolar cells. **Amacrine cells** create the same kind of horizontal connections in the inner plexiform layer. In most vertebrates there are ganglion cells that respond only on movement in one direction and do not on motion in the opposite direction. It is believed that amacrine cells play a key role in forming these receptive fields. In nocturnal species, large numbers of photoreceptor cells converge on a small number of interneurons and signals merge. Convergence decreases acuity, but increases sensitivity. Axons of **ganglion cells** form optic nerve, which conducts retina sensory output to the brain.

Sensory information is conveyed simultaneously through a few parallel pathways. One pathway projects visual signals to the superior colliculi in the midbrain that control eye gazing. The other pathway arises from special ganglion cells that are sensitive to the absolute brightness of light regardless of its pattern. This pathway projects to centers in the CNS that control smooth muscles contraction in the iris, which regulate amount of light enter the eye. This pathway also projects to suprachiasmatic nucleus, which plays critical role in regulation of circadian rhythms. The major visual projection in mammals is the **geniculostriate system**. The axons of the optic nerve (ganglion cells) form synapse in the thalamus region called the **lateral geniculate nucleus (LGN)**. From here visual information projects to the **primary visual cortex** in the occipital lobe of the cerebrum. In most mammals, the optic projections are only partially crossed at the optic chiasm: the phenomenon called **partial decussation**. In cats and primates, the projections of the medial (nasal) half of the retina cross to the contralateral side. The lateral (temporal) half of visual neurons projections do not cross and project ipsilateral. This mixing of input from the two eyes allows mammals with forward-facing eyes to merge binocular input for depth perception at the visual cortex (fig. 13.14).

The ability to distinguish color depends on the differential sensitivity of photopigments to light of different wavelength. Although many animals are color-blind, many other daytime active animals have well-developed color vision. In 1801, Thomas Young (1773–1829) proposed that

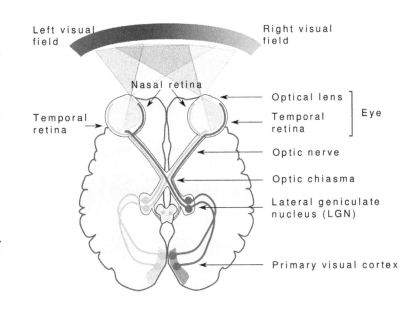

FIGURE 13.14   Visual Pathway.

human color perception is based on sensitivity to three light spectrums: red, green, and blue. Since that time this theory receives a significant experimental development. It was found that vertebrates with color vision may have up to four types of cone cells. The earliest vertebrates had all four cone types, which correspond to violet (370 nm), blue (445nm), green (508 nm), and orange (560 nm). Many fishes, turtles, lizards, and birds have four-color vision. Many amphibians lack color vision. However, some distinguish three colors. Almost all mammals are dichromatic. They have two types of cone cells sensitive to violet and orange. Scientists explain this loss of color vision among mammals by the fact that most mammals are nocturnal animals and do not benefit from color vision. Humans and other primates have three types of cone receptors, which got corresponding names: **red cones**, **green cones**, and **blue cones**.

The position of the eyes on the head is a result of a trade-off between the breadth of the visual field and depth of perception. Laterally located eyes can scan separate sectors of the surrounding world. The total field of view in that case is extensive. Vision in which the visual fields of both eyes do not overlap is called **monocular vision**. Monocular vision is most common among prey animals. It gives them a broad field of view and help in time to detect threads. Strictly monocular vision in which the visual field of both eyes are completely separated is rare and was found only in sharks, salamanders, penguins, and whales.

In animals with **binocular vision** the visual fields overlap. An extensive overlapping of visual fields is characteristic to human and apes. Overlapping in these species constitutes up to 90° of visual field and only 60° constitute monocular vision on each side. Birds have up to 70° and reptiles to 45° overlap of their visual fields. Within the overlap area, two visual fields merge into a single image, producing a sharp and deep **stereoscopic vision**. This vision gives a sense of depth, which comes from the way of processing of visual information. In binocular vision, each eye sees visual field separately. Half of each eye input goes to the same side, and the other half decussate via the optic chiasm to the opposite side of the brain. The result is that visual cortex areas on both sides receive information from both eyes. The brain compares the difference between two images. This difference in two images is called **parallax**. The nervous system takes advantage of the parallax resulted from the differences of both eyes positions. Each eye registers a slightly different image due to the distance between eyes. Although this difference is very small, it is enough to the nervous system to get a sense of depth from it. Accommodation also contributes to depth perception. The degree of accommodation required to bring an object into focus is used by the brain as an interpretation of the distance.

CHECK YOUR UNDERSTANDING

- Where is aqueous humor produced, and where is it drained?

- Why is the optic disc a blind spot of the eye?

- What is the role of rod and cone cells? What is the difference between them?

- What are the main refractive structures of the eye?

- What is the function of the iris and ciliary body?

13.4 Anatomy of the Ear and Physiology of Hearing

The sense of hearing is based on mechanoreception. This sense consists in transduction of mechanical movement of air molecules into sensory nerve impulses. The principal mechanoreceptors of hearing are **hair cells**. These cells got their name after hair-like microvilli on apical surface. The microvilli have constriction at their base and rest on a dense **terminal web** or **cuticular plate**. Hair cells are epithelial cells. They originate from embryo ectoderm and have no their own axons, but each cell is embraced by the dendrites of sensory neurons. The organ of hearing consists of three adjoining compartments: **external**, **middle**, and **inner ears**.

The **external ear** catches air waves and direct them toward the hearing receptors. It has three structures: **earlobe** (also called **auricle** or **pinna**), **external auditory canal** or **external acoustic meatus**, and **eardrum** or **tympanic membrane**. Pinna forms a surface that collects air waves. It is made of elastic cartilage covered by skin. Because cartilage tissues are avascular, clipping the earlobe or piercing do not bleed much. Size of the pinna indicates importance of hearing in animal life. As a rule, nocturnal animals that heavily rely on their hearing have a big pinna surface. The irregular shape and folds on the walls of the pinna helps to differentiate sounds coming from different directions. Paired ears provide stereophonic hearing. In many mammals, pinna serves for a regulation of body temperature. Many desert animals have big pinna, which increases radiation of body heat. Often pinna is mobile and rotates toward the source of the sound. Air waves captured by the pinna are directed toward the tympanic membrane via the external acoustic meatus. In primates the external acoustic meatus is a short straight tube, but in most mammals, it is L-shaped. The walls of the external acoustic meatus are lined by hairy epithelium with **ceruminous glands** that continuously secrete **cerumen** or **earwax** (see chapter 5, page 144). The coarse hairs and earwax protect the external acoustic meatus from fluids, dust, and parasites. Earwax lubricates and waterproofs the tympanic membrane, and keeps it soft and pliable. The external acoustic meatus is blindly ended by the tympanic membrane. The tympanic membrane is made of a thin sheet of epithelial and connective tissues. It is tightly stretched across the opening between the external auditory canal and middle ear cavity (fig. 13.15). The tympanic membrane has a shape of cone. Its tip pointing inside the middle ear and touches a tiny bone, the malleus. When air waves directed by walls of the external acoustic meatus strike the tympanic membrane, it begins to vibrate at the same frequency as the air.

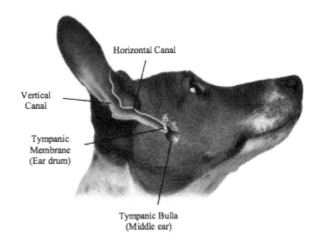

FIGURE 13.15   External Ear.

VETERINARY APPLICATION

Otitis externa is an inflammation of the skin of the external acoustic meatus that often occurs among dogs, cats, and rabbits. Usually, it is caused by parasites such as ear mites, bacterial or fungal infection. The irritation in the ear canal causes redness, pain, itching, and edema. The affected ear usually is red, moist, swollen, and painful, and often has a characteristic pungent odor. Inflammatory fluids drain downward and accumulate in the horizontal portion of the canal next to the tympanic membrane. Because topical medications are usually part of the treatment of otitis externa, the ear canals must be cleaned and discharges removed before the medications are applied. Because the ear canals are often swollen and painful, this process can be difficult for at least the first few days. Therapy for otitis externa often must be continued for many weeks to bring the condition under control.

The middle ear or **tympanic cavity** is a hollow chamber between the tympanic membrane and **oval window**. Oval window is an opening between middle and inner ears covered by a thin flexible membrane. Both middle and inner ears are located in cavity inside the petrous part of the temporal bone (Tympanic bulla). The tympanic cavity is lined by mucous membrane. The middle ear is filled with air and contains three tiny bones collectively called **auditory ossicles** (fig. 13.16). Ossicles are connected with each other by moveable synovial joints. They form bridge extended across the middle ear between the tympanic membrane and oval window. The first bone is called **malleus**. On one side malleus touches the tympanic membrane, and on the other side it joints with **incus**. It vibrates together with tympanic membrane when air waves strike it. Incus transmits vibrations from the malleus to the **stapes**. The stapes presses on the oval window and causes this membrane unison vibration. The tympanic membrane is ten times larger than membrane of oval window. The conversion of sound from large surface and focusing it on a much smaller area significantly amplifies force of air vibrations. The ossicles decrease the amplitude of the vibration, but increase their force; that is, **this mechanism works as an amplifier of the sound signal**.

Another main function of the middle ear is prevention of the damage to the supersensitive receptors in the inner ear from an abnormally loud sound. The preventive mechanism is termed **tympanic**

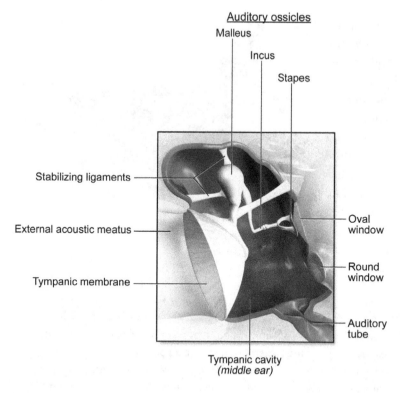

Auditory ossicles

Malleus

Incus

Stapes

Stabilizing ligaments

External acoustic meatus

Tympanic membrane

Oval window

Round window

Auditory tube

Tympanic cavity
(middle ear)

FIGURE 13.16   Middle Ear Anatomy.

reflex. The reflex circuit is initiated by the cochlear branch of the sensory vestibulocochlear nerve (VIII) and through the motor fibers of the facial nerve (VII) it activates effector organs: **stapedius** and **tensor tympani muscles**. The abnormally loud sounds trigger contraction of these muscles. The stapedius muscle pulls stapes and does not allow it to press on the oval window. At the same time, the tensor tympani muscle pulls the malleus and stops transmission of vibrations from the tympanic membrane to the malleus. Altogether contractions of both muscles cut off conduction of air vibrations toward the inner ear. This reflex may be triggered by chewing, loud vocalization, crying, or howling. Animals often use this mechanism to make extremely loud sounds less annoying and uncomfortable. Reflex does not protect from a sudden sound, like a gunshot: muscles contract slower than this sound, but it is very effective against a continuously increasing long-lasting sounds. These sounds cause dog to howl, when it hears a siren of an ambulance.

For the effective conduction of the air wave vibrations, air pressure on both sides of the tympanic membrane has to be equal. The air pressure in the middle ear is equalized through the **pharyngotympanic** (also called **auditory**, or **Eustachian**) **tube**. The auditory tube connects tympanic cavity with the nasopharynx: a part of the throat posterior to the nasal cavity. It is a soft collapsible tube. The entrance to the tube from the pharynx is guarded by a fold-shaped valve, which opens when the air pressure in the pharynx drops. For example, it opens when your cat yawns or swallows. The opening of the valve allows air to flow inside or outside of the middle ear and equalize air pressure across the tympanic membrane.

The inner ear accommodates structures associated with sensing of sound and equilibrium. It has three distinct regions: 1) the **cochlea** accommodates sensory receptors and structures associated with hearing; 2) the **vestibule**; and 3) **semicircular canals** are associated with vestibular sensations of body movement and head position (fig. 13.17). All structures are located in cavity inside the temporal bone. The cavity forms a network of tunnels called **bony labyrinth**. Bony labyrinth is filled with a fluid known as **perilymph**. The ionic composition of perilymph has a higher sodium ions concentration than potassium and is similar to an extracellular fluid. A continuous membrane called the **membranous labyrinth** lines inner walls of the bony labyrinth. The fluid inside the membranous labyrinth is called **endolymph**. In opposite to the perilymph, endolymph has higher concentration of potassium than sodium ions. Perilymph and endolymph are separated completely and normally do not mix. The difference in electrolyte concentration between perilymph and endolymph is important for generation of sensory impulses in the vestibulocochlear nerve.

The hearing portion of the inner ear is contained in a snail shell-shaped spiral cavity in the temporal bone called **cochlea**. Two openings: **oval** and **round windows** covered by membranes separate middle ear and cochlea. A spiral portion of membranous labyrinth known as the **cochlear duct** or **scala media**. The cochlear duct is filled with endolymph. The cochlear duct spirals around a screw-shaped core bone called **modiolus** and ends at the tip of the cochlea.

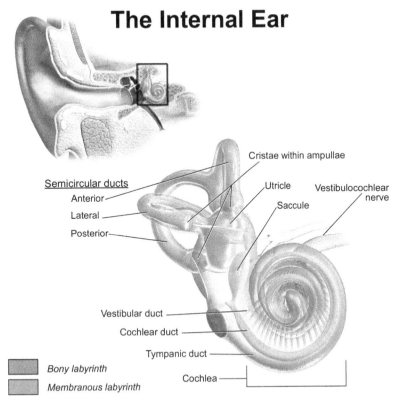

The Internal Ear

Cristae within ampullae

Semicircular ducts
Anterior
Lateral
Posterior

Utricle

Saccule

Vestibulocochlear nerve

Vestibular duct
Cochlear duct
Tympanic duct

Bony labyrinth
Membranous labyrinth

Cochlea

FIGURE 13.17   Anatomy of the Human Inner Ear.

Bony labyrinth is subdivided in two chambers, which spiral around the cochlear duct and are filled by perilymph: the **scala vestibuli** and the **scala tympani** sandwich the cochlear duct from both sides. On one side the scala vestibuli is closed by the oval window. On the other side, at apex of the cochlea, it has a narrow passage into the scala tympani called **helicotrema**. Beginning in helicotrema, scala tympani ends by round window closed by another soft elastic membrane. Morphologically the scala vestibuli and scala tympani create one continuous canal from both sides closed by two membranes in oval and round windows. This structural organization releases hydraulic pressure and allows perilymph fluid movement as sound is transmitted to the inner ear. Round window also damps sounds once they have made a first pass through the cochlea and prevents these waves from ricocheting around the inner ear. The scala vestibuli is separated from the cochlear duct by membrane called **vestibular membrane**. Vestibular membrane holds perilymph in the scala vestibuli off the endolymph in the cochlear duct and maintains ion balance in both fluids. A **basilar membrane** separates the cochlear duct from the underlying scala tympani. Basilar membrane is composed of collagenous connective tissue. Near the base of cochlea, it is stiff and narrow. At the cochlea apex, it is broad and flexible. This difference is important for transduction of vibrations onto receptor cells in the cochlear duct. An auditory sensor organ is called **spiral organ of Corti**. It is located inside the cochlear duct and rests on the basilar membrane. The vibrations of the basilar membrane are

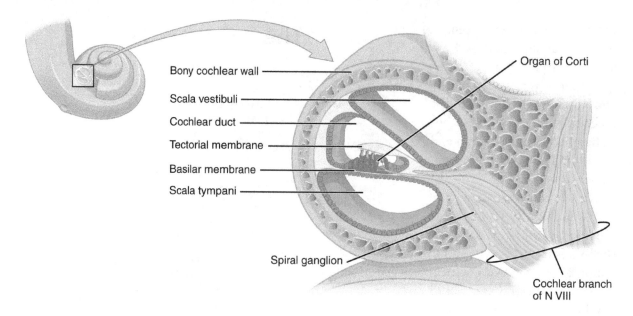

FIGURE 13.18   Cross Section through Human Cochlea.

detected by organ of Corti and transduced into the cochlear nerve impulses. At the base of the cochlea, there are a **spiral ganglion** that houses bodies of cochlear sensory neurons (fig. 13.18).

Sound is an air wave of a particular frequency. The air waves are generated by movement of air molecules. The movement of molecules is known as a kinetic energy. When molecule strikes the surface and stop, it lost this kinetic energy, which converts in other forms of energy: heat, chemical, or vibration of the surface. That is what happen, when air waves captured by the auricle reach tympanic membrane. Tympanic membrane begins to vibrate in unison with air. This vibration, through the auditory ossicles conducted to the stapes, which in its turn presses on oval window. The oval window vibrates at the same frequency as the tympanic membrane. However, when the ossicle transmits the force from the larger tympanic membrane to the much smaller oval window, the force of pressure is concentrated in a smaller area and for this reason it increases. The ossicle also acts as a lever system to amplify the vibration of the oval window. Vibration of the oval window press on the perilymph that fills the scala vestibuli. Vibration of the oval window generates pressure waves in the perilymph.

The pressure waves generated at the oval window travel through the perilymph of the vestibule to the scala vestibuli of the cochlea. High-frequency vibrations take shortcut through the cochlear duct to reach the scala tympani, they cause the endolymph and basilar membrane to vibrate. These vibrations occur close to the base of the cochlea, where the basilar membrane is narrow and stiff. Low-frequency vibrations travel farther into the cochlea and make the basilar membrane vibrate where it is wider and more flexible. For very low-frequency sounds that we cannot hear, the waves travel all the way to the tip of the cochlea, where the scala vestibuli connects with the scala tympani at the helicotrema. From the helicotrema waves travel back to the vestibule via the scala tympani, where they cause corresponding vibrations of the round window. The round window is essential. Without it the fluid would not move. As you know from the physics course, liquid cannot be compressed. When liquid is pushed from one area, it must move into another area. In the same way, as the oval window is pushed into the inner wear, perilymph moves and presses the round window, which bulges outward, and vice versa.

The spiral organ of Corti rests on the basilar membrane. The organ is composed of three components: **tectorial membrane**, **hair cells**, and **dendrites of cochlear nerve**, with which hair cells synapse. Tectorial membrane is a strong stiff plate made of regularly organized collagen fibers. It extends along the longitudinal length of the cochlea parallel to the basilar membrane (figs. 13.18–13.19). Hair cells are receptor cells. They rest on the basilar membrane and are organized in two rows: a single row of **inner hair cells**, and three rows of **outer hair cells**. Inner hair cells are responsible for sound detecting. Each hair cell has a set of microvilli called **stereocilia**. Stereocilia have different length. There are short and comparatively long stereocilia. Long stereocilia project from the cell and end very close, almost touching, the tectorial membrane. They are stiff, but can be bended at the base. All stereocilia are bound by an elastic filament termed **tip link** (fig. 13.20). When long stereocilia touch the tectorial membrane, they bend and via the tip link pull all other stereocilia bend at the same direction. Bending of stereocilia causes mechanically gated potassium channels in the plasma membrane of the hair cell to open. Because endolymph in the cochlear duct has a very high concentration of potassium, much higher than inside the hair cell, its ions move inside the cell and plasma membrane of the hair cell depolarizes. Depolarization of hair cell plasma membrane triggers release of neurotransmitters in the synaptic cleft between hair cell and cochlear nerve causing development of action potential. Hair cells are tuned into only a narrow range of frequencies (fig. 13.20). In mammals, differences in the orientation of hair cells in the inner and outer rows of the organ of Corti produce differences in sensitivity in different regions. Sequential grading of the tuned hair cells along the organ of Corti produces tone discrimination over a range of frequencies. The basilar membrane changes gradually in width. You can compare it with a harp in that each section of the membrane may resonate only to a distinctive range of frequencies. Thus, tones that enter the cochlea impart the greatest motion to the section of the basilar membrane that corresponds to their frequency. This way, specific tones stimulate specific sections of hair cells.

Pitch is determined by with area of the basilar membrane vibrates, whereas loudness is determined by how much the basilar membrane vibrates at that area. A loud noise produces sound waves with more energy, which in turn cause greater movement of the tympanic membrane, middle ear ossicles, and the perilymph and endolymph. Increased movement of these fluids produces greater vibration of the basilar membrane and stronger stimulation of nearby receptor cell.

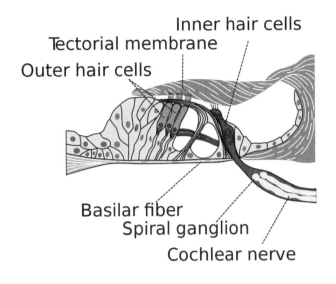

FIGURE 13.19   Organ of Corti.

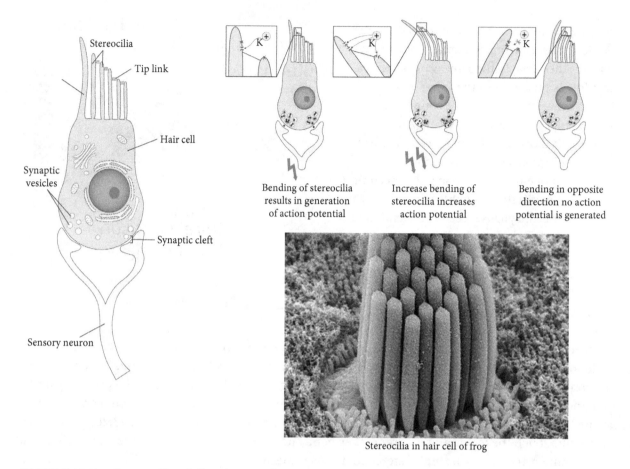

Bending of stereocilia results in generation of action potential

Increase bending of stereocilia increases action potential

Bending in opposite direction no action potential is generated

Stereocilia in hair cell of frog

FIGURE 13.20   Sensory Hair Cell and Stereocilia.

When basilar membrane moves back, away from the tectorial membrane, the stereocilia bend in opposite direction. The tip links are no longer stretched and the potassium ion channels close. Closing of ion channels causes hyperpolarization of the plasma membrane and cell stop to release neurotransmitters. Each inner hair cell contacts with many sensory neurons (fig. 13.20).

Approximately 90 percent of the sensory neurons are associated with inner hair cells, and only 10 percent of neurons contact outer hair cells. The function of outer hair cells is increase of sensitivity of the organ of Corti and amplification of vibrations. Outer hair cells can rapidly change their length in an oscillation fashion. Their jiggling enhances the movement of the basilar membrane hundred times.

Through the vestibulocochlear nerve, the neural signals proceed to the **cochlear nuclei** located at the junction between pons and medulla oblongata. Secondary sensory neurons from the cochlear nuclei synapse with neurons in the **superior olivary nucleus** in the pons. In superior olivary nucleus signals from both ears are compared to identify the location of the sound source. When the location of the sound source is found, the signal is sent to the inferior colliculi in the midbrain. Inferior colliculi are responsible for the

startle reflex. Startle reflex is responsible for head and body movement toward the source of a new sound. After that the signal proceeds to the thalamus. Neurons in inferior colliculi map an orderly representation of the auditory space around the head. Each neuron is space specific and responds only to the sounds from a particular direction. So, the outside world is mapped in inferior colliculi. This map computed by the brain, for example, allows a barn owl to locate mice in darkness within 1° of the sound source. Finally, the **primary auditory cortex** at the anterior parts of the temporal lobes receives auditory information via the thalamus.

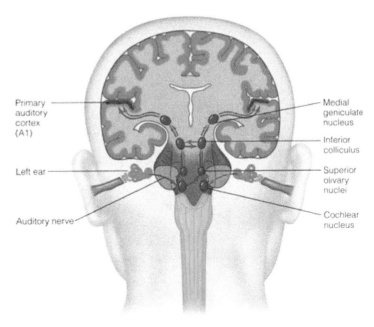

FIGURE 13.21   Auditory Sensory Input Pathway.

CHECK YOUR UNDERSTANDING

- Where is the primary auditory cortex located?

- What is the function of the tectorial membrane?

- What is the function of tip links?

- What is the role of the auditory tube?

- Which of three ossicles strikes the oval window?

- What is a tympanic reflex, and what effector organs are responsible for it?

13.5   Anatomy and Physiology of Vestibular Sensation

The sense of body balance depends on three sensory inputs: 1) visual, 2) proprioception of body skeletal muscles and tendons, and 3) vestibular sensations. As in hearing, vestibular sensation is also based on the mechanoreception. Its main receptors are hair cells. Vestibular apparatus occupies part of the bony labyrinth of the inner ear filled by perilymph. A membranous labyrinth is enclosed inside this bony labyrinth. Like in the cochlea, membranous labyrinth is filled by endolymph and both fluids do not mix. The inner ear contains organs that detect two types of equilibrium: static and dynamic. The vestibular organs consist of three **semicircular canals** and two **otolith organs: sacculus** and **utriculus**. Semicircular canals detect angular acceleration of the head and body; that is, they are sensors for dynamic equilibrium. Otolith organs detect linear movement and acceleration and can be considered as sensors for static equilibrium (fig. 13.22). All structures are lined by a vestibular epithelium.

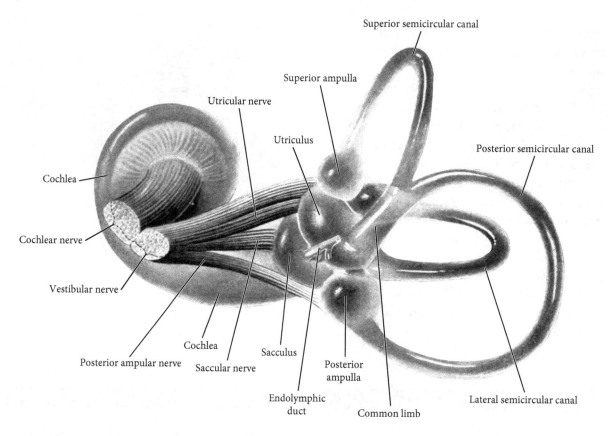

FIGURE 13.22   Human Vestibular Apparatus.

Utriculus and sacculus are parts of the big inner ear chamber known as a **vestibule**. Hair cells of these structures are organized in **macula**. Macula is located in epithelial lining and contains hair receptor cells. Hair cells of the vestibular apparatus are similar to those of the cochlea, except one detail: together with stereocilia, they also have a true cilium (see chapter 3, page 75) called **kinocilium**. In utriculus the macula is oriented approximately horizontally. In sacculus it is vertical. Hair cells in macula are covered by gelatinous **otolithic membrane**. Stereocilia and kinocilium are embedded in the gelatinous mass of otolithic membrane. Crystals of calcium carbonate lie on top of the otolithic membrane. The hair cells continuously secrete the neurotransmitter glutamate onto the dendrites of bipolar neurons that form a vestibular branch of the auditory nerve (VIII). When head moves, the crystals of calcium carbonate collectively called **otolith** by inertia leg behind, causing the otolithic membrane to slide against the microvilli and kinocilium of the hair cell (fig. 13.23). The stereocilia and kinocilium deflect and hair cell stop release of glutamate neurotransmitter. Glutamate stimulates sensory neurons to generate nerve impulses. When a hair cell stops releasing glutamate, the sensory neuron also stops generating nerve impulses.

Three semicircular canals oriented approximately at right angles toward each other. Each canal lies in one of three main planes of three directions of the space, which correspond to **anterior**, **posterior**, and **lateral**

ducts of the membranous labyrinth. All three ducts are connected to the utriculus. At the base, each canal is enlarged and forms a chamber called **ampulla**. Ampulla contains a cluster of hair cells termed **crista ampullaris**. Sterocilia and kinocilium of the crista ampullaris are embedded in a bell-shaped gelatinous mass called **cupula**. Acceleration of the head movement or its rotation causes the endolymph to slosh against the cupula, like water sloshing in a glass when glass is suddenly moved. This endolymph movement pushes against the cupula and deflects stereocilia and kinocilium, which results in altering release of the neurotransmitter onto the vestibular bipolar sensory neurons. Because for each of the three space directions there are two semicircular canals, one on each side of the head. Rotation of the head causes movement of endolymph on one side of the head in one direction and at the same time on the other side of the head—in opposite direction. This results in depolarization of the plasma membranes of the hair cells on one side of the head and hyperpolarization on the other. As a result, receptors from different sides of the head send different signals to the CNS for analysis and interpretation.

Through the vestibular branch of the auditory nerve (cranial nerve VIII), vestibular signals travel to the vestibular nuclei located at the pons–medulla oblongata junction. The vestibular nuclei forward the signals simultaneously to the thalamus, which relays them to next CNS centers: 1) inferior regions of the parietal lobe for consciousness awareness of the head and body position and

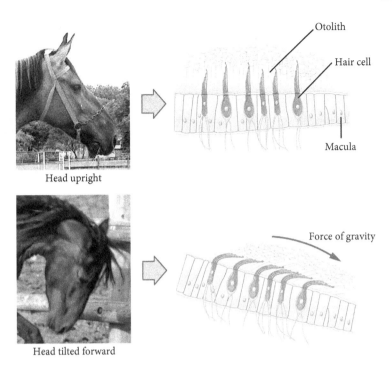

Head upright

Head tilted forward

FIGURE 13.23   Macula.

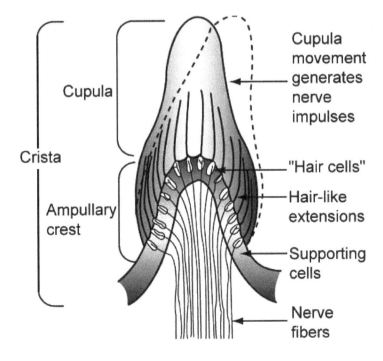

FIGURE 13.24   Crista Ampullaris.

movement; 2) nuclei of cranial muscles that control eye movement (oculomotor, trochlear, and abducens cranial nerves). The coordinated activity of these nerves allows the animal to watch the object in motion (for example, the cheetah continuously watches the antelope when chasing it); and 3) cerebellum and spinal cord to coordinate muscle contraction to maintain body balance.

CHECK YOUR UNDERSTANDING

- What is the difference between static and dynamic equilibrium?

- What role in body equilibrium do semicircular canals play?

- Why are the sacculus and utriculus considered to be mechanoreceptors?

- How do the hair cells in the crista ampullaris detect head rotation?

13.6   Integration of Senses

Special senses do not function in isolation. They collect and report information simultaneously and the CNS forms a cumulative sensation. The whole process of sensation and formation of an integral representation of the world proceeds in five principal steps:

1. Particular receptors detect and transduce stimuli onto associated sensory neurons.
2. Corresponding to the particular receptors cranial nerves transmit neural signals to the thalamus (except olfactory signals) in diencephalon of the brain.
3. The thalamus sorts signals and projects them to the appropriate centers in the primary sensory cortex. Olfaction travels through the olfactory tract directly to the primary olfactory cortex.
4. Primary sensory centers create awareness of the corresponding sensation. Thus, olfactory cortex in the temporal lobe allow to "feel" the aroma of the food. The primary gustatory cortex in the postcentral gyrus of the parietal lobe (primary sensory center) allows to taste food. A primary visual cortex in the occipital lobe forms a visual image of the food, and the primary auditory cortex in the temporal lobe forms auditory sensations that accompanied the meal.
5. Associative centers in the frontal lobes and limbic system integrate these separate sensations into a single meaningful sensation. The frontal lobe centers form the "rational awareness" of the food intake and environment accompanied this meal. The limbic system is responsible for the memories associated with previous meals, their taste, and emotions that accompany meals.

CHAPTER SUMMARY

- Special senses are different from general by complexity of sensory organs, location in the head, and concentration on external stimuli. They include taste, smell, vision, hearing, and body equilibrium. The modalities censored by special sensory organs include light, chemicals, and sound. The nerve impulses from these organs travel through cranial nerves to sensory nuclei via the thalamus, except olfactory signals.

- Olfaction is a chemoreception. All vertebrates have a main **olfactory system**. Terrestrial vertebrates also have a **vomeronasal system**. The receptive surface of the olfactory system is the **olfactory epithelium**. It has three cell types: **receptor cells**, **basal cells**, and **sustentacular cells**. Basal cells are progenitor cells that produce new receptor cells. Sustentacular cells are epithelial cells that secrete mucus and support olfactory sensory cells.

- Olfactory receptor cell is a bipolar neuron. It has a single narrow dendrite that extends into mucus-covered epithelial surface and ends by a **dendritic knob**. Apical surface of the dendritic knob carries a tuft of 20–30 plasma membrane projections called **olfactory cilia**.

- The axons of the olfactory sensory neurons are short and unmyelinated. They extend from the olfactory epithelium inside the cranium, where they synapse with neurons of **olfactory bulb**. There are several cell types within olfactory bulb, the most important of which are **mitral cells**. Axons of the mitral cells form the **olfactory tract** that bypasses the thalamus and conducts nerve impulses to the striatum and limbic system. Olfactory sensory neurons are only nerve cells exposed to the external environment. A regular olfactory sensory neuron has a life span of about 60 days before it degenerates. New neurons develop from **basal cells** in the nasal epithelium.

- The axon of olfactory neuron terminates within a globular cluster called a **glomerulus**. Glomerulus is a roll of terminal ends of many neurons that carry the same receptor protein sensitive to a specific odorant. Every glomerulus targets a particular odorant. All axons from the receptor cells that are sensitive to the same odorant converge and terminate at the same region of the olfactory bulb. In olfactory cortex, signals from different glomeruli converge and odors undergo integration.

- Most mammals (but not humans) have a second olfactory system called the **vomeronasal organ**. It is located below the main olfactory epithelium and forms a pouch usually isolated from the air breathed through the nose. The organ pumps air into lumen, where air wafts over receptor cells. In some reptiles, pheromones are delivered to the organ from the tongue.

- Sense of food is based on chemoreception. Gustation begins in a specialized receptor cells in **taste buds**. Taste bud contains cluster of 20 to 150 cells that includes: **receptor cells**, **basal cells**, and **supporting cells**. Receptor cells constitute only 5 to 15 percent. Life span of receptor cells is 5 to 15 days. Basal cells are located on the bottom of taste bud. They produce new receptor cells. An opening on the apex of the taste bud called **taste pore** allows dissolved food to enter taste bud and contact receptors.

- Taste buds are located on rounded projections called **papillae**. There are four groups of papillae: 1) **vallate or circumvallate papillae**, 2) **fungiform papillae**, 3) **foliate papillae**, and 4) **filiform papillae**. The sense of taste is based on detecting various chemicals, which fall in five groups: 1) **sweet**, 2) **sour**, 3) **salty**, 4) **bitter**, and 5) **umami**.

- Three cranial nerves—facial, glossopharyngeal, and vagus—conduct gustatory impulses from receptor cells in taste buds to the brain. Axons of these nerves terminate in the **solitary nucleus** in medulla oblongata, where they synapse with central sensory neurons in the thalamus. Vagus nerve in solitary nucleus is also synapse with motor neurons that control a reflexive secretion of saliva. From the thalamus signals go to the **primary gustatory cortex** in parietal lobes.

- Vertebrate eye focuses light on photosensitive cells. Accessory organs that facilitate visual sensation include: **eyelids**, **nictitating membrane**, **eyebrows**, **eyelashes**, **conjunctiva**, **lacrimal apparatus**, and **extrinsic muscles**.

- The **eyelids** are moved by **levator palpebrae superioris muscles** controlled via trigeminal and facial nerves. Circuit of these nerves constitute **blinking reflex**. An antagonist to the levator palpebrae superioris is **orbicularis oculi** that closes eye. The eyelid contains plate of a regular dense connective tissue called the **tarsal plate** that unclosed **tarsal** or **Meibomian glands**. Secretion of these glands is an oily fluid that prevents tear spillage, trapping tears between the oiled edge and the eyeball. Dysfunction of meibomian glands causes dry eyes. Tarsal glands open on the top of the eyelids. Both eyelids meet at the edges of the orbit at the medial and lateral **commissures** or **canthi**.

- **Nictitating membrane,** also called the **third eyelid,** protects and moisturize the eye. The gland of the third eyelid is called Harder's gland. It may secrete up to 50 percent of a tear film.

- The **conjunctiva** is a thin folded membrane. The fold of the conjunctiva that lines the eyelid is known as the **palpebral conjunctiva**. The **bulbar conjunctiva** covers sclera. Space between folds is termed the **conjunctival sac**. The conjunctiva protects eye and provides its smooth movement. The inflammation of the conjunctiva is called **conjunctivitis**.

- The **lacrimal apparatus** consists of **lacrimal glands** and system of ducts. Lacrimal glands release lacrimal and mucus into a conjunctival sac. Together with secretion of tarsal and Harder's glands, lacrimal fluids constitute tears. Tears moisturize and protect the cornea. Moving down by gravity, tears are collected in the medial canthi; through **lacrimal puncta** and canaliculi, they move to a lacrimal sac and into nasopharinx via a **nasolacrimal duct**.

- Six **extrinsic eye muscles**: four **rectus** and two **oblique muscles**, rotate eye. Extrinsic muscles are controlled by oculomotor (III), trochlear (IV), and abducens (VI) cranial nerves.

- The wall of a vertebrate eye has three layers or **tunics**. The outermost tunic is called **fibrous tunic**. It consists of a dense connective tissue. The middle layer is called **vascular tunic** or **uvea**. It carries blood vessels and provides oxygen and nutrients to eye tissues. The innermost layer is known as a **neural tunic** or **retina**. This layer is a brain outgrowth.

- The major portion of fibrous tunic is white colored **sclera**. Collagen fibers in sclera resist deformations and maintain eye shape. Fibers are arranged irregularly, which makes sclera opaque. Anteriorly is a transparent **cornea**. Junction between the cornea and sclera is called the **limbus**. Collagen fibers in the cornea are organized in regular parallel lines. Regular collagen organization, low water, and absence of blood vessels make the cornea translucent for light.

- The vascular tunic is composed of three distinct regions: the **choroid**, **ciliary body**, and **iris**. The choroid occupies middle and posterior regions. An extensive network of blood vessels provides oxygen and nutrients to all eye structures. The choroid is pigmented. In most domestic animals, except swine, choroid has a special reflective surface known as the **tapetum lucidum**.

- **Ciliary body** is a circle of smooth muscle termed **ciliary muscle. Suspensory ligaments** bind ciliary muscles with the lens. The process of adjusting lens curvature to focus light on retina is called **accommodation**. Contraction of ciliary muscles relaxes suspensory ligaments and elastic tissue rounds the lens. Relaxation of ciliary muscles increases tension of ligaments and flattens the lens. Secretory cells of ciliary body produce watery **aqueous humor**.

- The iris consists of pigmented smooth muscles. At the center the iris has an opening called the **pupil**. Relaxation and contraction of iris muscles reduce or enlarge pupil's diameter and regulate amount of light entering the eye.

- Retina has three layers: 1) outermost layer, close to the choroid, contains receptor **rod** and **cone cells**; 2) medial or **outer plexiform layer** contains bipolar and horizontal sensory neurons; 3) innermost **inner plexiform layer** is made of amacrine and ganglion neurons.

- The **lens** has three parts: the **lens capsule**, **lens epithelium**, and **lens fibers**. There are no nerves, blood vessels, or connective tissue in the lens. The lens capsule is a smooth, transparent basement membrane produced by the lens epithelium. Epithelium is a simple cuboidal epithelium located only on anterior side of the lens. Epithelial cells produce new lens fibers—long, thin, transparent cells arranged in concentric layers. Mature lens fibers are dead cells filled by transparent **crystalline**.

- Two cavities within the eye are **anterior chamber** located between posterior wall of the cornea and the iris and **posterior chamber**, a space between the iris and the lens. Both chambers are connected through the pupil and filled with an aqueous humor. To prevent buildup, the fluid is drained at the same rate as it is secreted. It is drained inside the anterior chamber into a blood vessel that circles the anterior edge of the iris, called the **scleral venous sinus** or **canal of Schlemm**. The third and largest chamber between the lens and retina is called the **vitreal chamber**. This chamber is filled by **vitreous humor**, which also often is called **vitreous body**, a thick transparent viscous gelatinous material. The vitreous humor presses the retina against choroid and guarantees retina's regular oxygen and nutrients supply.

- A photopigment **rhodopsin** consists of protein opsin and nonpeptide organic molecule **chromophore**—a special form of vitamin A. Absorption of light energy causes **photochemical reaction** that activates a G-protein signal-transduction cascade resulting in release of neurotransmitter in synapse with sensory neuron.

- The vertebrate retina contains **rod** and **cone photoreceptor cells** and a complex network of neurons: **bipolar cells, horizontal cells, amacrine cells**, and **ganglion cells**. A pigmented epithelium lies at the back of retina. It absorbs light not captured by the photoreceptors. It also controls the ionic environment around the rod and cone cells. Many retinas have central high-acuity region called **fovea centralis** that has the highest density of photoreceptors.

- Axons of retinal ganglion cells form optic nerve that exit eye at **optic disc**. Optic disc contains only axons. It has no receptors and is referred as a **blind spot**. Rod cells are more sensitive and used in dim light. Cones are less sensitive, but in a bright light they are used for color and high-acuity vision. Both cell types have two distinct regions: an **outer segment** containing photosensitive membranous structures, and **inner segment** containing nucleus, mitochondria, lysosomes, and so on. Distal end of the inner segment makes a synapse with retina neurons.

- Sensory impulses conveyed via three parallel pathways: 1) one pathway projects visual signals to superior colliculi in the midbrain that control eye movements; 2) another pathway projects to the CNS centers that control contraction of iris smooth muscles. This pathway also projects to suprachiasmatic nucleus, which regulates circadian rhythms; and 3) major visual projection in mammals is a **geniculostriate system**. The axons of the optic nerve form synapse in the thalamus region called **lateral geniculate nucleus** (LGN). From here visual information projects to the **primary visual cortex** in occipital lobe of cerebrum. In most mammals, the optic projections are only partially crossed at the optic chiasm: the phenomenon called **partial decussation**.

- Ability to distinguish color depends on differential sensitivity of photopigments to light of different wavelength. Although many animals are color-blind, many other animals with well-developed diurnal visual systems have color vision. Vertebrates with color vision may have up to four types of cone cells.

- The position of the eyes on the head is a result of a trade-off between breadth of visual field and depth of perception. Laterally located eyes can scan separate portions of the surrounding world. Vision in which the visual fields do not overlap is called **monocular vision**. In animals with **binocular vision** the visual field overlaps. Within the overlap area, two visual fields merge into a single image, producing a **stereoscopic vision**. In binocular vision, the visual field seen by each eye is divided: half of the input goes to the same side and the other half decussate to opposite side of the brain. Brain compares the difference between two images called **parallax**. Each eye registers a slightly different image, which gives a sense of depth.

- Principal mechanoreceptors of hearing are **hair cells**. These cells have apical surface covered by microvilli termed **stereocilia**. Stereocilia are rigid and rest on a dense **terminal web** or **cuticular plate**. This structure makes microvilli strong and able to band only at their base. Hair cells are epithelial cells embraced by dendrites of sensory neurons. The organ of hearing consists of three adjoining structures: **external**, **middle**, and **inner ear**.

- **External ear** includes **earlobe**, **external auditory canal**, and **tympanic membrane**. Pinna collects air waves. Its irregular shape helps to differentiate sounds from different directions and channel them into the external auditory meatus. The walls of external acoustic meatus are lined by hairy epithelium with **ceruminous glands** that secrete **cerumen**. Tympanic membrane is a thin and soft sheet of epithelium and connective tissue.

- The middle ear or **tympanic cavity** is a space between tympanic membrane and **oval window**. Oval window is covered by a thin flexible membrane. Tympanic cavity is filled with air and contains three bones called **auditory ossicles**. Ossicles are connected with each other by synovial joints. They form bridge between the tympanic membrane and oval window. Ossicles act as a system of levers that decreases the amplitude of vibration, but increases their force.

- Loud sound may damage receptor cells. Reflex that prevents this damage is termed **tympanic reflex**. The reflex circuit is initiated by the cochlear branch of the sensory vestibulocochlear nerve (VIII) and terminated by the facial nerve (VII) that activates **stapedius** and **tensor tympani muscles** to contract.

- Effective conduction of vibrations requires that air pressure on both sides of the tympanic membrane be equal. The air pressure is equalized via a **pharyngotympanic** (also called **auditory**, or **Eustachian**) **tube** that connects tympanic cavity with nasopharynx.

- The inner ear has three distinct regions: 1) the **cochlea**, responsible for hearing; 2) the **vestibule**; and 3) **semicircular canals** monitor body movement and head position. They are located in cavity inside temporal bone called **bony labyrinth**. Bony labyrinth is filled with a fluid known as **perilymph**. A continuous **membranous labyrinth** lines inner walls of the bony labyrinth and is filled by **endolymph**.

- A membranous labyrinth of cochlea is known as the **cochlear duct**. The cochlear duct spirals around a screw-shaped core bone called **modiolus**. Two chambers, the **scala vestibuli** and the **scala tympani**, parts of bony labyrinth, sandwich the cochlear duct from both sides. The cochlear duct is separated from the scala vestibuli by **vestibular membrane** and **basilar membrane** separates it from scala tympani. **Spiral organ of Corti,** located inside the cochlear duct, rests on basilar membrane. Organ of Corti detects vibrations of basilar membrane and converts them into nerve impulses.

- Organ of Corti has three components: **tectorial membrane, hair cells**, and **dendrites of cochlear nerve**. Tectorial membrane is a strong stiff plate extending parallel to the basilar membrane. Hair cells rest on the basilar membrane and are organized in two rows: a single row of **inner hair cells**, and three rows of **outer hair cells**. Inner hair cells detect sound. Their stereocilia have different length. Long stereocilia project from the cell and end close to the tectorial membrane. All stereocilia are bound by an elastic protein filament termed **tip link**. When long stereocilia touch the tectorial membrane, it bends and tip link pull all other stereocilia to bend at the same direction. Bending of stereocilia opens gated potassium channels in plasma membrane of hair cell and plasma membrane depolarizes.

- Neural signals proceed to the **cochlear nuclei** located at junction between pons and medulla oblongata. Secondary sensory neurons from cochlear nuclei synapse with neurons in **superior olivary nucleus** in the pons. In superior olivary nucleus signals from both ears are compared to identify the location of the sound source. When location of the sound source is found, the signal is sent to inferior colliculi in midbrain. Inferior colliculi are responsible for **startle reflex**: movement of head and body toward the sound source.

- Sense of body balance depends on three sensory inputs: 1) visual, 2) proprioception, and 3) vestibular sensations. The vestibular organs include three **semicircular canals** and two **otolith organs**: **sacculus** and **utriculus**. Semi-circular canals detect angular acceleration of the head and body; that is, they are sensors of dynamic equilibrium. Otolith organs detect linear movement and acceleration and can be considered as sensors for static equilibrium.

- Utriculus and sacculus are parts an inner ear chamber known as **vestibule**. Their hair cells are organized in **macula**. In utriculus macula is oriented approximately horizontally. In sacculus it is vertical. Hair cells in macula are covered by gelatinous **otolithic membrane**. Stereocilia and kinocilium are embedded in the gelatinous mass of otolithic membrane. Crystals of calcium carbonate lie on top of the otolithic membrane. The hair cells secrete the neurotransmitter glutamate continuously onto the dendrites of bipolar neurons that form a vestibular branch of the auditory nerve (VIII). When head moves, the crystals of calcium carbonate collectively called **otolith** by inertia leg behind, causing the otolithic membrane to slide against the microvilli and kinocilium of the hair cell. The stereocilia and kinocilium deflect and the hair cell stops releasing neurotransmitter, which causes sensory neurons to stop generating sensory signals.

- Three semicircular canals oriented approximately at right angles to each other. Each canal lies in one of three planes and are called **anterior**, **posterior**, and **lateral ducts**. All three ducts are connected to the utriculus. At the base, each canal forms a chamber called **ampulla** that contains a cluster of hair cells termed **crista ampullaris**. Sterocilia and kinocilium of the crista ampullaris are embedded in a bell-shaped gelatinous mass called **cupula**. Head rotation causes endolymph to slosh against the cupula and deflects stereocilia resulting in release of neurotransmitter onto the vestibular sensory neurons.

- Through the vestibular branch of cranial nerve VIII, vestibular signals travel to vestibular nuclei at the pons-medulla oblongata junction. Vestibular nuclei forward signals to the thalamus, which relays them to: 1) inferior regions of parietal lobe for conscious awareness; 2) nuclei of cranial muscles that control eye movement (oculomotor, trochlear, and abducens cranial nerves); and 3) the cerebellum and spinal cord to coordinate muscle contraction to maintain body balance and control muscle tension.

CHECK YOUR KNOWLEDGE

LEVEL 1. CHECK YOUR RECALL

1. The retina receives its oxygen supply from:
   A. Aqueous humor
   B. Vitreous body
   C. Choroid
   D. Pigmented epithelium
   E. Sclera venous sinus

2. The accessory glands that produce an oily secretion are:
    A. Conjunctiva
    B. Lacrimal glands
    C. Tarsal glands
    D. Ciliary bodies
    E. Ceruminous glands

3. The portion of the fibrous layer that is white and opaque is called:
    A. Choroid
    B. Cornea
    C. Retina
    D. Sclera
    E. Iris

4. Olfactory tract damage would probably affect the ability to:
    A. See
    B. Hear
    C. Feel pain
    D. Smell
    E. Find a body balance

5. Find the right sequence of air waves' pathway.
    A. Oval window → tympanic membrane → semicircular canals → Golgi tendon organ
    B. Organ of Corti → malleus → incus → stapes → auditory nerve → tympanic membrane
    C. Eustachian tube → round window → vestibular canal → tympanic canal → cochlear canal
    D. Basilar membrane → tectorial membrane → otoliths → utricle → saccule → malleus
    E. Pinna → tympanic membrane → malleus → incus → stapes → oval window → cochlear duct

6. The conjunctiva is a:
    A. Membrane that lines the inner surface of the eyelids and anterior surface of the eye
    B. Membrane that lines inner surface of the eyeball
    C. Membrane that constitute middle tunic of the eye
    D. Gel-like substance that fills the eyeball
    E. Connective tissue membrane that covered optic nerve

7. The hearing receptors are associated with the:
    A. Ampulla
    B. Organ of Corti
    C. Urticle
    D. Succule
    E. Auditory tube

8. Dogs can see in much dimmer light than humans because:
    A. Dogs have bigger eyes than humans.
    B. Dog eyes have a bigger lens than human eyes.
    C. Dog eye corneas may enlarge visual images better than human's corneas.
    D. Dog eyes have more cone cells than human eyes.
    E. Dog eyes have more rod cells than human eyes.

9. An ambulance siren in close proximity to a dog can cause the dog to howl. Which receptors are responsible for this response?
    A. Thermoreceptors and chemoreceptors
    B. Photoreceptors and nociceptors
    C. Mechanoreceptors and nociceptors
    D. Chemoreceptors and mechanoreceptors
    E. Photoreceptors and chemoreceptors

10. Stimuli from the vestibular apparatus are sent to all of the following centers, **except**:
    A. Vestibular nuclei
    B. Oculomotor nucleus
    C. Primary sensory center
    D. Cerebellum
    E. Trigeminal nucleus

11. The axons of the olfactory nerve terminate in the _____, where they synapse with _____.
    A. olfactory centers of temporal lobe; amacrine cells
    B. olfactory centers of temporal lobe; horizontal cells
    C. olfactory bulb; basal cells
    D. olfactory bulb; mitral cells
    E. olfactory tract; sustentacular cells

12. The primary olfactory cortex is located in the _____, whereas gustatory cortex is in the _____
    A. frontal lobe; parietal lobe
    B. parietal lobe; occipital lobe
    C. occipital lobe; temporal lobe
    D. frontal lobe; temporal lobe
    E. temporal lobe; parietal lobe

13. _____ depolarizes in darkness and are organized in batteries by _____.
    A. Rod cells; bipolar cells
    B. Cone cells; bipolar cells
    C. Rod cells; horizontal cells
    D. Con cells; horizontal cells
    E. Amacrine cells; bipolar cells

14. Sounds of high frequency are detected at the _____, whereas of low frequency are detected at the _____.

    A.   base of cochlea; apex of cochlea
    B.   apex of cochlea; base of cochlea
    C.   along the all cochlea; along the all cochlea

15. True or false: Hair cells in the organ of Corti depolarize or hyperpolarize, depending on the direction of the stereocilia inclination.
16. True or false: Vallate papillae are the largest papillae and have hundreds of taste buds.
17. True or false: Ora serrata is a border where the sclera meets the cornea.
18. True or false: Cone cells are best for vision in dim light.
19. True or false: Contraction of ciliary muscles makes a lens flat.
20. Match the taste with the chemical substance that generates it:

    _____ Sweet   a.   Hydrogen ions
    _____ Sour   b.   Glutamate
    _____ Salty   c.   Nitrogen containing compounds
    _____ Bitter   d.   Metal ions in food, such as Na^+, K^+, or Ca^{2+}
    _____ Umami   e.   Simple sugars

LEVEL 2. CHECK YOUR UNDERSTANDING

1. Explain how hair cells detect rotation of the head.
2. A brain trauma destroyed special pathway areas in the thalamus. Which special senses will not be affected and why?
3. If an animal suffers visual impairment only in one eye, why must the damage be located in the visual pathway prior to the optic chiasma?
4. You spin around few times. Why does the feeling of spinning remain when you stop?

LEVEL 3. APPLY YOUR KNOWLEDGE TO REAL LIFE

1. Which type of vision requires more muscular effort: close-up or far-away vision? Explain your answer.
2. If the lateral rectus muscle of a dog's eye was damaged and lost its ability to contract, what effect would it create in the affected eye?
3. What is the basic cause of motion sickness?

Chapter 14

The Endocrine System

LEARNING OBJECTIVES

The endocrine system is a master of control for body activities. Together with the nervous system, it controls all body organs. Even though the response from the endocrine system is not as fast as from the nervous system, its effect is very deep and long-lasting, sometimes continuing through the entire life span. In this chapter we will examine the principles of hormonal production, major groups of hormones, and mechanisms of their effect on target organs. The goal of this chapter is to give you the tools for analysis of hormone functions and their effects on an organism development and normal functioning. After reading this chapter, you will be able to do the following:

1. Describe what is common and what is different between the nervous and endocrine systems and how they coordinate their control over the organism.

2. Learn about different types of hormones and the mechanisms of their control of target cells.

3. Study the mechanisms that regulate hormone secretion.

4. Describe the diversity of endocrine glands and their specific role in maintaining body homeostasis.

5. Understand the role of the hypothalamus–pituitary gland axis in endocrine system functioning.

INTRODUCTION

The **endocrine system** consists of organs and secretory cells that produce chemical-signaling molecules and release them into the bloodstream. These signaling molecules are called **hormones**. They circulate through the blood or other body fluids and have a relatively long-lasting effect on distant target cells. Together with the nervous system, the endocrine system controls and regulates the activity of all body organs. The nervous system executes its regulatory functions through nerve impulses. The nervous system reacts instantaneously upon receipt of the stimulus. It is fast and causes a local short-lasting response (fig. 14.1.A). The endocrine system controls the organism through hormones. An endocrine response needs some time to release hormones into the blood flow and to reach sensitive cells known as **target cells** that are scattered over the body. The response lasts a comparatively long time (fig. 14.1.B).

Evolutionarily, the endocrine system is the oldest system, and its effect on the organism is more powerful than that of the nervous system. The means of control and the speed of the endocrine system are very different from those of the nervous system. The endocrine system influences metabolic activity of the organism and controls body homeostasis.

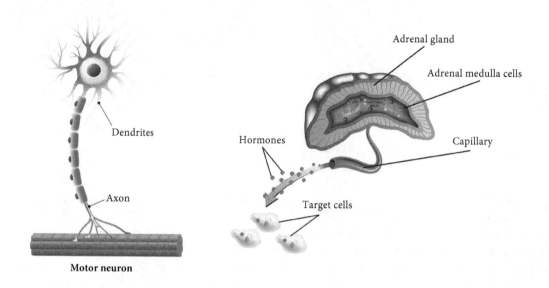

FIGURE 14.1   Comparison of the Nervous and Endocrine Systems.

Hormones influence a broad range of physiological processes. Every cell in an animal organism is a partner in some endocrine process. Most hormones participate in more than one physiological process. Altogether, this makes endocrinology—a science that studies organization and function of the endocrine system—a very complex, interesting, and intriguing discipline.

14.1   Overview of the Endocrine System

In the introduction to this chapter, we compared the immediate and precise responses of the nervous system on stimulus with the slow and general responses of the endocrine system. You may find that both systems use chemical signaling molecules: the nervous system uses neurotransmitters to conduct nerve impulse from the presynaptic to the postsynaptic neuron, whereas the endocrine system uses hormones to influence metabolism in target cells. The neurotransmitters diffuse a short distance across the synaptic cleft. Their short travel time ensures rapid, pinpointed control. The enzymatic breakdown or reuptake of neurotransmitters guarantees a quick termination of the nerve signal.

In contrast, hormones secreted from endocrine or neuroendocrine cells travel in long distances in the bloodstream to target cells, where they exert their effect. Whereas neurotransmitters from a neuron typically reach a single postsynaptic cell, hormone molecules carried through the blood can influence large populations of target cells. Therefore, transport of hormones over long distances permits very general and widespread responses. These responses are initiated slowly, relative to neural signals, but may last hours or days (tab. 14.1).

The functional units of the endocrine system are secretory cells that manufacture and secrete hormones. These cells may be organized in groups and form an **endocrine gland**. Very often, like G cells in gastric glands, cells are diffusely distributed and are not organized in clusters. In this case, an individual cell

TABLE 14.1   Comparison of the Nervous and Endocrine Systems

	Nervous System	**Endocrine System**
Definition	A system of nervous organs: brain, spinal cord, and peripheral nerves	A system of endocrine organs that secrete hormones
Composition	Composed of neurons and neuroglia cells	Composed of endocrine glands made of secretory cells
Nature of signal	Nerve impulses (waves of action potentials) and neurotransmitters	Hormones
Connectedness of the system	All neurons are organized into a continuous network	Organs not physically connected and system is discrete
Signal longevity	Short lasting	Long lasting
Signal speed	Fast	Slow
Signal transmission	Via neuron network	Via circulatory system

forms a unicellular endocrine gland. Endocrine glands, as a rule, are closely associated with the capillary system, so their secretions may quickly diffuse in the bloodstream.

CHECK YOUR UNDERSTANDING

- How do hormones move between the endocrine gland and a target organ?

- Compare and contrast the actions of the endocrine and the nervous systems to control body functions.

- How does the endocrine system differ from the nervous system with respect to their target cells?

Role of the Endocrine System in Regulation of Body Functions

Processes controlled by the endocrine system include water balance, metabolism, maintenance of mineral homeostasis, reproduction, and development. The endocrine system plays a very important role in animals' social behavior and the development of animal life cycles. The functions of the endocrine system may be classified in four groups:

1. **Regulation of cellular metabolism, organism growth, and development.** Hormones have a diverse impact on cell metabolism, both anabolic and catabolic processes. Alterations of the cell metabolism influence cell growth, division, and differentiation, which are foundations for organisms' growth and development.

2. **Maintenance of homeostasis of blood and other body fluids, and their volume and composition.** Hormones maintain homeostasis of substances dissolved in blood plasma, such as glucose, blood plasma proteins, amino acids, and so on. They control production of erythrocytes, leukocytes,

and platelets. Hormones are essential for maintaining a balance of electrolytes (Na+, K+, Ca2+) and other minerals in body fluids. Hormones control blood plasma osmotic pressure, the total volume of blood and interstitial body fluids.

3. **Control of food digestion and nutrient absorption.** Several hormones influence both the process of secreting substances necessary for digestion and activating absorption mechanisms.

4. **Control of animal reproduction and social behavior.** Hormones affect both development and function of the reproductive system as well as expression of sexual behaviors.

CHECK YOUR UNDERSTANDING

- Diabetes mellitus is characterized by a highly elevated glucose level. Which one of the main functions is most directly affected by this disease?

- Testosterone stimulates synthesis of new myofilaments and skeletal muscle growth. Which main function of the endocrine system does this hormone represents?

Difference between Endocrine and Exocrine Glands

There are many substances that influence cells' metabolism. However, not all of them can be called hormones. For examples, CO_2 dissolved in blood plasma changes blood pH and by that causes breathing and lung ventilation rate alteration. Thus, carbon dioxide influences pH of the blood and those mechanisms that maintain blood pH homeostasis. However, it cannot be regarded a hormone. As we identify a hormone, it is a compound secreted by special secretory cells that has an impact on target cells and is effective at a very low concentration. CO_2 is a metabolic by-product of all active cells. It is not produced by specialized secretory cells, and it is always present in the blood plasma in some substantial amount.

On the other hand, there are many secretory cells in the vertebrate organism whose secretions also cannot be called hormones. For example, chief cells of the gastric glands produce and release pepsinogen and gastric lipase—compounds essential for digestion of proteins and lipids in the stomach. These compounds are not hormones, and chief cells are not a part of the endocrine system. They are classified as **exocrine cells** that constitute the **exocrine gland**. The principal difference between endocrine and exocrine glands are:

1. Whereas endocrine glands are associated with the circulatory system and their secretions quickly diffuse through the interstitial fluids into the bloodstream, exocrine glands release their secretions into the ducts through which these compounds travel outside of the body or inside the body cavities, such as a lumen of the stomach (fig. 14.2).

2. Hormones produced by endocrine glands have a comparatively long life and exert their effect on remote target cells, whereas exocrine gland secretion has a local and comparatively short-term effect in the place of their release.

According to these definitions, the pituitary gland, pineal gland, adrenal glands are endocrine glands because they secrete hormones that travel with blood to the target cells. Salivary glands, sweat glands,

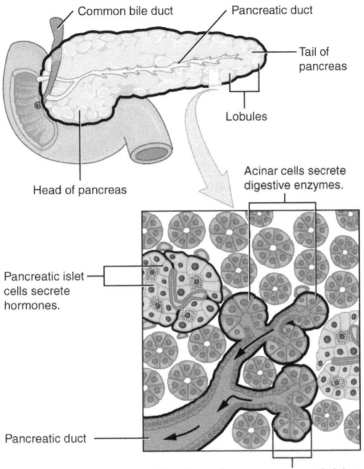

FIGURE 14.2   Endocrine and Exocrine Glands.

goblet cells, and lacrimal glands are exocrine glands, because they release their secretions into the system of ducts that deliver these compounds outside the body, like lacrimal gland secretions, or inside body cavities, like mucus or saliva.

CHECK YOUR UNDERSTANDING

- The gallbladder contains bile, which it releases to the duodenum through bile ducts. What type of gland is the gallbladder?

- CO_2 travel with blood and has an effect on many body cells. Why is CO_2 not considered a hormone?

- Why do we regard the pancreas as both an endocrine and an exocrine gland?

Classification of Chemical Signals

Hormones are signaling molecules through which the endocrine system controls body functions. However, there are many signaling molecules other than hormones. These signaling molecules may be classified in four groups: **intracrine**, **autocrine**, **paracrine**, and **pheromones**.

Intracrine signaling molecules are peptide growth factors that function inside the cell. The intracrine signaling consists of cell self-stimulation by its own product. An example of intracrine signaling molecule is fibroblast growth factor 2—a polypeptide that binds heparin and has broad mitogenic and angiogenic activities. This protein influences many processes, such as limb and nervous system development, wound healing, and tumor growth. Intracrine signaling molecules exert their effect exclusively inside the cell, in contrast to autocrine signals.

In autocrine signaling, a cell secretes a hormone or chemical messenger (called the autocrine agent) outside. After that, this agent binds to autocrine receptors in the plasma membrane of that same cell. This interaction between a cell receptor and its own product leads to various cellular responses or self-stimulation. An example of an autocrine agent is cytokine interleukin-1 in monocytes. These autocrine signaling molecules are produced by macrophages, monocytes, fibroblasts, dendritic cells, B lymphocytes, NK cells, and microglia; that is, critical immune system cells. When interleukin-1 is produced in response to external stimuli, it can bind to receptors in the plasma membrane of the same cell that produced it. This interaction of interleukin-1 with its own receptor generates an inflammatory response of the body against infection. Cytokines increase the expression of adhesion factors on endothelial cells to enable migration (called diapedesis) of immunocompetent cells (phagocytes, lymphocytes, and others) from the bloodstream to areas of infection or injury. They also affect the activity of the thermoregulatory center in the hypothalamus, which leads to a rise of body temperature (fever). That is why interleukin-1 is called an endogenous pyrogen.

Paracrine signaling molecules are also sometimes called local hormones. Cells secrete paracrine signaling factors that have a comparatively short life, diffuse on a short distance, and have effects on nearby cells. Cells release paracrine factors into the surrounding extracellular matrix. The effect of paracrine factors is proportional to their concentration gradient. Cells that are sensitive to paracrine signals are called **competent**. Bone morphogenetic protein, for example, induces bone formation and controls apoptosis, cell migration, division, and differentiation. Another example of paracrine signaling molecules are the **prostaglandins (PG)**—a group of lipid compounds called eicosanoids. Prostaglandins are powerful local vasodilators and inhibitors of blood clot formation. Through their role in vasodilation, prostaglandins are also involved in inflammation, smooth muscle contraction, and stimulation of pain signals.

Pheromones, also called ectohormones, are signaling molecules released outside of the body for communication among individuals in an animal population. There are alarm pheromones, sex pheromones, and many others that affect animal behavior and physiology.

CHECK YOUR UNDERSTANDING

- Damaged cells release leukotrienes, which cause smooth muscles in a nearby blood vessels to vasodilate and increase blood influx to the injured area. Is this an example of 1) intracrine, 2) autocrine, or 2) paracrine stimulation? Explain your answer.

Hormones

From all signaling factors, hormones differ by their long-distance effect on target cells, comparatively long life, and distribution inside the body through the bloodstream. Hormones include a large number of chemical compounds that fall into three classes: 1) **steroid hormones**, 2) **peptide** and **protein hormones**, and 3) **amine hormones**.

All steroid hormones are synthesized from cholesterol. In vertebrates, steroids are produced by gonads (testes and ovaries), the cortex of adrenal glands, and the placenta during pregnancy. Like cholesterol, all steroid hormones are lipid soluble and hydrophobic. They cannot be dissolved in blood plasma. Steroid hormones need special mechanisms for their transportation. The process of their interaction with target cells is also different from that of other hormones.

Peptide, protein, and amine hormones in contrast to steroid hormones are water soluble. They can be transported directly with blood flow, but cannot cross the target cell plasma membrane. Thus, their receptor protein has to be exposed outside on the membrane surface. That is why these hormones are combined in a group called **nonsteroidal hormones**. Peptide and protein hormones are different from each other in the number of amino acids and the complexity of their compound confirmation. In vertebrates these hormones include **antidiuretic hormone (ADH)**, **insulin**, and **growth hormone**. Amine hormones are modified amino acids. For example, **melatonin** originates from amino acid tryptophan, whereas **catecholamines** (**epinephrine, norepinephrine**, and **dopamine**) and **iodothyronines** (hydrophobic and lipid soluble) are products of amino acid tyrosine modification (tab. 14.2).

CHECK YOUR UNDERSTANDING

- What is the difference between steroid and nonsteroidal hormone transportation?

- Which chemical is a common precursor of all steroid hormones?

Mechanism of Regulation of Hormone Production

The effect of the hormone depends on its concentration in the blood. This means that the amount of each hormone has to be tightly regulated. Two processes influence hormone concentration: hormone synthesis and hormone elimination. Together they create a homeostasis of hormone levels in the animal body.

Synthesis and release of hormones into the bloodstream is regulated through the negative feedback mechanism. This mechanism may be executed through release of peripheral hormones. An example of such a sequence of hormone production with a negative feedback is the female reproductive cycle (fig. 14.3.A). In it, **gonadotropin-releasing hormone (GnRH)** stimulates **anterior pituitary gland** to secrete **follicle stimulating (FSH)** and **luteinizing (LH)** hormones. FSH in its turn stimulates development of follicles in the **ovaries** and secretion of **estrogens**. Estrogens, beside many different effects on the female organism, also inhibit the hypothalamus and anterior pituitary gland, which leads to a decrease of FSH production. Negative feedback also may be created by the action or response of an organism to the hormone stimulation. For example, cold air causes a decrease in body temperature, which leads to stress and the release of epinephrine by the adrenal glands. The epinephrine stimulates contraction of erector pili muscles

TABLE 14.2   Hormone Classes

Hormone Class	Components	Example(s)
Amine Hormone	Amino acids with modified groups (e.g., norepinephrine's carboxyl group is replaced with a benzene ring)	**Norepinephrine**
Peptide Hormone	Short chains of linked amino acids	**Oxytocin**
Protein Hormone	Long chains of linked amino acids	**Human Growth Hormone**
Steroid Hormones	Derived from the lipid cholesterol	**Testosterone** **Progesterone**

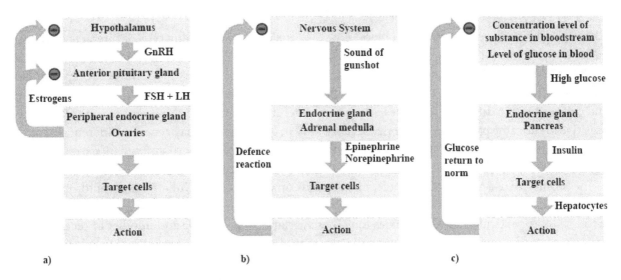

FIGURE 14.3   Negative Feedback Controls Hormone Production.

and raises up the hair. It also initiates vasomotion, which leads to a redistribution of the blood flow and a rise in body temperature. The return of body temperature to normal ends the stress reaction, and the level of epinephrine in the blood decreases (fig. 14.3.B). The hormones that control the level of chemical substances often are secreted in response to the concentration of a target substance. For example, **calcitonin** controls blood calcium ions level. The **thyroid gland** releases calcitonin when the concentration of Ca^{2+} in blood rises above the norm. The hormone stimulates osteoblast activity. Active osteoblasts absorb calcium from blood and deposit it in bone ECM. As a result, the concentration of calcium in blood decreases. When Ca^{2+} level returns to normal, the secretion of calcitonin is stopped (fig. 14.3.C).

Hormones are eliminated through three processes: 1) degradation by enzymes in liver; 2) excretion with urine by kidney; and 3) the uptake of hormones by target cells. The rate of hormone elimination depends on its concentration: the higher the hormone concentration, the faster it is eliminated from the blood. When the hormone level decreases, the rate of its elimination also decreases. The rate of hormone elimination is characterized by the hormone's half-life. The half-life is the time period during which the amount of the hormone is reduced within the bloodstream to one-half. As a rule, water-soluble hormones have a short half-life, from a few minutes to a few hours. Lipid-soluble hormones live longer, because carrying proteins protect them from degradation by enzymes. Thus, for example, **testosterone** has a half-life of around 12 days.

CHECK YOUR UNDERSTANDING

- What does the term *hormone half-life* mean?

- Explain why steroid hormones as a rule have a longer half-life?

14.2   Mechanism of Hormonal Effect on Target Organ

Although a hormone circulating with blood flow over the body passes many cells, it interacts only with particular cells known as target cells. A target cell responds to a particular hormone because it has special **receptor proteins** that interact with the hormone. A typical target cell has thousands of receptor molecules for a particular hormone. On the other hand, target cells have different types of receptor molecules and can respond to different hormones. Moreover, different cells may have different receptor molecules sensitive to the same particular hormone. Because of that, one hormone may generate different responses in different target cells. For example, norepinephrine increases the strength and rate of cardiac muscle contraction and inhibits smooth muscle contraction in the gallbladder and small intestine.

The sensitivity of a target cell to a hormone depends on the number of functional receptor molecules. The number of receptor protein molecules that recognize this hormone may vary and sensitivity of a target cell to a particular hormone varies too. These variations in the type and number of receptor proteins expressed by target cell contribute to the substantial versatility of hormonal regulation in animals.

Mechanism of Effect of Water-Soluble Nonsteroidal Hormones

Water-soluble hormones (peptide, proteins, and amines, except thyroid hormone) are polar molecules and unable to cross the plasma membrane. Their receptor proteins are located on the surface of the plasma membrane. The binding of a water-soluble hormone to its receptor initiates a series of biochemical reactions across the membrane called a **signal transduction pathway**. In this pathway, the hormone is the signaling molecule, or **first messenger**. Transduction pathway reactions generate other molecules within the cell called the **second messengers**. The second messengers then change target cell metabolism.

The signal transduction pathway functions through an internal plasma membrane protein complex known as a **G protein**. The binding of the hormone to a plasma membrane receptor causes a change in G protein confirmation. The activation of G protein triggers a cascade of enzymatic reactions associated with **adenylate cyclase** or **phospholipase C**. The target cell may have one or both cascades.

Adenylate cyclase activated by G protein forms second messenger molecules called **cyclic adenosine monophosphate (cAMP)** from ATP molecules. The cAMP then activates a **protein kinase** that phosphorylates (adds a phosphate group to) other molecules. Phosphorylation causes activation of these molecules (fig. 14.4).

Another membrane protein activated by the active form of G protein is a phospholipase C. Active phospholipase C produces two secondary messenger molecules: **diacylglycerol (DAG)** and **inositol triphosphate (IP$_3$)**. The DAG is a second messenger molecule similar to cAMP and, like cAMP, activates a protein kinase. Another secondary messenger, IP$_3$, diffuses into the cytosol and there increases intracellular concentration of Ca^{2+} by opening calcium channels in the plasma membrane and permitting Ca^{2+} to enter the cell from the extracellular fluid. Ca^{2+} plays the role of a third messenger, and it activates protein kinase enzymes. Hormones that use this pathway include epinephrine, oxytocin, and antidiuretic hormone.

Thus, one way or another, water-soluble hormones activate G protein, which through secondary (and tertiary) messengers causes activation of protein kinase. The protein kinase through phosphorylation of intracellular enzymes triggers a change in the metabolic activity of the target cell. For example, glucagon

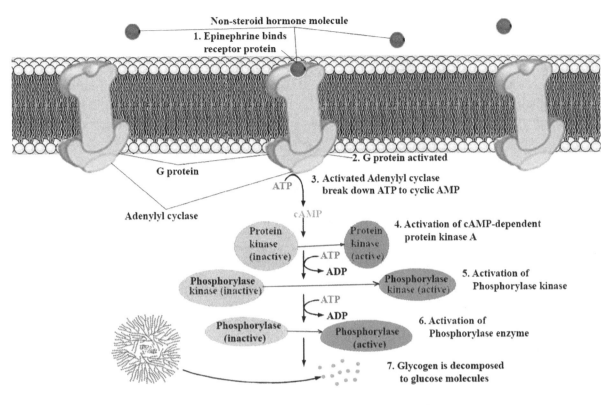

FIGURE 14.4   Mechanism of Nonsteroidal Hormone Effect on the Target Cell.

combined with G protein triggers the breakdown of glycogen molecules to glucose, which is released to the bloodstream. The mechanism of the intracellular enzyme cascade caused by water-soluble hormones has two important characteristics:

1.   It amplifies the signal at each step of this cascade of enzymatic reactions. Ultimately, it results in a massive response to the presence of a comparatively small amount of hormone.
2.   The multistep signaling pathway creates an opportunity to fine-tune and provides very precise control of the cellular response.

CHECK YOUR UNDERSTANDING

•   Why does the same hormone have different effects on different target cells?

•   Why are receptors of nonsteroidal hormones located on the surface of the cell membrane?

•   What is the specific role of cAMP in the signal transduction pathway?

Mechanism of Steroid and Other Lipid-Soluble Hormones' Effect on Target Organs

Lipid-soluble hormones are comparatively small and nonpolar. These properties make lipid-soluble hormones able to diffuse across the plasma membrane. The receptor proteins for these hormones have no need to be associated with the plasma membrane and, as a matter of fact, are dissolved in the cytosol or even karyoplasm of the cell. Thus, the lipid-soluble hormone, upon entering the cell, binds to the appropriate receptor protein inside the cytoplasm or karyoplasm and forms a **hormone-receptor complex**. The hormone-receptor complex then binds to a specific regulatory DNA sequence called the **hormone-response element (HRE)**. This attachment to the HRE results in transcription of mRNA and the activation of synthesis of a particular protein. Synthesis of new proteins changes cell organization or metabolic activity. For example, testosterone triggers synthesis of muscle contractile proteins and, as a result, building of bigger skeletal muscles than those in females (fig. 14.5).

CHECK YOUR UNDERSTANDING

- Why are receptor proteins of steroid hormones located inside the cell?

- As a rule, steroid hormones have a longer-lasting effect on target cells. Why?

- What main change in the target cell generates steroid hormone?

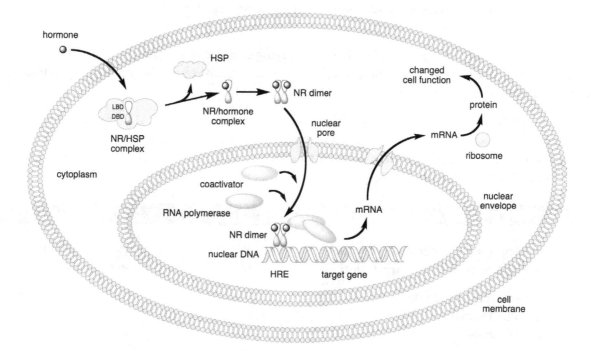

FIGURE 14.5   Mechanism of Steroid Hormone Effect on the Target Cell.

14.3   Overview of Endocrine Organs

Endocrine organs consist of secretory cells organized in structures. As a rule, they are closely associated with the circulatory system. Some endocrine organs function independent from other endocrine glands, and their activity is controlled through negative feedback by the final product or result of their activity. For example, the thyroid gland secretes calcitonin in response to a high calcium level in blood. When Ca^{2+} level returns to norm, calcitonin secretion stops. The hypothalamus plays a special role in endocrine system functioning. The hypothalamus has direct control over the pituitary gland and through it on other endocrine organs. This influence of the hypothalamus through the pituitary gland is called the **hypothalamic–pituitary gland axis**.

Hypothalamic–Pituitary Gland Axis

The hypothalamus is a part of the brain known as a diencephalon. It is located bellow the thalamus and is a part of the limbic system (see chapter 11, page 308). The hypothalamus consists of a number of small nuclei with various vital important functions. One of the most important functions of the hypothalamus is to link the nervous and endocrine systems via the pituitary gland. A special group of neurons in the hypothalamus is able to combine together reception of nerve impulses from other neurons, especially from the thalamus, and secrete hormones. For this property, these neurons are called **neuroendocrine cells**. Most of the hypothalamic hormones are called **release hormones** or **inhibitory hormones**. For example, **thyrotropin-releasing hormone**, **prolactin-releasing hormone**, **prolactin-inhibitory hormone**, or **growth hormone–inhibiting hormone**. Released into the hypothalamo-hypophyseal portal system, these hormones control activity of the **anterior pituitary gland**. The hormones secreted by the hypothalamus to control the anterior pituitary gland are as follows:

- **Thyrotropin-releasing hormone (TRH)** stimulates the release by the anterior pituitary gland of **thyroid-stimulating hormone (TSH)**. TSH, also called **thyrotropin**, stimulates the **thyroid gland** to release **thyroid hormone (TH)**. Thus, the sequence of released hormone is TRH → TSH → TH.

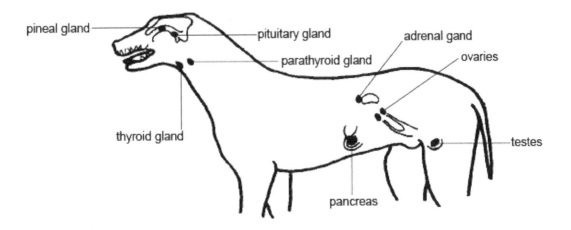

FIGURE 14.6   The Endocrine System of a Dog.

- **Prolactine-releasing hormone (PRH)** controls production and release of the **prolactin hormone (PRL)** from the anterior pituitary.
- **Prolactine-inhibiting hormone** inhibits release of prolactin hormone. Thus, production and release of PRL is regulated by two hypothalamic hormones: PRH and PIH.
- **Gonadotropin-releasing hormone (GnRH)** regulates secretion of **follicle-stimulating** and **luteinizing hormones** collectively known as **gonadotropins.**
- **Corticotropin-releasing hormone (CRH)** stimulates release of **adrenocorticotropin hormone (ACTH).**
- **Growth hormone–releasing hormone (GHRH)** stimulates anterior pituitary gland to release **growth hormone (GH)** or **somatotropin.**
- **Growth hormone–inhibiting hormone (GHIH)** inhibits secretion of GH.

The pituitary gland is also called the hypophysis. It is located bellow the hypothalamus, with which it is connected by a stalk called the infundibulum. The oval gland rests in the depression known as the sella turcica of the sphenoid bone. It consists of two structures different by origin, histology, and function, which are organized in one organ during the organism's embryo development: the anterior pituitary gland, also called the adenohypophysis; and the posterior pituitary gland, also known as the neurohypophysis.

As a matter of fact, the posterior pituitary gland is not an endocrine gland. It does not secrete its own hormones. In most mammals it constitutes one-fourth of the total mass of the pituitary gland. Its body consists of axon terminals of neuroendocrine cells located in the paraventricular and supraoptic nuclei of the hypothalamus. Approximately 10,000 neurons in these nuclei extend their unmyelinated axons through the infundibulum as the hypothalamo-hypophyseal tract where they are contact with a network of blood vessels called hypothalamo-hypophyseal portal system. The synaptic vesicles in the terminal of these axons are loaded with the hormones oxytocin and antidiuretic hormone (ADH), also called vasopressin. By demand, these hormones are released into the portal blood flow. The neurons of the supraoptic nucleus mostly produce ADH, whereas oxytocin is produced by the paraventricular nucleus (fig. 14.7).

ADH maintains body fluid balance, total blood volume, and

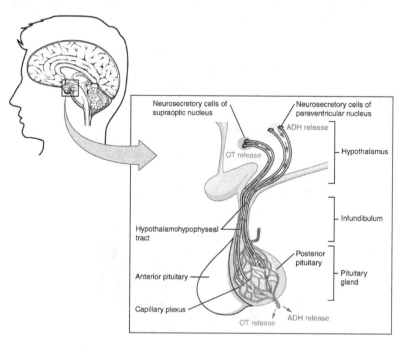

FIGURE 14.7   Relation between the Hypothalamus and the Posterior Pituitary Gland.

blood pressure. The hypothalamus monitors blood pressure and plasma concentration. The increased blood plasma concentration indicates a state of dehydration. In response to this change, axon terminals located in the posterior pituitary gland release ADH through the exocytosis. The target cells of the ADH include the kidneys, which increase reuptake of water from urine in collecting ducts and return it into the blood; high doses of ADH causes vasoconstriction. The secretion and release of ADH is controlled through the negative feedback and decreases with the increase of blood volume. There is a body of experimental data that shows ADH influence on formation of family bonds among voles. The high-density distributions of vasopressin receptors in the ventral forebrain regions of the prairie vole have been shown to facilitate and coordinate reward circuits during partner preference formation, critical for pair formation. In males this hormone triggers family defensive behavior, and in females it generates caring instincts.

Oxytocin stimulates contraction of smooth muscles. In females it stimulates contraction of the uterus's myometrium during childbirth. After the baby is born it causes milk flow by contraction of smooth muscles in the walls of lactiferous ducts. The production and release of oxytocin is regulated through the positive feedback: during the delivery its amount is increased in response to the increased pressure of the fetus on the walls of the birth canal and during breastfeeding, or suckling. In males, oxytocin facilitates sperm movement during ejaculation. Research has demonstrated that oxytocin is also released during physical contact between individuals, which causes mood improvement, lowers the level of stress hormones, reduces blood pressure, and increases pain tolerance. When petting your dog or cat, the posterior pituitary glands of both you and your pet release oxytocin.

The anterior pituitary gland is a true endocrine gland. It secretes a number of hormones collectively known as **stimulating** or **tropic hormones**, such as **thyroid stimulating hormone (TSH)** and **adrenocorticotropic hormone (ACTH)**. The secretions of the anterior pituitary gland are controlled by the hypothalamus and through negative feedback by the activity of the target organs or glands. For example, ACTH triggers release of glucocorticoid hormones by the adrenal cortex. The increased level of glucocorticoid hormones inhibits release of ACTH from the anterior pituitary gland. With the hypothalamus, the anterior pituitary gland communicates through the blood flow of the hypothalamic-pituitary portal system, which delivers hypothalamic hormones to secretory cells of the anterior pituitary gland. Thus, the anterior pituitary gland constitutes a second level of control in the hierarchic organization of the endocrine system (fig. 14.8).

The anterior pituitary gland hormones are (fig. 14.9):

1. **Adrenocorticotropic hormone (ACTH)**, also called **corticotropin**, stimulates the adrenal glands' development and production of multiple adrenal cortex steroid hormones. The hormone is produced by **corticotroph cells** in response to CRH from the hypothalamus.
2. **Follicle-stimulating hormone (FSH)** exerts its effect on gonads: testes in males and ovaries in female. In male FSH stimulates production of chemicals that bind and concentrate **testosterone**. In females it triggers maturation of ovarian follicles, development of oocytes, and secretion of **estrogens**. The hormone secretion is controlled by GnRH from the hypothalamus and the negative response of an increased level of estrogen.
3. **Luteinizing hormone (LH)**, like FSH, controls gonads. In males, LH stimulates testosterone secretion in testes. In females, this hormone stimulates production of estrogens and **progesterone**. It

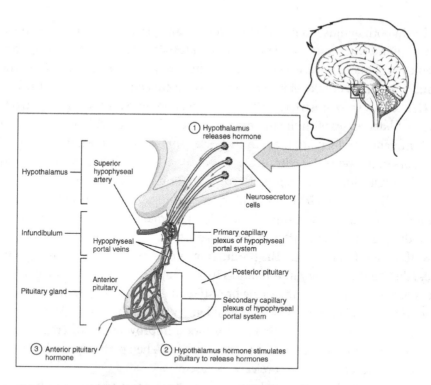

FIGURE 14.8   Relation between the Hypothalamus and the Anterior
Pituitary Gland.

also plays a crucial role in ovulation. Like FSH, it is produced by **gonadotroph cells** in response
to GnRH secretion by the hypothalamus.

4. **Growth hormone** influences all body cells, stimulating their growth and division. This function
    suggests another name of this hormone—**somatotropin**. It is produced by a group of cells known
    as **somatotrophs**. Somatotrophs release GH periodically throughout the day. The peak of secretion
    occurs during sleep. That is why young organisms grow quickly during sleep. Two hypothalamic
    hormones regulate its production: GHRH and GHIH. Primarily, GH influences fat breakdown
    (lipolysis), promotes synthesis of new glucose by the liver (gluconeogenesis), and inhibits glucose
    uptake by muscle fibers. These effects increase the concentrations of glucose and fatty acids in
    the blood, allowing cells to use them as fuel and raw materials for growth. Another effect of GH
    is stimulating the liver to produce **insulin-like growth factor (IGF)**, which is similar in its effect
    to **insulin** and triggers a rapid synthesis of proteins and cell division, leading to body growth.
5. **Melanocyte-stimulating hormones (MSH)**, also called **melanotropins** or **intermedins**, are a family
    of peptide hormones produced by a structure of anterior pituitary gland called **pars intermedia**.
    Acting in the hypothalamus, MSH inhibits the appetite center and contributes to sexual arousal.
6. **Prolactin** targets mammary glands. It stimulates mammary glands' growth and milk production
    after birth. The hormone is produced by **lactotroph cells**, which are stimulated by the prolactin-
    releasing hormone and inhibited by the prolactin-inhibiting factor from the hypothalamus.

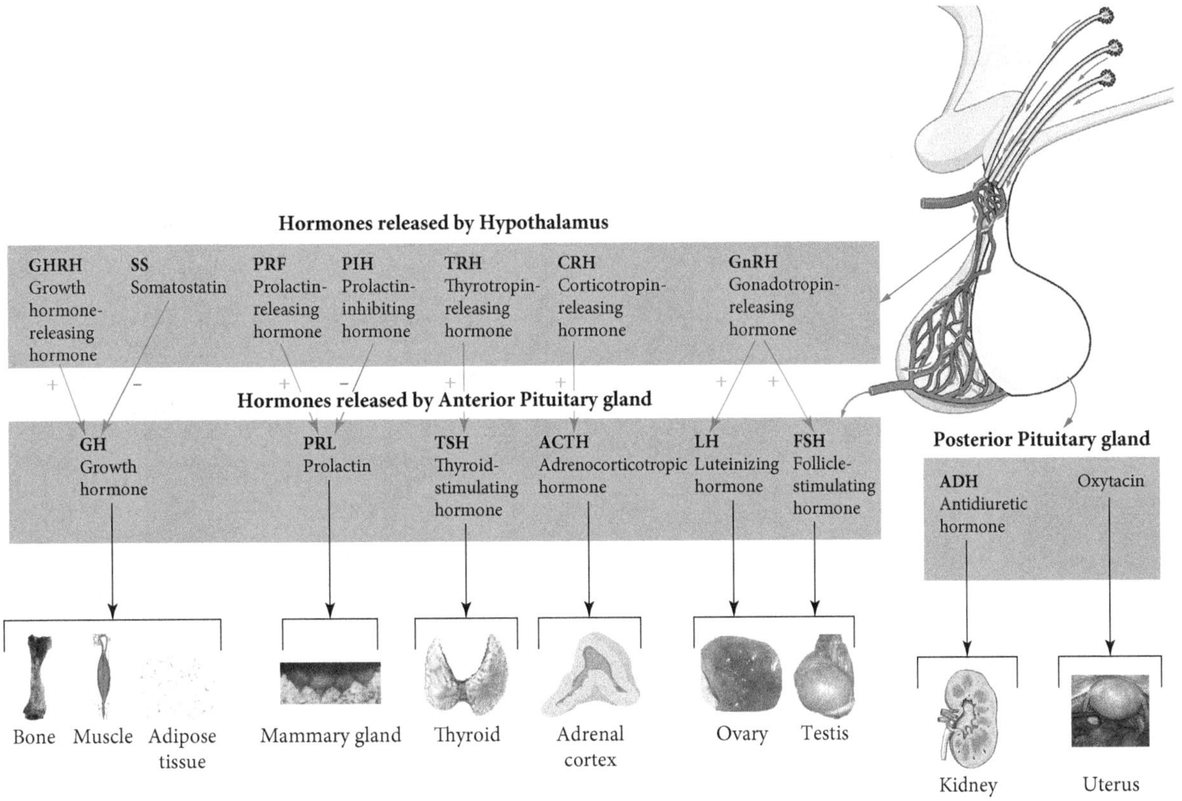

FIGURE 14.9 Hormones of the Hypothalamus and the Pituitary Gland.

7. **Thyroid-stimulating hormone** stimulates thyroid gland development and secretion of thyroid hormones. Cells called **thyrotrophs** produce this hormone in response to release of TRH by the hypothalamus.

CHECK YOUR UNDERSTANDING

- In your own words, describe the role of the hypothalamus in the endocrine system.

- What is the difference in the relationship of the anterior and posterior pituitary glands with the hypothalamus?

- How does the hypothalamus regulate release of ADH and oxytocin from the posterior pituitary gland?

- Explain how the hypothalamus controls the release of hormones from the anterior pituitary gland.

- What primary hormones are released from the anterior pituitary gland?

- Explain why fast-growing puppies and kittens are usually slender and often lose some fat.

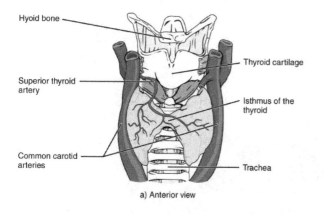

a) Anterior view

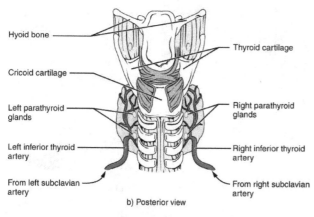

b) Posterior view

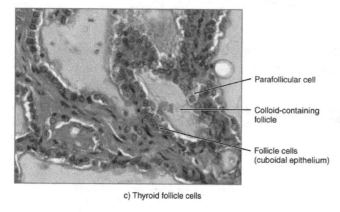

c) Thyroid follicle cells

FIGURE 14.10   Thyroid Gland.

Thyroid and Parathyroid Glands: Their Structure and Functions

The thyroid gland produces three hormones: two hormones that regulate body metabolism and one that participates in blood Ca^{2+} homeostasis. The hormones that control metabolic rate are called **permissive**, which means they "permit" target cells to be more responsive to stimulation by other hormones, the nervous system, or environmental factors. Hormones contain iodine. The **tetraiodothyronine** or **T4**, contains four iodine atoms, and **triiodothyronine**, or **T3**, contains three iodine atoms.

The thyroid gland develops from the cellular mass at the floor of the pharynx. It consists of two masses of secretory cells called **lobes** connected by a narrow bridge called an **isthmus** enclosed in a connective tissue capsule. The gland is subdivided into multicellular spherical structures known as **follicles**. Every follicle is made of a single layer of **follicle cells** that form a hollow sphere. The space inside this sphere is filled with a gelatinous **colloid**. The anterior pituitary gland through the TSH stimulate follicle cells to produce protein thyroglobulin and store it in colloid. On demand mobilized follicle cells reabsorb stored protein through endocytosis, convert it into active T_3 and T_4 hormones, and release into the bloodstream. Later much of the T_4 hormone is converted into the more active T_3 in the liver (fig. 14.10).

T_3 and T_4 hormones elevate oxygen consumption and heat production. They increase basal metabolic rate and growth in mammals and birds. Insufficient production of these hormones, known as a **hypothyroidism**, results in slow growth. In adult animals it causes lethargy. **Hyperthyroidism** or overproduction of T_3 and T_4 hormones results in hyperactivity, restless, nervousness, bulging eyes, and rapid weight loss, called **Graves' disease**. T_3 and T_4 hormones affect loss and replacement of hair in mammals and feather in birds. They promote sloughing or shedding of the skin. Deficit of these hormones in mammals or birds impair hair and feather growth and their depigmentation. In most vertebrates, elevation of T_3 and T_4 hormones correlates with gonad maturation, oogenesis in females or spermatogenesis in males.

The third hormone secreted by the thyroid gland is **calcitonin**. This hormone produced by cells that fill the space between follicles called **interstitial**, **parafollicular**, or **C-cells** and do not release their secretion into the colloid. The hormone regulates calcium and phosphorus metabolisms. Calcitonin production is directly controlled by blood Ca^{2+} level, and released when its level grows above the norm. Calcitonin (also known as **thyrocalcitonin**) is a linear polypeptide hormone that reduces blood Ca^{2+}. It lowers blood Ca^{2+} levels in two ways:

1. It inhibits osteoclast activity and favors to Ca^{2+} deposition in bones.
2. It inhibits reabsorption of Ca^{2+} and phosphate in kidneys and allows them to be excreted in urine.

VETERINARY APPLICATION

The medical condition with decreased production and secretion of the thyroid hormones is termed hypothyroidism. This disorder is most common in dogs but also develops rarely in other species, including cats, horses, and other domestic animals. In dogs, the most common cause of secondary hypothyroidism is destruction of pituitary thyrotrophic cells by an expanding, space-occupying tumor. Other rare forms of hypothyroidism in dogs include neoplastic destruction of thyroid tissue and congenital (or juvenile-onset) hypothyroidism. Although onset is variable, hypothyroidism is most common in dogs four to ten years old. It usually affects mid- to large-size breeds and is rare in toy and miniature breeds. Breeds reported to be predisposed include the golden retriever, Doberman pinscher, Irish setter, miniature schnauzer, dachshund, cocker spaniel, and Airedale terrier. There does not appear to be a sex predilection, but spayed females appear to have a higher risk of developing hypothyroidism than intact females.

Many of the clinical signs associated with canine hypothyroidism are directly related to slowing of cellular metabolism, which results in development of mental dullness, lethargy, exercise intolerance, and weight gain without a corresponding increase in appetite. Difficulty maintaining body temperature may lead to frank hypothermia; the classic hypothyroid dog is a heat-seeker. Alterations in the skin and coat are common. Dryness, excessive shedding, and retarded regrowth of hair are usually the earliest dermatologic changes.

Calcitonin protects bones from calcium loss during periods of calcium mobilization, such as pregnancy and lactation. The protective mechanisms include the direct inhibition of bone resorption and the indirect effect through the inhibition of the release of prolactin from the pituitary gland.

Parathyroid gland releases **parathyroid hormone (PTH)**, whose action is antagonistic to the calcitonin and elevates the blood calcium level. The name *parathyroid* points to the close association of this gland with the thyroid gland. It consists of one or two pairs of small oval bodies on the dorsal side of the thyroid gland. Mobility of the calcium is a life important to most vertebrates. When a bird secretes calcified eggshells or a deer grows a new rack of antlers, a large amount of calcium must be rapidly mobilized and transported. PTH raises blood calcium level through the following ways:

1. It promotes calcium retention by kidneys.
2. It activates vitamin D and, by that, facilitates calcium absorption across the small intestine walls.
3. It encourage osteoclasts to resorb bone matrix and release calcium into the bloodstream.

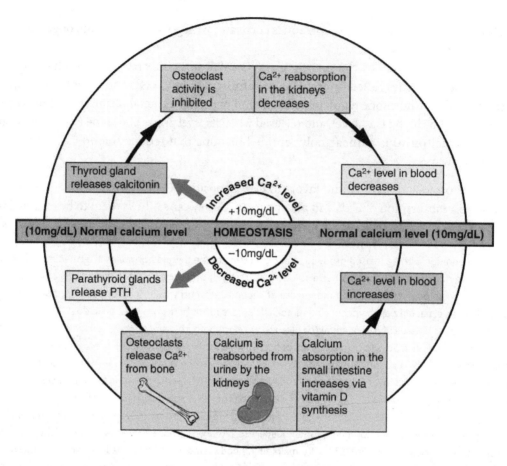

FIGURE 14.11   Blood Calcium Homeostasis Mechanism.

The two processes of bone deposition and bone decomposition take place simultaneously and in a healthy organism are dynamically balanced (fig. 14.11).

CHECK YOUR UNDERSTANDING

- What are the main functions of T_3 and T_4 hormones?

- What role do parafollicular cells play?

- Describe the structure and function of thyroid follicles.

- Describe the mechanism of regulation of T_3 and T_4 production.

- How does PTH effect the blood calcium level?

- Some dietary supplements that are designed to decrease body weight contain thyroid hormone. How would these supplements cause weight loss?

Adrenal Glands: Adrenal Cortex and Adrenal Medulla

Mammalian adrenal gland consists of two glands with different origins and functions. Like most organs, adrenal gland is enclosed in connective tissue membranous capsule. The layer beneath the capsule is formed by the **adrenocortical tissue** and constitutes **adrenal cortex**. The so-called **chromaffin tissue** forms the central part of the gland termed **adrenal medulla**.

The adrenal cortex produces and releases **corticosteroid hormones**. Corticosteroids derive from cholesterol. There are three main group of corticosteroids produced by adrenal cortex: 1) hormones involved in regulation of body water balance and sodium reabsorption in kidneys, called **mineralocorticoids**; 2) hormones that control carbohydrates' metabolism, called **glucocorticoids**; and 3) hormones involved in reproduction, or sex hormones (**estrogens**, **progestogens**, and **androgens**).

The adrenal cortex has three histologically distinctive layers: 1) **zona glomerulosa**; 2) **zona fasciculata**; and 3) **zona reticularis**. Zona glomerulosa creates the most superficial layer of the renal cortex. Cells in this zone are small and compact. They secrete mineralocorticoid hormones, such as **aldosterone**. Kidneys stimulate release of aldosterone by secreting protein **renin**. Mineralocorticoids stimulate sodium reabsorption in the walls of the nephron tubules. Reabsorbed sodium accumulates in the interstitial space and generates a gradient of concentration. Water simply follows sodium by osmosis, which reduces urine volume. The recovered water enters the blood and increases a total blood volume, which elevates blood pressure.

Zona fasciculata consists of cells organized in rows or stocks with blood sinuses between them. Cells of this zone produce glucocorticoids, such as **corticosterone** and **cortisol**. They are released in response to ACTH produced by the anterior pituitary gland. Cortisol constitutes up to 95 percent of the released glucocorticoids. About half of cortisol molecules are released during sleep, with its concentration reaching its maximum peak right before waking up. This rhythm of release is controlled by circadian rhythms detected by retina of the eye. Hormones of this zone effect carbohydrates metabolism and play an important role in defense and long-lasting stress reactions. Their actions resist stress and help repair injured or damaged tissues.

Cells of the zona reticularis are small and compact. They are sensitive to the ACTH and synthesize sex hormones together with an additional amount of glucocorticoids (fig. 14.12).

VETERINARY APPLICATION

Named after the neurosurgeon who first described the disease in 1912, Cushing's disease, also known as hyperadrenocorticism or hypercortisolism, is a hormone disorder that affects humans as well as dogs. The pituitary gland is a key part of a dog's endocrine system, responsible for controlling all of the hormone production throughout the dog's body. A tumor in the pituitary gland or an enlarged pituitary gland can lead to Cushing's disease. Cushing's disease specifically refers to an increased cortisol levels in a dog as a result of a benign tumor in the pituitary gland. Cortisol is one of the main stress hormones. There are generally two major forms of Cushing's syndrome in dogs: 1) **pituitary dependent**, affecting about 80 to 90 percent of dogs with Cushing's disease; it is caused by a tumor in the pituitary gland; and 2) **adrenal dependent:** about 15 to 20 percent of dogs with Cushing's disease are diagnosed with this type. In this form, Cushing's disease is caused by a tumor in one of the adrenal glands.

Adrenal gland tumors are more common in large dog breeds, while smaller breeds with Cushing's disease are more prone to pituitary tumors. Some dog breeds that generally have a higher chance of getting Cushing's disease include poodles, Yorkshire terriers, boxers, Staffordshire bull terriers, Boston terriers, beagles, Jack Russell terriers, and German shepherds. In both cases, the tumors are usually benign. If the tumor causing the disease has not spread to other parts of the dog's body, it can be removed through surgery.

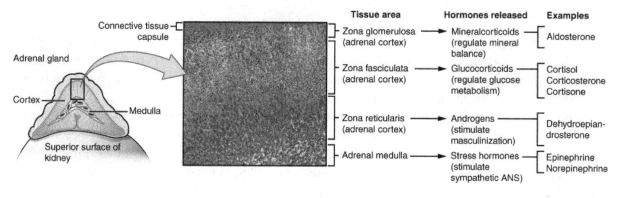

FIGURE 14.12   Adrenal Glands.

In many mammals, including primates, there is additional peripheral layer known as a **fetal zone**. The fetal zone produces molecules precursors of estrogens. Transported to the placenta, these molecules are converted into estrogens, which promotes maintenance of pregnancy and prevent initiation of a new reproductive cycle. Failure of the fetal zone to function terminates gestation and results in premature birth. After the birth, the fetal zone reduces and may completely disappear.

Adrenal medulla produces two short-term stress hormones: **epinephrine** and **norepinephrine**. Their release is triggered by the sympathetic nervous system. About 80 percent of all secretions of the adrenal medulla is an epinephrine. Both hormones help facilitate the fight-or-flight response.

CHECK YOUR UNDERSTANDING

- What hormones are produced by the middle zona fasciculate of the adrenal cortex?

- What is the relationship among CRH, ACTH, and cortisol?

- What two hormones are produced by the adrenal medulla?

- What three main hormone groups are produced by the adrenal cortex?

Endocrine Pancreas and Its Role in Regulation of Blood Glucose

The pancreas is a composite gland that consists of exocrine and endocrine components. Acinar cells constitute the exocrine part of the pancreas. These cells secrete pancreatic digestive enzymes and discharge them into pancreatic ducts. The endocrine part consists of **pancreatic islets** also known as **islets of Langerhans** (fig. 14.13). They constitute 1 to 2 percent of the pancreas volume and receive 10 to 15 percent of pancreatic blood flow.

Pancreatic islets contain five cell types:

1. **Alpha cells** constitute 20 percent of pancreatic islets. They produce the hormone **glucagon**.
2. **Beta cells** constitute 70 percent of pancreatic islets. They secrete the hormones **insulin** and **amylin**.
3. **Delta cells** constitute less than 10 percent. They produce the hormone **somatostatin**.

4. **Epsilon cells** constitute less than 1 percent. These cells produce the hormone **ghrelin**.
5. **PP cells**, also called **gamma cells**, constitute less than 5 percent of total mass of pancreatic islets. Their secretion is **pancreatic polypeptide (PP)**.

Glucagon mobilizes stored glycogen and triggers process of its breakdown. Liberated from glycogen, glucose molecules enter bloodstream. It also has an effect on breakdown of lipids in the liver and elevation of fatty acids in the blood. Glucagon is one of several hyperglycemic hormones. It especially important among herbivores and in fasting carnivores. In birds and lizards, it is more important than insulin for carbohydrates metabolism. Its production and release are controlled by the blood glucose level.

Insulin is a hormone antagonist to the glucagon. It controls the overall metabolism of carbohydrates, fats, and proteins. Insulin promotes, sometimes indirectly, conversion of end products of carbohydrate, protein, and fat digestion into storage forms. One action of insulin is to inhibit fat

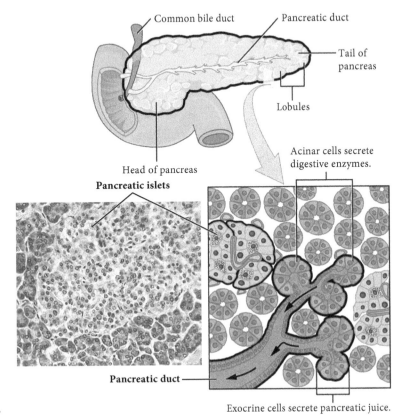

FIGURE 14.13 Pancreas.

breakdown, promote fat synthesis, and lower the level of fatty acids in the blood. Insulin facilitates glucose metabolism and inhibits the breakdown of glycogen in the liver. The most important insulin function is promotion of glucose entry inside cells, especially into skeletal and cardiac muscle cells. Thus, insulin decreases the level of glucose in blood. A low or insufficient insulin production decreases the ability of cells to consume glucose. Glucose blood level grows, and kidneys excrete it with urine. A medical condition of presence glucose in urine is called diabetes. Production and release of insulin is controlled by the blood glucose level.

Amylin is another hormone secreted by beta cells. It plays a role in glycemic regulation by slowing gastric emptying and promoting satiety, thereby preventing a rapid increase in the blood glucose level after meal. Thus, it functions as a synergist partner of insulin. Like the two previous hormones, amylin is released according to the level of glucose in the blood (fig. 14.14).

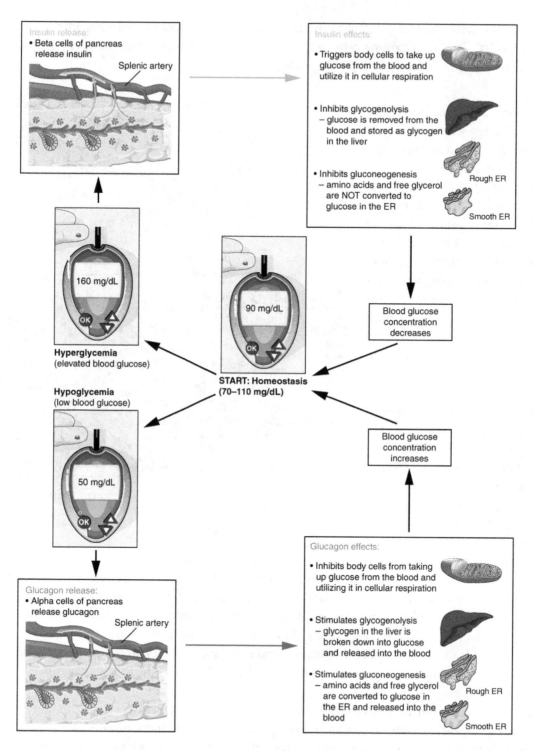

FIGURE 14.14   Homeostatic Regulation of Blood Glucose.

Somatostatin, also known as **growth hormone–inhibiting hormone (GHIH)**, is produced by D cells. It is a peptide hormone. It suppresses pancreas endocrine cells and inhibits secretion of insulin and glucagon. Release of this hormone is induced by low pH, when acidic chime from the stomach enters the duodenum. In the stomach, somatostatin acts directly on the acid-producing parietal cells of the gastric glands. Indirectly, somatostatin inhibits secretion of gastrin, secretin, and histamine, which dramatically reduces gastric digestion. It also decreases the rate of gastric emptying and reduces smooth muscle contractions and blood flow within the intestine.

Ghrelin, often called the "hunger hormone" and also known as **lenomorelin**, is a peptide hormone. Ghrelin regulates appetite. An empty stomach secretes ghrelin, which acts on receptors of the hypothalamus's hunger center. The presence of ghrelin and its increase in blood flow generates a feeling of hunger and increases appetite. It also increases secretion of gastric acid and gastrointestinal motility to prepare the body for food intake. When the stomach fills with food and its walls become stretched, the ghrelin secretion stops and causes hunger to end and the appetite to lower. This hormone also plays an important role in regulation of energy distribution and usage. Ghrelin receptors are found in dopamine neurons that link the ventral tegmental area to the nucleus accumbens (a center that plays a role in processing sexual desire, reward, and reinforcement, and in development of addictions). Thus, ghrelin is associated with the reward system and plays an important role in generation of rewarding euphoric emotions.

Pancreatic polypeptide is usually released into the blood following a protein-rich or fat-rich meal. The function of PP is to self-regulate pancreatic secretion activities (endocrine and exocrine). It also has effects on hepatic glycogen level and gastrointestinal secretions. It stimulates the gastric juice secretion. It is the antagonist of cholecystokinin and inhibits the pancreatic secretion which is stimulated by cholecystokinin. Glucose and fats also induce PP secretion.

VETERINARY APPLICATION

Diabetes mellitus is a chronic disease resulting from insufficient insulin production or target cell insulin resistance. Diabetes affects 1 in 230 cats. Eighty to 95 percent of diabetic cats experience something similar to type 2 diabetes. The condition is treatable, and treated properly, the cat can have a normal life expectancy. In type 2 cats, effective treatment may lead to diabetic remission, in which the cat no longer needs injected insulin. Cats generally show a gradual onset of the disease over a few weeks or months. The first outward symptoms are a sudden weight loss (or gain), accompanied by excessive drinking and urination. Appetite is suddenly either ravenous or absent, because of the inability to use glucose as an energy source. The back legs become weak and the gait becomes stilted or wobbly, due to diabetic neuropathy, which is caused by damage to the myelin sheath of the peripheral nerves due to glucose toxicity and cell starvation caused by chronic hyperglycemia. The cat displays a plantigrade stance, standing on its hocks instead of on its toes as normal. The cat may also have trouble walking and jumping, and may sit down after a few steps. In the final stages, the cat becomes lethargic. Untreated, diabetes leads to coma and then death.

A fasting glucose blood test will normally be suggestive of diabetes. The same home blood test monitors used in humans are used on cats, usually by taking blood from the ear or paw pads. As the disease progresses, ketone bodies will be present in the urine, which can be detected with the same urine strips as for humans.

Pineal Gland

The pineal gland is located on the dorsal side of the midbrain (see Chapter 11, page 308). In some recent and fossil vertebrates, the pineal gland is inserted into an opening in the bony cranium, known as the pineal foramen, and covered only by a thin layer of integument. This allows the pineal gland to respond to changes in photoperiod (fig. 14.15). In mammals this gland is involved in detecting seasonal or daily light changes. It also regulates reproductive cycles in many vertebrates. The hormone produced by this gland is known as **melatonin**. Available experimental data suggests that melatonin influences melanin production.

Gonads (Ovaries and Testes)

The primary function of gonads is production of sex cells: sperm cells in males and egg cells in females. Beside germinal cells, gonads have secretory cells that produce a number of sex hormones. All sex hormones produced by gonads are steroids.

The hormone of the testes is called **testosterone**. Testosterone is considered a male hormone. However, female ovaries and adrenal glands also produce some small amount of this hormone. Testosterone production is regulated by a multilevel negative feedback loop that involves the hypothalamus and the anterior pituitary gland. The hypothalamus GnRH triggers release of FSH and LH. The LH stimulates testosterone synthesis, and FSH stimulates production of a protein that binds testosterone and concentrates it in the testes. Production of the testosterone inhibits hypothalamic secretion of the GnRH, which leads to decrease of LH and FSH production by the anterior pituitary gland.

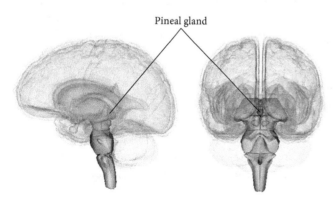

Pineal gland

FIGURE 14.15   Pineal Gland.

Like all steroid hormones, testosterone easily crosses the plasma membrane of target cells and binds to intracellular receptors that influence gene expression. Testosterone generates two main effects on target cells: 1) **anabolic effects**, which consist of stimulating bone growth and increasing muscle mass; and 2) **androgenic effects**, which include secondary male characteristics.

Ovaries produce female sex hormones: **estrogens** and **progesterone**. As with the testosterone, female sex hormones are controlled through the negative feedback loop, which includes GnRH from the hypothalamus, and FSH and LH from the anterior pituitary gland. Estrogens stimulate the development of female secondary characteristics, such as breasts and skin vascularization; regulate reproductive cycles; and so forth.

Progesterone production reaches its peak after ovulation and during pregnancy. It prepares the female body for pregnancy and supports fetal development. It influences the state of smooth muscles, body temperature, blood-clotting process, bones, and metabolism.

CHECK YOUR UNDERSTANDING

- What are the target tissues and effects of melatonin?

- What are the target tissues and main effects of testosterone and estrogens?

The Kidneys as an Endocrine Gland

Beside their major function to maintain body fluid homeostasis and remove waste materials from an organism, the kidneys are also an important endocrine organ (fig. 14.16). Their endocrine role includes:

1. **Regulation of red blood cell production.** There are certain cells in kidneys sensitive to blood oxygen level. The decrease of blood oxygen triggers production and release by these cells of hormone **erythropoietin**, or **EPO**. Target cells of the EPO are erythrocyte progenitor cells in red bone marrow. Stimulated by EPO, these cells divide and develop in new erythrocytes that increase blood oxygen–carrying capacity.

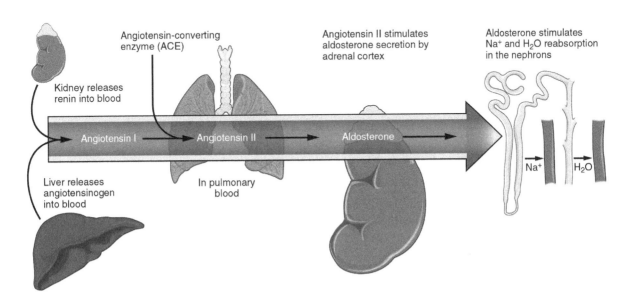

Angiotensin-converting enzyme (ACE)

Angiotensin II stimulates aldosterone secretion by adrenal cortex

Aldosterone stimulates Na^+ and H_2O reabsorption in the nephrons

Kidney releases renin into blood

Angiotensin I → Angiotensin II → Aldosterone →

Na^+ H_2O

Liver releases angiotensinogen into blood

In pulmonary blood

FIGURE 14.16   Renin-Angiotensin System.

2. **Control of water and electrolyte body balance.** A special group of nephrons called juxtaglomer-ular nephrons monitor blood pressure in incoming afferent arterioles. The low blood pressure stimulates release in blood of the protein enzyme hormone **renin** that converts the plasma protein angiotensinogen to angiotensin I. It is the first step in a chain of chemical reactions called the renin-angiotensin-aldosterone system, which results in retention of sodium ions from urine. Reabsorption of sodium increases osmotic pressure of interstitial fluid and, consequently, movement of water back from nephron tubules into the interstitial space.

3. **Conversion of vitamin D to its active form.** In the kidneys vitamin D is converted into its hormonally active form, called **calcitriol**. Calcitriol increases the level of Ca^{2+} in the blood through the 1) increase of the uptake of calcium from the small intestine into the blood; 2) reabsorption of calcium by the kidneys, which reduce the loss of calcium in the urine; and 3) release of calcium into the blood from bone through an activation of bone resorption by osteoclasts.

CHECK YOUR UNDERSTANDING

- Why is kidney failure always associated with anemia?

- What role do the kidneys play in regulation of blood pressure?

The Thymus

The thymus is located in the mediastinum, posterior to the sternum and between the lungs. The thymus secretes a group of hormones, including **thymulin**, **thymopoietins**, and **thymosins**, which affect production and differentiation of T lymphocytes. These hormones mainly act locally as paracrine compounds in immune response development.

Adipose Tissue

Adipose tissue is scattered throughout the body. The cells that create this tissue are known as adipocytes. The prime function of adipocytes is to store fat. Together with fat storage, these cells produce a number of hormones, including:

1. **Adiponectin.** This is a protein hormone, which is involved in regulating glucose levels as well as fatty acid breakdown. It modulates a number of metabolic processes, including glucose regulation and fatty acids' oxidation. Adiponectin is secreted from adipose tissue (and also from the placenta in pregnancy) into the bloodstream and is very abundant in plasma relative to other hormones. Many studies have found adiponectin to be inversely correlated with body mass index. Concentration of circulating adiponectin increases under caloric restricted diet in animals and humans. Transgenic mice with increased adiponectin show reduced adipocyte differentiation and increased energy expenditure associated with mitochondrial uncoupling. The hormone may result in diabetes type 2, obesity, and atherosclerosis. Adiponectin in combination with leptin has been shown to completely reverse insulin resistance in mice. Adiponectin automatically self-associates into larger structures. Three adiponectin molecules bind together to form a trimer. The trimers

continue to self-associate and form hexamers or dodecamers. There is a sexual dimorphism in presence of different types of large adiponectin structures. Females have increased proportions of the high-molecular weight forms. Recent studies showed that the high-molecular weight form may be the most biologically active form regarding glucose homeostasis. High-molecular-weight adiponectin was further found to be associated with a lower risk of diabetes. Adiponectin exerts some of its weight reduction effects via the brain. This is similar to the action of **leptin**. The two hormones perform complementary actions and have synergistic effects.

2. **Resistin.** Resistin is produced and released from adipose tissue to serve endocrine functions involved in insulin resistance. Resistin level increases with obesity in humans, rats, and mice.

3. **Leptin.** This is a protein, but it is able to cross the blood-brain barrier to interact with its main target cells: neurons in the hypothalamus satiety center. Leptin induces satiety, a feeling of fullness, and prevents obesity. Leptin secretion directly depends on the amount of fat stored in adipose tissue. With the increase in fat storage, leptin secretion grows and appetite decreases.

4. **Estradiol (E2).** Adipose tissue in both males and females contributes to the production of estradiol. The estradiol generates development of female secondary sex characteristics, such as development of breasts and specific feminine body shape, bones, joints, and feminine fat deposition in the breasts, hips, thighs, and buttocks, maturation of the vagina and vulva, and closure of epiphyseal plate (thereby limiting final height) in both sexes. In the female, estradiol acts as a growth hormone for tissue of the reproductive organs, supporting the lining of the vagina, the cervical glands, the endometrium, and the lining of the fallopian tubes. It enhances growth of the myometrium. Estradiol appears necessary to maintain oocytes in the ovary. During the menstrual cycle, estradiol produced by the growing follicles triggers, via a positive feedback system, the hypothalamic-pituitary events that lead to the luteinizing hormone surge, inducing ovulation. In the luteal phase, estradiol, in conjunction with progesterone, prepares the endometrium for implantation. During pregnancy, estradiol increases due to placental production. The estradiol, together with estrone and estriol promote uterine blood flow, myometrial growth, stimulate breast growth, and at term, promote cervical softening and expression of myometrial oxytocin receptors. In baboons, blocking of estrogen production leads to pregnancy loss, suggesting estradiol has a role in the maintenance of pregnancy. Bone structure is affected also, resulting in early osteopenia and osteoporosis. The estrogen receptor, as well as the progesterone receptor, have been detected in the skin, including in keratinocytes and fibroblasts. The decrease of estradiol causes atrophy, thinning, and increased wrinkling of the skin and a reduction in skin elasticity, firmness, and strength. These skin changes constitute an acceleration in skin aging and are the result of decreased collagen content, irregularities in the morphology of epidermal skin cells, decreased ground substance between skin fibers, and reduced capillaries and blood flow. The positive and negative feedback loops of the menstrual cycle involve ovarian estradiol as the link to the hypothalamic-pituitary system to regulate gonadotropins.

Estrogen has been found to increase the secretion of oxytocin and to increase the expression of the oxytocin receptor in the brain. A single dose of estradiol has been found to be sufficient to increase circulating oxytocin concentration. Estradiol has been tied to the development and progression of cancers such as breast cancer, ovarian cancer, and endometrial cancer. Estradiol affects target tissues mainly by interacting with two nuclear receptors called estrogen receptor α (ERα) and estrogen receptor β (ERβ).

One of the functions of these estrogen receptors is the modulation of gene expression. Once estradiol binds to the ERs, the receptor complexes then bind to specific DNA sequences, possibly causing damage to the DNA.

In males, estradiol prevents apoptosis (physiological self-destruction) of sperm cells. Males with low estradiol or other estrogens are tall and eunuchoid, as epiphyseal closure is delayed or may not take place. There is evidence that the programming of adult male sexual behavior in many vertebrates is largely dependent on estradiol produced by adrenal cortex and adipose tissue during prenatal life and early infancy.

CHECK YOUR UNDERSTANDING

- What are the hormones of the thymus? What are their target tissues?

- How does increased fat storage affect the appetite?

- What is the function of the hormone resistin?

CHAPTER SUMMARY

- The functional units of the endocrine system are secretory cells that manufacture and secrete hormones. These cells may be organized in groups and form organ **endocrine gland,** or diffusely distributed and form unicellular endocrine gland.

- The endocrine system performs four major functions: 1) regulation of cellular metabolism, organism growth, and development; 2) maintenance of homeostasis of blood and other body fluids, their volume, and composition; 3) control of food digestion and nutrient absorption; and 4) control of animal reproduction and social behavior.

- There are many signaling molecules other than hormones that are classified in four groups: **intracrine**, **autocrine**, **paracrine**, and **pheromones**. From other signaling factors, hormones differ by their long-distance effect on target cells, comparatively long life, effect on only cells that have receptor proteins, and blood distribution.

- Hormones fall into three chemical classes: 1) **steroid hormones**; 2) **peptide** and **protein hormones**; and 3) **amine hormones**.

- Steroid hormones are lipids. In vertebrates, these hormones are produced by gonads, cortex of adrenal glands, and placenta. Steroids are lipid soluble and hydrophobic.

- Peptide, protein, and amine hormones are water soluble. They are transported directly with blood flow, but cannot cross the target cell plasma membrane. Their receptor protein has to be exposed outside on the membrane surface. These hormones cumulatively are called **nonsteroidal hormones**.

- The effect of a hormone depends on its concentration in the blood. Two processes influence hormone concentration: hormone synthesis and hormone elimination. Synthesis and release of hormones into the bloodstream is regulated through negative feedback. The hormone is eliminated through three processes: 1) hormone degradation by enzymes in the liver; 2) excretion of the hormone by the kidneys; and 3) uptake of the hormone by the target cells. The rate of hormone elimination depends on its concentration: the higher its concentration, the faster it is eliminated from the blood. The rate of hormone elimination is characterized by the hormone's half-life. The half-life is the time period during which an amount of the hormone within the bloodstream is reduced to one-half. Water-soluble hormones have a short half-life, from a few minutes to a few hours. The lipid-soluble steroid hormones live longer, because carrying proteins protect them from degradation by enzymes.

- A target cell responds to a hormone because it has **receptor proteins** that interact with the hormone. A target cell has thousands of receptor molecules for a particular hormone and may have different types of receptor molecules, which allows it to respond to different hormones. Different cells may have different receptor molecules that are sensitive to the same hormone. Because of that, responses in different target cells on the same hormone may be different.

- Water-soluble hormones are polar molecules and unable to cross the plasma membrane. Their receptor proteins are located on the surface of the plasma membrane. The binding of a water-soluble hormone to its receptor initiates a series of biochemical reactions across the membrane called a **signal transduction pathway**. In this process, the hormone functions as a **first messenger**. Transduction pathway reactions within the cell generate **second messengers**. The second messengers then change target cell metabolism.

- The mechanism of an intracellular enzyme cascade caused by water-soluble hormones 1) amplifies the signal at each step of enzymatic reactions and 2) creates an opportunity to precisely control the cellular response.

- Lipid-soluble hormones are able to diffuse across the plasma membrane. Receptor proteins for them are located in cytosol, where they form a **hormone-receptor complex**. The hormone-receptor complex then binds to a regulatory DNA sequence called **hormone-response elements (HREs)** and affects gene expression.

- The hypothalamus has direct control over the pituitary gland and through it over other endocrine organs. This influence is termed the **hypothalamic–pituitary gland axis**. The hormones of the hypothalamus are called **release hormones** or **inhibitory hormones**: **thyrotropin-releasing hormone (TRH)**; **prolactin-releasing hormone (PRH)**; **prolactin-inhibiting hormone**; **gonadotropin-releasing hormone (GnRH)**; **corticotropin-releasing hormone (CRH)**; **growth hormone–releasing hormone (GHRH)**; **growth hormone–inhibiting hormone (GHIH)**.

- The pituitary gland is connected with the hypothalamus by a stalk called the **infundibulum**. It consists of two structures that are different in origin, histology, and function: the **anterior pituitary** and **posterior pituitary glands**. With the hypothalamus, the anterior pituitary gland is connected by blood flow of hypothalamo-pituitary portal system.

- The posterior pituitary gland is not an endocrine gland. It does not produce hormones, but consists of axon terminals of neuroendocrine cells located in paraventricular and supraoptic nuclei of the hypothalamus. Synaptic vesicles in axons' terminals are loaded with the hormones **oxytocin** and **antidiuretic hormone (ADH)**.

- ADH maintains body fluid balance, total blood volume, and blood pressure. Target cells of ADH include the kidneys, which increase reuptake of water from urine in collecting ducts and return it into the blood; high doses of ADH cause vasoconstriction. ADH influences formation of family bonds among voles. The high-density distribution of vasopressin receptors in ventral forebrain regions of the prairie vole facilitate and coordinate reward circuits during partner pair formation. In males this hormone triggers family defensive behavior; in females it generates caring instincts.

- Oxytocin stimulates smooth muscle contraction. In females, it stimulates contraction of the uterus's myometrium during childbirth and milk ejection by lactiferous ducts. In males, oxytocin facilitates ejaculation. Oxytocin released during physical contact between individuals improves mood, lowers stress, reduces blood pressure, and increases pain tolerance.

- Anterior pituitary gland hormones are known as **stimulating** or **tropic hormones**: **adrenocorticotropic hormone (ACTH)** or **corticotropin**; **follicle-stimulating hormone (FSH)**; **luteinizing hormone (LH)**; **growth hormone**; **melanocyte-stimulating hormones (MSH)** also called **melanotropins** or **intermedins**; **prolactin**; **thyroid-stimulating hormone**.

- The thyroid gland produces three hormones: two hormones that regulate body metabolism and one that regulates blood Ca^{2+} homeostasis. The gland consists of two **lobes** connected by an **isthmus**. Multicellular spherical structures known as **follicles** are made of a single layer of **follicle cells** that form a hollow sphere filled with a gelatinous **colloid**.

- T_3 and T_4 hormones elevate oxygen consumption and heat production. They increase basal metabolic rate and growth in mammals and birds. Insufficient production causes **hypothyroidism**, which results in slow growth and lethargy. **Hyperthyroidism**, or overproduction of T_3 and T_4 hormones, results in hyperactivity, restless, nervousness, bulging eyes, and rapid weight loss, called **Graves' disease**. T_3 and T_4 hormones affect loss and replacement of hair in mammals and feathers in birds. They promote sloughing or shedding of the skin. A deficit of these hormones in mammals or birds impairs hair and feather growth and their depigmentation.

- **Calcitonin** is produced by **interstitial**, **parafollicular**, or **C-cells**. It regulates calcium and phosphorus metabolisms. Calcitonin production is directly controlled by blood Ca^{2+} level and released when its level grows above the norm.

- The parathyroid gland releases **parathyroid hormone (PTH)**, which is an antagonist to calcitonin and increases the blood calcium level.

- The mammalian adrenal gland consists of two glands with different origins and functions: **adrenal cortex** and **adrenal medulla**.

- The adrenal cortex produces three groups of **corticosteroid hormones**: 1) hormones involved in regulation of body water balance and sodium reabsorption in kidneys, called **mineralocorticoids**; 2) hormones that control carbohydrates' metabolism, called **glucocorticoids**; and 3) sex hormones (**estrogens**, **progestogens**, and **androgens**).

- The adrenal cortex has three histologically distinctive layers: 1) **zona glomerulosa**; 2) **zona fasciculata**; and 3) **zona reticularis**. The zona glomerulosa is the most superficial layer of renal cortex. Its cells secrete mineralocorticoid hormones, such as **aldosterone**. Cells in the zona fasciculata produce glucocorticoids, such as **corticosterone** and **cortisol**. They are released in response to ACTH released by the anterior pituitary gland. Cells of the zona reticularis are small and compact. They are sensitive to the ACTH and synthesize sex hormones together with an additional amount of glucocorticoids.

- The adrenal medulla produces **epinephrine** and **norepinephrine**. Their release is triggered by the sympathetic nervous system. Both hormones facilitate the fight-or-flight response.

- The pancreas has exocrine and endocrine components. The endocrine part consists of **pancreatic islets**, also known as **islets of Langerhans**. They constitute 1 to 2 percent of the pancreas and receive 10 to 15 percent of its blood flow. Pancreatic islets contain five cell types: 1) **alpha cells** produce the hormone **glucagon**; 2) **beta cells** secrete the hormones **insulin** and **amylin**; 3) **delta cells** produce **somatostatin**; 4) **epsilon cells** produce **ghrelin**; and 5) **gamma cells** secrete **pancreatic polypeptide (PP)**.

- The pineal gland is located on the dorsal side of the midbrain. This gland is involved in detecting seasonal or daily light changes. It also regulates reproductive cycles in many vertebrates. The hormone produced by this gland is known as **melatonin**.

- The hormone of the testes is called **testosterone** and has two main effects: 1) **anabolic effects**, which consist of stimulating bone growth and increasing muscle mass; and 2) **androgenic effects**, which include development of secondary male characteristics.

- Ovaries produce **estrogens** and **progesterone**. Estrogens stimulate development of female secondary characteristics and regulate reproductive cycles. Progesterone production reaches its peak after ovulation and during pregnancy. It prepares the female body for pregnancy and supports fetal development. It influences the state of smooth muscles, body temperature, blood-clotting process, bones, and metabolism.

- The kidneys secrete a number of hormones, whose functions are 1) **Regulation of red blood cells production**. Kidneys produce **erythropoietin** (**EPO**) that stimulates erythrocyte progenitor cells in red bone marrow to divide and develop in new erythrocytes; 2) **Control of water and electrolyte body balance**. Kidney release in blood protein enzyme hormone **renin** that convert plasma protein angiotensinogen to angiotensin I. It is a first step in chain of chemical reactions called renin-angiotensin-aldosterone system, which results in retention of sodium ions from urine, reabsorption of water, and increase of blood pressure; 3) **Conversion of vitamin D to an active form**. In the kidneys, vitamin D is converted into its hormonally active **calcitriol** that increases Ca^{2+} blood level by: a) increase of the uptake of calcium from the small intestine; b) reabsorption of calcium by the kidneys, which reduces the loss of calcium in the urine; and c) release of calcium into the blood from bone by activation of bone resorption by osteoclasts.

- Adipocytes produce a number of hormones, including adiponectin, resistin, leptin, and estradiol.

CHECK YOUR KNOWLEDGE

LEVEL 1. CHECK YOUR RECALL

1. How do steroid hormones differ from polypeptide and most amino-acid-derived hormones?
   A. Steroids are lipid soluble and cross the plasma membrane easily.
   B. Polypeptide and amino-acid-derived hormones are longer lived in the bloodstream and, thus, amplify signals higher.
   C. Polypeptide hormones are the most structurally complex and induce permanent changes in target cells.
   D. Only polypeptide hormones directly affect genes' activity.
   E. Steroid hormones bind to receptors in the plasma membrane, whereas polypeptide hormones bind to receptors in cytoplasm.

2. All steroid hormones are synthesized (originate) from:
    A. Proteins
    B. Amino acids
    C. Fatty acids
    D. Nucleic acids
    E. Cholesterol

3. Synthesis of hormones is regulated mostly through the:
    A. Reflex arch
    B. Negative feedback
    C. Positive feedback
    D. Diurnal rhythms
    E. Biological clock

4. A special protein called _____ makes the target cell sensitive to hormone.
    A. antigen
    B. ligand
    C. receptor protein
    D. acceptor protein
    E. transport protein

5. Which of these organs is an endocrine gland?
    A. Salivary gland
    B. Thyroid gland
    C. Sweat gland
    D. Sebaceous gland
    E. Mammary gland

6. All of the following are endocrine glands **except**:
    A. Adrenal gland
    B. Pineal gland
    C. Pituitary gland
    D. Pancreas
    E. Lacrimal gland

7. Which of the following is **not** a peptide hormone?
    A. Insulin
    B. Testosterone
    C. Adrenocorticotropic hormone
    D. Oxytocin
    E. All of them are peptide hormones.

8. The hormone aldosterone regulates blood pressure through:
    A.   Reabsorption of sodium
    B.   Secretion of sodium
    C.   Reabsorption of potassium
    D.   Secretion of potassium
    E.   Secretion of calcium

9. Why does a hormone (for example, epinephrine) generate different reactions in different target cells (for example, in smooth muscle cells)?
    A.   Because the reaction of the cell depends on the amount of the hormone.
    B.   Because of the influence of environment on the cell; for example, body temperature.
    C.   Because cells have different receptor proteins; say, α- and β-receptors.
    D.   It depends on the circumstances; sometimes cell reacts one way, sometimes another.
    E.   It depends on the influence of other surrounding cells.

10. Hormones that act on the same target cells yet have opposite effects are said to be:
    A.   Synergists
    B.   Hydrophilic hormones
    C.   Antagonists

11. What is a major function of the endocrine system?
    A.   The endocrine system communicates directly with target cells through the neurotransmitters.
    B.   The endocrine system releases hormones into the bloodstream to reach receptors on target cells.
    C.   The endocrine system produces immediate, short-lasting effects.
    D.   The endocrine system secretes products into ducts that lead to body surfaces or cavities.

12. When the concentration of thyroid hormone in blood increases, it:
    A.   Inhibits thyroid stimulating hormone secretion by the pituitary gland
    B.   Stimulates secretion of thyroid releasing hormone secretion by the hypothalamus
    C.   Stimulates the pituitary gland to secrete thyroid releasing hormone
    D.   Stimulates the pituitary gland to secrete thyroid stimulating hormone
    E.   Activates a positive feedback homeostatic loop

13. All of the following are hormones of the anterior pituitary gland **except**:
    A.   Growth hormone (GH)
    B.   Follicle-stimulating hormone (FSH)
    C.   Thyroid-stimulating hormone (TSH)
    D.   Parathyroid hormone (PTH)
    E.   Prolactin

14. Oxytocin is a hormone produced in the _____ and released through the _____.
    A. anterior pituitary gland; posterior pituitary gland
    B. anterior pituitary gland; hypothalamus
    C. hypothalamus; anterior pituitary gland
    D. hypothalamus; posterior pituitary gland
    E. posterior pituitary gland; hypothalamus

15. Which of the following organs combines exocrine and endocrine glands?
    A. Pineal gland
    B. Thyroid gland
    C. Pancreas
    D. Adrenal gland
    E. Ceruminous gland

16. Which of the following is secreted by nerve fibers in the posterior pituitary gland?
    A. Thyroid-stimulating hormone
    B. Adrenocorticotropic hormone
    C. Luteinizing hormone
    D. Anti-diuretic hormone
    E. Follicle-stimulating hormone

17. Releasing hormones are produced by:
    A. The anterior pituitary gland
    B. The posterior pituitary gland
    C. The hypothalamus
    D. The ovaries and testes
    E. It depends on which releasing hormone you are talking about.

18. The hormone calcitonin _____, whereas parathyroid hormone (PTH) _____
    A. decreases blood concentration of Ca^{2+}; increases blood concentration of Ca^{2+}
    B. increases blood concentration of Ca^{2+}; decreases blood concentration of Ca^{2+}
    C. decreases blood concentration of glucose; increases blood concentration of glucose
    D. increases blood concentration of glucose; decreases blood concentration of glucose

19. Oxytocin has a strong effect on:
    A. Water retention and urea production by kidneys
    B. Growth of somatic cells and mitosis
    C. Oogenesis in females and spermatogenesis in males
    D. Contractions of uterus and release of milk by mammary glands
    E. Metabolism of carbohydrates and proteins

20. Prolactin is a hormone that is produced by the _____ and has an effect on the _____.
    A. thyroid gland; secretion of milk by mammary glands
    B. anterior pituitary gland; secretion of milk by mammary glands
    C. posterior pituitary gland; secretion of milk by mammary glands
    D. hypothalamus; concentration of glucose in blood
    E. parathyroid gland; growth of hair and hair color

21. With which gland does the hypothalamus have a close anatomical and physiological relationship?
    A. Pineal gland
    B. Adrenal gland
    C. Thyroid gland
    D. Pituitary gland

22. What connects the hypothalamus and pituitary gland?
    A. Vermis
    B. Isthmus
    C. Infundibulum
    D. Medulla oblongata
    E. Fornix

23. In mammals:
    A. The pineal gland controls both male and female reproductive cycles.
    B. Estrogen is produced by the hypothalamus to control ovulation.
    C. Melatonin controls anabolic steroid production.
    D. GnRH stimulates LH to control production of testosterone.
    E. The anterior pituitary gland produces and releases ADH.

24. Insulin:
    A. Decreases concentration of glucose in blood
    B. Increases glucose concentration in blood
    C. Increases the rate of breakdown of glycogen to glucose
    D. Stimulates the kidneys to secrete glucose into urine
    E. Stimulates hepatocytes to release glucose into the bloodstream

25. Which hormone exerts its effect primarily on the reproductive organs?
    A. Anti-diuretic hormone
    B. Follicle-stimulating hormone
    C. Prolactin-releasing factor
    D. Adrenocorticotropic hormone
    E. Epinephrine

26. Calcium concentration in blood is controlled by:
    A. Hypothalamus and anterior pituitary gland
    B. Thyroid and parathyroid glands
    C. Adrenal and pineal glands
    D. Adrenal cortex and adrenal medulla
    E. Anterior and posterior pituitary glands

27. Two antagonistic hormones are:
    A. Calcitonin and parathyroid hormone
    B. Melatonin and follicle-stimulating hormone
    C. Aldosterone and epinephrine
    D. ADH and GnRH
    E. Oxytocin and prolactin

28. The adrenal cortex produces only:
    A. Polypeptide hormones
    B. Corticosteroid hormones
    C. Amine-derived hormones
    D. Glucagon
    E. Prolactin

29. The target organ for luteinizing hormone (LH) is:
    A. Liver
    B. Kidneys
    C. Pancreas
    D. Gonads
    E. Thyroid gland

30. Adrenal medulla produces only:
    A. Aldosterone and cortisol
    B. Glucagon and insulin
    C. Epinephrine and norepinephrine
    D. Prolactin and oxytocin
    E. Estrogen and progesterone

31. Insulin and glucagon are products of:
    A. Hypothalamus
    B. Anterior pituitary gland
    C. Adrenal medulla
    D. Adrenal cortex
    E. Pancreas

32. Melatonin is a hormone secreted by the _____, and it regulates _____.

    A.   posterior pituitary gland; level of the blood sugar
    B.   pineal gland; diurnal and seasonal rhythms of animal activity
    C.   ovaries; pregnancy
    D.   thymus; immunity
    E.   adrenal cortex; balance of electrolytes in body fluids, such as sodium or potassium

33. What element is necessary for the production of triiodothyronine (T_3) and thyroxine (T_4)?
    A.   Magnesium
    B.   Potassium
    C.   Calcium
    D.   Iodine
    E.   Sodium

LEVEL 2. CHECK YOUR UNDERSTANDING

1. Explain why the effects of steroid hormones have a long latent period (are seen after a longer delay) than the effect of peptide hormones.
2. In patients receiving cortisone drug therapy, adrenocorticotropic hormone (ACTH) secretion decreases, and adrenal glands shrink. Explain why patients experience these changes.
3. Certain dietary supplements that are prescribed for weight loss contain thyroid hormone. How would these supplements cause weight loss? Would these products generally be safe?
4. What is the relationship between the adrenal medulla and the sympathetic nervous system?
5. Females with an adrenal medulla tumor may develop male secondary characteristics. Explain why this happens.

LEVEL 3. APPLY YOUR KNOWLEDGE TO REAL LIFE

1. Using your knowledge of the stress response, explain why the physiological changes of the stress response are important to survival in the short term and become destructive when they persist over long periods.
2. Tumors of the parathyroid gland often secrete excessive parathyroid hormone (PTH). Predict the effects of such a tumor.
3. Pitocin and syntocinon facilitate labor contractions. In what situations may these drugs need to be used?

Chapter 15

The Cardiovascular System

LEARNING OBJECTIVES

The main function of the cardiovascular system is to transport substances through the body. It consists of the heart, blood vessels, and blood. The heart is an "engine" that pumps blood through a network of blood vessels. Blood vessels and blood constitute the circulatory system, which is part of the cardiovascular system. In this chapter you will learn about:

1. The structural and functional organization of the blood-moving engine—the heart.

2. Tissue that forms the heart and its organization in the organ.

3. Blood flow through the heart and the mechanism of cardiac wall contraction.

4. Factors that affect the heart's performance and health.

INTRODUCTION

The heart is a muscular organ. It pumps blood through the blood vessels. Its walls are made of muscles that rhythmically contract and propel blood. These rhythmic contractions have an internal origin and do not need external excitation from motor neurons. The ability of autonomic contraction is a principal property of cardiac muscle. The heart begins to contract from the very first days of its development in embryogenesis and never stops until the last days of life. Such nonstop coordinated and rhythmic work creates special requirements for heart organization and functioning, which we will now analyze.

15.1   Overview of the Cardiovascular System

The term *circulatory system* describes a network of blood vessels and other passages, and blood that circulates inside this network. The circulation is a pressure-driven blood flow through a system. The principal purpose of this flow is to deliver oxygen, nutrients, hormones, immune agents, heat, and other commodities to all cells of the body and remove waste products of cellular metabolism, such as carbon dioxide, nitrogenous compounds, and so on. Which forces drive animal evolution to develop a cardiovascular system? The answer is in fact that there are only two methods of oxygen transportation: 1) diffusion—a passive movement of oxygen down its gradient of concentration, and 2) convection—a passive movement of oxygen over long distances, carrying with it media, such as blood or other fluids. There is no mechanism of active oxygen transport. For multicellular organisms bigger than 1–2 mm, the diffusion is too slow a process to satisfy its interior structures with needed nutrients and oxygen. Organisms larger than 1 mm need some circulation that transport oxygen over body to provide cells with an adequate amount of needed oxygen and other commodities. The data supporting this idea show that in most modern vertebrates, metabolic intensity is strongly correlated with the oxygen-carrying capacity of their circulatory system. Thus, the process of evolutionary development of big active multicellular organisms inevitably leads to development of a cardiovascular system.

The term *cardiovascular system* includes the circulatory system and heart. The heart is a pumping organ, driving the blood through vessels. In vertebrates the heart may have a very different construction and be composed of two to four compartments called chambers.

Organization of Body Blood Flow

Blood vessels that deliver blood to the heart are called **veins**. The chambers of the heart that receive blood from veins are called **atria** (singular **atrium**). Blood vessels that take blood from the heart are known as **arteries**. Chambers which push blood out of the heart into arteries are called **ventricles**.

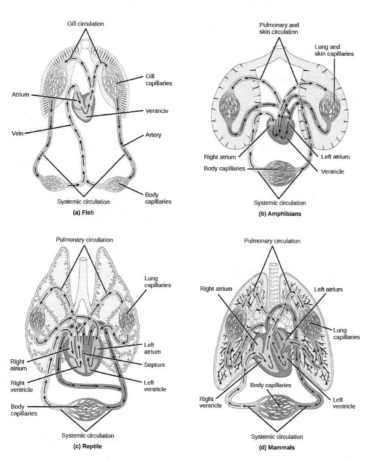

FIGURE 15.1   Comparative Anatomy of Vertebrate Circulatory System.

There are two principal patterns of blood circulation in vertebrates: **single circulation** and **double circulation**. At the first circuit type, blood passes the heart only one time, when it makes a complete circuit. It is characteristic of fishes. In a double circulation system, blood passes through the heart twice to make a complete circuit. This type of circulation is characteristic of all amniotes. It was a major evolutionary leap, which opened the opportunity for vertebrates to leave the water and populate the land. The double circuit consists of a **systemic circuit** that serves to deliver oxygen to all body cells, and a **pulmonary circuit** that consists of blood vessels that move poorly oxygenated blood (termed **deoxygenated**) to the lungs and take oxygenated blood back to the heart for its further moving into the systemic circuit. Development of a pulmonary circuit requires development of the lungs. This process took a long time in the history of vertebrates and left a number of intermediate circuit conditions characteristic of lungfishes, amphibians, and reptiles (fig. 15.1).

Heart and blood vessels arise from the embryonic mesoderm. The embryonic heart is tubular and from the very first steps of development has autonomic rhythmic contractions. These contractions drive blood through the circulatory system and facilitate development of the network of blood vessels. Fishes have a two-chambered heart and two enlarged blood vessels that deliver and take blood away.

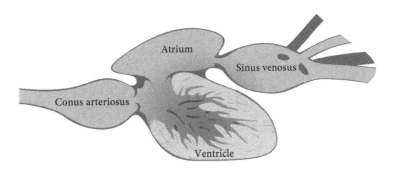

FIGURE 15.2   Two-Chambered Heart of Fish.

Together they constitute a muscular tube separated into the **sinus venosus**, **atrium**, **ventricle**, and the last in this sequence, **conus arteriosus** (fig. 15.2). Cells of the sinus venosus generate autonomic rhythmic contractions that propagate along heart chambers. With gradual development of the intermediate circuit in lungfishes and amphibians, a single atrium splits into two atria, but the ventricle remains single. These animals have three chambers in their heart. In reptiles the process of subdivision of the heart interior in chambers continues, and the wall, called the **interventricular septum**, separates this single ventricle. Even though it does not completely separate the pulmonary and systemic circuits, it provides effective functional separation of the oxygenated and deoxygenated bloodstreams, as is observed among crocodiles. Mammals and birds have a four-chambered heart, which provides complete separation of the pulmonary and systemic circuits and significantly elevates the metabolic level of these animals.

CHECK YOUR UNDERSTANDING

- Describe the difference between pulmonary and systemic circuits.

- Why was development of the interventricular septum a big leap in the evolution of terrestrial animals?

15.2   The Heart

The heart of birds and mammals has four chambers: two atria and two ventricles. In birds, the sinus venosus is reduced to a small but clearly visible structure. The conus arteriosus presents only in the embryo. Later it splits into the pulmonary trunk and aorta. In mammals, the sinus venosus is reduced to a patch of fiber cells that form the **sinoatrial node**, in the wall of the right atrium. It functions as a pacemaker, generating the waves of contractions that spread across the heart. Structurally similar, bird and mammalian hearts arose independently from a different group of tetrapod ancestors and are an example of so-called convergent evolution.

The heart is located in the mediastinum and is slightly shifted to the left side. Ventrally, it is protected by the sternum, dorsally by the vertebral column, and laterally by the ribs. It has the shape of a cone. The

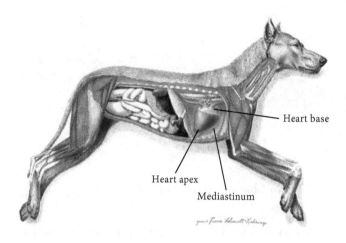

Heart base

Heart apex

Mediastinum

FIGURE 15.3   Location of the Dog Heart.

sharp region of this cone is called the **apex**, and the broad flattened part that is associated with major blood vessels is known as the **base**. The base of the heart is oriented toward the head. The apex is tilted to the left and is directed caudally (fig. 15.3).

The primary function of the heart is pumping blood. It is a tireless and enduring organ that never stops throughout the whole lifetime. The heart pumps blood by two processes. It pushes blood through the blood vessels by creating a positive pressure and sucks blood from veins through negative pressure. The heart of the slow-moving dogfish shark moves 7.5 liters of blood per hour. The heart of a resting hen moves 24 L/h, a human heart 280 L/h, and the heart of giraffe almost 1,200 L/h. The increased heart rate is termed **tachycardia**, whereas a decreased heart rate is called **brachycardia**.

Along with this main function, the heart also plays a principal role in a blood pressure homeostasis. Increase or decrease of the **heart rate** and **cardiac output** are the main factors that influence blood pressure. The atrial regions of the heart also produce the hormone **atrial natriuretic peptide (ANP)** that lowers blood pressure by decreasing sodium ion retention in the kidneys. Sodium is removed from body fluids with urine. It decreases blood osmotic pressure and reduces water reabsorption. This results in total blood volume decrease, which causes lowering of the blood pressure.

CHECK YOUR UNDERSTANDING

- The heart is in the mediastinum. What is the mediastinum?

- Describe how the atrial natriuretic peptide regulates blood pressure.

Pericardium

On the outside, the heart is covered by two strong connective tissue membranes: **fibrous pericardium** and **serous pericardium**. Fibrous pericardium creates an external capsule. It is tough and made up of dense and loose connective tissues. It protects the heart, anchors it to the surrounding structures, and prevents it from overfilling with blood. Fibrous pericardium is continuous with the external adventitial layer of the nearby great blood vessels: **vena cava**, **pulmonary trunk**, and **aorta**.

The serous pericardium is a thin membrane constructed as all serous membranes (see chapter 5, page 134). On one side it consists of secretory epithelium, whose cells secrete serous fluid. On the other side, it is made of areolar connective tissue, which makes membrane resilient and elastic. The serous pericardium folds in two wings in such a way that the epithelium occupies the inner walls of both wings, and areolar tissue creates the external surface. The areolar layer of one wing fuses to the fibrous

The Heart Wall

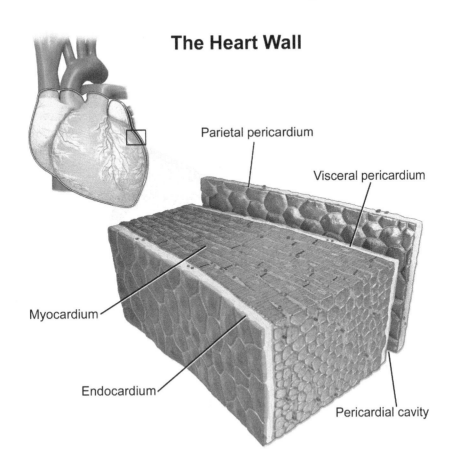

Parietal pericardium

Visceral pericardium

Myocardium

Endocardium

Pericardial cavity

FIGURE 15.4   Serous Pericardium.

pericardium and is called the **parietal pericardium**. The other wing sticks to the walls of the heart. It is called the **visceral pericardium** or **epicardium**. The space between the parietal and visceral pericardia is filled with serous fluid and is called the **pericardial cavity** (fig. 15.4). The serous fluid acts as a lubricant that guarantees smooth frictionless movement of the heart. The visceral pericardium firmly fuses with the heart and is considered a superficial layer of heart walls. The areolar layer of the visceral pericardium contains some amount of adipose tissue, which tends to accumulate fat, especially in the **atrioventricular** and **interventricular salci**.

CHECK YOUR UNDERSTANDING

- What is the purpose of the serous fluid inside the pericardial cavity?

- What major blood vessels are associated with the heart?

- Which structures form the pericardial cavity?

Anatomy of the Heart

Beneath the visceral pericardium lays a thick muscular layer called the **myocardium**. The myocardium has two components: 1) cardiac muscle tissue and 2) fibrous skeleton. Cardiac muscle tissue consists of **cardiac muscle cells** or **cardiomyocytes**. Cardiomyocytes are attached and interwoven with the fibrous skeleton, which is composed of irregular dense connective tissue. The fibrous skeleton creates a structural support for cardiac muscle attachment. The collagen of the fibrous skeleton insulates atria from ventricles. As a result, electric impulses generated in the sinoatrial node pass from atria to ventricles with a delay, which is important for coordinated heart contraction.

VETERINARY APPLICATION

Dilated cardiomyopathy (DCM) is a disease characterized by dilation or enlargement of the heart chambers resulting in an abnormally large heart. This disease eventually results in heart failure, since the damaged heart muscle is too weak to efficiently pump blood to the rest of the body. DCM is very common in dogs, representing the most common reason for congestive heart failure (CHF). The left ventricle is most always involved. Since the myocardium cannot work effectively to pump blood out of the heart, subsequent backup of blood into the left atrium and ultimately into the lungs occurs. This backup of blood into the lungs results in pulmonary edema and is a sign of congestive heart failure.

Symptoms of DCM include 1) shortness of breath; 2) fainting; 3) pulmonary edema and elevated jugular venous pressure and low pulse pressure. Often present are signs of mitral and tricuspid regurgitation.

The treatment of dogs with dilated cardiomyopathy varies with the severity of heart failure and specific organ damage. Treatment may include oxygen administration, fluid therapy, and administration of drugs (bronchodilators) that improve breathing, and drugs that modify heart function, such as control arrhythmias. If low doses of anti-arrhythmic drugs are effective, the heart often can be stabilized.

The third and thin layer of the heart wall is the **endocardium**. The endocardium is composed of a simple squamous epithelium similar to that of the lining lumen of blood vessels and several layers of connective tissue. Epithelial cells of the endocardium are called **vascular endothelial cells**. These cells have unique functions, such as developing blood-heart barrier and helping regulate electrolyte concentration, neutrophil recruitment, and hormone trafficking.

Heart chambers that receive blood from veins are known as atria. The right atrium receives blood from three major veins: the **anterior vena cava**, which collects blood from the head, neck, and first limbs; the **posterior vena cava** that collects blood from the hind limbs, abdomen, and chest; and the **coronary sinus** that collects blood from the blood vessels of the heart. The right atrium is larger than the left and has also thinner wall. This allows the right atrium accommodate more blood. The left atrium receives blood from four **pulmonary veins**: two of which take oxygenated blood from the right lung and two of which take blood from the left lung. Externally, both atria have a muscular pouch called an **auricle** (fig. 15.5). The right auricle is larger than the left. The internal surface of the right atrium has muscular ridges on the ventral side called **pectinate muscles**. Atria are separated from each other by a thin wall called the **interatrial septum**. A small depression in the interatrial septum known as a **fossa ovalis** is a memoir of a passage between atria called the **foramen ovale** that exists in the fetus but closes after birth. Fetus lungs are closed. All oxygen the fetus receives from the mother, and the foramen ovale creates a bypass of oxygenated blood from the right atrium to the left for further distribution through the systemic circuit. After birth, the lungs open and the newborn organism begins to use its own pulmonary circuit. Opening of the lungs causes a decrease of pressure in the right atrium, and the foramen ovale closes, but in its place remains the fossa ovalis. The inability of the foramen ovale to close after birth is termed **patent foramen ovale**. With the growth of the organism, its heart also grows, and the patent foramen ovale increases in size. Later it may cause inappropriate clot formation.

Ventricles push blood out of the heart. The right ventricle pushes blood into the **pulmonary trunk** that carries deoxygenated blood to lungs. The left ventricle moves oxygenated blood into an **aorta** that distributes blood among smaller arteries of the systemic circuit. Ventricles have stronger walls than

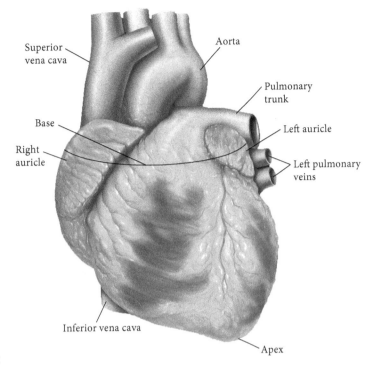

FIGURE 15.5   Human Heart, External View.

atria. The walls of the left ventricle are much thicker than the walls of the right ventricle. The left ventricle pushes blood into the systemic circuit, which transports it to all body parts, whereas the right ventricle pushes blood a comparatively shorter distance to the lungs, located on both sides of the heart. Ventricles are larger than atria. The left ventricle is bigger in diameter and longer than the right ventricle. Walls of both ventricles have a ridged surface formed by cardiac muscles collectively referred to as **trabeculae carneae**. A thick muscular wall called the **interventricular septum** separates ventricles from each other.

Atria are connected with corresponding ventricles by **atrioventricular foramens**, guarded by **atrioventricular (AV) valves**. These valves promote blood movement only in one direction—from atrium to ventricle—and prevent its backflow. The valve between the right atrium and right ventricle is called the **tricuspid valve**. The valve between the left atrium and the left ventricle is called the **bicuspid valve**. For its shape similar to a headwear ancient kings of the Middle East, it is also called the **mitral valve**. Both valves have soft flaps or **cusps**. The cusp is composed of an endocardium fold that covers the passage between the atrium and ventricle. This fold is soft and bends inside the ventricle, when atrium walls contract and blood pressure in the atrium becomes higher than in the ventricle. As their names imply, a tricuspid valve has three cusps, whereas a bicuspid valve has only two. Every cusp on the top is attached to a group of tough, tendinous strands referred to as **chordae tendineae**. Chordae tendineae are anchored to the muscles in the wall of the ventricle. These muscles protrude over the surface of the ventricle wall

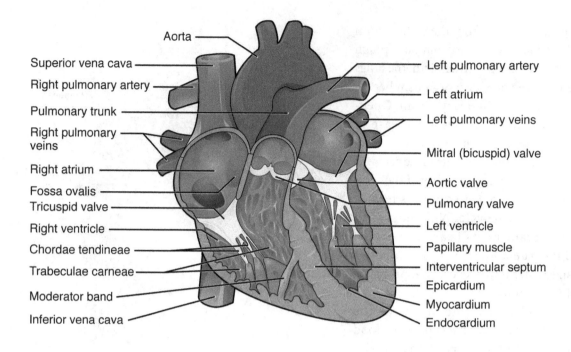

Aorta

Superior vena cava

Right pulmonary artery

Pulmonary trunk

Right pulmonary veins

Right atrium

Fossa ovalis

Tricuspid valve

Right ventricle

Chordae tendineae

Trabeculae carneae

Moderator band

Inferior vena cava

Left pulmonary artery

Left atrium

Left pulmonary veins

Mitral (bicuspid) valve

Aortic valve

Pulmonary valve

Left ventricle

Papillary muscle

Interventricular septum

Epicardium

Myocardium

Endocardium

Anterior view

FIGURE 15.6   Frontal Section through the Human Heart.

and are called **pupillary muscles** (fig. 15.6). When ventricle walls contract, papillary muscles also contract and pull on the chordae tendineae. This maneuver does not allow cusps bend backward inside the atrium and keeps the valve closed when the blood pressure in ventricle is higher than in the atrium.

VETERINARY APPLICATION

Hypertrophic cardiomyopathy (HCM) is a disease of heart muscle. It characterized by an increased thickness of the walls of the left ventricle (hypertrophy). The hypertrophy of the left ventricle may be caused by other diseases, such as systemic hypertension, or it can be a primary disease in itself. HCM is diagnosed when hypertrophy is not caused by other disease.

HCM changes heart structure and can impair its functioning in several ways: 1) ventricular chamber size may be reduced, which decreases its ability to fill with blood; 2) ventricular walls become stiff, which impairs the ability of the ventricle to relax and does not allow it to fill efficiently; 3) there may be an increase in ventricular pressure during diastole, causing blood to back up into the vessels of the lungs. This backflow may cause congestive heart failure, which includes pulmonary edema and/or pleural effusion.

Because the left ventricle is unable to fill adequately, less blood is pumped out to the body with each heartbeat. If the blood supply to other vital organs is inadequate, heart rate may increase to compensate for the decreased oxygen supply. A decrease in blood flow to the kidneys can result in an increased release of renin, which increases blood volume and, consequently, blood pressure on the left side of the heart and contributes to congestive heart failure.

Contraction of ventricles propels blood into two major arteries: the pulmonary trunk that takes blood from the right ventricle, and the aorta that receives blood from the left ventricle. The entrance to both arteries is guarded by **semilunar valves**. These valves prevent blood backflow from the pulmonary trunk and aorta, when both ventricles relax and their blood pressure become lower than in arteries. Semilunar valves have three cusps shaped like a half-moon and composed of collagen core, covered by endocardium. The semilunar valves do not attached to chordae tendineae or papillary muscles. Every valve is named according the vessel it guards. The pulmonary trunk carries the **pulmonary valve**, and the aorta has the **aortic valve**. Thus, the blood flow through the heart in both sides (pulmonary and systemic circuits) is controlled by a system of two valves. On the right side it is the tricuspid and pulmonary valves; on the left side it is the bicuspid and aortic valves. This anatomic organization guarantees a one-way movement of the blood through the heart.

To work effectively, all four valves have to be firmly anchored in the heart walls and their shape has to not be distorted during the powerful contractions of the cardiac walls. The **fibrous skeleton of the heart** forms a support frame for valve attachment and prevents valve passages from collapsing under high pressure. It is a high-density plate made of regular dense connective tissue, which forms and anchors the valves and controls the forces exerted on them. The plate consists of four circular bands of dense connective tissue, which encircle the bases of all four valves. These fibrous rings are called **annuli fibrosi cordis**. In youth, this collagen structure is free of calcium and is quite flexible. With aging some calcium can accumulate on this skeleton. This accumulation contributes to the delay of the wave of cardiac muscle depolarization between AV node and bundle of His.

Many cardiac muscle are anchored to opposite sides of the valve rings. The atrioventricular rings serve for the attachment of the muscular fibers of the atria, ventricles, bicuspid, and tricuspid valves. The left atrioventricular ring is connected with the aortic arterial ring. A triangular mass of fibrous tissue, known as a **fibrous trigone**, connects rings in one structure. It is the strongest part of the fibrous skeleton of the heart (fig. 15.7). The fibrous rings surrounding the arterial orifices serve for the attachment of the great vessels and semilunar valves are known as the **aortic annulus**.

In some animals, the fibrous trigone can undergo increasing mineralization with age, leading to the formation of an **os cordis** (heart bone), or two: left **os cordis sinister** and right **os cordis dexter**. It is found in male red deer and oxen, and occasionally observed in goats and some other animals, such as otters.

CHECK YOUR UNDERSTANDING

- Which side of the heart acts as the pulmonary pump? The systemic pump?

- What is the role of the chordae tendineae and papillary muscles?

- What is the heart skeleton, and what is its function?

- Describe the position and role of tricuspid and bicuspid valves.

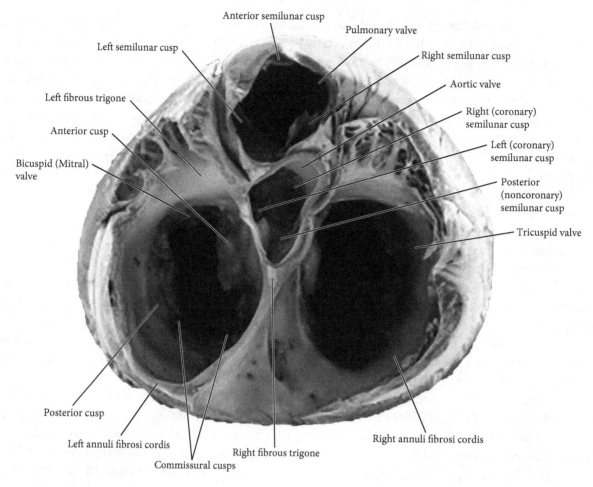

FIGURE 15.7   Fibrous Skeleton in Dog Heart.

Heart Blood Flow

The heart is a pumping center for both the pulmonary and the systemic circuits. Here both circuits receive their impulse for blood movement. For simplicity and ease of understanding, these circuits will be described separately. After that the total picture of blood circulation through the heart will be presented.

Cardiac pulmonary circuit. Deoxygenated blood is collected into three major veins: anterior vena cava, posterior vena cava, and coronary sinus, which drains blood from coronary veins. At this time the muscular wall of the right atrium is relaxed and is ready to accommodate incoming blood. Incoming blood pressure expands the right atrium. When right atrium expands to its maximum, muscles in its wall contract and blood exerts its pressure on the cusps of the tricuspid valve. Under blood pressure, the cusps bend, the valve opens, and blood moves from the right atrium into the right ventricle. The right ventricle expands when it receives blood from the right atrium. After ejecting blood, the right atrium relaxes. Hydrostatic pressure in the right atrium drops, whereas in the right ventricle it rises. The blood in the ventricle presses on the cusps, the tricuspid valve closes, and blood is trapped in the ventricle. Further increase of blood pressure in the right ventricle opens the semilunar pulmonary valve, and blood enters the pulmonary trunk. Blood accumulated in the pulmonary trunk presses on the cusps of the semilunar pulmonary valve and closes it. From this point blood has only one direction to go—toward the lungs, where it releases carbon dioxide and loads with oxygen.

Cardiac systemic circuit. Oxygenated blood returns to the heart through four pulmonary veins: two veins from each lung. The dilated left atrium accommodates this oxygenated blood. At the next step, atrial walls contract and blood is forced through the bicuspid valve to the left ventricle. The mechanism of opening and closing the bicuspid valve is the same as for the tricuspid. Walls of the left ventricle dilate, and blood fills the ventricular space. Following this, contraction of the muscles in walls of the left ventricle propels blood into the aorta through the semilunar aortic valve. Increased blood pressure in the aorta shuts the aortic valve, and blood moves into blood vessels of the systemic circuit.

Total view of blood flow through the heart. As a matter of fact, both sides of the heart propel blood at the same time and in a coordinated way. Heart relaxation and contraction pass in waves from the atria to ventricles. The relaxation of cardiac muscular walls is called **diastole**, and their contractions are known as a **systole**. The process of cardiac blood flow is divided into four steps (fig. 15.8).

1. At the very beginning, all heart chambers are relaxed. This period may be termed heart diastole (**AD+VD**). Both relaxed atria receive blood influx together.

2. When blood fills both atria, they contract. At this moment ventricles remain relaxed. The blood pressure in both ventricles is lower than in the atria, and blood is pushed from the atria into the ventricles. This second step can be termed atrial systole and ventricular diastole (**AS+VD**).

3. The emptied atria relax, whereas the ventricles filled with blood contract, and blood enters the pulmonary trunk and aorta. This third step is characterized by atria diastole and ventricular systole (**AD+VS**).

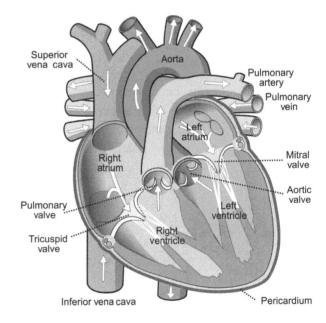

FIGURE 15.8 Blood Flow through the Human Heart.

4. After the ventricles empty, they relax, and the heart returns to the first state of complete heart diastole (**AD+VD**), and the whole process can be repeated again.

Symbolically, the total sequence of events may be presented as:

(**AD+VD**) → (**AS+VD**) → (**AD+VS**) → (**AD+VD**) → ...

CHECK YOUR UNDERSTANDING

- What are systole and diastole?

- How do the heart valves create one-way blood flow?

- What will happen if the atria and ventricles contract together?

Electrophysiology of the Heart

From chapter 8 (page 225) you learned that cardiac muscles have special properties expressed in their autonomous contraction. The group of cardiac muscle cells that lead this process is known as a heart **pacemaker**. In a healthy heart, the pacemaker is a group of cardiac muscle cells in the wall of the right atrium known as the **sinoatrial node (SAN)**. The cardiomyocytes of the SAN generate changes in their membrane potentials that spread along the heart and create waves of heart walls contraction. These waves of cardiac muscle contractions are rhythmic and involve all cardiac muscles at every cycle. Each wave of contraction has a special pattern that facilitates blood flow through the heart. Four principal anatomic properties support successful heart performance: 1) cardiac muscle cell structure, 2) special type of junctions between adjacent muscles cells, 3) **Purkinje fibers** that facilitate rapid transmission of electrical signals, and 4) heart fibrous skeleton that provides electrical isolation of cardiac conductive pathways.

The myocardium is composed of cardiac muscle tissue. Cardiomyocytes usually have one single nucleus. They have a striated appearance and contract involuntary (see chapter 9, page 268). Striation of the cardiac muscle demonstrates sarcomere organization of its contractile units. Cells are short and often are branched. Their sarcoplasmic reticulum has less cisterna, and cardiac muscles depend on influx of Ca^{2+} from outside of the cell for their contraction. Cells contain a large amount of mitochondria that constitute about 25 percent of all sarcoplasmic content (compare this with 2 percent in a skeletal muscle). Their involvement in the process of blood moving guarantees them a very good blood supply. However, their sarcoplasm is also very rich with myoglobin and creatine kinase (an enzyme that catalyzes the transfer of the phosphate group to ADP and conversion of it into ATP and creatine). Myoglobin, intensive blood supply, and a large amount of mitochondria in the cell together support great demand of the heart for energy. Thus, cardiac muscle cells can rely exclusively on aerobic cellular respiration, which makes these muscles fatigue resistant or tireless. These muscles can be classified as oxidative fatigue resistant type 1 muscles. Cardiomyocytes are also very versatile in using different types of fuel for oxidation reactions, from carbohydrates to fat molecules and proteins. When, for example, highly active skeletal muscles produce an increased amount of a lactic acid, cardiac muscle cells absorb it and use as an energy source, breaking lactic acid up to water and carbon dioxide. Of course, this strong dependence on oxidative reactions makes cardiac muscle cells very sensitive to low oxygen, a condition termed **ischemia**.

Special cells of the SAN have unique properties that make them capable of rhythmically generating action potentials, called autorhythmicity. Evolutionarily, the SAN of mammals originates from the sinus venosus. The heart, whose contraction impulses are generated by its muscle cells, are termed myogenic. All vertebrates have a myogenic heart. Usually, they are well innervated, but they continue to beat even when all nervous connections are removed. Cells of the SAN have a poorly developed contractile apparatus. Their critical property is a high frequency of spontaneous depolarization. By initiating a wave of depolarization that spreads throughout the heart, they impose their rhythm of depolarization on the heart as a whole. The pacemaker cells have no voltage-gated sodium channels, and because of that, their sarcolemma depolarizes slowly. The membrane potential of these cells has no resting stage but undergoes continuous cyclic changes. This oscillation of membrane potential is generated by the opening of slow potassium voltage-gated channels when the membrane potential reaches its minimum level.

The complete cycle of polarization, depolarization, and repolarization is divided in a few steps or phases. Pacemaker cells are never at rest and cycles continuously follow one another.

1. Beginning from the short period, when the muscle cell is relaxed, it has a membrane potential also known as the **pacemaker potential**. The pacemaker potential is due to a group of special voltage-gated channels. These channels open when the membrane potential reaches its minimum negative voltage, about −85 to −90 mV. At this time the muscle cell is maximally relaxed. Slow potassium channels open first. In addition, there also is a slow continuous influx of leaking sodium ions called the "funny" or pacemaker current. Exit of K^+ and influx of Na^+ ions depolarizes membrane until it reaches a set value around −40 mV, known as the **threshold potential**. Another hypothesis is based on the idea of a "calcium clock." According to this hypothesis, calcium is released from the sarcoplasmic reticulum within the cell. This calcium increases activation of the sodium-calcium exchanger. The sodium-calcium exchanger moves sodium inside the cell and calcium out, resulting in the increase in membrane potential.

2. The next phase begins with a rapid depolarization lasting 10–20 ms. It occurs due to an increased net flow of positively charged ions into the cell. In pacemaker cells, the increase in membrane voltage is mainly due to activation of calcium channels that allow Ca^{2+} to enter the cell.

3. The last phase is known as a "rapid repolarization." It begins with the closure of the Ca^{2+} channels. The slow K^+ channels remain open, and potassium continues to leak out of the cell. The continued exit of K^+ results in a net outward positive current and restoration of negative charge inside the cell. This net outward positive current repolarizes the cell. The K^+ channels close when the membrane potential is returned to −85 to −90 mV. Ionic pumps—the sodium-calcium exchanger and sodium-potassium pump—restore ion concentrations back to the state of pre-action potential. This means that the intracellular calcium is pumped out. In chapter 9 you learned that Ca^{2+} is responsible for muscle cell contraction. Once the Ca^{2+} is pumped out and its concentration inside the cell decreases, the contraction stops and cardiomyocyte cells relax. When the membrane potential reaches its lowest negative level (pacemaker potential), potassium voltage gated channels immediately open, and the cycle repeats (fig. 15.9).

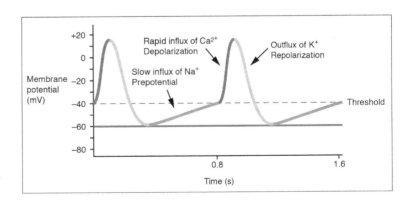

FIGURE 15.9   SAN Pacemaker Potential.

A specific organization of voltage-gated channels in cardiac cells influences their ability to be stimulated by incoming electrical stimuli. Cardiac muscle cells have two refractory periods. The first is called the **absolute refractory period**. During this period cardiomyocyte remains absolutely unresponsive to any incoming action potential, no matter how strong it is. The absolute refractory period in cardiac muscle cells is very long and develops immediately followed the development of pacemaker potential, until the closure of sodium and calcium channels. The following short **relative refractory period** allows a stronger-than-usual stimulus to generate new action potential. The relative refractory period is due to the leaking of potassium ions, which makes the membrane potential more negative (hyperpolarized). That is why a stronger stimulus than normal is required (fig. 15.10).

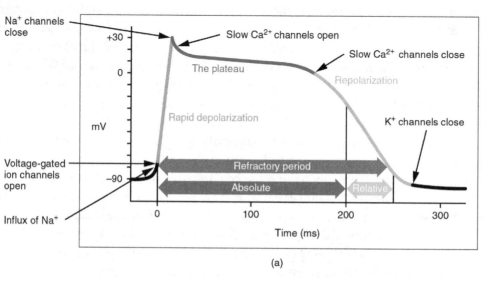

(a)

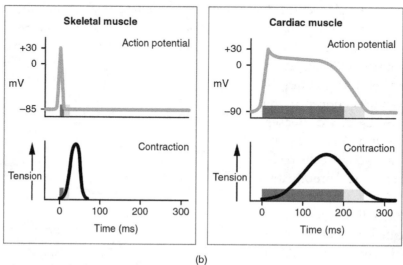

(b)

FIGURE 15.10   Comparison of Refractory Periods of Cardiac and Skeletal Muscles.

Another important structural characteristic of myocardium is that cardiomyocytes are connected to each other by **intercalated discs**. Intercalated discs allow the action potential to be transferred from one cell to the next. Cells united by intercalated discs contract together as one unit, termed a **syncytium**. An intercalated disc is a special type of junction between adjacent cells, made of a combination of gap junctions with desmosomes. The intercalated disc allows fast transition of electrical impulses from one cell to another nearby (fig. 15.11). This property of the cardiomyocytes is termed **electrical coupling**. The gap junctions are made of a special protein known as **connexin**. Connexins firmly hold cells close and form a pore through which ions (including Na^+, Ca^{2+}, and K^+) can pass. As potassium is highest within the cell, it is mainly potassium that passes through. This increased potassium in the neighbor cell causes the membrane potential to lightly increase. The increase of the membrane potential activates the sodium channels and initiates development of an action potential in the cell. A brief chemical gradient driven efflux

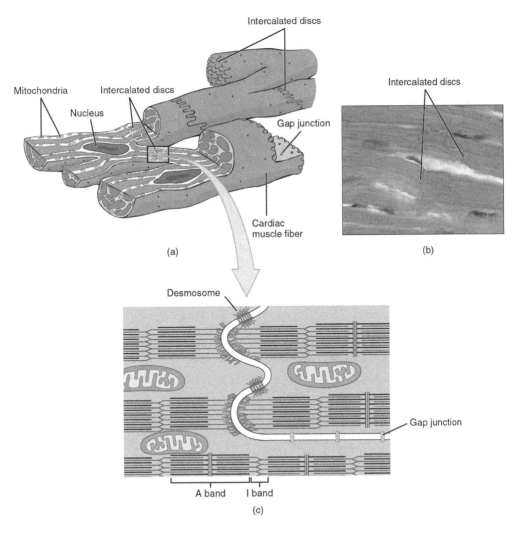

FIGURE 15.11   Intercalated Discs between Cardiomyocytes.

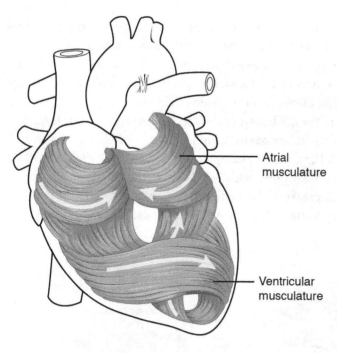

Atrial musculature

Ventricular musculature

FIGURE 15.12   Orientation of Muscle Cells in the Myocardium.

of Na+ through the connexon at peak depolarization causes the conduction of cell-to-cell depolarization, not potassium. These connections allow for the rapid conduction of the action potential throughout the heart and are responsible for allowing all of the cells in the atria to contract together. All gap junctions that connect cardiomyocytes in one single contractile unit are strongly oriented in one direction. This facilitates conduction of the myocardial electrical current in one direction and in a particular sequence. Uncoordinated contraction of heart muscles is the basis for arrhythmia and heart failure.

The myocardium has an elegant and complex pattern of orientation of its muscle cells. Muscle cells swirl and spiral around the heart chambers and are organized in two layers. The outer muscular layer forms a figure-eight pattern around the atria and bases of the great blood vessels (pulmonary trunk and aorta). The inner muscular layer forms a figure-eight pattern around the ventricles and proceeds toward the apex. This complex swirling pattern allows the heart to pump blood very effectively (fig. 15.12).

The **Purkinje fibers** are located in the inner ventricular walls, just beneath the endocardium in a space called the subendocardium. The Purkinje fibers are specialized conducting fibers composed of electrically excitable cells, which are larger than regular cardiomyocytes. They have much less myofibrils but a large number of mitochondria. The Purkinje fibers are characterized by numerous fast voltage-gated sodium channels. These cells conduct cardiac action potentials more quickly and efficiently than any other cells in the heart. Purkinje fibers allow the heart's conduction system to create synchronized contractions of ventricles and are therefore essential for maintaining a consistent heart rhythm. They are influenced only by electrical discharge from the sinoatrial node. During the ventricular contraction the Purkinje fibers carry the electrical impulse from both the left and right branches of interventricular bundles or bundles of His to the myocardium of the ventricles. This causes the muscle tissue of the ventricles to contract together and eject blood into the pulmonary trunk and aorta.

Purkinje fibers can also fire electrical impulses at a rate of 15–40 beats per minute, in contrast to the SAN, which in a normal state can fire at 60–100 beats per minute. The slow Purkinje fibers' waves of action potentials are masked by the stronger and faster waves generated by the SAN and are normally suppressed. Thus, they serve as the last resort when other heart pacemakers fail. When a Purkinje fiber does fire, it is called a premature ventricular contraction or PVC.

The atria and ventricles are electrically divided by the collagen protein fibers of the heart fibrous skeleton. Collagen is a good insulator and impermeable to electrical current. The only pathway for electricity

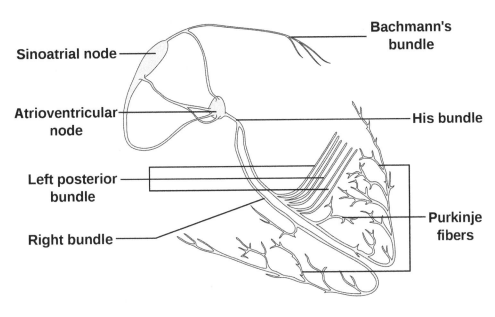

Sinoatrial node

Bachmann's bundle

Atrioventricular node

His bundle

Left posterior bundle

Right bundle

Purkinje fibers

FIGURE 15.13   Conduction System of the Heart.

through this collagen barrier left by the heart fibrous skeleton is a sinus that opens up to the interventricular node and exits to the bundle of His. The sinus consists of group of three narrow bridges between right atrium and ventricular myocardium (fig. 15.13). This narrow bridge slow down the rate of electrical impulse. As a result, ventricles contract with some delay after atria. Organization of myocardium muscles in swirling layers and spatial distribution of electric impulses promote sequential opening and closing of heart valves and, finally, continuous blood flow in one direction.

VETERINARY APPLICATION

Canine heartworms, ***Dirofilaria immitis***, are common in the hearts and major blood vessels of dogs. They also can infect cats, wolves, coyotes, jackals, foxes, ferrets, bears, seals, and sea lions. There are very rare records of their infestation in humans. *Dirofilaria immitis* is a round filarial worm. The female adult worm is about 30 cm in length, and the male is about 23 cm, with a coiled tail. Females cause most of the damage. The worms are transferred from dog to dog through an infected mosquito. Mosquitoes transfer microscopic larva with their saliva, when they bite. Larva migrate through the body and several month later accumulates in the pulmonary trunk. Here they mature into adult worms.

The first sign of heartworm disease is often early aging. Dogs gray prematurely around the muzzle and forelegs. Dog's activity level decreases and their coats lack luster. Further progression of the disease results in a chronic dry cough most noticeable at night, when the dog is at rest. At the same time, the dog's heart and pulmonary arteries enlarge due to mechanical obstruction of the worms. Major arteries become inflamed and their valves are damaged.

To cure dogs infected by heartworms, medicine that contains arsenic is used. Melarsomine is sold under the brand name Immiticide and has a greater efficacy and fewer side effects than the previously used thiacetarsamide, sold as Caparsolate, which makes it a safer alternative for dogs with late-stage infections.

CHECK YOUR UNDERSTANDING

- What is the importance of the extended refractory period in cardiac muscle cell?

- What is the path of an action potential through the conduction system of the heart?

- What anatomic features slow the conduction rate of the action potential as it passes through the AV node? What is the function of this delay?

- Describe the steps for SAN cells to spontaneously depolarize and serve as pacemaker cells.

Cardiac Cycle and Electrocardiogram

A **cardiac cycle** includes all changes within the heart from the beginning of one heartbeat to the beginning of the next. One heartbeat includes the contraction and relaxation of the heart chambers.

The process of spreading a depolarization wave across the myocardium is called **conduction**. Structures of the heart that generate, support, and provide a pathway for electrical current constitute the cardiac **conduction system**. The SAN is an area where the electrical waves are initiated. Cardiomyocytes electrically coupled by gap junctions rapidly spread electric current across both atria. Stimulated by this electrical current, cells in both atria synchronously contract. However, there is no gap junction coupling among cardiomyocytes of atria and ventricles. Moreover, the myocardium of atria and ventricles are isolated by fibrous skeleton. The only opening through it is a specialized group of muscle cells in the right atrial wall called the **atrioventricular node** or **AV node**. A bundle of cells called the **atrioventricular bundle** or **bundle of His** passes through the fibrous layer and enters the interventricular septum. Inside the wall of the interventricular septum, the atrioventricular bundle separates into the right and left **bundle branches**, which travel along the right and left surfaces of the septum. The bundle branches are connected with a system of Purkinje fibers that form a network in the walls of both ventricles (fig. 15.13).

The electrical current spreads across the atria and travels through the AV node relatively slowly. When electricity reaches the atrioventricular bundle and Purkinje fibers, its speed of propagation increases. These properties of the heart conduction system allow the atria to contract together, before the ventricles. This maneuver propels blood from the atria to the ventricles and then from the ventricles to the main heart arteries, because the atria-ventricular valves prevent backflow from the ventricles to the atria and blood has only this one exit.

Regular rhythmic generation and propagation of waves of electricity across the walls of the heart set up ionic currents in the interstitial fluid of surrounding heart tissues. This induces voltage variations in the body that reach various parts of the body surface. The process of measuring and recording these voltage variations over time is known as an **electrocardiogram** or **EKG** (or **ECG**). The depolarization, and consequently contraction, of the atria corresponds to the first rise of the curve and is termed a **P wave**. Q, R, and S waves are organized into one continuous **QRS complex** and result from depolarization of both ventricles. The repolarization of two ventricles generates a **T wave** (fig. 15.14).

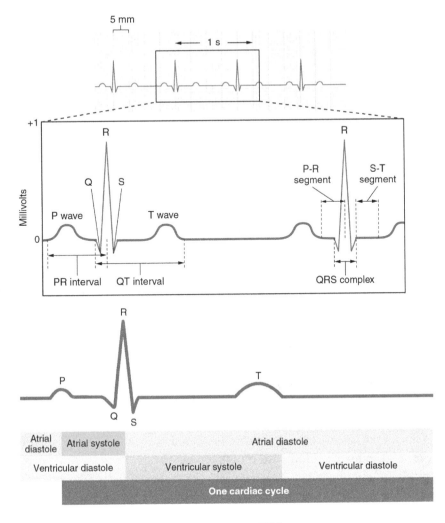

FIGURE 15.14   Electrocardiogram. Human EKG.

CHECK YOUR UNDERSTANDING

- What event in the heart is indicated by the P wave?

- What event in the heart is indicated by the T wave?

- What events in the heart are indicated by the QRS complex?

Mechanical Physiology of the Heart

Blood influx to the heart has to be equal to blood output into the main blood vessels. This means that in a healthy heart the right and left ventricles eject equal blood volumes. Because the blood flow is easier to measure in the systemic circuit, the descriptions of basic characteristics of heart mechanic performance are given next for the left ventricle.

The total number of heart contractions in a minute is called **heart rate**. There is a rule, according to which the heart rate is higher among small animals and slows with the increase in animal size. A left ventricle ejects blood in the aorta and via it into the systemic circuit. The amount of blood ejected into the aorta in one stroke is known as a **stroke volume**. Three variables identify stroke volume: 1) **venous return**; 2) **preload**; and 3) **afterload**.

Venous return is the volume of blood returned to the heart via the great veins. Since the amount of blood that enters the heart has to be equal to the blood volume that left it, the stroke volume strongly depends on venous return. The venous return determines the preload of the heart.

A preload is the ability of the heart walls to stretch to accommodate blood load from main veins. This stretch is just prior to heart muscle contraction. The ventricle filling with blood creates a tension in the ventricular myocardium.

Afterload is the amount of blood that remains during the ventricle systole. Afterload is a result of arteries' resistance to the incoming blood. It is measured by the pressure that must be applied to eject blood into the aorta.

The relationship between these three characteristics is described by the **Frank-Starling law**. This law states that the higher the volume of the blood entering the heart becomes (venous return), the greater is the stretch of the heart walls (preload) and the stronger is its contraction. A stronger ventricular contraction generates greater stroke volume. The relation between venous return and cardiac output reveals through the next sequence of events: 1) increased preload causes increased force of contraction; 2) physical activity increases venous return and stretches the myocardium; 3) cardiomyocytes generate more tension during contraction; and 4) increased cardiac output matches increased venous return. This relation plays a central role in enabling the heart to match blood output to its input.

A **cardiac output** is an amount of blood ejected into the systemic circuit in one minute expressed in liters per minute. Cardiac output is determined by stroke volume and heart rate:

$$\textbf{Cardiac output} = \textbf{Stroke volume} \times \textbf{Heart rate}$$

A change in heart rate, stroke volume, or both changes cardiac output. A **cardiac reserve** is the difference between maximum and resting cardiac outputs. Cardiac reserve is a measure of the level and duration of physical effort in which an organism can engage.

CHECK YOUR UNDERSTANDING

- What are two factors that determine cardiac output?

- Which of the following increases stroke volume: (a) increased venous return; (b) increased Ca^{2+} in sarcoplasm; (c) afterload? Explain your answer.

- If both heart rate and stroke volume increase, how will this affect cardiac output?

- Is the relationship between stroke volume and heart rate, on one side, and cardiac output, on the other, direct or inverse?

Regulation of Heart Activity

Cardiac output is directly influenced by heart rate and stroke volume. In their turn, both heart rate and stroke volume are affected by a number of factors, among which are nervous signals and hormones.

The heart rate can be altered by external factors that influence the SAN and AV node. The factors that change heart rate are called **chronotropic agents**. Chronotropic agents may increase or decrease heart rate. According this different effect on heart rate, they are divided into two groups: 1) positive chronotropic agents that increase heart rate and 2) negative chronotropic agents that decrease heart rate. The autonomic nervous system (both the sympathetic and parasympathetic divisions) and varying levels of some hormones are among these chronotropic agents.

Positive chronotropic agents cause an increase in heart rate and include sympathetic nerve stimulation and some hormones. Sympathetic axons release the neurotransmitter norepinephrine (NE). This hormone acts directly on the cells of the SAN. The sympathetic nerves also stimulate the adrenal medulla to release epinephrine (EPI) and NE. Both EPI and NE bind to β_1-adrenergic receptors of the cardiomyocytes. The binding initiates an intracellular pathway involving G protein that activates enzyme adenylate cyclase. Adenylate cyclase initiates production of the secondary messenger cAMP that activates protein kinase (see chapter 14, page 398). The protein kinase phosphorylates Ca^{2+} channels and opens them. Positively charged Ca^{2+} enters the cells of the SAN. Their cellular membranes depolarize. When depolarization reaches threshold level of depolarization, the cells fire action potential. AV node cells also increase calcium influx and increase the rate of electrical current conduction. Together, this increases heart rate.

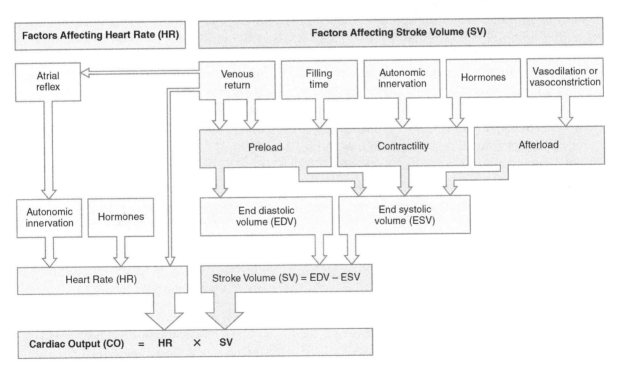

FIGURE 15.15   Factors Affecting Cardiac Output.

Thyroid hormone also has a positive effect on heart rate. It increases sensitivity of SAN cells to NE and EPI by increasing the number of β_1-adrenergic receptors. Some substances can increase heart rate. Nicotine and cocaine both increase the amount of NE present in the synaptic cleft. Nicotine stimulates an increase of NE release, whereas cocaine inhibits reuptake of NE from the synaptic cleft. Caffeine inhibits the breakdown of the cAMP.

Negative chronotropic agents decrease heart rate. The parasympathetic nervous system plays a key role in this process. Postsynaptic axons release acetylcholine that binds to muscarinic receptors on the membrane of cardiac muscle cells. Muscarinic receptors are K^+ channels. The opening of these channels allows potassium ions to leave muscle cells and results in sarcolemma repolarization. Blockage of these channels causes membrane hyperpolarization. Hyperpolarization makes cells of SAN less capable of generating new electric impulses. It takes a longer period to these cells to reach the threshold level and the heart rate decreases. Another effective negative chronotropic agent is beta blockers. Beta blockers interfere with binding of NE and EPI and are used to treat high blood pressure.

The ability of the autonomic nervous system to influence heart rate is termed an **autonomic reflex**. The cardiac center in the medulla oblongata monitors blood pressure through baroreceptors and the level of carbon dioxide with H^+ concentration through chemoreceptors. The cardiac center reflexively responds to this sensory input by altering nerve signals relayed through sympathetic and parasympathetic neurons. The **atrial reflex**, for example, protects the heart from overfilling.

Another way to control cardiac output is change stroke volume. The factors that influence stroke volume are called **inotropic agents**. Inotropic agents alter contractility of cardiac muscle cells. An increase or a decrease in the force of contraction is generally due to a change in the available Ca^{2+} in the sarcoplasm. Changes in Ca^{2+} concentration alter the number of cross bridges formed and thus the force of contraction generated.

Positive inotropic agent increases Ca^{2+} concentration, which results in formation of additional cross bridges. Positive inotropic agents include NE and EPI. These ligands bind to β_1-adrenergic receptors, cause an increase of Ca^{2+} level inside muscle cell. Thyroid hormone is also a positive inotropic agent. It increases the number of β_1-adrenergic receptors in cardiac muscle cells.

Negative inotropic agent decreases contractility by decreasing available Ca^{2+}, and fewer cross bridges are formed. Electrolyte imbalances, including an increase of K^+ or H^+, act as negative inotropic agents. Certain drugs, for example nifedipine that blocks Ca^{2+} channels, are negative inotropic agents and decrease cardiac output. That is why, they are often prescribed to treat high blood pressure.

CHECK YOUR UNDERSTANDING

- Which of the following increases stroke volume: (a) increased venous return; (b) increased Ca^{2+} in sarcoplasm; or (c) afterload? Explain your answer.

- Describe the difference between positive and negative chronotropic agents.

- Describe the atrial reflex, which involves baroreceptors within the atria, the cardiac center, and the heart.

- If a patient is given a Ca^{2+} channel blocker, how will this affect heart rate and force of contraction? Explain your answer.

CHAPTER SUMMARY

- The term **circulatory system** describes a network of blood vessels and blood that circulates inside them. Blood delivers oxygen, nutrients, hormones, immune agents, heat, and other commodities to all cells of the body and removes waste products. The **cardiovascular system** includes the circulatory system and heart.

- Blood vessels that deliver blood to the heart are called **veins**. The chambers of the heart which receive blood from veins are called **atria** (singular **atrium**). Blood vessels that take blood from the heart are **arteries**. Chambers that push blood out of the heart into arteries are **ventricles**.

- There are two principal patterns of blood circulation in vertebrates: **single circulation** and **double circulation**. At the first circuit type, blood passes the heart only one time, when it makes a complete circuit. This is characteristic of fishes. In a double circulation system, blood passes through the heart twice to make a complete circuit. The double circuit consists of a **systemic circuit** that serves to deliver oxygen to all body cells, and a **pulmonary circuit** that consists of blood vessels that move poorly oxygenated blood (termed **deoxygenated**) to the lungs and take oxygenated blood back to the heart.

- In fishes with single circulation, the heart is a muscular tube separated into the **sinus venosus**, **atrium**, **ventricle**, and **conus arteriosus**. With development of an intermediate circuit in lungfish and amphibians, a single atrium splits into two atria, but the ventricle remains single. These animals have a heart with three chambers. In reptiles the process of subdivision of the heart interior continues and the **interventricular septum** separates the ventricle. Mammals and birds have a four-chambered heart with complete separation of pulmonary and systemic circuits.

- The heart is located in the mediastinum and shifted to the left side. Ventrally, it is protected by the sternum; dorsally by the vertebral column; and laterally by the ribs. It has the shape of a cone. The sharp region of this cone is called the **apex**, and a broad flattened part that is associated with major blood vessels is known as the **base**.

- The heart plays a principal role in blood pressure homeostasis. An increase or decrease of the **heart rate** and **cardiac output** is the main factor that influences blood pressure. The atrial regions of the heart produce the hormone **atrial natriuretic peptide (ANP)** that lowers blood pressure by decreasing sodium ion retention in the kidneys. Sodium is removed from the body fluids with urine, which decreases blood osmotic pressure and reduces water reabsorption. This decreases blood volume and lows blood pressure.

- The heart is covered by two membranes: **fibrous** and **serous pericardium**. Fibrous pericardium is made up of dense and loose connective tissues. It protects the heart, anchors it to the surrounding structures, and prevents it from overfilling with blood. It is continuous with an external adventitial layer of the nearby great blood vessels: the **vena cava**, **pulmonary trunk**, and **aorta**.

- The serous pericardium consists of the secretory epithelium that secrete serous fluid. On the other side, the serous pericardium is made of areolar connective tissue, which makes it resilient and elastic. The areolar layer of one side fuses to the fibrous pericardium and is called the **parietal pericardium**, and on the other side fuses to the heart and is called the **visceral pericardium** or **epicardium**. Space between the parietal and visceral pericardia is filled with serous fluid and is called the **pericardial cavity**. The serous fluid acts as a lubricant that guarantees smooth heart movement.

- Beneath the visceral pericardium is the **myocardium,** made of cardiac muscle tissue and fibrous skeleton; the **endo-cardium** is composed of a simple squamous epithelium similar to that of lining lumen of blood vessels and several layers of connective tissue. Cardiac muscle tissue consists of **cardiac muscle cells** or **cardiomyocytes**. Cardio-myocytes are attached and interwoven with the fibrous skeleton, which is composed of irregular dense connective tissue. The fibrous skeleton creates a frame for attachment and anchoring cardiomyocytes; when they contract, this gives structural support to the heart walls and insulates cardiac electric pathways. Epithelial cells of the endocardium are called **vascular endothelial cells**. These cells have unique functions, such as developing blood-heart barrier, helping regulate electrolyte concentration, recruiting neutrophil, and trafficking hormones.

- The right atrium receives blood from three veins: 1) the **anterior vena cava**, which collects blood from head, neck, and forelimbs; 2) the **posterior vena cava**, which collects blood from the hind limbs, abdomen, and chest; and 3) the **coronary sinus**, which collects blood from the blood vessels of the heart. The right atrium is larger than the left and has thinner wall. This allows the right atrium to accommodate more blood. The left atrium receives blood from four **pulmonary veins**: two of which take oxygenated blood from the right lung and two others from the left. Externally, both atria have a muscular pouch called an **auricle**. The right auricle is larger than the left. The internal surface of the right atrium has muscular ridges on the ventral side called **pectinate muscles**. The atria are separated from each other by a thin wall called the **interatrial septum**. A small depression in the interatrial septum is known as a **fossa ovalis**. This depression is what remains from a passage between atria called the **foramen ovale** that functions in the fetus, but closes after birth.

- The right ventricle pushes blood into the **pulmonary trunk** which carries deoxygenated blood to the lungs. The left ventricle moves oxygenated blood into the **aorta**. Ventricles have stronger walls than atria. Walls of the left ventricle are thicker than of the right ventricle. Walls of both ventricles have a ridged surface formed by cardiac muscles referred to as **trabeculae carneae**. A thick **interventricular septum** separates ventricles from each other.

- Atria are connected with corresponding ventricles by **atrioventricular foramens**, guarded by **atrioventricular (AV) valves**. The valve between the right atrium and right ventricle is called the **tricuspid valve**. The valve between the left atrium and left ventricle is called the **bicuspid valve** or **mitral valve**. Both valves have soft flaps or **cusps**. The cusp is composed of endocardium. Every cusp bends inside the ventricle, when the atrium walls contract and blood pressure in the atrium is higher than in the ventricle. Every cusp on the top is attached to a group of tough strands referred to as **chordae tendineae**. Chordae tendineae are anchored to the muscles in the wall of the ventricle called **pupillary muscles**. Papillary muscles contract together with ventricular myocardium and pull chordae tendineae. This maneuver does not allow cusps to bend inside the atrium and keeps the valve closed when blood pressure in the ventricle is higher than in the atrium.

- Contraction of ventricles propels blood into two major arteries: pulmonary trunk and aorta. Their entrances are closed by **semilunar valves**: **pulmonary valve**, and **aortic valve**.

- Heart valves are anchored in the **fibrous skeleton of the heart**: a high-density plate. The plate consists of four circular bands of dense connective tissue, which encircle the bases of all four valves. These fibrous rings are called **anuli fibrosi cordis**. A triangular mass of fibrous tissue, known as a **fibrous trigone**, connects rings in one structure. It can undergo increasing mineralization with age, leading to the formation of one **os cordis** or two: left **os cordis sinister** and right **os cordis dexter** heart bones.

- Heart relaxation and contraction pass in waves from atria to ventricles. Relaxation of cardiac muscular walls is called **diastole**, and their contractions are called **systole**. Cardiac blood flow is divided in four steps: 1) beginning from the moment when all heart chambers are relaxed, called heart diastole, when both atria receive blood from veins; 2) atria filled with blood contract, whereas ventricles remain relaxed. The blood pressure in both ventricles is lower than in atria, and blood is pushed from atria into ventricles. This second step can be termed atrial systole and ventricular diastole; 3) empty atria relax, whereas ventricles filled with blood contract, and blood enters the pulmonary trunk and aorta. This third step is characterized by atria diastole and ventricular systole; 4) empty ventricles relax and the heart returns to a state of heart diastole.

- A group of cardiac muscle cells in the **sinoatrial node (SAN)** that generate waves of cardiac muscle contraction is called a **pacemaker**. The waves of contraction are rhythmic and involve all cardiac muscles at every cycle. These waves have a special pattern resulting in a regular alteration of diastole and systole of atria and ventricles. Four heart anatomic properties support its performance: 1) cardiac muscle cells structure, 2) special type of junctions between adjacent muscles cells, 3) **Purkinje fibers** that facilitate rapid conduction of electrical signals, and 4) heart fibrous skeleton that provides electrical isolation of conductive pathways.

- The cells of myocardium have a large amount of mitochondria (about 25 percent of their sarcoplasmic content). Cells have a good blood supply. However, their sarcoplasm is rich with myoglobin and creatine kinase. Cardiac muscle cells rely exclusively on aerobic cellular respiration and are fatigue-resistant. They are also very versatile in using different types of fuel for oxidation reactions, from carbohydrates to fat molecules and proteins. The dependence from oxidative reactions makes cardiomyocytes sensitive to low oxygen, a condition termed ischemia.

- The complete membrane potential cycle includes: 1) beginning from period of complete relaxation, when it has a membrane potential called **pacemaker potential**. The pacemaker potential is due to a group of voltage-gated channels, which open at very negative voltages, developed by the Na^+/K^+ pump. Sodium channels open first. The influx of positive ions of Na^+ depolarizes membrane, until it reaches a set value around –40 mV, known as the **threshold potential**. Another hypothesis is based on idea of a "calcium clock." According this hypothesis, calcium is released from the sarcoplasmic reticulum, within the cell. This calcium increases activation of the sodium-calcium exchanger. The sodium-calcium exchanger moves sodium inside the cell and calcium out, causing an increase of membrane potential; 2) the next phase begins with a rapid depolarization lasting 10–20 ms due to an increased net flow of positively charged ions into the cell. In pacemaker cells, the increase in membrane voltage is mainly due to activation of calcium channels that allow Ca^{2+} enter the cell. 3) The last phase is known as "rapid repolarization." It begins with the closure of Ca^{2+} channels. Slow K^+ channels remain open, and potassium continues to leak out of the cell. The continued exit of K^+ results in a net outward positive current and restoration of a negative charge and cell repolarization. K^+ channels close when the membrane potential is returned to –60 mV. Ionic pumps restore pre-action potential concentration of ions. Once the Ca^{2+} is pumped out and its concentration inside the cell decreases, the muscle cells relax. When the membrane potential reaches its lowest negative level, the cycle repeats.

- The **absolute refractory period** is characterized by a complete unresponsiveness of the cell to any incoming action potential. It is long and develops together with the pacemaker potential. The short **relative refractory period** allows a stronger-than-usual stimulus to generate new action potential. The relative refractory period is due to potassium ion leakage, which hyperpolarizes membrane potential. That is why a stronger stimulus than normal is required.

- Cardiomyocytes are connected by **intercalated discs**, a combination of gap junctions and desmosomes. Intercalated discs allow an action potential to be transferred between cells. This property is termed **electrical coupling**.

- **Purkinje fibers** are located in the inner ventricular walls, beneath the endocardium. The Purkinje fibers are specialized conducting fibers composed of electrically excitable cells, which are larger than regular cardiomyocytes. They have much fewer myofibrils, but a large number of mitochondria. Purkinje fibers are characterized by numerous fast voltage-gated sodium channels. These cells conduct cardiac action potentials more quickly and efficiently than any other cells in the heart. Purkinje fibers allow the heart's conduction system to create synchronized contractions of ventricles.

- A **cardiac cycle** includes all changes within the heart from the beginning of one heartbeat to the beginning of the next.

- The process of spreading depolarization wave across the myocardium is called **conduction**. Structures of the heart that generate, support, and provide a pathway for electrical current constitute cardiac **conduction system**. Cardiomyocytes of atria and ventricles do not bind by gap junctions. Atria and ventricles are electrically isolated by collagen protein fibers of the heart fibrous skeleton. The only opening through it is a specialized group of muscle cells in the right atrial wall called the **atrioventricular node** or **AV node**. A bundle of cells called the **atrioventricular bundle** or **bundle of His** passes through the fibrous layer and enters the interventricular septum. Inside the wall of the interventricular septum, the atrioventricular bundle separates into the right and left **bundle branches**, which travel along the right and left surfaces of the septum. The bundle branches are connected with Purkinje fibers that form a network in the walls of both ventricles.

- The measuring and recording of cardiac voltage changes is called **electrocardiogram** or **EKG** (or **ECG**). The depolarization, and consequently contraction, of the atria corresponds to the first rise of the curve, termed a **P wave**. Q, R, and S waves are organized into one **QRS complex** that results from depolarization of ventricles. Repolarization of ventricles generates a **T wave**.

- Blood influx to the heart has to be equal to blood output into main blood vessels. This means that in a healthy heart the right and left ventricles eject equal blood volumes.

- The heart rate is the number of heart contractions in a minute. The left ventricle ejects blood in the aorta. The amount of blood ejected into the aorta in one stroke is known as the **stroke volume**. Three variables identify stroke volume: 1) **venous return**; 2) **preload**; and 3) **afterload**.

- Venous return is the volume of blood returned to the heart via the great veins. Since the amount of blood that enters the heart has to be equal to the amount of blood that left it, the stroke volume strongly depends on venous return.

- A preload is the ability of the heart walls to stretch to accommodate blood from main veins.

- Afterload is the amount of blood that remains during the ventricle systole. Afterload results from arteries' resistance to blood injection.

- The relationship between venous return, preload, and afterload is described by the **Frank-Starling law**, which states that there is a positive relation among venous return increases, preload, and strength of contraction. A stronger ventricular contraction generates a bigger stroke volume: 1) increased preload increases force of contraction; 2) physical activity increases venous return and stretches the myocardium; 3) cardiomyocytes generate higher tension; and 4) increased cardiac output elevates venous return.

- **Cardiac output** is the amount of blood ejected into the systemic circuit in one minute expressed in liters per minute. It depends on the stroke volume and heart rate: **cardiac output = stroke volume × heart rate**. **Cardiac reserve** is the difference between maximal cardiac output and resting cardiac output. It is a measure of maximal physical effort in which an organism can engage.

- Factors that affect heart rate are called **chronotropic agents**.

- **Positive chronotropic agents** increase heart rate. They include sympathetic nerve stimulation and some hormones. Sympathetic axons release norepinephrine (NE), hormones from adrenal medulla: epinephrine (EPI) and NE bind to β_1-adrenergic receptors and initiate opening of Ca^{2+} channels. Ca^{2+} influx increases heart rate. Thyroid hormone increases sensitivity of SAN cells to NE and EPI by increasing the number of β_1-adrenergic receptors.

- **Negative chronotropic agents** decrease heart rate. Postsynaptic axons of the parasympathetic nervous system release acetylcholine that binds to muscarinic receptors. Muscarinic receptors are K^+ channels, whose blockage causes membrane hyperpolarization and makes the SAN less capable of generating electric impulses. Beta blockers interfere with binding of NE and EPI and are used to treat high blood pressure.

- The ability of the autonomic nervous system to influence heart rate is termed an **autonomic reflex**. The cardiac center in the medulla oblongata monitors blood pressure through baroreceptors and carbon dioxide with H^+ concentration in the blood, and responds by altering nerve signals via the ANS. The **atrial reflex** protects the heart from overfilling.

- Factors that influence stroke volume are called **inotropic agents**. They alter cardiac contraction via availability of Ca^{2+} in sarcoplasm that inhibits formation of cross bridges.

- Positive inotropic agent increases Ca^{2+} concentration, which results in formation of additional cross bridges. Positive inotropic agents include NE and EPI. These ligands bind to β_1-adrenergic receptors, cause an increase of Ca^{2+} level inside muscle cell. Thyroid hormone is also a positive inotropic agent. It increases the number of β_1-adrenergic receptors in cardiac cells.

- A negative inotropic agent decreases contractility by decreasing available Ca^{2+}, resulting in fewer cross bridges formation. Electrolyte imbalance, including an increase in K^+ or H^+, acts as a negative inotropic agent.

CHECK YOUR KNOWLEDGE

LEVEL 1. CHECK YOUR RECALL

1. Which of the following is a right blood pathway from the vena cava to the pulmonary circuit?
   - A. Right atrium → pulmonary valve → right ventricle → tricuspid valve
   - B. Right atrium → tricuspid valve → right ventricle → pulmonary valve
   - C. Tricuspid valve → right atrium → pulmonary valve → right ventricle
   - D. Pulmonary valve → right atrium → tricuspid valve → right ventricle
   - E. Right atrium → right ventricle → tricuspid valve → pulmonary valve

2. Blood pressure is determined by:
    A. Cardiac output
    B. Peripheral resistance
    C. Viscosity
    D. All of the above
    E. None of the above

3. Stroke volume is the:
    A. Volume of blood discharged from the left ventricle with each contraction
    B. Volume of blood discharged from ventricle in a minute
    C. Systolic blood pressure
    D. Diastolic blood pressure
    E. Strength of the pulse

4. The normal pacemaker of the heart is the:
    A. Purkinje fibers
    B. Bundle of His
    C. Sinoatrial node
    D. Atrioventricular node
    E. Ventricular syncytium

5. **Chordae tendinae** are connective tissue fibers that:
    A. Transmit cardiac impulses through cardiac muscles
    B. Create skeleton of the heart
    C. Prevent blood backflow from ventricles to atria
    D. Generate excitation signal for cardiac muscles contraction
    E. Create internal lining of blood vessels

6. The right atrium receives blood directly from the:
    A. Pulmonary veins only
    B. Superior vena cava and inferior vena cava only
    C. Superior vena cava, inferior vena cava, and coronary sinus only
    D. Superior vena cava, inferior vena cava, and pulmonary veins only

7. The correct pathway of cardiac impulse is:
    A. AV node → SA node → Purkinje fibers → AV bundle
    B. AV node → AV bundle → Purkinje fibers → SA node
    C. SA node → AV node → AV bundle → Purkinje fibers
    D. SA node → Purkinje fibers → AV node → AV bundle

8. Which part of the electrocardiogram would **most** be affected by abnormally slow depolarization of the ventricles?
    A. P wave
    B. QRS wave
    C. T wave
    D. R-T interval

9. What is the cause of arrhythmia?
    A. Coronary atherosclerosis
    B. Pacemaker conduction system is malfunctioning
    C. Ischemia to myocardium
    D. Nerve impulses that disrupt propagation of excitation wave across the myocardium
    E. Hormonal influence, for example epinephrine and norepinephrine

10. What is the stroke volume if cardiac output is 4,200 ml and heart rate is 100 beats in 60 seconds?
    A. 70 ml
    B. 60 ml
    C. 42 ml
    D. It cannot be determined.

11. The right atrium receives blood from the _____, whereas the left atrium from the _____.
    A. anterior vena cava, posterior vena cava, and coronary sinus; four pulmonary veins
    B. four pulmonary veins; anterior vena cava, posterior vena cava, and coronary sinus
    C. anterior and posterior vena cava; four pulmonary veins
    D. anterior and posterior vena cava; coronary sinus
    E. pulmonary sinus; four pulmonary veins

12. In an electrocardiogram, the P wave corresponds to _____ and the T wave to _____.
    A. atria walls depolarization; atria walls repolarization
    B. atria walls depolarization; ventricle walls depolarization
    C. atria walls repolarization; atria walls depolarization
    D. atria walls repolarization; ventricle walls repolarization
    E. atria walls depolarization; ventricle walls repolarization

13. Chronotropic agents are those that influence _____, and inotropic agents influence _____.
    A. cardiac output; stroke volume
    B. heart rate; stroke volume
    C. cardiac output; heart rate
    D. stroke volume; heart rate
    E. heart rate; cardiac output

14. True or false: When ventricles are in systole, atrioventricular valves are closed and semilunar valves are open.

15. True or false: Purkinje fibers can generate their own electrical impulses, but impulses from the SAN are stronger and suppress them.

16. True or false: The AV node increases the speed of electric waves from atria to ventricles.
17. Match the term with its description:

_____ Venous return   a. Cardiac center prevents heart overfilling

_____ Preload   b. Amount of blood ejected by heart in aorta in one minute

_____ Afterload   c. Number of heart cycles in one minute

_____ Cardiac output   d. Blood volume ejected during ventricle systole

_____ Stroke volume   e. Blood remaining in systolic ventricle

_____ Heart rate   f. Ability of the heart walls to stretch to take blood

_____ Atrial reflex   g. Blood volume returned to the heart via great veins

LEVEL 2. CHECK YOUR UNDERSTANDING

1. When the SAN fails, the AV node takes over pacing the heart and produces a rhythm known as a junctional rhythm. Explain why an electrocardiogram of the heart with this rhythm has no P wave.
2. Explain what will happen if venous return is bigger that cardiac output.
3. What will happen with the heart rate if cardiac output remains unchanged and stroke volume decreases?

LEVEL 3. APPLY YOUR KNOWLEDGE TO REAL LIFE

1. Your dog has a SAN failure. Are the atria in the heart of your dog stimulated to contract? Explain your answer.
2. A patient has been diagnosed with mitral valve insufficiency, which causes the valve not to close properly. Predict the signs and symptoms you can expect from this disease.

Chapter 16

The Circulatory System II

Blood Vessels

LEARNING OBJECTIVES

The circulatory system transports substances through the body. Anatomic construction of blood vessels is designed for transportation of gases, nutrients, and waste compounds. Their walls prevent development of blood clots and are able to organize transportation of white blood cells to damaged body tissues. Blood vessels regulate blood flow, control blood pressure, and secrete a variety of chemicals. Mammalian blood vessels are organized in two circuits: pulmonary and systemic. This chapter discusses:

1. Structural organization and classification of blood vessels.

2. Functional organization of the mammalian circulatory system.

3. Dynamics of blood flow and mechanisms of its control.

4. Mechanisms of control of blood pressure and chemistry.

INTRODUCTION

Blood vessels transport gases. The circulatory system adjusts an organism to changes in pressure on or within the body. For example, whales dive to depth of 2,000 meters and feed there for an hour. At that time, a whale experiences an external pressure over 16 million Pa (atmosphere air pressure at sea level) per square meter of its body. Blood transports excess heat produced within the body to the skin to dissipate it. Reptiles accumulate the heat of the sun and through blood vessels transport it to deep body parts to warm them. Nutrients are carried to active organs for metabolic use or temporary storage. The circulatory system transports hormones to target organs and waste compounds to the kidneys. Blood transports agents of the immune system to defend the organism. The total network of body blood vessels constitutes the organism's **vasculature**.

16.1 Overview of Blood Vessels

Blood vessels form a network with tubes of different diameters, wall elasticity, and permeability for carrying substances. Some vessels carry oxygenated blood while others carry deoxygenated blood. Blood vessels known as capillaries are responsible for exchange of gases and other chemical compounds with interstitial fluids.

The Structure of an Artery Wall

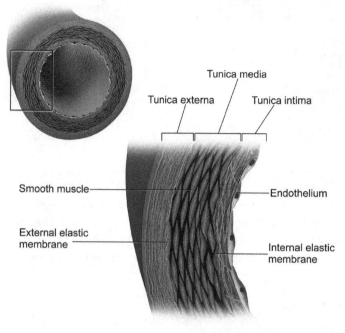

FIGURE 16.1   Structure of an Artery Wall.

Despite these differences, there are anatomic characteristics common to them all. Every blood vessel has a space inside called the **lumen**. Blood moves inside this lumen. Walls of blood vessels are composed of three different tissue type layers called **tunics**. These three tunics are the **tunica interna**, **tunica media**, and **tunica externa**.

The tunica interna is often called the **tunica intima**. It is the innermost layer that surrounds the lumen. The tunica intima consists of two layers: the **endothelium** and **internal elastic lamina** (fig. 16.1). The endothelium consists of a very tiny sheet of simple squamous epithelium. It is continuous with the endocardium of the heart. Endothelial cells facilitate frictionless blood flow and prevent formation of a thrombus. Endothelial cells secrete many chemicals—for example, nitric oxide, collagen, and clotting factors. Beneath the endothelium, the tunica intima carries the internal elastic lamina. The internal elastic lamina consists of elastic connective tissue. Its matrix contains type IV collagen fibers—soft, distensible, and elastic. This tissue is easy stretched and recoiled back to its original size. The internal elastic lamina is responsible for elasticity of blood vessels. Accumulation of calcium in this layer with aging causes decrease of blood vessels' elasticity, increase of vessels' resistance to blood flow, and elevation of blood pressure.

The tunica media constitutes the middle layer of the wall of blood vessels. It also consists of two layers: a layer of smooth muscles and underlying it, the **external elastic lamina**. Smooth muscle cells are arranged in circles around the lumen. They control the diameter of the vessel and, thus, the amount of blood that flows through it. Smooth muscles are innervated by sympathetic nerves called **vasomotor nerves** and hormones, such as epinephrine and norepinephrine.

Vasomotor nerves stimulate contraction of smooth muscles and decrease of blood vessel diameter, termed **vasoconstriction**. When stimulation of smooth muscles stops, muscle relax. The relaxation of smooth muscles of the tunica media leads to an increase in vessel diameter, called **vasodilation**. Vasoconstriction and vasodilation are major antagonistic processes that control blood pressure and blood flow through the vessel. The external elastic lamina, like the internal elastic lamina, is made of elastic connective tissue. It is responsible for blood vessel elasticity. External and internal elastic lamina tend to recoil when hydraulic blood pressure decreases. This elasticity allows the diameter of the blood vessel to adjust to exerted blood pressure.

The tunica externa is also known as an **adventitia**. It constitutes the outermost part of the blood vessel wall. The adventitia is composed of irregular dense connective tissue. It is strong and resistant to stretching. These properties of the adventitia make the tunica externa strong supportive layer that prevents blood vessel from overstretching and injury.

CHECK YOUR UNDERSTANDING

- Describe functional differences among the three types of blood vessels.

- Describe the structural organization and principal function of the tunica interna.

- What is the composition and role of the tunica media?

- Define the terms *vasoconstriction* and *vasodilation*.

Classification of Blood Vessels

Blood vessels are classified in three major groups (fig. 16.2): **arteries**, **veins**, and **capillaries**. In addition to that, there are groups of supporting blood vessels, known as **vasa vasorum** and **anastomosis**.

Arteries receive blood from the heart. They maintain stable blood flow to organs and play a principal role in control of blood pressure. Blood is ejected into arteries under high pressure. To hold and withstand the pressure of incoming blood, arteries have to be strong, distensible, and elastic. In general, arteries have

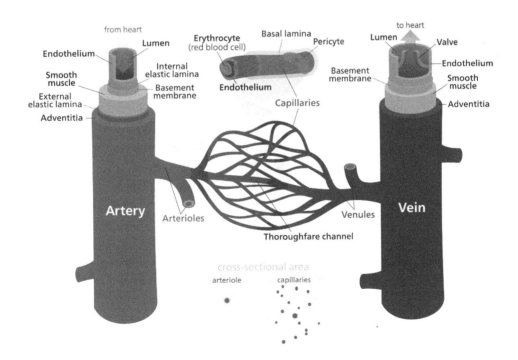

FIGURE 16.2   Major Blood Vessels of the Circulatory System.

a strong tunica media with a thick muscular layer and extensive internal and external elastic laminae. The thickness of the arterial wall depends on the artery's size and function. According to these characteristics, arteries are classified in three classes: **elastic**, **muscular**, and **arterioles**.

Veins are blood vessels that drain blood from all body regions and organs and deliver it to the heart. Veins that collect blood from a group of capillaries are called **venules**. **Postcapillary venules** are the smallest venules that drain blood from individual capillaries.

Capillaries are the smallest blood vessels, located between arteries and veins. They are the blood vessels responsible for exchange of gases, nutrients, and waste compounds between the circulatory system and body tissues. On one side capillaries receive blood from arterioles, and on the other side they transport it to venules. Capillaries are organized in a network known as a **capillary bed**.

The **vasa vasorum** is a network of a very tiny blood vessels that supply the walls of large blood vessels, such as elastic arteries (pulmonary tract, aorta) and large veins (venae cavae, brachiocephalic, or subclavian veins). These small vessels serve to provide blood supply and nourishment for the tunica externa (adventitia) and some layers of the tunica media of large vessels. Vasa vasorum are more frequent in veins than in arteries. Studies of pig and human arteries have shown that there are three different types of vasa vasorum:

1. **Vasa vasorum internae** originate directly from the main lumen of the artery and then branch inside the artery wall.
2. **Vasa vasorum externae** originate from branches of the main artery and then from the outside dive back into the vessel wall of the main artery.
3. **Venous vasa vasorae** originate within the vessel wall of the artery but then drain into the main lumen or branches of nearby veins.

Vascular anastomoses are pathways between big blood vessels, formed by so-called **collateral vessels**. There are three types of vascular anastomoses:

1. **Arterial anastomosis** is found in many organs and body parts, such as the heart, brain, joints, and so on. Arterial anastomoses are very dynamic. The old anastomoses may degenerate and new ones develop, depending on sufficiency of tissue blood supply. Tissues that are insufficiently perfused with blood are deprived of oxygen. Suffering low-oxygen cells (the condition is termed *hypoxia*) secrete signaling chemicals that trigger growth of new blood vessels. The process of growing new blood vessels is called angiogenesis. New blood vessels connect parts of circulation via collaterals and increase blood flow to the tissue.
2. **Venous anastomosis** is the most numerous type of anastomoses. These connect two veins by small collateral vessels. Small veins are often so interconnected by collaterals that they form a network, well visible, for example, in the skin.
3. **Arteriovenous anastomosis** connects arteries with veins. Anastomosis makes a direct connection between arteries and veins and allows blood to bypass the capillary bed. This anatomic structure allows distribution of blood flow among tissues that need oxygen most. Examples of arteriovenous anastomoses are found in the skin and in fetal circulation, where blood needs to be shunted between the arterial and venous systems to bypass certain organs, such as lungs (in a fetus lungs are not functional).

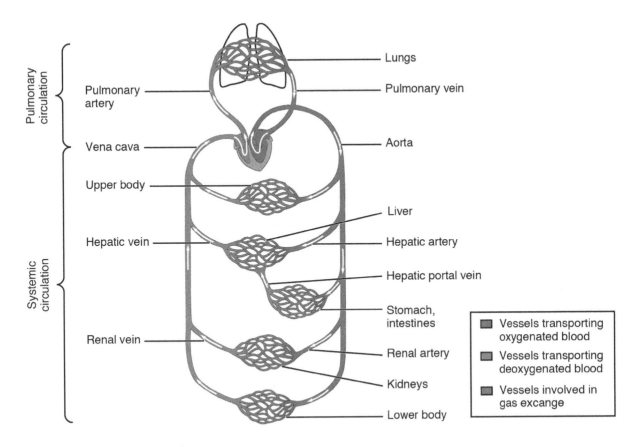

FIGURE 16.3   Portal System.

There is a special type of blood vessel arrangement known as a **portal system**. In it, blood flows through the sequence of two capillary beds and a **portal vein** between them (fig. 16.3). In a portal system blood moves from the artery into the first capillary bed; from here it is drained into the portal vein that delivers blood to the second capillary bed; the last capillary bed donates blood to veins, which transport blood to the heart. The hypothalamo-hypophyseal portal system (see chapter 14, page 401) and hepatic portal system (see chapter 19, page 572) are examples.

CHECK YOUR UNDERSTANDING

- What is an anastomosis?

- What is a portal system?

- Why do big arteries need the vasa vasorum?

Anatomy and Function of Arteries

Elastic arteries are the largest arteries. Often, they are named **conducting arteries** because they conduct blood from the heart to all body parts. Walls of elastic arteries have a large proportion of elastic connective

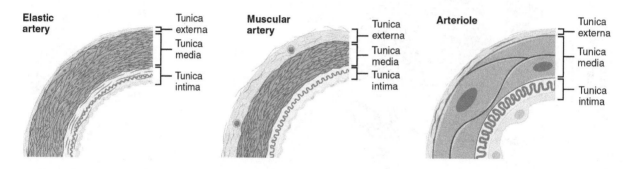

FIGURE 16.4   Structure of Different Types of Arteries.

tissue. Elastic tissue allows an artery to stretch and accommodate blood ejected from the heart during the ventricular systole and to recoil back during ventricular diastole. Aorta, pulmonary trunk, brachio-cephalic, common carotid, subclavian, and common iliac arteries are examples of elastic arteries. Elastic arteries branch into smaller muscular arteries (fig. 16.4).

Muscular arteries have a medium-sized diameter and often are referred as **distributing arteries**. They distribute blood among body regions and organs. Muscular arteries have a thick muscular layer in the tunica media. Their elastic laminae are restricted to internal and external elastic laminae. The relatively greater amount of muscle makes them capable of vasodilation and vasoconstriction. A lesser amount of elastic tissue limits their ability to stretch. Most arteries—for example, brachial, anterior tibial, internal coronary, and inferior mesenteric—belong to this class. Muscular arteries give rise to arterioles.

Arterioles are the smallest arteries. They have less than six layers of smooth muscles in the tunica media. The number of tunics in arterioles also varies. The largest arterioles have all three tunics, whereas the smallest arterioles have only the tunica intima surrounded by a single layer of smooth muscles. Smooth muscle cells in arterioles are in a state of continuous partial contraction called **vasomotor tone**. These muscles are controlled by the vasomotor center in the medulla oblongata. The center receives sensory input from central chemoreceptors that monitor pH of the cerebrospinal fluid and peripheral chemore-ceptors in aorta and carotid arteries that monitor blood oxygen level. An increase of carbon dioxide level in CSF causes a decrease of pH. When it receives the signal about low pH, the vasomotor center via the SNS stimulates vasodilatation, especially in the brain. Peripheral chemoreceptors inform the vasomotor center about blood oxygen level. Low oxygen also triggers vasodilation and an increase of blood flow first of all to the brain. Arterioles play an important role in regulating systemic blood pressure and distribution of blood flow among body regions.

CHECK YOUR UNDERSTANDING

- Describe the three types of arteries.

- How does the difference in structure of elastic and muscular arteries affect their functions?

- Which type of artery controls blood flow to organs? Which type controls blood flow to tissue?

Anatomy and Function of Veins

Veins outnumber arteries. They have a larger average diameter of the lumen and as a result contain more blood than arteries. Up to 70 percent of blood may be accumulated in veins. This makes veins a major body blood reservoir. In an emergency situation, such as profound bleeding, this blood can be injected in the bloodstream to maintain blood pressure. Veins have thinner walls than arteries, with much less smooth muscle in the tunica media. Because of that, their walls are less elastic and often have a collapsed appearance. Their ability to vasodilate and vasoconstrict is comparatively low.

The postcapillary venules, as a rule, have only endothelium surrounded by a tiny layer of connective tissue. Thanks to that, postcapillary venules are able to exchange gases and other chemicals with the surrounding interstitial fluid in the same way as it happens in capillaries. Bigger venules have all three tunics.

Blood in veins has a low pressure and moves slowly. One-way movement of the blood is secured by **venous valves**. These valves are folds of endothelium. Inside, the lumen folds overlap. Closure of venous valves prevents backward blood flow. They are especially numerous in the veins of the legs, where they prevent blood from moving down due to gravity (fig. 16.5).

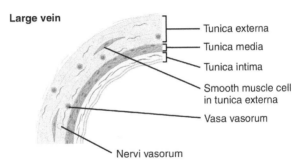
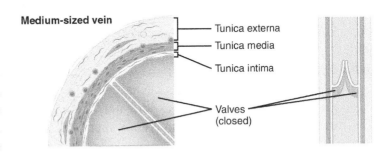
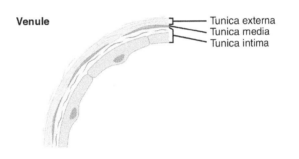

FIGURE 16.5 Structure of Walls, Different Veins.

CHECK YOUR UNDERSTANDING

- Describe the main structural differences between veins and arteries.
- What is the role of venules in vasculature?
- What is the function of venous vales?

Anatomy and Function of Capillaries

Capillaries are the smallest blood vessels, at 5–10 μm in diameter. They bind arterial and venous blood flows. Their wall is only one endothelial cell (simple squamous epithelium) thick. These vessels are the site for exchange of substances between the circulatory system and interstitial fluid. Capillaries are organized in networks termed a **capillary bed**. There are three types of capillaries: 1) **continuous**, 2) **fenestrated**, and 3) **sinusoid** (fig. 16.6).

In continuous capillaries the endothelial cells create an uninterrupted lining. Their endothelial cells are not connected by tight junctions like most cells in the simple squamous epithelium. There are always narrow gaps between endothelial cells in the capillary wall called **intercellular clefts**. An intercellular cleft allows small molecules, such as water and ions, to pass through the capillary wall. Lipid-soluble molecules, such as cholesterol and fatty acids, can passively diffuse through the endothelial cell membranes following concentration gradient. At the same time, big protein molecules, such as albumins, blood cells, and cellular fragments, are too big to pass through these gaps and stay inside the bloodstream.

Fenestra in Latin means "window." Fenestrated capillaries have pores about 60–80 nm in diameter. These fenestrae are created by radially oriented fibrils in the cell body that allow small molecules and some proteins to come through. Both continuous and fenestrated capillaries have continuous basal lamina (basal membrane). Fenestrated capillaries are found in endocrine glands, intestines, pancreas, and glomeruli of the kidney.

Sinusoid capillaries are also known as **discontinuous**. These are a special type of open-pore capillary that have a 30–40 μm diameter opening in the endothelium. This capillary type allows red and white blood cells with a diameter of 7.5 μm to 25 μm and serum protein molecules to pass. Sinusoid capillaries are characteristic of the red bone marrow, lymph nodes, and adrenal glands. Some sinusoids are distinctive in that they do not have the tight junctions between cells. They are called **discontinuous sinusoid capillaries**. This type of capillary is characteristic of the liver and spleen, where greater movement of cells and materials is necessary. Discontinuous sinusoid capillaries allow not only big protein molecules but also blood cells to pass.

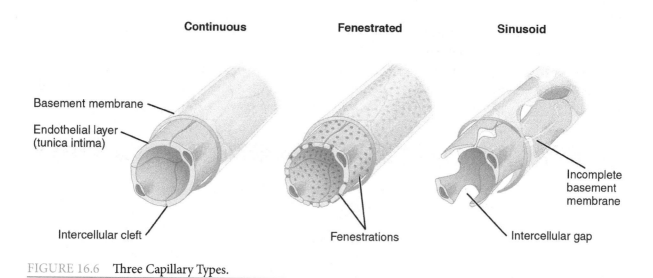

FIGURE 16.6   Three Capillary Types.

The capillary wall performs an important function by allowing nutrients and waste substances to pass. Molecules larger than 3 nm, such as albumin and other large proteins, are transported through the tiny endothelial squamous cells via **transcellular transportation**. Molecules smaller than 3 nm—such as water, ions, and gases—cross the capillary wall through the space between cells in a process known as **paracellular transport**. Capillaries that form part of the blood-brain barrier allow only transcellular transport.

Capillary beds control their blood flow via autoregulation. Autoregulation is based on a direct local negative feedback and allows an organ to maintain constant flow despite a change in central blood pressure. This negative feedback is formed by a specific response of smooth muscles in arteriole wall known as a **myogenic response**. High blood pressure stretches the arteriole wall. To counteract the increased pressure, smooth muscles in the arteriole contract (a phenomenon known as a **Bayliss effect**) and blood flow to capillary decreases.

Vessels called **true capillaries** branch from the metarterioles and make up the bulk of the capillary bed. At the origin of each true capillary, a smooth muscle ring called a **pericapillary sphincter** controls blood flow. Sphincter relaxation increases, whereas its contraction decreases blood flow. When the pericapillary sphincter is closed, blood flows from the metarteriole directly to the postcapillary venule and bypasses the capillary bed (fig. 16.7). Smooth muscles of the pericapillary sphincter demonstrate autorhythmicity. They rhythmically contract and relax at a rate of about five to ten cycles per minute. These cycles are referred to as **vasomotion**. At any given time, only about one-fourth of the capillary beds are

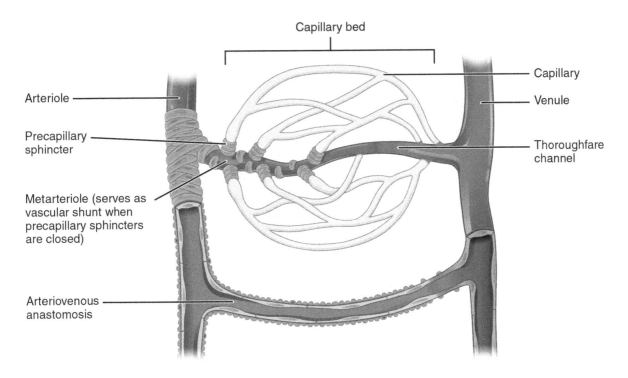

FIGURE 16.7   Capillary Bed.

open. There is not enough blood available to fill all capillaries at the same time. The specific amount of blood entering capillaries per unit time per gram of tissue is called **perfusion**. Perfusion is measured in milliliters per minute per gram (ml/min/g).

CHECK YOUR UNDERSTANDING

- Describe the general anatomic structure and function of capillaries.

- What type of capillary is the most permeable? Where in the body are these capillaries found?

- What is the myogenic response, and how does it influence blood perfusion?

16.2   Hemodynamics—A Physiology of Blood Flow

The main force that drives blood through the blood vessels is a **blood pressure** gradient created by heart and blood vessels. Blood pressure gradient is the difference between high pressure in areas close to the heart and low pressure in the peripheral vasculature. Blood pressure is measured in millimeters of mercury (mm Hg), which is the force exerted by a one-millimeter column of mercury. Thus, the blood pressure 120 mm Hg is equal to that generated by a 120 mm column of mercury height. Blood pressure varies dramatically along the vasculature. It is highest in the large systemic arteries and close to 0 in the large systemic veins (fig. 16.8).

The magnitude of the blood pressure gradient is one main factor that determines **blood flow**, or the volume of blood that flows per minute. Generally, blood flow matches cardiac output. It is directly proportional to the pressure gradient. When blood pressure gradient increases, the blood flow grows and vice versa. Three main factors influence blood pressure: **cardiac output**, **resistance**, and **blood volume**. Cardiac output (**CO**) (see chapter 15, page 432) and peripheral resistance (**PR**) are the two main factors that determine the pressure gradient (ΔP) that drives blood: $\Delta P = CO \times PR$.

Resistance is determined by three variables: 1) **blood vessel radius**, 2) **viscosity of blood**, and 3) **blood vessel length**. Mammals and birds need a high rate of blood flow to maintain a high demand in O_2 supply. The oxygen delivery in the systemic circuit may be described as:

O_2 delivery rate = cardiac output × (arterial O_2 concentration – venous O_2 concentration).

High resistance of blood vessels in the systemic circuit can be overridden only by an exceptionally high blood pressure.

The radius of the vessel significantly affects resistance. There is a reverse relation between a vessel's radius and its resistance: the smaller the blood vessel radius, the higher its resistance to blood flow and vice versa. If the cross section is a ring, then the **cross-sectional area** of the blood vessel is equal: $S = \pi r^2$, where **r** is the radius of the blood vessel. The **total cross-sectional area** is estimated as the aggregate radii across the total number of a given type of vessel (artery, capillary, or vein): **total radius = $r_1 + r_2 + r_3 + \ldots + r_n$**. Thus, the total cross section of all blood vessels is $S_{Total} = \pi(r_1 + \ldots + r_n)^2$. The equation demonstrates that the total radius grows slower than total cross section. An individual capillary has a very small cross-sectional area, but

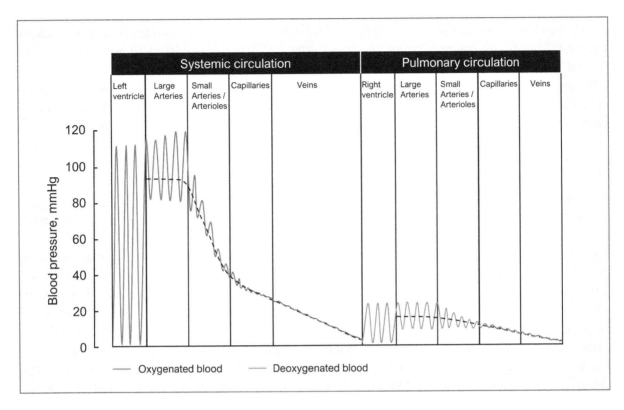

FIGURE 16.8   Human Circulation Blood Pressure.

the total cross-sectional area of all capillaries is much larger than total cross-sectional areas of arteries and veins. This difference is physiologically very important, because it has a significant influence on the velocity of the blood flow. **Blood flow velocity** is the rate of blood transportation per unit of time and is measured in centimeters per second (cm/s). The velocity of blood flow is largely determined by the cross-sectional area of the blood vessel. As the arterial system branches into more, progressively smaller vessels, the total cross-sectional area increases. This increase in area causes the velocity of blood flow to decrease. For this reason, the velocity of blood flow is fastest in the aorta and slowest in the capillaries. Thus, blood flow velocity changes as it moves through the different vessels: velocity of blood flow is fast in the arteries. It slows down in the capillaries, then speeds up again in veins. The slow blood flow rate secures enough time for efficient capillary exchange of respiratory gases, nutrients, wastes, and hormones between body tissues and blood.

Viscosity is a measure of fluid liquidity or thickness. It is a resistance of fluid to flow. Viscosity is a result of friction among molecules in blood. The higher the viscosity of the liquid, the higher its resistance. Thus, resistance directly depends on viscosity. Blood has a relatively high viscosity due to the proteins (first of all albumins) and blood cells. Blood viscosity varies depending on the concentration of proteins, blood cells, or amount of water. Peripheral resistance especially varies when the concentration of substances transported in the blood changes due to diffusion between body tissues and capillaries.

The length of a blood vessel also influences resistance. The longer the blood vessel, the greater its resistance. More pressure is needed to propel blood through a long vessel than a short one. This is one reason why resistance in the pulmonary circuit is so low. The shorter pulmonary vessels generate less resistance to blood flow. This also explains in part why blood pressure rises with obesity: with body size increase, the total length of blood vessels and their resistance grow proportionally.

The total volume of blood is directly related to blood pressure. As blood volume increases, blood pressure increases too. The ability of vessels to stretch due to an increase of blood volume is termed blood vessel **compliance**. Veins are the most compliant vessels. They easily stretch to accommodate an additional amount of blood without significant increase of blood pressure. When the veins become unable to accommodate additional blood, the extra blood moves to the arteries. However, arteries are much less compliant vessels, and when blood volume in arteries increases, blood pressure rises. Anything that decreases the compliance of arteries or veins, such as changes of elasticity of blood vessels with aging, makes the vasculature less able to adapt to increases in blood volume. So, when compliance decreases, even small increases in blood volume can raise blood pressure.

The pressure in the pulmonary circuit is lower than in the systemic circuit. The cardiac output of the right and left ventricles is equal. This means that the volume of blood passing through the pulmonary circuit per unit of time is the same as the volume passing through the systemic circuit. However, the resistance in the systemic circuit is much higher than that in the pulmonary circuit. For this reason, the pressures in the two circuits are very different. The pressure in the pulmonary circuit is very stable and remains low from the pulmonary artery to the pulmonary veins. The low blood pressure in the pulmonary circuit prevents any loss of fluid from the plasma across the capillary walls by filtration. The abnormal high pulmonary blood pressure will force fluids out of capillary flow and their accumulation in lungs: the life-threatening medical condition called **pulmonary edema**. Blood pressure in the systemic circuit changes dramatically. The aorta and elastic arteries have the highest blood pressure, and it declines as it spreads throughout the muscular arteries (fig. 16.8).

Because the heart has both contraction (systole) and relaxation (diastole) periods, the blood is injected in the circuit in pulses. These pulsed injections result in regular sequential variation of blood pressure gradient. It rises during ventricular systole and declines at ventricular diastole. Thus, there are two different pressures: **systolic pressure** corresponds to a maximum value reached during ventricle contraction, and **diastolic pressure** is a minimal blood pressure value during ventricle relaxation. The **arterial mean pressure** is an average blood pressure over the entire cardiac cycle. It is not equal the average of the systolic and diastolic pressures, because systole and diastole have different durations. The difference between the systolic and diastolic pressures is termed **pulse pressure**. The most dramatic decline of blood pressure in the systemic circuit takes place in the arterioles. The sharp decrease in pulse pressure is due to the sharp increase in peripheral resistance in the arterioles.

At the capillary bed, blood pressure continues to decrease and reaches a minimum at the venule side of the capillary bed. In veins blood pressure declines even further and finally reaches 0 mm Hg in the right atrium. The low pressure is largely due to the high compliance of veins and the declining resistance as these vessels merge and become larger. Venous blood must be returned to the heart at the same rate as it is pumped into the arteries. But the venous circuit is under such low pressure that there is not enough strong driving force to propel venous blood back to the heart. Veins have a higher cross-sectional area than arteries, which decreases the venous blood flow compare with that in the arteries. In some veins blood potentially can flow backward. For example, in the legs it may move backward, forced by gravity. An important mechanism that prevents blood backflow and moves blood in veins is called the **skeletal muscle pump.** Deep veins of the legs are surrounded by skeletal muscles. Contraction of these muscles squeezes veins and propels blood upward. Valves inside the veins prevents this blood from flowing backward (fig. 16.9).

Another mechanism is in the thoracic and abdominopelvic cavities. Veins in these cavities are not surrounded by skeletal muscle. This mechanism is known as the **respiratory pump.** The respiratory pump is driven by the rhythmic changes in pressure in the thoracic and abdominopelvic cavities associated with respiratory cycles of lungs' ventilation. Inspiration increases pressure in the abdominopelvic

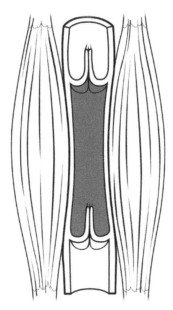
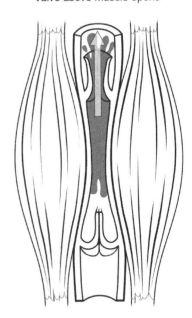

Muscles relaxed, valves closed

Muscles contracted, valve above muscle opens

FIGURE 16.9   Skeletal Muscle Pump.

cavity and decreases pressure in the thoracic cavity. This gradient of the pressure between abdominopelvic and thoracic cavities propels blood from the abdominal veins into veins in the thorax. During the expiration, abdominopelvic pressure drops, veins expand and fill with blood, while thoracic veins are squeezed and emptied into the right atrium.

CHECK YOUR UNDERSTANDING

- What is the blood pressure and blood pressure gradient?

- What is compliance?

- What is the role of the skeletal muscle pump in blood movement?

Regulation of Blood Pressure

A particular pressure gradient must be present at all times for blood flow to meet the body's needs. Homeostasis of blood pressure is maintained by a multilevel organized mechanism that includes local, nervous, and hormonal regulations. These regulatory mechanisms are classified as short-term and long-term.

Short-term control of blood pressure includes control from the nervous system and certain hormones. These short-term effects are generally achieved by adjustment of resistance and cardiac output.

Specialized baroreceptors in the atria, vena cava, common carotid artery, and aortic arch monitor blood pressure. The last two play a leading role and are known as the **carotid sinus** and **aortic sinus**, respectively.

These receptors depolarize and fire rapid action potentials in response to pressure exerted on the arterial wall. The signals from baroreceptors trigger the **baroreceptor reflex**, based on the reflex arch that involves the ANS. Signals from carotid sinus baroreceptors travel through the glossopharyngeal nerve (cranial nerve IX). Signals from the aortic sinus travel with the vagus nerve (cranial nerve X). All signals travel to the brain stem, where centers of both sympathetic and parasympathetic neurons are located. Both the sympathetic (SNS) and parasympathetic (PNS) divisions of the autonomic nervous system (ANS) have immediate effects on blood pressure. The SNS prepares the body for stress. Postganglionic axons of the SNS release the neurotransmitters norepinephrine and epinephrine into cardiac and smooth muscle cells in the blood vessels. Both neurotransmitters generate two immediate responses: 1) an increase of heart rate and contractility, which increases cardiac output; and 2) vasoconstriction of all types of vessels, but especially arterioles, which increases peripheral resistance. Both responses elevate blood pressure.

The parasympathetic nervous system has the opposite effect on blood pressure. The axons of the vagus nerve release acetylcholine onto SAN and A-V node cells. This slows the heart rate and decreases cardiac output and blood pressure. The increased activity of the parasympathetic nervous system inhibits activity of the sympathetic nerves. Inhibition of the sympathetic nervous system allows smooth muscles in walls of blood vessels to relax and vessels to dilate. Together, this decreases blood pressure (fig. 16.10).

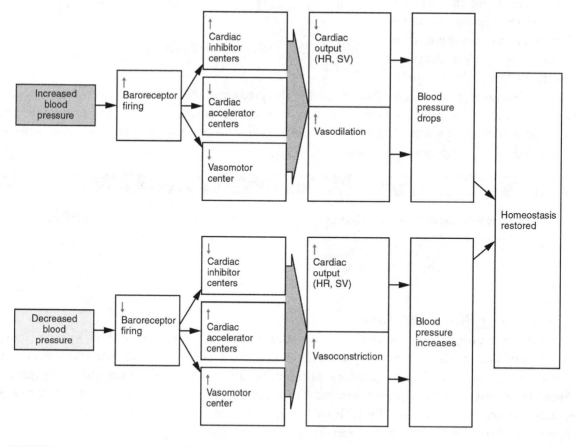

FIGURE 16.10   Baroreceptor Reflex.

There are two groups of chemoreceptors known as the **peripheral chemoreceptors** and **central chemoreceptors** (see chapter 20, page 646). The peripheral chemoreceptors primarily play a role in the regulation of breathing, but they also affect blood pressure. These receptors respond mostly to the level of oxygen in the blood. A significant decrease in the blood oxygen level triggers a negative feedback response that stimulates an increase in heart rate and causes vasoconstriction. Central chemoreceptors in the medulla oblongata respond to the pH of the interstitial fluid in the brain. The low pH (increased blood acidity) stimulates increase of sympathetic neurons' activity, which results in vasoconstriction and raises blood pressure.

Epinephrine, norepinephrine, and thyroid hormone increase cardiac output. The effect of epinephrine and norepinephrine is similar to that of the SNS. Thyroid hormone has an indirect effect on cardiac output. It stimulates cardiac muscle cells to produce more receptor proteins sensitive to epinephrine and norepinephrine and thereby increase impact of these compounds on cardiac output.

Epinephrine and norepinephrine also cause vasoconstriction, which elevates a vessel's peripheral resistance. Another powerful vasoconstrictor hormone is angiotensin II, a part of the renin-angiotensin-aldosterone system (RAAS). The hormone natriuretic peptide (ANP) (see chapter 15, page 432) is an antagonist to epinephrine, norepinephrine, and angiotensin II. It stimulates vasodilation, especially in renal circulation, which causes a decrease of peripheral resistance and blood pressure.

There are a number of vasoactive chemicals released by damaged tissues that have a short-term effect on local blood flow. They constitute part of the body defense mechanism. Thus, **histamine** and **bradykinin** are inflammatory mediators. They are released in response to a trauma, an allergic reaction, or infection. These chemicals cause vasodilation by either directly stimulating arteriole vasodilation or indirectly by stimulating endothelial cells of the vessel to release nitric oxide. **Nitric oxide** is a very powerful but short-term vasodilator that increases blood flow. **Endothelin, prostaglandins**, and **thromboxanes** are released by injured tissues and cause vasoconstriction. They prevent massive blood loss from the damaged vessel.

Long-term control of blood pressure is based on regulation of water amount and total blood volume in the body. The long-term control of blood pressure is executed by kidneys and hormones that affect their performance. The mechanism consists of regulation of water amount in urine, which affects total blood volume.

The endocrine system regulates blood volume through the ANP, angiotensin II, ADH, and aldosterone (see chapter 14). The ANP blocks sodium channel proteins and decreases sodium reabsorption in the nephron tubular system. Sodium ions are retained in filtrate and removed with urine. Sodium concentration in blood decreases, and blood osmotic pressure drops too. Low blood osmotic pressure results in a decrease of blood pressure. Other hormones cause an increase in blood pressure using different mechanisms. ADH increases blood volume by retaining water in nephrons' distal convoluted tubules and collecting ducts through synthesis of new aquaporin proteins. It also stimulates vasoconstriction. That is why it is also named vasopressin. Aldosterone causes water retention through reabsorption of sodium ions in distal convoluted tubules, increase of interstitial osmotic pressure, and by that diffusion of water molecules from urine back to the bloodstream. Angiotensin II is a part of the RAAS. It is also a powerful vasoconstrictor.

- What mechanism constitutes the short-term regulation of blood pressure?

- Which hormone decreases blood pressure?

- What are prostaglandins, and how do they affect bleeding?

Physiology of Capillary Blood Flow and Blood Perfusion

The blood flow to a tissue through a capillary bed is known as **tissue perfusion**. Capillaries are very tiny blood vessels. Their walls are made of a single layer of squamous epithelial cells about 0.2 μm in thickness. Some capillaries have specialized contractile epithelial cells called **pericytes**. Pericytes participate in control of blood flow through capillaries. The average diameter of capillaries is almost equal to the diameter of a red blood cell.

Capillary walls are designed to facilitate exchange of gases, nutrients, ions, and wastes between the bloodstream and body tissues. The movement across capillary walls is called **capillary exchange**. There are three main mechanisms of capillary exchange: 1) **diffusion and osmosis through gaps and fenestrations**; 2) **diffusion through the membranes of endothelial cells**; and 3) **transcytosis**.

1. Junctions between endothelial cells are incomplete and have gaps. Some capillaries have fenestrations. Small molecules, like water, monosaccharides, and amino acids, can pass through these openings.
2. Lipid-soluble compounds, such as oxygen, carbon dioxide, cholesterol, and fatty acids, can easily diffuse across the membranes of endothelial cells.
3. Large molecules, like lipids and proteins, are transported through the layer of endothelial cells by transcytosis (see chapter 3, page 74).

Tissue perfusion, first of all, depends on arterial blood pressure. Other principal factors that influence tissue perfusion are local factors. Local factors allow fine adjustment of blood supply to meet tissues' needs. There are two local control mechanisms of tissue perfusion: the **myogenic mechanism** and **metabolic control**.

The myogenic mechanism is based on the state of smooth muscles in the arterioles that supply the capillary bed with blood. Increases in arteriolar pressure open stretch-sensitive channels in the arteriolar smooth muscle cells. This initiates a depolarization in the membranes of these cells that results in their contraction; that is, an increase in arteriolar pressure leads to their vasoconstriction. When arteriolar pressure decreases, the arteriolar smooth muscles relax.

Blood is present in capillaries only one second. During this time blood has to release oxygen and nutrients into surrounding tissues and absorb carbon dioxide and wastes. When the velocity of blood flow increases, less capillary exchange takes place. When velocity decreases, flow is inadequate and blood that has already undergone capillary exchange remains in the capillary longer then it is needed.

The myogenic mechanism regulates blood flow by altering arteriolar resistance. The velocity of blood flow is inversely related to resistance. The increase of resistance decreases velocity and vice versa. The myogenic mechanism slows blood flow by increasing resistance when arteriolar pressure rises, and it speeds up blood flow by decreasing resistance when arteriolar pressure lowers. Both changes maintain local tissue perfusion at a constant level and ensure that gases and other substances continue to be exchanged in adequate amounts even in the face of fluctuating blood pressure.

Metabolic control is based on regulation of cellular metabolism. Metabolically active tissues generate waste materials. The more active tissue is, the more wastes it generates. One of the major waste products is carbon dioxide, which in combination with water produces carbonic acid: $CO_2 + H_2O = H_2CO_3$. Carbonic acid dissolved in water dissociates on hydrogen and bicarbonate ions: $H_2CO_3 = H^+ + HCO_3^-$. The active tissues, for example skeletal muscles, have a low concentration of oxygen and increased acidity, because of the increased amount of hydrogen ions in interstitial fluid. These conditions stimulate smooth muscles in local arterioles to relax. The dilation of arterioles increases tissue perfusion and ensures adequate oxygen and nutrient delivery to the actively metabolizing cells. Cells with low metabolic activity consume much less oxygen and generate a comparatively small amount of waste. As a result, they have a comparatively high level of oxygen and low concentration of hydrogen ions. These conditions cause constriction of smooth muscles in local arterioles and a decrease in tissue perfusion.

Blood vessels that provide heart tissues with oxygen and nutrients constitute **coronary circulation**. Coronary circulation is a part of the systemic circuit. It receives around 5 percent of total cardiac output. In the systemic circuit, tissue perfusion reaches its maximum during ventricular systole and is minimal at ventricular diastole. In contrast to that, the myocardium perfusion is high during the ventricular diastole and decreases to minimum during systole. This reverse perfusion pattern is a result of squeezing of cardiac blood vessels during the powerful myocardium contraction and vasodilation of cardiac vessels during myocardium diastole. This is one reason why extreme increases in heart rate and/or force of contraction can be dangerous. Such conditions can lead to a situation in which the heart does not have enough time in diastole and the myocardium is not adequately perfused. The main local autoregulatory mechanism of cardiac muscle tissue is based on monitoring of oxygen concentration in the cardiac interstitial fluid. A low oxygen level in the interstitial fluid during intensive physical activity triggers the production of chemicals called vasodilators. These chemicals dilate the arterioles serving the myocardium and so greatly increase perfusion.

Nervous tissue is the most metabolically active tissue in the body. It requires a constant sufficient oxygen and glucose supply. A sudden decrease in nervous tissue perfusion results in loss of consciousness within a few seconds. In vertebrates the brain accounts for less than 2 percent of the total body mass, but it receives about 15 percent of the total cardiac output. Active neurons consume more oxygen and generate more carbon dioxide. Together, they force cerebral blood vessels in active areas of the brain to dilate, and their perfusion increases. Active neurons communicate through neurotransmitters. Some neurotransmitters are strong vasodilators. Astrocytes (see chapter 10, page 291) form the brain-blood barrier. They monitor oxygen and carbon dioxide transport between the blood and brain. Deviation of these substances from a normal concentration stimulates astrocytes to release vasodilators that open arterioles and increase perfusion of the brain's active regions.

An artery that enters a skeletal muscle is called a **feed arteriole**. Feed arterioles branch into multiple arterioles and end in **terminal arterioles** that supply a capillary bed. At rest, resistance in the feed arteries is relatively high, and many of the terminal arterioles are constricted, which limits tissue perfusion.

Physical activity increases skeletal muscle metabolism. The consumption of O_2 grows, and release of CO_2 leads to an increase in interstitial fluid acidity. Smooth muscles in terminal arterioles relax, and skeletal muscle perfusion increases. If this new perfusion level is not sufficient, the vessels proximal to the terminal arterioles also dilate. If this is still not enough, feed arterioles dilate and blood flow to the muscle rise up to 50-fold.

The skin is the largest organ of the mammalian body. Its blood supply is located in the dermis. Nutrients and oxygen diffuse from the dermis into the epidermis. Blood vessels in skin are sensitive to many factors and especially to temperature. An increase in temperature causes vasodilation of the dermis blood vessels. A decrease in temperature forces blood vessels to constrict. This mechanism is important for body temperature homeostasis. Another important mechanism of regulation skin blood flow is control of it by the SNS. Signals from sympathetic nerves may dilate or constrict dermis vessels and alter skin perfusion.

Water does not move between the bloodstream and interstitial fluids by diffusion or transcytosis. It moves through the gaps between endothelial cells by **filtration**. Water filtration in the capillary bed is driven by a gradient of water pressure between blood and interstitial fluid. This gradient is formed by the **blood hydrostatic pressure** and **interstitial fluid hydrostatic pressure**.

Hydrostatic pressure (HP) is a force exerted on the wall of the vessel. Blood hydrostatic pressure is a force generated by the blood. It pushes water out of the blood vessel. Interstitial fluid also has hydrostatic pressure that forces water from interstitial fluid inside the blood vessel. The difference between hydrostatic pressure of the blood and that of the interstitial fluid forms a **hydrostatic pressure gradient**. Normally, blood hydrostatic pressure is higher than that of interstitial fluid, and the gradient of hydrostatic pressure directs water from the blood vessel into interstitial space.

Osmosis is a process of water movement across the semipermeable plasma membrane from a solution with a lower solute concentration to a solution with a higher solute concentration. The pressure created by moving water is called **osmotic pressure**. The osmotic pressure is proportional to solute the concentration (see chapter 2, page 39). Blood plasma contains much more chemicals than interstitial fluid and normally has a higher solute concentration than interstitial fluid. Globular proteins collectively known as **albumins** play a special role in formation of high blood plasma osmotic pressure. Their concentration is crucial for maintaining a comparatively high blood osmotic pressure. The difference between a high blood osmotic pressure and a comparatively low interstitial osmotic pressure creates an osmotic pressure gradient known as **colloid osmotic pressure**. Colloid osmotic pressure drives water molecules from interstitial fluid to enter the bloodstream.

The capillary water filtration is called a **net filtration pressure (NFP)**. It is determined by two opposite forces: the hydrostatic pressure gradient that forces blood out of circulation and the colloid osmotic pressure (COP) that drives blood inside the capillary. The final result of the capillary water filtration is a compromise between these forces. Blood enters into the capillary bed under comparatively high pressure created by the heart, whereas colloid osmotic pressure is comparatively low. The high hydrostatic pressure gradient at the arteriolar site forces water to leave the bloodstream, and net filtration pressure has a positive value: **NFP = BHP − (IHP + COP)**. At the venular capillary end, the blood hydrostatic pressure gradient decreases. At the same time, because blood lost a significant amount of water, but blood cells and big protein molecules such as albumins cannot come through small gaps between

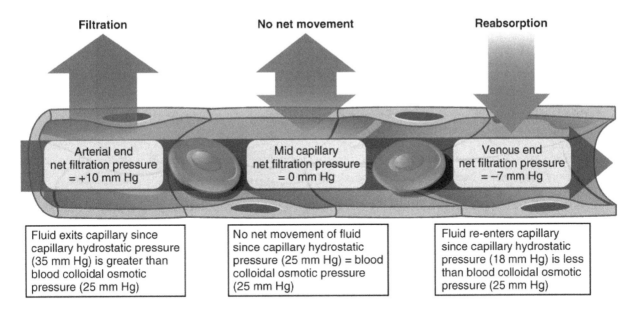

FIGURE 16.11 Capillary Exchange.

endothelial cells and remain inside capillaries, the colloid osmotic pressure increases and overrides the hydrostatic pressure gradient. This causes water to enter back into the blood flow, and net filtration pressure becomes negative (fig. 16.11).

CHECK YOUR UNDERSTANDING

- What is tissue perfusion?

- How is the coronary circulation pattern different from that of other systemic circuits?

- What is net filtration pressure?

- Explain how low blood albumin may affect net filtration pressure.

CHAPTER SUMMARY

- Blood vessels are organized in tubular networks. Walls of blood vessels are composed of three layers called **tunics**: the **tunica interna**, **tunica media**, and **tunica externa**.

- The tunica interna or **tunica intima** consists of two layers: the **endothelium** and **internal elastic lamina**. The endothelium is a simple squamous epithelium layer continuous with the endocardium of the heart. Endothelial cells secrete many chemicals: nitric oxide, collagen, and clotting factors. The internal elastic lamina is beneath the endothelium. It is made of elastic connective tissue containing soft, distensible, and elastic collagen type IV.

- The tunica media consists of a layer of smooth muscles and, underlying it, an **external elastic lamina**. Smooth muscles are arranged in circles around the lumen. They control the diameter of the vessel. Smooth muscles are controlled by sympathetic **vasomotor nerves** and hormones, such as epinephrine and norepinephrine. Vasomotor nerves stimulate contraction of smooth muscles and decrease of blood vessel diameter, termed **vasoconstriction**. Relaxation of smooth muscles is called **vasodilation**. Vasoconstriction and vasodilation constitute major mechanisms of controlling blood pressure and flow. The external elastic lamina is made of elastic connective tissue and is responsible for blood vessel elasticity.

- The tunica externa or **adventitia** is composed of irregular dense connective tissue. It is strong, is resistant to stretching, and prevents overstretching of blood vessels.

- Blood vessels are classified in three major groups: **arteries**, **veins**, and **capillaries**. In addition to that, there are supporting blood vessels, known as **vasa vasorum** and **anastomosis**.

- Arteries receive blood from the heart. Blood is ejected into arteries under high pressure. To hold and withstand the pressure of incoming blood, arteries have distensible and elastic walls, with strong tunica media having a thick muscular layer and extensive elastic lamina. Arteries are classified in three classes: **elastic**, **muscular**, and **arterioles**.

- Veins drain blood from organs and deliver it to the heart. Veins that collect blood from the **capillary bed** are called **venules**. The smallest venules that drain blood from individual capillaries are known as **postcapillary venules**.

- **Vasa vasorum** are very tiny blood vessels that supply oxygen and nourishment for the tunica externa and some layers of the tunica media of large blood vessels. They are more frequent in veins than arteries. There are three types of vasa vasorum: 1) **vasa vasorum interna**; 2) **vasa vasorum externae**; and 3) **venous vasa vasora**.

- **Vascular anastomoses** are pathways between big blood vessels, formed by **collateral vessels**. There are three types of vascular anastomoses: 1) **Arterial anastomosis** is found in many organs and areas, such as the heart, brain, joints, and so forth. Insufficiently perfused tissues secrete signaling chemicals that trigger growth of new blood vessels called **angiogenesis**. 2) **Venous anastomosis** is the most numerous type of anastomoses. It connects two veins by small collateral vessels. 3). **Arteriovenous anastomosis** connects arteries with veins bypassing the capillary bed.

- The **portal system** consists of two capillary beds connected by a **portal vein**. The hypothalamo-hypophyseal portal system and hepatic portal system are examples of the portal system.

- Elastic arteries are the largest arteries, with a large proportion of elastic connective tissue, which allows an artery to stretch and accommodate a large amount of high-pressure blood ejected by the heart. The aorta, pulmonary trunk, brachiocephalic, common carotid, subclavian, and common iliac arteries are elastic arteries.

- Muscular arteries have a medium-sized diameter and often are referred as **distributing arteries**. The relatively greater amount of muscle and lesser amount of elastic tissue make them capable of vasodilation and vasoconstriction and restricted ability to stretch.

- Arterioles are the smallest arteries. The number of tunics in arterioles varies depending on the size of the vessel. The largest arterioles have all three tunics, whereas the smallest have only the tunica intima surrounded by a single layer of smooth muscles. Smooth muscle cells in arterioles are in a continuous state of partial contraction called

vasomotor tone. These muscles are controlled by the vasomotor center in the medulla oblongata. An increase of CO_2 level in central chemoreceptors stimulates vasoconstriction. An increase of CO_2 in tissues causes vasodilatation.

- Veins outnumber arteries. They have a bigger average diameter and contain a major amount of blood. In an emergency situation this blood can be injected into the bloodstream to maintain blood pressure and oxygen delivery. Veins have thinner walls than arteries and much less smooth muscle. Their walls are less elastic and often are collapsed.

- Postcapillary venules have only endothelium surrounded by a tiny layer of connective tissue. They are able to exchange gases and other chemicals with interstitial fluid.

- Blood in veins has low pressure and moves slow. **Venous valves** are folds of endothelium that prevent backward blood flow.

- **Capillary** are the smallest blood vessels, at 5–10 µm in diameter. Capillary walls are made of a single layer of endothelial cells. These vessels are the site of exchange of substances between the blood and interstitial fluid. Capillaries are organized in networks termed a **capillary bed**. There are three types of capillaries: 1) **continuous**, 2) **fenestrated**, and 3) **sinusoid**.

- In continuous capillaries the endothelial cells create an uninterrupted continuous lining. Their endothelial cells are not connected by tight junctions and have narrow gaps called **intercellular clefts**. An intercellular cleft allows small molecules to pass.

- Fenestrated capillaries have pores about 60–80 nm in diameter in endothelial cells created by radially oriented fibrils that allow small molecules and some proteins to diffuse. The fenestrated capillaries are found in endocrine glands, intestines, pancreas, and kidney glomeruli.

- Sinusoid or **discontinuous** capillaries have pores 30–40 µm in diameter open in the endothelium. These capillaries allow red and white blood cells with a diameter of 7.5 µm to 25 µm and serum proteins to pass. Sinusoid are characteristic of red bone marrow, lymph nodes, and adrenal glands. Some sinusoids in the liver and spleen do not have tight junctions between cells. They are called **discontinuous sinusoid capillaries**.

- Molecules larger than 3 nm, such as albumins, are transported through the endothelial cells via transcellular transportation. Molecules smaller than 3 nm, such as water, ions, and gases, cross the capillary wall through the space between cells via **paracellular transport**. Capillaries that form part of the blood-brain barrier allow only transcellular transport.

- The autoregulation of capillary blood flow is based on a specific response of smooth muscles known as a **myogenic response**. When blood pressure rises, arterioles counteract the high pressure by an increase in blood flow.

- Vessels called **true capillaries** branch from metarterioles and make up the capillary bed. A smooth muscle ring called the **pericapillary sphincter** controls blood entrance into capillaries. Sphincter contraction directs blood flow from the metarteriole to postcapillary venule and bypasses the capillary bed. At any given time, only about one-fourth of the capillary beds are open. The specific amount of blood entering capillaries per unit of time per gram of tissue is called **perfusion**.

- The main force that drives blood through the blood vessels is a **blood pressure** gradient created by the heart and blood vessels. Three main factors influence blood pressure: **cardiac output**, **resistance**, and **blood volume**. Resistance is determined by three variables: 1) blood vessel radius, 2) blood vessel length, and 3) blood viscosity.

- There is a reverse relation between a vessel's radius and its resistance: a decrease of vessel radius increases its resistance and vice versa. An individual capillary has a very small cross-sectional area, but the total cross-sectional area of all capillaries is larger than the total cross-sectional areas of arteries and veins. **Blood flow velocity** is the rate of blood transportation. The velocity with which blood flows is largely determined by the cross-sectional area of the blood vessel. As the arterial system branches into more, progressively smaller vessels, the total cross-section area increases, and velocity of blood flow decreases; that is, the velocity of blood flow is fastest in the aorta and slowest in capillaries. The length of a blood vessel increases resistance. A higher pressure is needed to propel blood through long vessel than a short one.

- Viscosity is a resistance of fluid to flow. Blood has a relatively high viscosity due to proteins and blood cells. Blood viscosity may vary, especially at the periphery where the concentration of transported substances changes due to diffusion between blood and tissues.

- Cardiac output (**CO**) and peripheral resistance (**PR**) are the two main factors that determine the pressure gradient (Δ**P**) that drives blood: Δ**P = CO × PR**.

- As blood volume increases, blood pressure increases. The ability vessels to stretch is termed blood vessel **compliance**. Veins are the most compliant vessels. They stretch to accommodate additional blood volume without a rise in blood pressure. Arteries are much less compliant vessels, and when blood volume in arteries increases, blood pressure rises.

- Cardiac output of right and left ventricles is equal, but resistance in the systemic circuit is much higher than that in the pulmonary circuit. For this reason, the pressures in two circuits are different. Pulmonary circuit pressure is stable and low. In the systemic circuit, blood pressure is highest in the aorta and elastic arteries and declines along muscular arteries.

- Blood is injected in the circuit in pulses. These pulsed injections result in regular variation of blood pressure. It rises during ventricular systole and declines at ventricular diastole. Thus, there are **systolic** and **diastolic pressure**. The difference between systolic and diastolic pressures is termed **pulse pressure**. The most dramatic drop in blood pressure in the systemic circuit takes place in arterioles. This decrease is due to an increase of arteriolar peripheral resistance.

- At the venule side of the capillary bed, blood pressure continues to drop and finally reaches 0 mm Hg in the right atrium. The low pressure in veins is largely due to their high compliance and low resistance. Venous blood under such a low pressure has no driving force to propel it to the heart. A mechanism that moves blood in veins is called the **skeletal muscle pump**: veins are surrounded by skeletal muscles, whose contraction squeezes veins and propels blood forward.

- Another mechanism is in the thoracic and abdominopelvic cavities. This mechanism is known as the **respiratory pump**. It is driven by rhythmic changes in pressure in the thoracic and abdominopelvic cavities caused by respiratory cycles. Inspiration increases abdominopelvic pressure and decreases thoracic pressure. The gradient of pressure between cavities propels blood from abdominal into thoracic veins. During expiration the abdominopelvic pressure drops, veins here expand and fill with blood, while thoracic veins are squeezed and emptied into the right atrium.

- Homeostasis of blood pressure is maintained by a multilevel mechanism that includes local, nervous, and hormonal regulations that are classified as short-term and long-term mechanisms.

- **Short-term control of blood pressure** is formed by the nervous system and certain hormones. These short-term effects are generally achieved by adjustment of resistance and cardiac output.

- Sympathetic (SNS) and parasympathetic (PNS) divisions of the autonomic nervous system (ANS) have immediate effects on blood pressure. The SNS postganglionic axons release norepinephrine and epinephrine that immediately results in 1) an increase in heart rate and contractility, which increases cardiac output; and 2) vasoconstriction of all vessels, especially arterioles, which increases peripheral resistance. Both changes increase blood pressure.

- Axons of the vagus nerve release acetylcholine onto SAN and A-V node cells. This slows the heart rate and decreases cardiac output and blood pressure. The increased activity of the PNS inhibits activity of the SNS. Inhibition of the SNS allows smooth muscles in the walls of blood vessels to relax, vessels to dilate, and blood pressure to drop.

- Blood pressure is monitored by baroreceptors in the atria, vena cava, common carotid artery, and aortic arch. The last two are known as the **carotid sinus** and **aortic sinus**. These receptors fire rapid action potentials in response to pressure exerted on arterial walls and are part of the **baroreceptor reflex**.

- There are two groups of chemoreceptors known as the **peripheral chemoreceptors** and **central chemore-ceptors**. The peripheral chemoreceptors primarily play a role in regulation of breathing, but they also affect blood pressure. These receptors respond mostly to the blood oxygen level. A decrease in blood oxygen triggers a negative feedback response that stimulates an increase in heart rate and vasoconstriction. Central chemoreceptors in the medulla oblongata respond to pH of brain interstitial fluid. The decrease of pH stimulates an increase in sympathetic neurons' activity, which results in vasoconstriction and a rise in blood pressure.

- Epinephrine, norepinephrine, and thyroid hormone increase cardiac output. The effect of epinephrine and norepinephrine is similar to that of sympathetic neurons. Thyroid hormones stimulate cardiac muscle cells to produce more receptors for epinephrine and norepinephrine.

- Epinephrine and norepinephrine also cause vasoconstriction and increase peripheral resistance. Angiotensin II is another vasoconstrictor hormone. The hormone atrial natriuretic peptide (ANP) causes vasodilation, especially in the renal circulation, which causes a decrease in peripheral resistance and blood pressure.

- A number of vasoactive chemicals released by damaged tissue have a short-term impact on local blood flow. They constitute part of the body defense mechanism. **Histamine** and **bradykinin** are inflammatory mediators. They are released in response to trauma, an allergic reaction, or infection. These chemicals cause vasodilation either directly by stimulating arterioles or indirectly by stimulating endothelial cells of the vessel to release nitric oxide. **Nitric oxide** is a very powerful but short-term vasodilator that increases blood flow. Other vasoactive chemicals are **endothe-lin**, **prostaglandins**, and **thromboxanes**. They are released by injured tissues and cause vasoconstriction, which prevents blood loss from the damaged vessel.

- **Long-term control of blood pressure** is based on regulation of water amount and blood volume. It is executed by the kidneys and is based on regulation of water amount in urine, which affects total blood volume.

- The hormones ANP, angiotensin II, ADH, and aldosterone regulate blood pressure. ANP helps remove Na^+ with urine. Water follows Na^+, and blood pressure drops. ADH increases blood volume by retention of water and vasoconstriction. Aldosterone causes water retention via reabsorption of Na^+ in distal convoluted tubules that facilitates reabsorption of water from urine back to blood. Angiotensin II is a strong vasoconstrictor.

- Movement of substances across capillary walls is called **capillary exchange**. It includes 1) **diffusion and osmosis through gaps and fenestrations**; 2) **diffusion through the membranes of endothelial cells**; and 3) **transcytosis**. Small molecules—water, monosaccharides, and amino acids—pass through gaps and fenestrae. Lipid-soluble compounds—oxygen, carbon dioxide, cholesterol, and fatty acids—diffuse across membranes of endothelial cells. Large molecules are transported by transcytosis.

- Tissue perfusion depends on arterial blood pressure and local factors. Two mechanisms control local perfusion: **myogenic** and **metabolic mechanisms**.

- The myogenic mechanism is based on the state of arteriolar smooth muscles. An increase in blood pressure opens stretch-sensitive channels in arteriolar smooth muscles and initiates arteriolar vasoconstriction. A decrease in blood pressure relaxes arteriolar smooth muscles and increases blood flow.

- Active tissues generate waste materials. They have low concentration of oxygen and increased acidity. These conditions cause smooth muscles in local arterioles to relax and increase tissue perfusion. Cells with low metabolic activity have a high oxygen level and a low concentration of H^+. These conditions constrict smooth muscles in local arterioles and decrease tissue perfusion.

- Water filtration in the capillary bed is driven by a gradient of water pressure formed by **blood hydrostatic pressure gradient** and **colloid osmotic pressure**.

- Hydrostatic pressure is a force exerted on walls of the vessel. The difference between hydrostatic pressure of the blood and that of interstitial fluid forms a hydrostatic pressure gradient that directs water from blood vessels.

- Osmosis is water movement across a semipermeable membrane from a solution with a lower solute concentration to a solution with a higher solute concentration. Blood plasma has high osmotic pressure due to globular proteins called **albumins**. The difference between high blood osmotic pressure and low interstitial osmotic pressure creates an osmotic pressure gradient called **colloid osmotic pressure** that drives water molecules from interstitial fluid to the blood.

- Capillary water filtration, called **net filtration pressure (NFP)**, is determined by blood hydrostatic pressure (BHP), interstitial hydrostatic pressure (IHP), and colloid osmotic pressure (COP): **NFP = BHP − (IHP + COP)**.

CHECK YOUR KNOWLEDGE

LEVEL 1. CHECK YOUR RECALL

1. Which hormone decreases blood pressure?
   A. Antidiuretic hormone
   B. Aldosterone
   C. Epinephrine
   D. Norepinephrine
   E. Atrial natriuretic peptide

2. Which of the following is **not** a characteristic of a capillary?
   A. A capillary wall consists of an endothelium and a basement membrane only.
   B. Fenestrated capillaries allow for larger amounts of materials to be exchanged.
   C. Sinusoid capillaries are the main type of capillary around the brain.
   D. Capillaries often are arranged in a capillary bed that is supplied by an arteriole.
   E. The capillaries are the only site of tissue perfusion.

3. Which statement about veins is true?
   A. Veins always transport deoxygenated blood.
   B. Veins transport blood under high pressure.
   C. Veins drain into smaller vessels called venules.
   D. The largest tunic in a vein is the tunica externa.
   E. Veins have less space in their lumen than that of an artery.

4. Vasa vasorum are found in the tunica _____ of a large blood vessel.
   A. intima
   B. media
   C. externa
   D. All of these are correct.
   E. None of these is correct.

5. Which of the following decreases perfusion of a tissue?
   A. Decreased blood flow
   B. Vasodilation
   C. Angiogenesis
   D. Increase of tissue activity
   E. Increased carbon dioxide, decreased pH, and low oxygen

6. Which of these is a blood vessel with the lowest pressure gradient that must be overcome by skeletal muscle contraction and breathing?
   A. Arteriole
   B. Artery
   C. Vein
   D. Venule
   E. Capillary

7. Resistance is increased with:
   A. Length of blood vessels
   B. Increase of blood vessel diameters
   C. Blood flow velocity
   D. Decrease of colloid osmotic pressure
   E. Increase of cardiac output

8. Which of the following statements is correct?
    A. Total blood flow increases with a decrease in pressure gradient.
    B. Total blood flow decreases with an increase in resistance.
    C. Total blood flow increases with an increase in viscosity.
    D. Total blood flow increases with an increase in total blood vessel length.
    E. All of the above are correct.

9. Velocity of blood flow is lowest in:
    A. Elastic arteries
    B. Muscular arteries
    C. Arterioles
    D. Capillaries
    E. Veins

10. Capillary walls consist of:
    A. Three tunics: tunica interna, middle tunic, and tunica externa
    B. Only two tunics: tunica interna and tunica externa
    C. Three tunics, but there is no external elastic lamina in middle tunic
    D. Tunica interna covered by a thin layer (less than six cells) of smooth muscles
    E. One layer of endothelial cells covered by a basal lamina

11. Which of the following factors increases peripheral resistance?
    A. Increase in total blood volume
    B. Increase in blood flow velocity
    C. Decrease in blood vessel length
    D. Increase in blood vessel radius
    E. Vasodilation

12. Blood vessel connections that bypass capillary bed are known as:
    A. Anastomosis
    B. Vasa vasorum
    C. Portal system
    D. Arterioles
    E. Venules

13. In arteries blood is moved by the _____, whereas in veins it is moved by the _____.
    A. respiratory pump; skeletal muscle pump
    B. skeletal muscle pump; respiratory pump
    C. respiratory pump; heart
    D. heart; respiratory pump
    E. skeletal muscle pump; heart

14. As a rule, blood pressure gradient drives blood _____, whereas colloid osmotic pressure drives blood _____.

   A.   into arteries; into veins
   B.   from arterioles into capillaries; from capillaries into venules
   C.   from capillaries into interstitial fluid; from interstitial fluid into capillaries
   D.   from interstitial fluid into capillaries; from capillaries into interstitial fluid.

15. The internal elastic lamina is a part of the _____, whereas the external elastic lamina is a part of the _____.

   A.   adventitia; middle tunic
   B.   middle tunic; tunica intima
   C.   tunica intima; adventitia
   D.   adventitia; tunica intima
   E.   tunica intima; middle tunic

16. Elastic arteries have _____, whereas veins have _____.
   A.   the thickest muscular layer; the thickest adventitia
   B.   the thickest adventitia; the thickest tunica intima
   C.   the thickest tunica intima; the thickest muscular layer
   D.   no muscular layer; no adventitia
   E.   no adventitia; no tunica intima

17. True or false: Venous valves are endothelial folds that prevent backward flow of blood.
18. True or false: Discontinuous sinusoid capillaries are characteristic of endocrine glands and kidney glomeruli.
19. True or false: Capillaries in the brain allow only paracellular transport.
20. True or false: The myogenic response controls capillary blood flow through pericapillary sphincters.
21. Match the term with its description:

   _____ Vasomotion   a.   Inflammatory mediator that causes vasodilation
   _____ Resistance   b.   Receptors in medulla oblongata sensitive to pH
   _____ Pressure gradient   c.   Difference between systolic and diastolic pressure
   _____ Perfusion   d.   Receptor sensitive to pressure in aorta
   _____ Pulse pressure   e.   Difference between pressure in aorta and remote arteries
   _____ Aortic sinus   f.   Total blood supply of an organ or tissue
   _____ Central chemoreceptors   g.   Increases when blood viscosity increases
   _____ Bradykinin   h.   Vasodilation and vasoconstriction cycles

LEVEL 2. CHECK YOUR UNDERSTANDING

1. Explain why it is easier take blood from a vein than an artery.
2. Explain why a giraffe has higher blood pressure than a dog.
3. Why does a fat dog have higher blood pressure than the same breed of dog with a normal weight?
4. Explain why total blood volume can never fill all capillaries in the body.

LEVEL 3. APPLY YOUR KNOWLEDGE TO REAL LIFE

1. One of the outcomes of liver cirrhosis is a significant decrease in production of albumins. Explain the outcome of low albumin production. Which symptoms does it cause?

2. You and your dog spend a lot of time outside on a very hot day. You feel thirsty, and you see that your dog has the same feeling. At this time, how do you think there is change in your blood pressure? What about the blood pressure of your dog? Explain your answer.

Chapter 17

The Circulatory System III

Blood

LEARNING OBJECTIVES

Blood is a media that transports almost everything the mammalian body needs. Blood connects all body parts, providing them with nutrients and oxygen. It collects and removes waste compounds produced by cells. These processes affect blood composition. That is why clinicians examine blood more often than any other tissue in search of disease signs and causes.

In this chapter, you will find information on composition and functions of blood. It is expected that after reading this chapter, you will be able to:

1. Explain what components constitute blood.

2. Describe the formed elements of blood and their specific functions.

3. Describe the mechanisms that control blood cell production.

4. Understand what processes prevent blood loss.

5. Explain what we have to know in order to make a safe blood transfusion.

INTRODUCTION

The science that studies blood, blood forming tissues, and blood-related disorders is called **hematology**. Blood forms the media whose responsibilities include three main functions: transportation, regulation, and protection.

Blood transports gases, first of all: O_2 and CO_2 between the lungs and all body tissues. It transports nutrients between the digestive system and tissues; and wastes between tissues and the urinary system. Hormones are transported from endocrine glands to target cells.

Blood plays a major role in maintaining homeostasis. It controls and regulates pH of the body fluids. Blood distributes heat and regulates body temperature. The osmotic colloid pressure of blood plasma is a key component of tissue fluid and electrolyte balance essential for normal activity of neurons and muscle cells.

White blood cells are the principal elements of an organism's immune system. Besides that, blood plasma carries numerous compounds that protect organisms from blood loss, toxins, and pathogenic agents, such as viruses, bacteria, fungi, or parasites.

17.1   Overview of Blood

Blood is a special type of connective tissue. Like all other connective tissues, it has two major components: formed elements and matrix (see chapter 4, page 100). Formed elements of the blood are blood cells and cellular fragments called **platelets** or **thrombocytes**. Blood matrix is called **blood plasma**. Blood plasma has two components: 1) straw-colored fluid and 2) blood plasma proteins. Fibrinogen is a fibrous protein in blood plasma. It is a water-soluble protein that constantly circulates with blood. Under special conditions it is enzymatically converted into water-insoluble fibrin, which precipitates and creates a blood clot. A group of globular proteins, known as **albumins**, form colloid osmotic pressure.

Hematocrit

The hematocrit is a percentage of red blood cells in the total blood volume. In the laboratory hematocrit is evaluated by precipitation of blood formed elements. Precipitation may be performed under gravity or by spinning a blood sample in centrifuge. A fast-spinning blood sample in a centrifuge is separated into three fractures. The light fracture, called blood plasma, accumulates on the top. This fracture forms about 55 percent of total blood volume. The heaviest fracture, which contains red blood cells, concentrates at the bottom and accounts for 44 percent. This fracture has the dark red color characteristic of erythrocytes. Between the pale-yellow plasma coat and dark red erythrocyte coat, there is a tiny, around 1 percent of total volume, **buffy coat** that consists of white blood cells and platelets (fig. 17.1).

The hematocrit is a very important blood characteristic. It directly correlates with the ability of the blood to transport oxygen, called the **blood oxygen carrying capacity**. The increase of the hematocrit corresponds with the increase of the blood oxygen carrying capacity and vice versa. The hematocrit varies among different species. It also varies among individuals of the same species and the same individual. As a rule, the hematocrit is high among youngsters and decreases with aging. Adult males have a hematocrit higher than females, because testosterone stimulates the kidneys to produce a hormone called **erythropoietin (EPO)**, which facilitates erythrocyte production. A dehydrated organism, as a rule, has an elevated hematocrit. A high hematocrit also can indicate some medical conditions, such as particular forms of anemia. A high hematocrit is characterized by an abnormally high total amount of red blood cells. This increases blood viscosity and resistance and, as a result, increases the working load on the heart, which may cause heart failure. An increase of the hematocrit elevates blood oxygen carrying capacity and improves skeletal muscles' oxygen supply and performance. Purposeful increase of the hematocrit (for example, by injection of an additional amount of red blood cells in the bloodstream) is called **doping**.

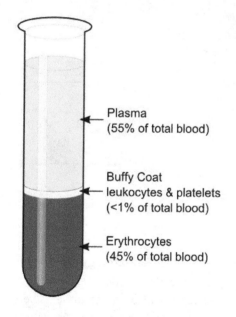

Plasma
(55% of total blood)

Buffy Coat
leukocytes & platelets
(<1% of total blood)

Erythrocytes
(45% of total blood)

FIGURE 17.1   **Main Blood Components Separated after Centrifugation.**

CHECK YOUR UNDERSTANDING

- Which substances does blood transport through the body?

- What does the term *blood oxygen carrying capacity* mean?

- Why does the hematocrit correspond with the blood oxygen carrying capacity?

- Why is a high hematocrit dangerous?

Blood Plasma

Blood plasma is a yellow-colored liquid. It is an extracellular matrix of blood tissue. It constitutes about 55 percent of the total blood volume. Water makes up 92 to 95 percent of blood plasma volume. Proteins (serum albumins, globulins, and fibrinogen) constitute 6 to 8 percent of blood plasma. Other blood plasma components include glucose, clotting factors, electrolytes (Na^+, Ca^{2+}, Mg^{2+}, HCO_3^-, Cl^-, etc.), hormones, respiratory gases (carbon dioxide and oxygen), and wastes (urea). Blood plasma also serves as a reserve of proteins. It plays a vital role in intravascular osmotic pressure. The presence of a higher protein concentration in blood plasma than in intracellular fluids makes blood osmotic pressure always higher. This helps keep electrolyte concentration balanced and protects the body from infection and toxins.

Blood plasma composition is similar to that of interstitial fluid. Both have similar concentration of electrolytes, nutrients, and wastes, except proteins. Blood has special proteins that are found only in the blood plasma and because of that are cumulatively called **plasma proteins**. A homogeneous liquid, which consists of large protein molecules or ultramicroscopic particles dispersed in a water, is called **colloid**. Colloid blood plasma is denser than water and has a high viscosity. If you put a drop of blood in pure water, it will sink, because its density approximately is 1025 kg/m^3, or 1.025 g/ml.

Plasma proteins form blood osmotic pressure, which is always higher than osmotic pressure of an interstitial fluid. The difference between these two osmotic pressures is known as **colloid osmotic pressure**. Colloid osmotic pressure is responsible for drawing water from an interstitial space inside the capillary bloodstream (see chapter 16, page 476). Malnutrition or some medical conditions can cause a decrease in plasma proteins' level. This results in loss of blood water and accumulation it in the interstitial space: a condition known as **edema**.

The most abundant plasma proteins are **albumins**. They make up 58 percent of all plasma proteins. Albumins are the smallest plasma proteins and are mainly responsible for formation of the colloid osmotic pressure. These proteins also serve as a transport protein and carry ions, hormones, and lipid molecules with the blood flow.

The second-largest group of plasma proteins are **globulins**. They constitute about 37 percent of all plasma proteins. The smallest **alpha globulins** and the larger **beta globulins** serve as carrier molecules that transport hydrophobic compounds, such as lipids, steroid hormones, some metals, and ions. **Gamma globulins** are also called **immunoglobulins** or **antibodies**. They are an important part of the vertebrate immune system.

Fibrinogen is a fibrous protein that constitutes about 4 percent of the total amount of plasma proteins. Together with other clotting proteins, it is responsible for blood clot formation. A small group of plasma proteins (less than 1 percent) are known as **regulatory proteins**, whose function is controlling the rate of chemical reactions in the blood.

Formed Elements

The term *formed elements* is a collective name of all blood cells and cellular fragments. Formed elements include red blood cells, also called **erythrocytes**; white blood cells, collectively called **leucocytes**; and fragments of cells known as **platelets** or **thrombocytes**. Clinicians study formed elements in a specially prepared thin sample on microscope slide glass called a **blood smear**. A blood smear is a film made by placing a drop of blood on one end of a slide glass. With a cover glass, blood is dispersed over the slide surface. The slide is dried in the air and fixed to the glass by a brief treatment with methanol. To distinguish different types of cells from each other, the slide is stained with different colors (fig. 17.2).

Regulation of Blood Production

Blood formed elements have a relatively short life span. The process of new blood cells' production is called **hemopoiesis** or **hematopoiesis**. In developing embryos, blood formation occurs in aggregates of blood cells in the yolk sac, called **blood islands**. The fetus produces new blood in the spleen, liver, and lymph nodes. Eventually, all hematopoiesis concentrates in the **red bone marrow**, mainly in the pelvis, cranium, vertebrae, and sternum. With aging the total amount of red bone marrow decreases and is restricted to the long bones, such as the femur and tibia. In some vertebrates, hematopoiesis can occur wherever there is a loose stroma of connective tissue and slow blood flow; for example, in the gut, spleen, or kidney.

The process of hematopoiesis starts with hematopoietic stem cells called **hemocytoblasts**. Hemocytoblasts are considered multipotent cells, meaning that they can differentiate and develop into many different cell types. Hemocytoblasts produce two blood lines: **myeloid**

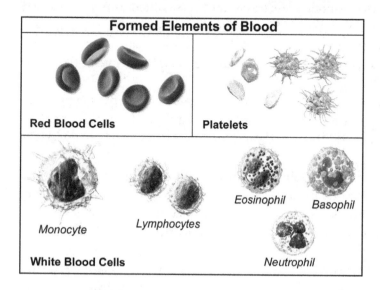

Formed Elements of Blood

Red Blood Cells

Platelets

Monocyte

Lymphocytes

Eosinophil

Basophil

Neutrophil

White Blood Cells

FIGURE 17.2   Formed Elements of Blood.

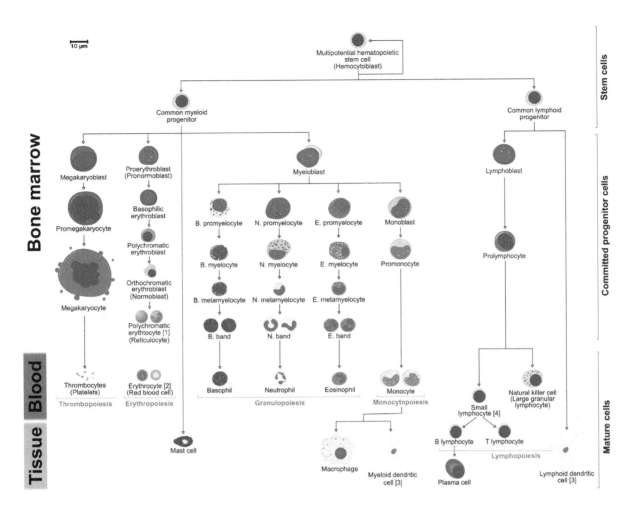

FIGURE 17.3   Hematopoiesis Diagram.

and **lymphoid lines**. Myeloid cells produce red blood cells, white blood cells (except lymphocytes), and platelets. Lymphoid cells produce all types of lymphocytes (fig. 17.3).

The development of hematopoietic cells is controlled by **colony-stimulating factors (CSFs)**. Production of different types of formed elements is controlled by different CSFs. Depending on the type of produced blood cells, there are three processes of formed elements production: **erythropoiesis, leucopoiesis**, and **thrombopoiesis**. The key players in self-renewal and development of hematopoietic cells are glycoprotein growth factors known as **interleukins (IL-2, IL-3, IL-6, IL-7)**. The other three factors that specifically stimulate the production of committed cells are **granulocyte-macrophage CSF (GM-CSF), granulocyte CSF (G-CSF)** and **macrophage CSF (M-CSF)**. The hormone **erythropoietin (EPO)** is required for a myeloid progenitor cell to become an erythrocyte. A **thrombopoietin** stimulates myeloid progenitor cells to differentiate to megakaryocytes.

CHECK YOUR UNDERSTANDING

- What changes happen with hematopoietic tissue with an organism's aging?

- Which substances regulate hematopoiesis?

17.2 Erythrocytes

Erythrocytes, or red blood cells (RBCs), are responsible for transport of oxygen and carbon dioxide between the lungs and body tissues. They make up more than 99 percent of all blood formed elements. Erythrocytes lack a nucleus and organelles. Rather, they are considered formed elements, like platelets, but historically it happened that they were called cells, and this label has stuck to them. The process of erythrocytes' production is called **erythropoiesis**. Erythropoiesis is controlled by the hormone EPO, which stimulates red bone marrow to increase erythrocyte production.

Erythrocyte Structure and Function

Erythrocytes are very small (4–8 μm), usually biconcave, flexible cells. The biconcave shape increases the cell's surface area by 20 to 30 percent, thereby increasing the rate of oxygen diffusion inside the RBC. The absence of a nucleus and organelles frees space for the red-pigmented protein **hemoglobin**, responsible for transport of oxygen. The absence of organelles means that erythrocytes cannot perform most of the processes associated with oxygen consumption, and they deliver all oxygen accumulated inside the cell to tissues without leaving something for themselves. Thus, the absence of a nucleus and organelles enables erythrocytes to carry respiratory gasses more efficiently. Erythrocytes of reptiles and birds are different from mammalian. They are ovoid and have a nucleus (fig. 17.4).

The biconcave shape helps erythrocyte be very flexible and allows them to squeeze through the smallest capillaries. A special protein called **spectrin** forms a soft elastic lattice frame in an erythrocyte's plasma membrane, which makes this membrane flexible and able to withstand rupture when the erythrocyte is folded. All these allow erythrocytes to stack and line up in a single line inside the capillary. This single file of erythrocytes is called a **rouleau**.

There are three types of hemoglobin: embryonic, fetal and adult. Embryonic hemoglobin is present in the early stages of fetal development. Fetal hemoglobin has a higher affinity for oxygen than adult hemoglobin and is replaced by adult hemoglobin shortly after birth. Dogs do not have fetal or embryonic hemoglobin.

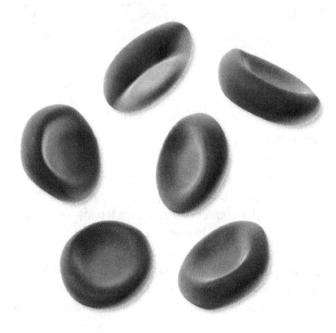

FIGURE 17.4   Red Blood Cells.

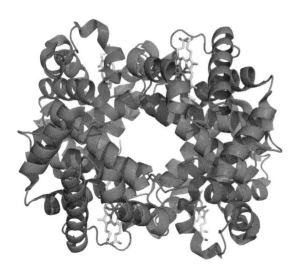

FIGURE 17.5   Hemoglobin.

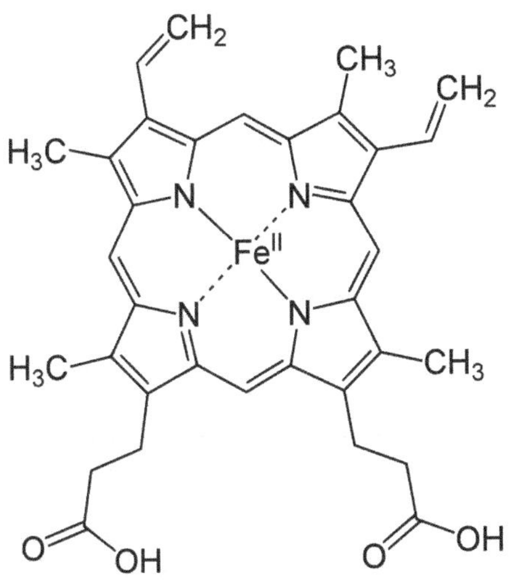

FIGURE 17.6   Heme Group.

Horses do not have embryonic hemoglobin, and their fetal hemoglobin is structurally identical to adult hemoglobin, and therefore some would say that there is no fetal hemoglobin. Pig (and horse) fetal hemoglobin has the same affinity to oxygen as their adult hemoglobin.

Hemoglobin is a protein molecule made of four subunits called **globin**. Two subunits are termed **alpha (α) globin** (or **α chain**), and the other two are known as **beta (β) globin** (or **β chain**) (fig. 17.5). Every globin has a so-called **heme group**; a coordinated compound composed of a **porphyrin ring** with an iron ion (**Fe^{2+}**) in the center (fig. 17.6). Iron creates ionic bonds with an oxygen molecule. Four globin chains altogether have four porphyrin groups with iron in their center. **Fe^{2+}** binds one molecule of oxygen. Thus, one hemoglobin molecule can bind four oxygen molecules and carry them from the lungs to body tissues. Molecules of hemoglobin associated with oxygen are called **oxygenated** or **oxyhemoglobin**. Hemoglobin that carries maximal four oxygen molecules is called **fully saturated**, whereas hemoglobin molecules with one to three oxygen molecules are called **partially saturated**. Hemoglobin without oxygen is termed **deoxygenated** or **deoxyhemoglobin**.

Globin molecule also can create weak chemical bonds with carbon dioxide. Carbon dioxide binds to the amino group (-NH$_2$) at one end of the globin molecule. It does not bind with Fe^{2+} and thus does not compete with oxygen. This means that oxygen and carbon dioxide are transported independently and do not interfere with each other's transport.

CHECK YOUR UNDERSTANDING

- What advantage does an erythrocyte get when it loses its nucleus and organelles?

- Why do oxygen and carbon dioxide transports not affect each other?

- How many molecules of oxygen can carry one molecule of hemoglobin?

Life Span of Erythrocytes

The absence of a nucleus and organelles in an erythrocyte results in its inability to maintain cellular homeostasis and repair damage. As a result, erythrocytes have a comparatively short life span and cannot reproduce through mitosis. A normal erythrocyte life span varies among species. In mice it is 20–30 days; in cats 68 days; and in pigs 85 days. Dogs and humans have an average erythrocyte life span of 120 days, horses and sheep 150 days, and cows 160 days.

The process of erythrocytes aging is called **senescence**. It is characterized by the decrease of enzymes' activity and loss of cell membrane elasticity. About 1 percent of cells reach their terminal age and are removed from circulation daily. There are two processes of erythrocyte destruction: **extravascular** and **intravascular**. Extravascular destruction of erythrocytes takes place in the liver, spleen, and lymph nodes by the mononuclear phagocyte system. Macrophages of the mononuclear phagocyte system phagocytize around 90 percent of aged erythrocytes. The aging red blood cell undergoes changes in the plasma membrane, making it susceptible to selective recognition by macrophages and subsequent phagocytosis. The other 10 percent are destroyed intravascular. This process takes place inside blood vessels. Erythrocytes undergo a process termed **eryptosis**, a special mechanism of programmed cell death. In a healthy organism, eryptosis has the same rate as erythrocyte production, which secures a balance of circulating red blood cells.

Hemoglobin from the phagocytized erythrocyte is decomposed into heme and globin. Globin is a protein that is hydrolyzed into amino acids that later are reused for synthesis of other proteins. The heme group is decomposed into Fe^{2+} and a green pigment **biliverdin**. The enzyme **biliverdin reductase** converts biliverdin into a yellow pigment called **bilirubin**. Bilirubin is excreted into the bloodstream, where albumin transports it to the liver. In the liver it is conjugated and excreted into bile, which in turn is excreted into the small intestine. In the small intestine bilirubin is converted to **urobilinogen**. Some amount of the urobilinogen is converted in the large intestine to **stercobilin**, a brown pigment that gives its color to feces. Another part of urobilinogen is reabsorbed back to the blood flow. In the kidneys, this compound is converted to **urobilin**, which becomes a component of urine.

Iron is a very valuable element. Its absorption from nutrients is a complex and slow process. That is why an organism is "interested" in conserving available iron and preventing its loss. The iron from heme is released and transported by a globulin protein called **transferrin** to the liver or spleen. Here iron is bound by the proteins **ferritin** and **hemosiderin** for storage. **Transferrin** also transports iron to the red bone marrow for reuse in erythropoiesis. A small amount of iron is lost every day in sweat, urine, and feces. Iron also may be lost in injury with bleeding and menstruation. This iron has to be replaced by dietary iron (fig. 17.7).

CHECK YOUR UNDERSTANDING

- How are erythrocytes and hemoglobin recycled?

- What is the fate of iron after hemoglobin decomposition?

- Describe the difference between extravascular and intravascular erythrocyte decomposition.

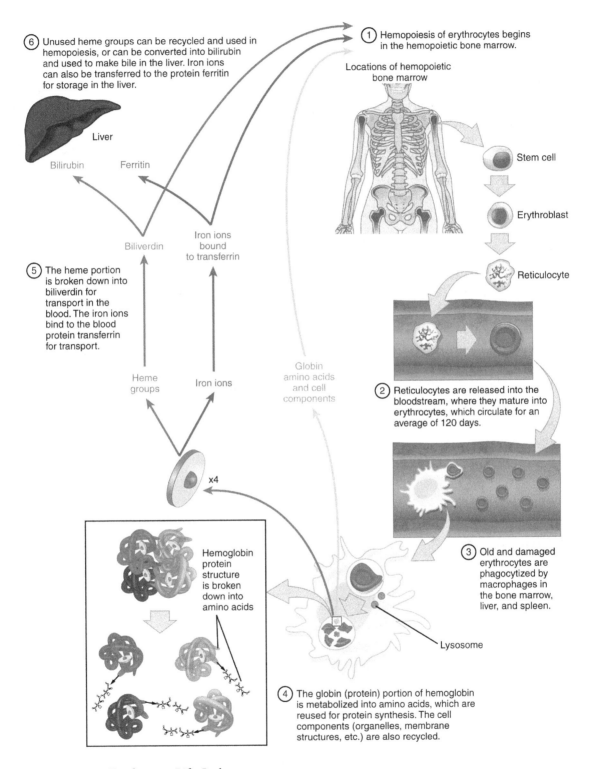

⑥ Unused heme groups can be recycled and used in hemopoiesis, or can be converted into bilirubin and used to make bile in the liver. Iron ions can also be transferred to the protein ferritin for storage in the liver.

Liver

Bilirubin   Ferritin

Biliverdin

Iron ions bound to transferrin

⑤ The heme portion is broken down into biliverdin for transport in the blood. The iron ions bind to the blood protein transferrin for transport.

Heme groups   Iron ions

Globin amino acids and cell components

x4

Hemoglobin protein structure is broken down into amino acids

① Hemopoiesis of erythrocytes begins in the hemopoietic bone marrow.

Locations of hemopoietic bone marrow

Stem cell

Erythroblast

Reticulocyte

② Reticulocytes are released into the bloodstream, where they mature into erythrocytes, which circulate for an average of 120 days.

③ Old and damaged erythrocytes are phagocytized by macrophages in the bone marrow, liver, and spleen.

Lysosome

④ The globin (protein) portion of hemoglobin is metabolized into amino acids, which are reused for protein synthesis. The cell components (organelles, membrane structures, etc.) are also recycled.

FIGURE 17.7   Erythrocyte Life Cycle.

Erythropoiesis

Erythropoiesis is a process of erythrocyte production. Erythrocytes constitute 99 percent of the total amount of all formed elements. The rate of the process is controlled by the hormone erythropoietin. The EPO production is triggered by low oxygen in the blood flow. Chemoreceptors in the kidneys monitor oxygen concentration and, when its level drops below the norm, stimulate EPO release. Erythrocyte production requires iron, vitamin B, and amino acids.

At the beginning, the myeloid stem cell, stimulated by the numerous CSFs, forms a progenitor cell. The progenitor cell develops into a **proerythroblast**, which is a large, nucleated cell. The proerythroblast develops into the smaller **erythroblast**. The erythroblast begins to actively produce hemoglobin, and its nucleus is expelled out of the cell in a process termed **denucleation**. Finally, when the nucleus is expelled and cytoplasm becomes loaded with hemoglobin, the erythroblast develops into a **normoblast**. The next stage of erythrocyte development is called a **reticulocyte**. The reticulocyte loses most of its organelles, except the endoplasmic reticulum and associated with this reticulum ribosomes. Ribosomes continue to produce hemoglobin. The development of the myeloid stem cell into reticulocyte takes about five days. The reticulocyte enters the bloodstream, where it circulates one to two days before it becomes a mature erythrocyte. The whole process may be described by the following sequence of transformations: **myeloid stem cell → proerythroblast → erythroblast → normoblast → reticulocyte → erythrocyte** (fig. 17.3).

Reticulocytes that enter the bloodstream constitute 0.5 to 2.0 percent of circulating red blood cells. A reticulocyte percentage higher than "normal" can be a sign of anemia. The number of reticulocytes is a good indicator of bone marrow activity: it represents recent production and allows for the determination of reticulocyte count and the reticulocyte production index. When there is an increased production of red blood cells to overcome chronic or severe loss of mature red blood cells, such as in hemolytic anemia, there is often a markedly high number and percentage of reticulocytes. A very high number of reticulocytes in the blood can be described as **reticulocytosis**. Abnormally low numbers of reticulocytes can be attributed to aplastic anemia, pernicious anemia, bone marrow malignancies, problems of erythropoietin production associated with kidney disorder, various vitamin or mineral deficiencies (iron, vitamin B_{12}, and folic acid), and other causes of anemia due to poor RBC production.

CHECK YOUR UNDERSTANDING

- What hormone influences erythropoiesis?

- Erythrocytes originate from which hematopoietic line?

- What is the difference between reticulocyte and erythrocyte?

17.3   Leukocytes

Role of White Blood Cells in an Organism

Leukocytes are white blood cells that form an organism's immune system. Their major function is defending an organism against pathogens. Leukocytes constitute less than 1 percent of blood formed elements. They are 1.5–3 times larger than erythrocytes, have a nucleus and all organelles, and do not have hemoglobin. Most leukocytes are wandering cells and are remarkably flexible. Many of them spend a short time in the blood flow. Eventually, they leave the bloodstream and populate tissues. Flexible leukocytes squeeze through gaps between endothelial cells in walls of blood vessels, a process termed **diapedesis**. Leukocytes move into the tissue, attracted by chemicals produced by damaged, dead, infected cells, or pathogens. Attraction of motile cells by chemicals is termed **positive chemotaxis**.

Leukocyte are classified in two distinguish classes: **granulocytes** and **agranulocytes**. These terms reflect the presence or absence of visible granules in their cytoplasm. These granules are vesicles containing chemicals that serve to facilitate special functions performed by these cells.

An abnormal number of leukocytes is characteristic of different pathological processes in an organism. A low leukocyte count, known as a **leukopenia**, compromises the organism's ability to defend from infectious diseases. The abnormally high number of white blood cells is called **leukocytosis**. Leukocytosis is characteristic of an infected or highly stressed organism. A **differential count**, or **white blood cell differential count**, is a measure of the amount of each type of white blood cells in blood. Infection, tissue necrosis, red bone marrow failure, and cancers all affect the total amount of white blood cells and the number of particular leukocytes. That is why a differential blood cell count is a very important part of any diagnostic procedure. For example, acute infection and tissue necrosis are characterized by an increased neutrophil count. Decreased neutrophil count called **neutropenia** may be a result of a high rate of neutrophil usage or destruction faster than the bone marrow can produce them; or when their production in the bone marrow is reduced. In the first case it may be a chronic infection or autoimmune disease. In the second case it can be a sign of red bone marrow cancer. The increased eosinophil count may be caused by parasite worms, allergy, or some autoimmune diseases. High basophil count is characteristic of inflammatory reactions during immune response, allergic diseases, or stress reactions. The monocyte number increases in some chronic inflammatory disorders. Abnormally low monocytes may result from steroid therapy, for example, or long usage of prednisone drugs. Lymphocytes fight different pathogenic agents, but their primary targets are viruses. That is why an abnormally high lymphocyte count suggests the presence of viral infection. A decreased lymphocyte count can be the result of HIV infection, leukemia, or sepsis.

CHECK YOUR UNDERSTANDING

- What are the main functions of white blood cells?

- What two main classes of leukocytes do you know?

- What does differential count mean, and how is it clinically useful?

Granulocytes

Granulocytes are leukocytes that after special staining have well-visible granules in their cytoplasm. Different granulocytes have an affinity to different stains, and according to this affinity, granulocytes are classified in three groups: **neutrophils**, **eosinophils**, and **basophils**.

Neutrophils

Neutrophils are the most numerous leukocytes. They constitute 50 to 70 percent of the total number of leukocytes. Neutrophils got their name from their neutral or pale-colored granules. A neutrophil is around 1.5 times larger than an erythrocyte. Their nucleus has varying shape and is divided into three to five well-visible lobes connected by narrow nucleoplasm bridges (fig. 17.8). This specific characteristic has suggested another name for these white blood cells—**polymorphonuclear leukocytes**. They are the most active phagocytes and usually arrive first at the area of an infection or injury. A white-yellow, yellow, or yellow-brown exudate formed at the site of inflammation during bacterial or fungal infection, called **pus**, contains mostly neutrophils.

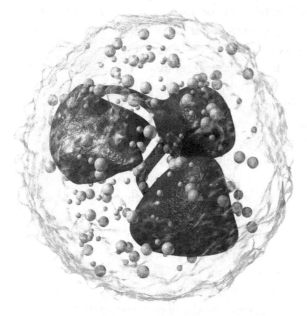

FIGURE 17.8   Neutrophil.

Neutrophils usually remain in circulation for about 10 or 12 hours before they exit the blood vessels and enter the tissue. Neutrophils are the most active type of white blood cell. They arrive first, attracted by cytokines produced by the activated endothelium, mast cells, macrophages, damaged or infected cells, and pathogenic organisms, especially bacteria. In their turn, neutrophils release cytokines, which amplify the inflammatory reaction of other white blood cells. Their number grows dramatically during bacterial infection. In addition to recruiting and activating other cells of the immune system, neutrophils play a key role in the front-line defense against invading pathogens, especially bacteria. Neutrophils attack microorganisms in three ways: **phagocytosis** (ingestion; fig. 17.9), **degradation** (release of anti-microbial compounds), and generation of **neutrophil extracellular traps (NETs)**.

Neutrophils ingest a large amount of microorganisms or organic particles and often become stuffed with digested microorganisms. To be recognized, bacteria must be coated by antibody proteins called **opsonins**, a process known as **antibody opsonization**. Ingested bacteria enter the neutrophil cytoplasm through phagocytosis (see chapter 3, page 73) inside a phagosome. Reactive chemicals

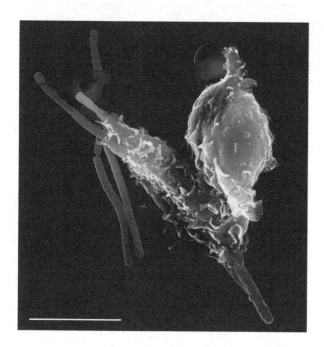

FIGURE 17.9   Neutrophils Engulfing Anthrax Bacteria.

that contain oxygen, called **reactive oxygen species**, and hydrolytic enzymes are secreted inside the phagosome and digest bacteria.

The consumption of oxygen during the generation of reactive oxygen species has been termed the **respiratory burst.** The respiratory burst generates large quantities of superoxide, a reactive oxygen species. Superoxide decays spontaneously or is broken down via enzymes to hydrogen peroxide. Hydrogen peroxide then is converted to hypochlorous acid (HClO). HClO is a weak acid, but its bactericidal properties are enough to kill bacteria. HClO is also necessary for the activation of proteases—enzymes that break down protein molecules.

Neutrophils also release an assortment of proteins in three types of granules (**azurophilic granules**, **specific granules**, and **tertiary granules**) by a process called **degranulation**. The contents of these granules have antimicrobial substances and help combat infection.

Active neutrophils produce neutrophil extracellular traps (NETs): a web of fibers composed of chromatin and serine proteases that trap and kill bacteria. It is suggested that NETs provide a high local concentration of antimicrobial components and bind, disarm, and kill microbes independent of phagocytic uptake. In addition to their possible antimicrobial properties, NETs may serve as a physical barrier that prevents further spread of pathogens. Trapping of bacteria may be a particularly important role for NETs in sepsis. In addition, NETs participate in thrombus formation.

Eosinophils

Eosinophils contain red or pink-orange granules in the cytosol. Typically, they constitute 1 to 4 percent of the total leukocyte number. Their nucleus is subdivided in two lobes, connected by a thin bridge. An eosinophil is about 1.5 times larger in diameter than an erythrocyte. Eosinophils phagocytize numerous antigen-antibody complexes or allergens. They play a special role in defending an organism from parasitic worms. Eosinophils manufacture a number of chemical mediators that attach to worms and immobilize them. An abnormally high number of eosinophils may be a sign of parasitic worm infestation (fig. 17.10).

Basophils

Basophils are 1.5 times larger than erythrocytes. They are the least numerous granulocytes. Basophils have a bilobed nucleus and numerous deep blue-violet granules in the cytosol (fig. 17.11). The primary components of basophil granules are histamine and heparin. Histamine is a strong vasodilator. It also increases capillary permeability, especially at the arterioles side. The heparin is an anticoagulant that prevents blood clot formation.

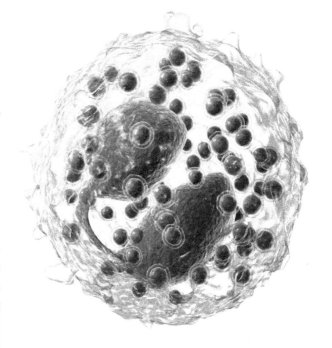

FIGURE 17.10 Eosinophil.

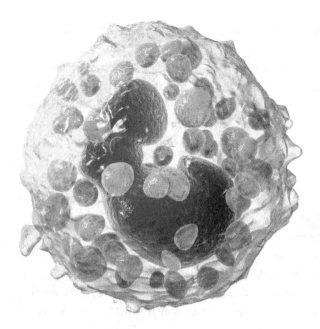

FIGURE 17.11   Basophil.

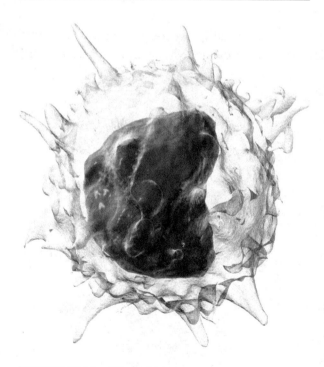

FIGURE 17.12   Monocyte.

Together, both chemicals play a principal role in inflammatory reaction, characterized by swelling, itching, and accumulation of fluids in affected tissue.

Agranulocytes

Agranulocytes also have granules, but these granules are so small that they are almost invisible in light microscope. There are two types of agranulocytes: **lymphocytes** and **monocytes**.

Monocytes

Monocytes are the biggest blood cells. They are three times as large as erythrocytes. Monocytes constitute 2 to 8 percent of the total number of leukocytes. They are easily distinguished from other leukocytes by a kidney-bean shaped nucleus (fig. 17.12). Monocytes circulate within blood about three to five days; after that they exit the bloodstream and move into tissues, where they transform into large phagocytes termed **macrophages**. All macrophages in the body originate from monocytes. They are major housekeepers in an organism that maintain body tissues and keep them clean of bacteria, viruses, dead cells, cellular fragments, and different contaminants. These large phagocytes are found in all tissues, where they patrol for pathogens by amoeboid movement. Macrophages include phagocytes such as dendritic cells, Kupffer cells, alveolar macrophages, microglia, and others. Together, they constitute the **mononuclear phagocyte system**. Macrophages that encourage inflammation are called **M1 macrophages**. They phagocytize microbes and initiate an immune response. M1 macrophages produce nitric oxide (NO) or reactive oxygen intermediates (ROI) to protect against bacteria and viruses. Macrophages that decrease inflammation, promote collagen synthesis, and encourage tissue repair are called **M2 macrophages**.

Additionally, macrophages activate other cells of the immune system. They display antigens of the phagocytized pathogenic agents and by that signal about the presence of this pathogen. Microbial fragments that remain after pathogen digestion are incorporated into a special complex of molecules called the **major histocompatibility complex** or **MHC**. The MHC together with pathogen antigen is exposed at the monocyte cell surface (and macrophages and dendritic cells). This process is called **antigen presentation.** Presented antigen triggers a special immune reaction, when it becomes recognized by T cells (see chapter 18, page 543).

Lymphocytes

Lymphocytes constitute 20 to 40 percent of the total number of white blood cells. Their main residency is lymphatic organs: lymphatic nodes, spleen, thymus, and so on (see chapter 18, page 531). Lymphocytes are comparatively small blood cells with a spherical dark-stained nucleus that occupies almost all space inside the cell and leaves only a narrow rim of light blue cytoplasm. There are three groups of lymphocytes: **T lymphocytes (T cells), B lymphocytes (B cells),** and **natural killer (NK) cells.**

NK cells are so-called cytotoxic lymphocytes. They directly attack and destroy pathogenic cells. They are especially effective in destruction of cancerous cells. NK cells provide rapid responses to virus-infected cells, acting around three days after infection, and respond to tumor formation. NK cells detect the MHC presented on infected cell surfaces and trigger release of cytokines—proteins that cause lysis of a pathogenic cell or its apoptosis. NK cells have a unique ability to recognize stressed cells in the absence of antibodies and the MHC. This ability gives them a very fast immune reaction. They are called "natural killers" because they do not require activation to kill cells that are missing "self" markers of MHC I. This role is especially important because harmful cells that are missing MHC I markers cannot be detected and destroyed by other immune cells, such as T lymphocytes (fig. 17.13).

B and T cells are structurally very similar, but their role in the immune system is different. Active B cells produce and release in blood flow proteins collectively called **antibodies**. Antibodies travel with blood flow and, when they meet an antigen, bind to it. Binding of antibodies to antigens on the surface of pathogenic cells leads to destruction or deactivation of these cells. B cells form functional groups.

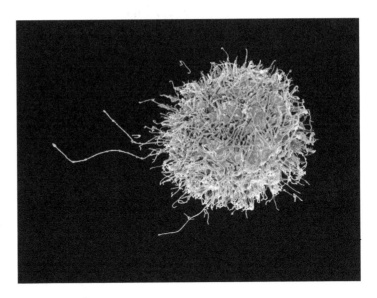

FIGURE 17.13   Natural Killer (NK) Cell.

Each group of B cells produces a particular antibody that binds only to a particular antigen and does not react to others. This ability guarantees a precise specific immune response. T cells also demonstrate specific reaction on particular antigens. Some T cells directly attack cells that carry alien antigens. They are called **cytotoxic T cells**. Another group of T cells does not attack pathogenic invaders, but activates a particular group of B cells that produces an antibody for antigens found by these T cells. They are called **helper T cells** for their ability to facilitate B cells' immune reaction (fig. 17.14; see chapter 18, page 549).

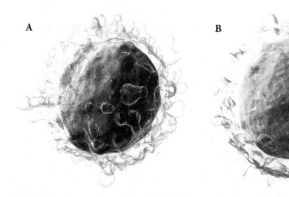

A   B

FIGURE 17.14   Lymphocytes. A. T Cell; B. B Cell.

CHECK YOUR UNDERSTANDING

- How do granulocytes and agranulocytes differ?

- Which type of granulocytes is most numerous, and what is its function?

- What is the function of monocytes?

- How do T cells and B cells differ?

- What type of leukocytes will be increased in an acute bacterial infection?

- What is the unique characteristic of NK cells?

- What leukocytes have an abnormally high count during an acute allergic reaction?

Leukopoiesis

Leukocytes make up less than 0.01 percent of formed elements. Their production is called **leucopoiesis**. Because *leukocyte* is a common name of three different lines of white blood cells, there are three pathways of leukocytes production: **granulocytopoiesis**, **monocytopoiesis**, and **lymphocytopoiesis** (fig. 17.3).

Granulocytopoiesis is a process of production and maturation of granulocytes: neutrophils, eosinophils, and basophils. The process begins within the red bone marrow and proceeds through the next steps (fig. 17.3): **pluripotent hematopoietic stem cell → myeloblast → promyelocyte → eosin/neutron/basophilic myelocyte → metamyelocyte → band cell → granulocytes (eosino/neutron/basophil)**. All three types of granulocytes are derived from myeloid stem cells. This stem cell is stimulated by multi-CSF and GM-CSF to form a progenitor cell. The granulocyte line develops when the progenitor cell forms a **myeloblast** under the influence of G-CSF. The myeloblast ultimately differentiates into one of the three types of granulocytes (fig. 17.3).

Like granulocytes, monocytes are also derived from myeloid stem cells. The myeloid stem cell differentiates into a progenitor cell, and under the influence of M-CSF this cell forms a **monoblast**. This is the monocyte line. Eventually, the monoblast forms a **promonocyte** that differentiates and matures into a **monocyte** (fig. 17.3).

Lymphocytes are derived from **lymphoid stem cells** through the lymphoid line. The lymphoid stem cell differentiates into **B lymphoblasts** or **T lymphoblasts**. B lymphoblasts develops, into B cells and T lymphoblasts develops into T cells. Some lymphoid stem cells differentiate into NK cells (fig. 17.3).

17.4 Platelets

Platelets are not cells. They are cellular fragments. Platelets are the smallest formed elements involved in the process that prevents blood loss from an injured blood vessel, called **hemostasis**. Platelets have no nucleus and organelles. They cannot reproduce by mitosis and are produced de novo from specialized cells known as **megakaryocytes**. Platelets contain different types of granules that house clotting factors and enzymes, a small number of mitochondria, and glycogen, which is necessary to maintain oxidation reactions for production of ATP. They also have a cytoskeleton made of actin and myosin filaments.

Platelet Formation

Formation of platelets begins from hematopoietic stem cells. Their precursor cells are **megakaryoblasts**. Megakaryoblasts belong to the myeloid blood cell line. Megakaryoblasts develop into megakaryocytes. Megakaryocytes are giant cells. Their name reflects the fact that megakaryocytes have a massive nucleus. Megakaryocytes regularly undergo mitosis. Their mitosis is limited by duplication of DNA and duplication of chromosomes, and is not accompanied by cytokinesis (see chapter 3, page 89). As a result, their nucleus becomes large and contains multiple DNA copies.

Some hormones, such as **thrombopoietin**, stimulate megakaryocytes to develop long cytoplasmic extensions filled with cytosol, granules, and some organelles. These extensions protrude through clefts in the bone marrow sinusoids inside the bloodstream. The force of the blood coursing past the arms lops off small pieces that become platelets (fig. 17.15).

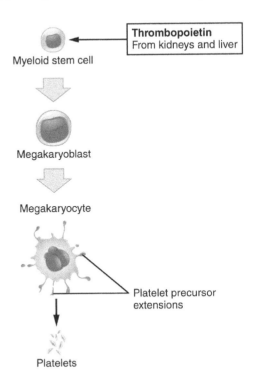

Myeloid stem cell

Thrombopoietin
From kidneys and liver

Megakaryoblast

Megakaryocyte

Platelet precursor extensions

Platelets

FIGURE 17.15   Platelet Formation.

Each arm can give rise to thousands of platelets. Most remain in general circulation, where they have a life span of only seven to ten days. Once platelets have reached old age, the liver and spleen remove them from circulation.

CHECK YOUR UNDERSTANDING

- How are platelets produced?

17.5 Hemostasis

The mechanism that prevents massive blood loss from injured blood vessels is known as **hemostasis**. Hemostasis is organized in a series of events that form a **blood clot**, which "plug" the broken vessel. The process includes five steps: 1) **Vascular spasm** → 2) **platelet plug formation** → 3) **coagulation** → 4) **clot retraction** → 5) **thrombolysis** (fig. 17.16).

Vascular Spasm

Vascular spasm is the first immediate reaction of the blood vessel to injury. Vascular spasm is a result of two processes: vasoconstriction and increase of an interstitial fluid hydrostatic pressure.

Vasoconstriction is produced by vascular smooth muscle cells, and is a first response to injury. When a blood vessel is damaged, an immediate reflex, initiated by local sympathetic pain receptors,

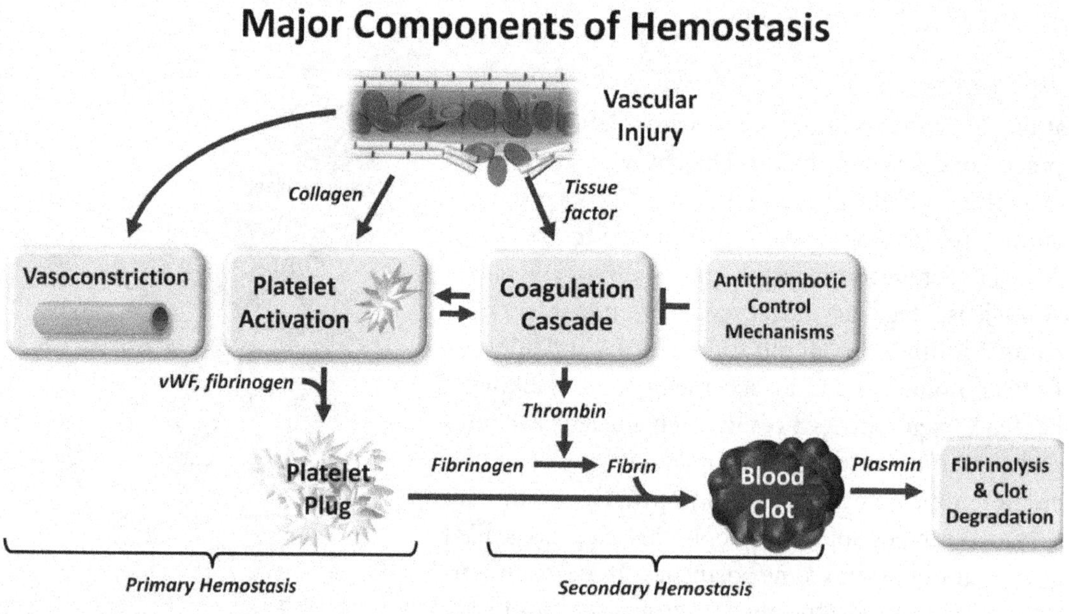

FIGURE 17.16   Hemostasis.

Major Components of Hemostasis

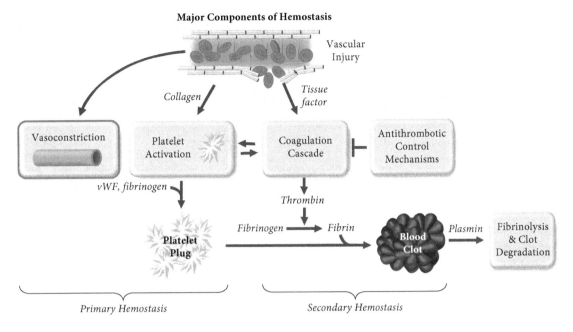

FIGURE 17.17   Vascular Spasm—the First Step of Hemostasis.

causes contraction of smooth muscles in the wall of the injured blood vessel. Normally, endothelial cells release prostacyclin and nitric oxide (NO), which induce relaxation of the smooth muscle cells in the walls of blood vessels. Platelets in blood flow secrete thromboxane A2 and serotonin. Both stimulate smooth muscle cell contractions. In a healthy, undamaged blood vessel, the relaxation prevails. However, damaged endothelial cells cannot produce a sufficient amount of prostacyclin and NO. Platelets accumulated at the injured area increase production of serotonin. As a result, the contraction overcomes relaxation, and smooth muscles in the damaged blood vessel contract. Both sympathetic and chemical influences cause a decrease in blood vessel diameter and diminished blood flow (fig. 17.17).

The damaged vessel loses blood, which accumulates in surrounding tissues, a condition called **hemorrhage**. The tissues fill with blood. The hydrostatic pressure in the surrounding tissue grows and presses from outside on the blood vessel. Both vasoconstriction and high external hydrostatic pressure compress the blood vessel and stop blood from flowing through it (fig. 17.18).

Injury. A blood vessel is injured. Blood with all its content (erythrocytes, white blood cells, etc.) are leaking out of the breaks into an interstitial space.

Vascular spasm. The smooth muscle in the vessel wall contracts near the injury point. Blood hemorrhage, accumulated around breaks presses from outside on the vessel wall. Altogether, it decreases vesseldiameter and reduce blood loss.

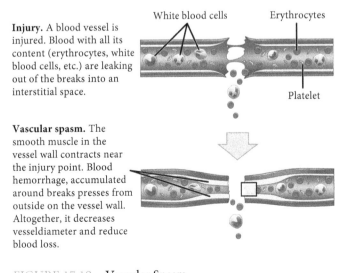

FIGURE 17.18   Vascular Spasm.

CHECK YOUR UNDERSTANDING

- What are two factors that cause vasoconstriction?

- What are the factors that cause smooth muscle contractions?

- How does blood loss affect vessel constriction?

Plug Formation

A vasospasm minimizes blood loss from injured blood vessels. It can completely stop bleeding from the smallest arterioles for a while, but it cannot stop bleeding entirely, especially from a big blood vessel. The next step of hemostasis is a **platelet plug formation (primary hemostasis)** (17.19). Normally, platelets do not stick to each other. However, damaged endothelial cells release a glycoprotein called a **von Willebrand factor (vWF)**. The adventitia of the injured blood vessel exposes its collagen fibers. Contact of platelets with collagen and vWF triggers a series of changes within platelets termed **platelet activation**. Activated platelets release ATP, ADP, serotonin, calcium, clotting factors, and other chemicals from their granules by exocytosis. These factors attract and activate nearby platelets and make them clump together or **aggregate** to form a **platelet plug**. This plug seals the injured vessel temporarily. When platelets come across the injured endothelium cells, they change shape, release granules, and become

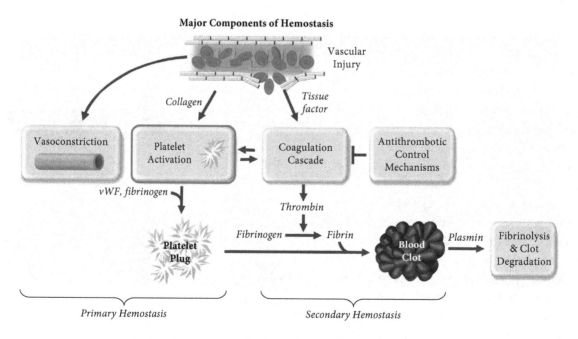

FIGURE 17.19   Platelet Plug Formation—the Second Step of Hemostasis.

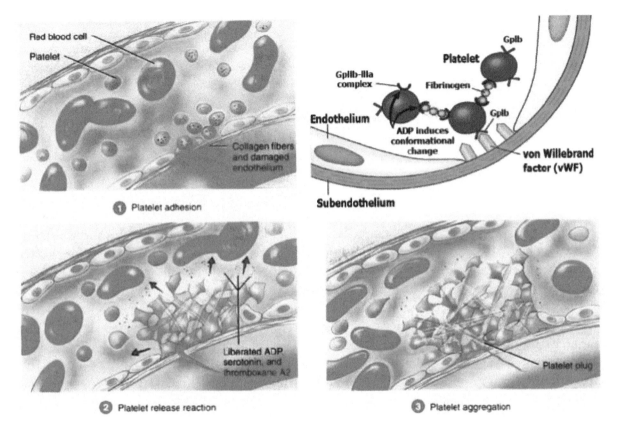

FIGURE 17.20   Plug Formation.

"sticky." Platelets express certain receptors, some of which are used for the adhesion of platelets to collagen. Activated platelets express glycoprotein receptors, which interact with other platelets. Platelets aggregate and adhere to each other. At the same time, they release cytoplasmic granules' chemicals, such as adenosine diphosphate (ADP), serotonin, and thromboxane A2. The ADP attracts more platelets to the affected area; serotonin is a vasoconstrictor; and thromboxane A2 assists in platelet aggregation, vasoconstriction, and degranulation. As more chemicals are released, more platelets stick and release their chemicals. Platelet plug formation proceeds and is maintained through a positive feedback loop (fig. 17.20).

CHECK YOUR UNDERSTANDING

- Describe the role of platelets in hemostasis.

- What factors trigger platelets' aggregation?

Coagulation

The substance that binds platelets, endothelial cells, and other formed elements together and creates a strong clot is a protein called **fibrin**. Fibrin converts the soft, liquid platelet plug into a solid mass by a process of **coagulation** (fig. 17.21). Fibrin is a product of enzymatic transformation of **fibrinogen** (or **factor I**). Fibrinogen is a hydrophilic dissolved in blood plasma glycoprotein. It is produced by hepatocytes in the liver (see chapter 19, page 598) and released to the blood. Some amount of fibrinogen is absorbed and stored in vesicles by megakaryocytes and, from them, transits into platelets. During coagulation the fibrinogen in blood plasma and platelets is converted into fibrin through a series of chemical reactions termed **coagulate cascade** reactions. The process takes place at the surface of damaged endothelial cells. Healthy endothelial cells do not allow platelets to attach. But injured cells get sticky. Platelets aggregate around them and form a plug. The enzymes that maintain the coagulation cascade are collectively known as **clotting factors**. Most of these clotting factors are produced in an inactive form by hepatocytes and constantly circulate in blood. Each factor is named with Roman numeral. Thus, there are clotting factors I–XIII. Historically, each factor got its number in the order of its discovery, but not in the order they participate in the coagulate cascade. That is why the reactions do not proceed in a numerical sequence (fig. 17.22).

Synthesis of factors II, VII, IX, and X requires vitamin K and are known as a vitamin K–dependent factors. Vitamin K is a group of structurally similar, fat-soluble vitamins that are essential for production of the active forms of these clotting factors. Most modern drugs that prevent blood clot formation are designed to prevent conversion of vitamin K in active clotting factors.

There are two pathways of coagulation cascade: the **extrinsic pathway** and the **intrinsic pathway**. In the end both pathways converge and proceed through a **common pathway**, which leads to fibrin formation and its precipitation in blood clot.

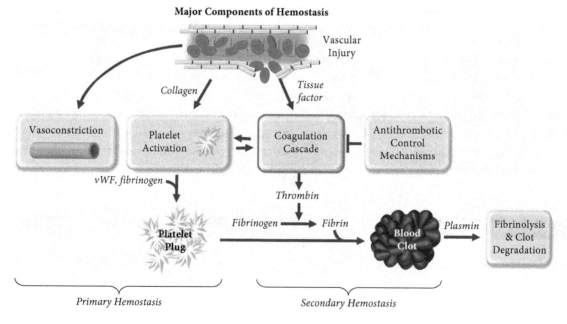

FIGURE 17.21   Third Step of Hemostasis—Coagulation Cascade.

The **extrinsic pathway** got its name because its initiation factor is located outside of the blood flow, or "extrinsic to" it, and for this reason is called the **tissue factor**. The main role of the tissue factor pathway is to generate a thrombin burst, a process by which thrombin, the most important constituent of the coagulation cascade in terms of its positive feedback activation roles, is released very rapidly in 15 seconds. The process develops very quickly in three steps (fig. 17.22):

1. Damaged subendothelial cells secrete tissue factor, also known as **thromboplastin** or **factor III**, and display it in their plasma membrane.
2. The tissue factor binds and forms a complex with an inactive form of **factor VII** and Ca^{2+} circulating in the bloodstream, which converts factor VII into an active **factor VIIa**.
3. The formed complex plays the role of an enzyme, which cleaves inactive **factor X** into active **factor Xa**.

The **intrinsic pathway** (also called the **contact activation pathway**) is less significant to hemostasis under normal physiological conditions than the extrinsic pathway. It is triggered by the damage inside, or "intrinsic to," the injured blood vessel and initiated by platelets. This pathway takes approximately three to six minutes. It requires more clotting factors (VIII, IX, X, XI, and XII) and proceeds through more steps (fig. 17.22):

1. Platelets adhering to a damaged blood vessel wall release **factor XII**. The released factor XII binds with every negatively charged surface and becomes active (**factor XIIa**). The damaged wall of the blood vessel exposes negatively charged collagen fibers, which attract and activate factor XII.
2. Factor XIIa is an enzyme that activates another clotting factor, **factor XI**.

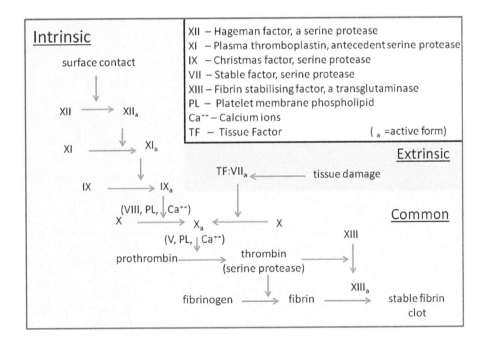

FIGURE 17.22   Blood Coagulation Cascade.

3. Active factor XIa in its turn activates clotting **factor IX**.
4. **Factor IXa** with **Ca²⁺** and platelet factor 3 (**PF₃**) forms a large enzyme complex that converts inactive **factor VIII** into its active form (**factor VIIIa**).
5. In a last step of the intrinsic pathway, factor VIIIa converts inactive factor X to active factor Xa.

From this point the intrinsic and extrinsic pathways proceed to the end through a **common pathway**. In reality, both pathways depend on each other to be completed. A deficiency in any clotting factor can disrupt the entire coagulation cascade. It is also very important to note that the intrinsic pathway is not activated by just collagen fibers, but by the exposure to any negatively charged surface, including a glass test tube. For this reason, before usage a blood test tube has to be treated with anticoagulant (heparin, for example) to prevent clot formation.

The **common pathway** finalizes the clot formation with production of fibrin. It proceeds through four steps (fig. 17.22):

1. **Factor Xa** combines with **factors II** and **V, Ca²⁺**, and platelet factor 3 (**PF₃**) to form **prothrombin activator**.
2. Prothrombin activator converts inactive **prothrombin** into active enzyme thrombin.
3. Thrombin transforms blood-soluble fibrinogen into insoluble fibrin.
4. **Factor XIII** is activated in the presence of **Ca²⁺**. Activated **factor XIIIa** stabilizes fibrin monomers and binds them into a network of fibrin polymer, which forms a framework of a developing clot. This fibrin web-like network traps big protein molecules and blood formed elements.

Like a platelet plug formation, the clotting cascade is controlled by a positive feedback. Thus, thrombin activates factors V and VIII. These factors' activity results in production of thrombin. The increased amount of thrombin leads to activation of more factors V and VIII, and amplification of the clot formation. The initiated intrinsic or extrinsic pathway continues until the final step, clot formation, is reached. The size of the clot is limited. Thrombin is either depleted by being trapped in the clot or quickly degraded by enzymes and, thus, removed from the process (fig. 17.23).

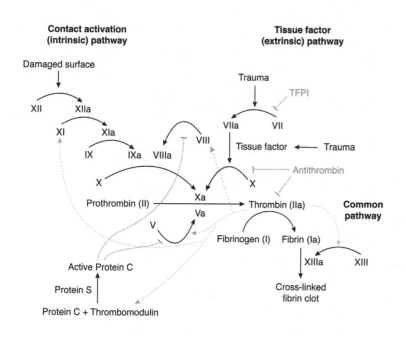

FIGURE 17.23   Regulation of Coagulation Cascade.

- What are the main elements of the coagulation cascade?

- How do the intrinsic and extrinsic pathways differ?

- What is the final step of the common pathway?

Clot Retraction

Formation of a blood clot is necessary to stop bleeding and prevent blood loss. However, the clot cannot remain forever. To return to a normal state, the blood clot has to be removed and blood flow has to be restored. The elimination of the blood clot from the blood vessel includes two processes: **clot retraction** and **thrombolysis**.

Platelets have a cytoskeleton made of a contractile actin and myosin proteins. It makes platelets able to contract. Trapped by a fibrin web, platelets contract and squeeze serum out of the clot. This makes the clot smaller and dryer. The small clot pulls the sides of the blood vessel closer, which facilitates the blood wall healing.

Thrombolysis

When the blood vessel is healed, the clot has to be removed to restore normal blood flow.

The process of dissolving a blood clot is called **thrombolysis** (fig. 17.24). Thrombolysis begins with the breakdown of the fibrin network that cements the clot together, a process known as **fibrinolysis** (fig. 17.25):

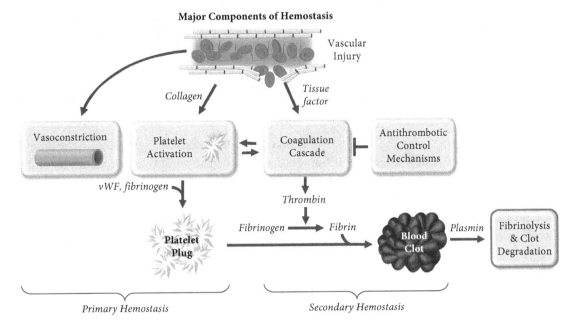

FIGURE 17.24   Clot Degradation Is the Last Step of Hemostasis.

1. Endothelial cells release an enzyme called **tissue plasminogen activator**, or **tPA**.

2. An inactive form of protein called **plasminogen** constantly circulates in the bloodstream. This protein has a high affinity and actively creates chemical bonds with fibrin molecules. Within a few days after clot formation, it becomes saturated with plasminogen molecules bound to fibrin. The tPA released by endothelial cells transforms inactive plasminogen into an active **enzyme plasmin**.

3. Plasmin break down both fibrin and fibrinogen molecules. Degraded fibrin

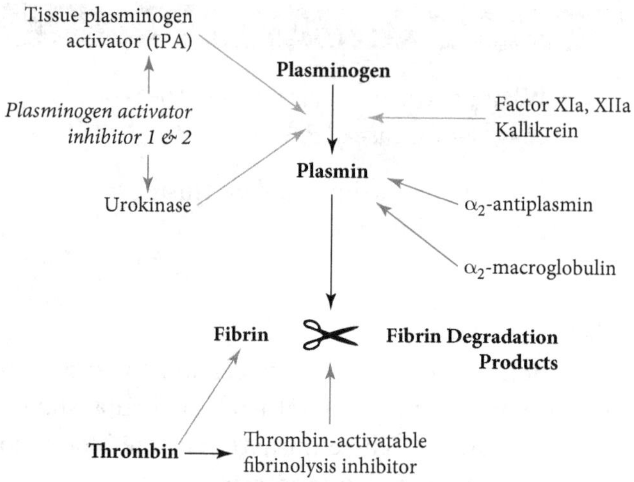

FIGURE 17.25   Fibrinolysis.

does not hold the clot, whose components fall apart and dissociate from the endothelial cells. Dissolved clot components are moved out by the blood flow.

Thus, the whole hemostasis process consists of a number of sequential steps, the principal of which are: **vascular spasm → platelet plug formation → coagulation → clot retraction → thrombolysis**.

CHECK YOUR UNDERSTANDING

- What is the mechanism of clot retraction?

- What are the roles of tPA and plasmin in thrombolysis?

Factors Regulating Blood Clotting

Blood clotting is tightly controlled. Different substances are required for the proper functioning of the coagulation cascade. Ca^{2+} and phospholipids are required for formation of the prothrombin complex to function. Calcium mediates the binding of the complexes on factor Xa and factor IXa to the phospholipid surfaces expressed by platelets. Vitamin K is essential for synthesis of factors II, VII, IX, and X. The enzyme **vitamin K epoxide reductase (VKORC)** restores vitamin K back to its active form. VKORC is pharmacologically important as a target of anticoagulant drugs, such as warfarin and different forms of coumarins (for example, acenocoumarol, phenprocoumon, ducumarol). These drugs create a deficiency of reduced vitamin K by blocking VKORC and inhibit production of clotting factors.

Endothelial cells produce chemicals that regulate the first and second stages of clot formation. Two of these chemicals are **prostacyclin**, which inhibits platelet activation, and **nitric oxide**, which causes vasodilation. Prostacyclin belongs to a large group of chemicals known as prostaglandins. It inhibits platelet activation and is also an effective vasodilator. Like many other prostaglandins, prostacyclin causes

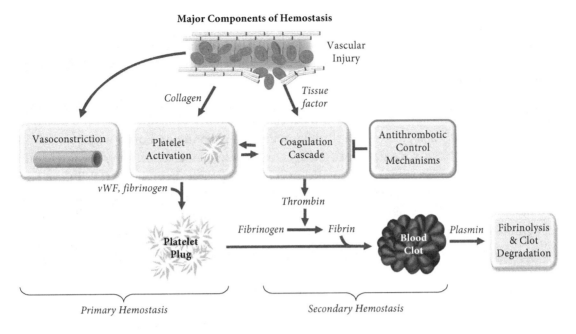

FIGURE 17.26   Control of the Thrombus Formation.

inflammation. Anti-inflammatory drugs such as ibuprofen inhibit prostaglandin formation. Thus, usage of these drugs may increase risk of clot formation, and their intake has to be stopped before surgery.

Endothelial cells and hepatocytes also produce a number of chemicals collectively called **anticoagulants** that inhibit coagulation. Anticoagulants include **antithrombin III**, **heparan sulfate**, and **protein C**. Antithrombin III binds and inhibits the activity of both factor Xa and thrombin. It inhibits thrombin that has already formed and prevents the formation of new thrombin. Heparan sulfate is a polysaccharide that stimulates antithrombin III activity. Active protein C catalyzes reactions that break down factors Va and VIIIa. This protein is activated by another enzyme, **protein S** (fig. 17.23).

CHECK YOUR UNDERSTANDING

- How does prostacyclin regulate hemostasis?

- What is the function of antithrombin III?

- Why does blockage of VKORC by warfarin prevent clot formation?

Disorders of Blood Clotting

A medical condition characterized by inability to control blood clot formation is termed a **clotting disorder**. A clotting disorder can be classified in two principal groups: 1) **bleeding disorders** characterized by inability or low ability of clot formation, and 2) **hypercoagulation disorders** characterized by improper clot formation when there are no healthy reasons for it.

Bleeding disorders increase blood loss. Often, they are associated with clotting proteins' deficiency. For example, **hemophilia A** is caused by a shortage of factor VIII, and **hemophilia B** by low factor IX. Most of these diseases result from mutations in gene-coded clotting factors and are inheritable. They can be treated by replacement of the missing clotting factor with periodic infusions.

Hypercoagulation disorders are characterized by inappropriate clot formation, a medical condition called **thrombosis**. The clot, or **thrombus**, obstructs blood flow and can completely stop it, causing an ischemic effect. In addition, a piece of the thrombus, called a **thromboembolus**, may detach from the thrombus and move with the blood flow until it lodges in a smaller blood vessel. The place where a thrombus most often develops is in leg veins, a condition called **deep vein thrombosis (DVT)**. An embolus originated in DVT can move through the vena cava to the heart, lodge in the pulmonary arteries, and cause a dangerous condition called **a pulmonary embolism**. Other emboli can occlude blood vessels in the brain and cause **stroke**, or stick into a coronary artery and cause a **myocardial infarction**.

VETERINARY APPLICATION

Von Willebrand's disease is a blood disease caused by a deficiency of von Willebrand factor (vWF), an adhesive glycoprotein involved in platelet plug formation. The condition causes excessive bleeding following an injury.

vWF is an autosomal trait, which both males and females express and transmit genetically and with equal frequency. This is the most common hereditary blood-clotting disorder in dogs, occurring with more frequency in some breeds, including German shepherds, Doberman pinschers, standard poodles, Shetland sheepdogs, and golden retrievers.

Symptoms include spontaneous hemorrhage from mucosal surfaces, bleeding nose, blood in the feces (black or bright red blood), blood in urine, bleeding gums, bleeding from the vagina (excessively), bruising of skin, prolonged bleeding after trauma, and blood loss anemia.

A clinical diagnosis of von Willebrand disease is based on a specific measurement of plasma vWF concentration bound to the antigen. The length of time that it takes for platelets to plug a small injury is measured with a test called the buccal mucosa bleeding time (BMBT).

Von Willebrand disease can't be cured. But it can be managed. The treatment includes controlling bleeding, reducing the number of bleeding events, and correcting any underlying conditions that might be contributors to the disorder.

Blood Typing

A blood type refers to the presence, absence, or variation of glycoproteins on the surface of red blood cells. Glycoproteins on the plasma membrane, which are signaling molecules that play a role in self-recognition, are known as **antigens**. At the same time, blood plasma may contain chemicals called **antibodies** that have affinity with antigens and create with them chemical bonds, a process called **agglutination**. There is a rule: blood that has erythrocytes with particular antigens on their membranes never has antibodies that forms chemical bonds (**agglutinate**) with these antigens. Thus, every blood contains one or another combination of antigens and antibodies called **blood type**. Humans, for example, have four main blood types and a number of additional types (fig. 17.27). In veterinary practice there are many different blood types. In dogs, more than a dozen blood types have been identified. In cats there have been three blood groups described but there are likely to be more.

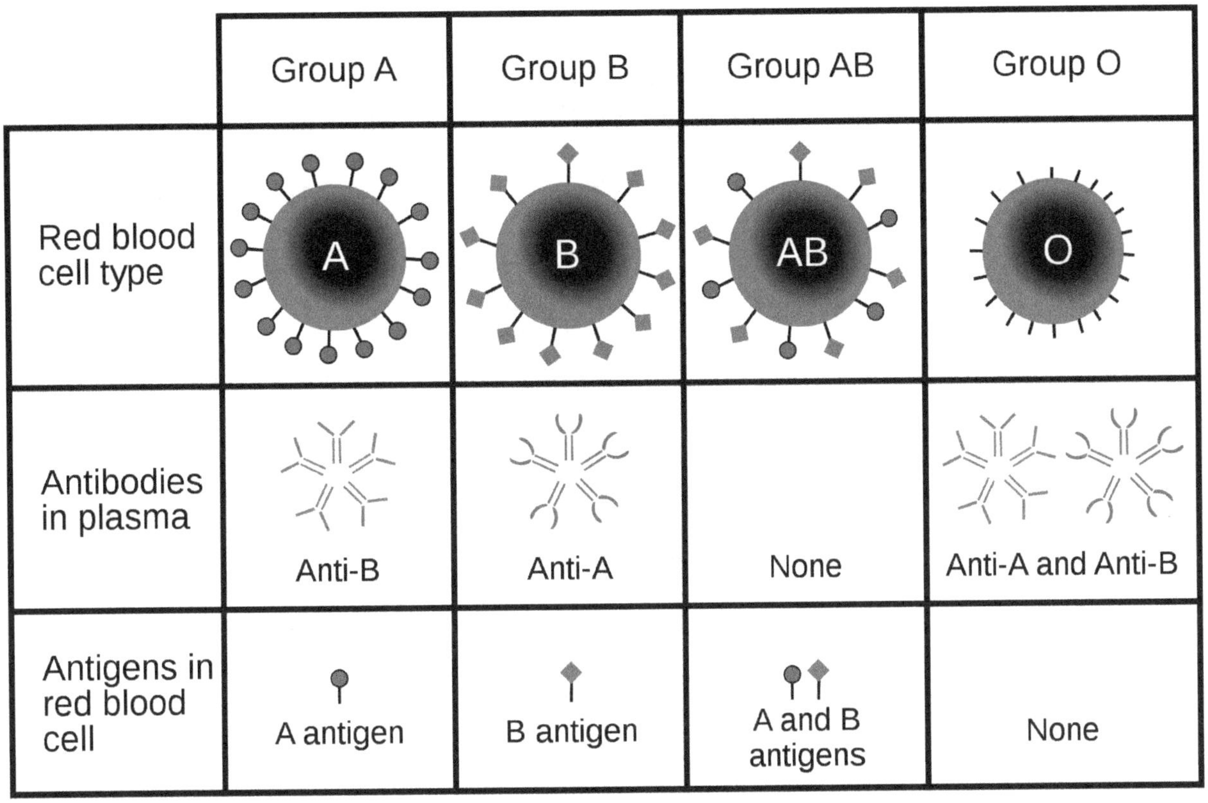

	Group A	Group B	Group AB	Group O
Red blood cell type	A	B	AB	O
Antibodies in plasma	Anti-B	Anti-A	None	Anti-A and Anti-B
Antigens in red blood cell	A antigen	B antigen	A and B antigens	None

FIGURE 17.27   Human Blood Types.

The most widely used blood grouping system in dogs is the **dog erythrocyte antigen (DEA) system**. There are eight blood groups within this system: DEA 1 (DEA 1.1 and DEA 1.2) and DEA2–DEA 7. The condition of a particular blood type presence is termed positive. When it is absent, the condition is termed negative. Often, rottweilers, Labrador retrievers, and golden retrievers have DEA 1.1 or DEA 1.2 positive blood types, and Greyhounds and German shepherds are frequently DEA 1.1 and DEA 1.2 negative. For this reason, greyhounds are commonly used as donors. The reason blood types are considered important is that the immune system of DEA-negative dogs recognizes DEA-positive as a foreign substance and attacks it. This can lead to severe transfusion reactions if a negative dog receives blood from a DEA-positive donor. Dogs do not have natural antibodies against other blood groups. There is no major risk for the first transfusion. Compatibility tests are not required for a dog's first blood transfusion. Antibodies form within five to seven days of the first transfusion, and consequently, if a second transfusion is required five days later than the original transfusion, compatibility tests are necessary. Dogs can be positive for one DEA 1.1 or DEA 1.2 or negative for both DEA 1.1 and DEA 1.2. DEA 1.1 and DEA 1.2 are the most antigenic, and hence ideally a donor would be DEA 1.1 and DEA 1.2 negative. Transfusion reactions can occur when DEA 1.1- and DEA 1.2-negative dogs receive DEA 1.1- or DEA 1.2-positive blood.

Neonatal isoerythrolysis is a veterinary condition when a DEA-negative female who has previously been sensitized to DEA 1.1-positive blood is mated to a DEA 1.1-positive male.

Cats have an **AB** blood group system and inherit blood types as a simple dominant trait, where A is dominant over B. Cats have three blood groups: **type A**, **type B**, or **type AB**. Group A, which can be either A/A or A/B, is the most common blood type of domestic short- and long-haired cats. Group B, which is always B/B, is very common in Devon rex, Persians, British shorthair, Somali, Himalayan, and Birman breeds. Rarely, cats can also be group AB. Cats with blood type A have antibody B in their blood plasma. Cats with blood type B have A antibody in blood plasma; and cats with blood type AB have no circulating antibodies in their blood plasma. Antibody A reacts only on antigen A, and antibody B agglutinates only antigen B. A mismatched blood transfusion can lead to a life-threatening reaction immediately after a first transfusion. Group A cats have low titres of anti-B antibodies; hence, giving group A cats group B blood will cause destruction of red blood cells and a mild transfusion reaction. Group B cats have high titres of anti-A antibodies, and giving group B cats type A blood can result in a potentially fatal transfusion reaction. Type AB cats do not have anti-A or anti-B alloantibodies and can receive type A/B or A blood (table 17.1).

TABLE 17.1   Blood Group Incompatibility in Cats

Donor Group	Recipient Group	Transfusion Reaction
A	A	None
B	B	None
B	A	Slight
A	B	Potentially fatal
AB	AB	None
A	AB	None

Antibodies can be transmitted in milk, putting kittens at risk if they are a different blood type from their mother. Even a few drops of AB mismatched blood can be fatal to a cat. This is also important when breeding cats, as kittens with type A blood can have a fatal reaction (called **neonatal isoerythrolysis**) if they drink milk containing antibodies from a type B queen.

CHECK YOUR UNDERSTANDING

- What determines blood type?

- What is the difference between dog and cat blood types?

- How it possible for a queen with blood type B to have a kitten with blood type A?

CHAPTER SUMMARY

- The science that studies blood forming tissues, blood, and disorders related to it is called **hematology**. Blood has three main functions: transportation, regulation, and protection.

- Blood is a special type of connective tissue. It has formed elements—blood cells and cellular fragments called **platelets** or **thrombocytes,** and matrix called **blood plasma**.

- The hematocrit is a percentage of erythrocytes in blood. Fast spinning of blood sample in a centrifuge separates it in three fractures: 1) a light fracture, called blood plasma, accumulates on the top; it forms about 55 percent of total blood volume; 2) erythrocytes precipitate at the bottom and account for 44 percent; 3) white blood cells and platelets sandwich between them and form a tiny **buffy coat**.

- The hematocrit correlates with ability of the blood to transport oxygen, called **blood oxygen carrying capacity**. An increase of the hematocrit causes an increase in the oxygen carrying capacity and vice versa. The hematocrit varies among different species and even the same individual. It is high among young organisms and decreases with aging. Adult males have a hematocrit higher than females.

- Water makes up 92 to 95 percent of blood plasma. Proteins constitute 6 to 8 percent. Other components include glucose, clotting factors, electrolytes, hormones, respiratory gases, and wastes.

- Plasma proteins create blood osmotic pressure. It is always higher than interstitial fluid osmotic pressure. The difference between them is called **colloid osmotic pressure**. Colloid osmotic pressure draws water from the interstitial space into capillaries. The decrease of plasma proteins' level results in accumulation of water in the interstitial space, known as **edema**.

- **Albumins** make up 58 percent of plasma proteins. Albumins are responsible for the colloid osmotic pressure. They also serve as transport proteins that carry ions, hormones, and lipid molecules.

- **Globulins** constitute about 37 percent of plasma proteins. **Alpha globulins** and **beta globulins** are carriers that transport hydrophobic compounds: lipids, steroid hormones, some metals, and ions. **Gamma globulins** are also called **immunoglobulins** or **antibodies**. They are part of the immune system. **Fibrinogen** is a fibrous protein that constitutes about 4 percent of plasma proteins. Together with other clotting proteins, it is responsible for blood clot formation. **Regulatory proteins**—a small, less than 1 percent— group of plasma proteins, control chemical reactions in blood.

- Production of new blood cells is called **hematopoiesis**. It concentrates in **red bone marrow**, mainly in the pelvis, cranium, vertebrae, and sternum. With aging the total amount of red bone marrow decreases and is restricted to the long bones of the axial skeleton, such as the femur and tibia.

- Hematopoiesis starts with stem cells called **hemocytoblasts**. Hemocytoblasts produce two groups of cells: **myeloid** and **lymphoid lines**. Red blood cells, white blood cells (except lymphocytes), and platelets originate from myeloid cells; lymphocytes originate from lymphoid cells.

- Hematopoietic cells development is controlled by **colony-stimulating factors (CSFs)**. Three processes— **erythropoiesis**, **leucopoiesis**, and **thrombopoiesis**—lead to development of different blood cells. Key players in hematopoiesis are glycoprotein growth factors, called **interleukins**. Other factors are 1) **granulocyte-macrophage CSF (GM-CSF)**, 2) **granulocyte CSF (G-CSF)**, and 3) **macrophage CSF (M-CSF)**. The hormone **erythropoietin** (**EPO**) is required for a myeloid cell to become an erythrocyte. A **thrombopoietin** stimulates development of megakaryocytes.

- Erythrocytes transport oxygen and carbon dioxide. They make up more than 99 percent of all blood formed elements. Erythrocytes are usually small, biconcave, flexible cells without a nucleus or organelles. Erythrocytes of reptiles and birds are ovoid and have a nucleus.

- The biconcave shape makes an erythrocyte flexible and allows it to squeeze through the smallest capillaries. Protein **spectrin** forms a soft elastic lattice frame in plasma membrane that makes the membrane flexible and able to withstand rupture when the erythrocyte is folded.

- Protein hemoglobin has four subunits: 2 **alpha (α) globin** (or α chain) and 2 **beta (β) globin** (or β chain). Every globin has **heme group**: a **porphyrin ring** with Fe^{2+} in the center. Fe^{2+} binds one molecule of oxygen. One hemoglobin molecule can bind four oxygen molecules. Hemoglobin loaded with oxygen is called **oxygenated** or **oxyhemoglobin**. Hemoglobin that carries four O_2 molecules is called **saturated**, whereas hemoglobin with one to three O_2 molecules is called **unsaturated**. Hemoglobin without oxygen is termed **deoxygenated** or **deoxyhemoglobin**.

- Erythrocytes' life span varies among species. In mice it is 20–30 days; in cats 68 days; and in pigs 85 days. Dogs and humans have an average erythrocyte life span of 120 days; horses and sheep 150 days; and cows 160 days. Their aging is called **senescence**. There are two processes of erythrocytes' destruction: **extravascular** and **intravascular**. Extravascular destruction takes place in the liver, spleen, and lymph nodes. Around 90 percent of erythrocytes are destroyed extravascular by macrophages. The aging erythrocyte undergoes changes in the plasma membrane, making it susceptible to selective recognition by macrophages and subsequent phagocytosis. The other 10 percent are destroyed intravascular by **eryptosis**, a special process of programmed cell death.

- After erythrocyte death, hemoglobin is decomposed into heme and globin. Globin is a protein that is hydrolyzed into amino acids. The heme group is decomposed into Fe^{2+} and a green pigment **biliverdin**. An enzyme called **biliverdin reductase** converts biliverdin in **bilirubin**. Bilirubin is excreted into the blood and transported to the liver. In the liver it is conjugated and together with bile excreted into the small intestine. In the small intestine bilirubin is converted to **urobilinogen**. Some amount of the urobilinogen in the large intestine is converted into **stercobilin**, a brown pigment that gives its color to feces. Another part of urobilinogen is reabsorbed back to the blood. In the kidneys, this compound is converted to **urobilin** and excretes with urine.

- The iron from heme is transported by the protein **transferrin** to the liver or spleen. Here it is bound by the protein **ferritin** and **hemosiderin** for storage. **Transferrin** also transports iron to red bone marrow for erythropoiesis. A small amount of iron is loss in sweat, urine, and feces.

- Erythropoiesis begins with the myeloid stem cell. Stimulated by numerous CSFs, the stem cell develops in a **proerythroblast** and later in an **erythroblast** that produces hemoglobin and expels the nucleus. The erythroblast becomes a **normoblast** and later a **reticulocyte**. The reticulocyte still continues to produce hemoglobin and enters the bloodstream, where it circulates for one to two days before it becomes a mature erythrocyte.

- Reticulocytes that enter the bloodstream constitute 0.5 to 2.0 percent of circulating red blood cells. The number of reticulocytes is an indicator of bone marrow activity: it represents a reticulocyte production index. A high reticulocyte count is called **reticulocytosis**. An abnormally low number of reticulocytes can be attributed to aplastic anemia, pernicious anemia, bone marrow malignancies, kidney disorder, and various vitamin or mineral deficiencies.

- Leukocytes defend an organism against pathogens. They constitute less than 1 percent of blood formed elements. They are larger than erythrocytes, have a nucleus and organelles, but do not have hemoglobin. Most leukocytes are wandering cells and are remarkably flexible. Many of them spend a short time in the blood flow. Flexible leukocytes squeeze between endothelial cells in the walls of blood vessels, a process termed **diapedesis**. Leukocytes move into the tissue, attracted by chemicals produced by damaged, dead, infected cells or pathogens.

- Leukocytes are classified in two classes: **granulocytes** and **agranulocytes**. A low leukocyte count, known as a **leukopenia**, compromises immune system defense ability. An abnormally high number of white blood cells is called **leukocytosis**. Leukocytosis is characteristic of an infected or highly stressed organism. A **differential count**, or **white blood cell differential count**, is a measure of the amount of each type of white blood cells in blood.

- Granulocytes are classified in three groups: **neutrophils**, **eosinophils**, and **basophils**.

- Neutrophils constitute 50 to 70 percent of the total leukocyte number. They are the most active phagocytes and arrive first at the area of infection or injury, attracted by cytokines released by endothelium, mast cells, macrophages, damaged or infected cells, and pathogenic organisms, especially bacteria. Neutrophils release cytokines, which amplify inflammatory reaction and recruit other immune system cells. They attack microorganisms in three ways: **phagocytosis**, **degradation**, and generation of **neutrophil extracellular traps (NETs)**.

- Ingested bacteria are digested by chemicals called **reactive oxygen species** and hydrolytic enzymes. The consumption of oxygen during the generation of reactive oxygen species has been termed the **respiratory burst**. The respiratory burst generates large quantities of superoxide, a reactive oxygen species. Superoxide decays to hydrogen peroxide. Hydrogen peroxide then is converted to hypochlorous acid (HClO). The HClO kills bacteria. A **neutrophil extracellular trap** (**NET**) is a web of fibers composed of chromatin and serine proteases. An NET provides a high local concentration of antimicrobial components and binds, disarms, and kill microbes. It also serves as a physical barrier that prevents further spread of pathogens.

- Eosinophils constitute 1 to 4 percent of the total leukocyte number. Eosinophils phagocytize numerous antigen-antibody complexes or allergens. They defend organism from parasitic worms.

- Basophils are the least numerous granulocytes. The primary components of basophil granules are histamine and heparin. Histamine is a strong vasodilator. It also increases capillary permeability, especially at the arterioles side. The heparin is an anticoagulant that prevents blood clot formation. Both play principal role in inflammatory reaction, characterized by swelling, itching, and accumulation of fluids in affected area.

- There are two types of agranulocytes: **lymphocytes** and **monocytes**.

- Monocytes are the biggest blood cells. They are three times as large as erythrocytes. Monocytes constitute 2 to 8 percent of the total number of leukocytes. Monocytes circulate within blood about three to five days, then exit bloodstream and move into tissues, where they transform into large phagocytes, called **macrophages**. Macrophages constitute the **mononuclear phagocyte system**. **M1 macrophages** phagocytize microbes and initiate the immune response. They produce nitric oxide (NO) and reactive oxygen intermediates (ROI) against bacteria and viruses. **M2 macrophages** decrease inflammation, promote collagen synthesis, and encourage tissue repair.

- Macrophages activate other cells of the immune system. Microbial fragments that remain after pathogen digestion are incorporated into a special molecular complex called the **major histocompatibility complex**, or **MHC**. The MHC with pathogen antigen is exposed at the monocyte cell surface. This process is called **antigen presentation.** Presented antigen triggers an immune reaction when it becomes recognized by T cells.

- Lymphocytes constitute 20 to 40 percent of the total number of white blood cells. Their main residency is lymphatic organs: the lymphatic nodes, spleen, thymus, and so forth. There are three groups of lymphocytes: **T lymphocytes (T cells), B lymphocytes (B cells),** and **natural killer (NK) cells**.

- NK cells are cytotoxic lymphocytes. They directly attack and destroy pathogenic cells. They are especially effective in destruction of cancerous cells. NK cells provide rapid responses to virus-infected cells. NK cells detect the MHC present on infected cell surfaces and trigger release of cytokines, proteins that cause lysis of pathogenic cell or its apoptosis. NK cells have a unique ability to recognize stressed cells in the absence of antibodies and the MHC.

- B and T cells are structurally very similar, but their role in the immune system is different. Active B cells produce **antibodies** that bind to antigens on the surface of pathogenic cells and destroy or deactivate them. B cells form functional groups or clones. Each group of B cells produce a particular antibody that binds only to a particular antigen. T cells also have specific reaction on particular antigens. Some T cells directly attack cells that carry alien antigens. They are called **cytotoxic T cells**. T cells that activate a particular group of B cells are called **helper T cells**.

- Leukocyte production is called **leucopoiesis**. There are three pathways of leukocytes production: **granulocyto- poiesis, monocytopoiesis,** and **lymphocytopoiesis.**

- Granulocytopoiesis produces neutrophils, eosinophils, and basophils. All granulocytes originate from myeloid stem cells. These stem cells, stimulated by multi-CSF and GM-CSF, form progenitor cells. The granulocyte line develops when the progenitor cell forms a **myeloblast** under the influence of G-CSF: **stem cells → myeloblasts → promyelocytes → eosin/neutron/basophilic myelocytes → metamyelocytes → band cells → granulocytes**.

- A myeloid stem cell stimulated by M-CSF develops into a **monoblast**. The monoblast forms a **promonocyte** that becomes a **monocyte**.

- **Lymphoid stem cells** produce **B lymphoblasts** or **T lymphoblasts**. B lymphoblasts develop in B cells; T lym- phoblasts in T cells. Some lymphoid stem cells differentiate into NK cells.

- Platelets are cellular fragments involved in prevention of blood loss, called **hemostasis**. Platelets have no nucleus and organelles. They are produced de novo from **megakaryocytes**.

- **Thrombopoietin** stimulates a megakaryocyte to develop long cytoplasmic extensions filled with cytosol, granules, and some organelles. These extensions protrude through the clefts in bone marrow sinusoids and expose in the bloodstream. The force of the blood coursing past the arms lops off small pieces that become platelets. Each arm can give thousands of platelets that remain in circulation for seven to ten days and then are removed by the liver or spleen.

- Hemostasis is organized in a series of events that form a **blood clot**: 1) **vascular spasm** → 2) **platelet plug formation** → 3) **coagulation** → 4) **clot retraction** → 5) **thrombolysis**.

- Vascular spasm includes 1) vasoconstriction and 2) increase of interstitial fluid hydrostatic pressure. Pain receptors in damaged blood vessel initiate immediate reflective vasoconstriction via sympathetic nerves. Endothelial cells release prostacyclin and nitric oxide (NO), which induces relaxation of smooth muscles in the walls of blood vessels. Platelets secrete thromboxane A2 and serotonin, which stimulate smooth muscle contraction. In healthy blood vessel, the relaxation prevails, but damaged endothelial cells cannot produce enough prostacyclin and NO to override increased production of serotonin and contraction overcomes relaxation. Lost blood accumulates in surrounding tissues, causing **hemorrhage**. Hydrostatic pressure in surrounding tissue presses on the blood vessel wall. Both vasoconstriction and high external hydrostatic pressure compress blood vessel and stop blood from flowing through it.

- The next step of hemostasis is a **platelet plug formation (primary hemostasis)**. Damaged endothelial cells release glycoprotein—**von Willebrand factor (vWF)**. Adventitia of the injured blood vessel exposes collagen fibers. Contact of platelets with collagen and vWF triggers **platelet activation**. Activated platelets release ATP, ADP, serotonin, calcium, clotting factors, and other chemicals that stimulate platelets to **aggregate** and form a **platelet plug**.

- Fibrin converts the soft liquid platelet plug into a solid mass by **coagulation**. It is a product of enzymatic transformation of **fibrinogen** (or **factor I**). **Coagulation cascade** reactions convert soluble fibrinogen into hydrophobic fibrin. Enzymes that maintain coagulation cascade are known as **clotting factors**. Most of these clotting factors are produced in inactive form in the liver and constantly circulate in blood.

- Synthesis of factors II, VII, IX, and X requires vitamin K and are known as a vitamin K–dependent factors. Vitamin K is a group of structurally similar, fat-soluble vitamins.

- There are two pathways of coagulation cascades: **extrinsic** and **intrinsic**. At the end both pathways converge and proceed via a **common pathway**, which leads to formation of a blood clot.

- The **extrinsic pathway** is initiated by a factor developing outside the blood flow, called **tissue factor**. The process proceeds in: 1) damaged subendothelial cells secrete tissue factor, known as a **thromboplastin** or **factor III**, and display it in plasma membrane; 2) tissue factor binds with circulating in bloodstream inactive **factor VII** and Ca^{2+} and converts factor VII into an active **factor VIIa**; 3) factor VIIa cleaves inactive **factor X** into active **factor Xa**.

- The **intrinsic pathway** is triggered by a damage inside blood vessel. It proceeds through the following steps: 1) platelets adhering to a damaged blood vessel wall releases **factor XII**, which binds with every negatively charged particle and becomes active **factor XIIa**; 2) factor XIIa activates **factor XI**; 3) **factor XIa** activates **factor IX**; 4) **factor IXa**, Ca^{2+} and **platelet factor 3** form a large enzyme complex that converts inactive **factor VIII** into active **factor VIIIa**; 5) factor VIIIa converts inactive factor X to active factor Xa.

- The **common pathway** finalizes clot formation by production of fibrin. It proceeds through four steps: 1) **factor Xa** combines with **factors II, V**, Ca^{2+}, and platelet factor 3 and forms **prothrombin activator**; 2) prothrombin activator converts inactive **prothrombin** into active enzyme **thrombin**; 3) thrombin transforms blood-soluble fibrinogen into insoluble fibrin; 4) **factor XIII** is activated in presence of Ca^{2+}. Activated **factor XIIIa** stabilizes fibrin monomers and binds them into a network of fibrin polymer, which forms the framework of a developing clot. The network of fibrin traps big protein molecules and blood formed elements.

- The clotting cascade is controlled via positive feedback. Thrombin activates factors V and VIII. These factors stimulate production of thrombin. The increased amount of thrombin activates more factors V and VIII, and amplifies clot formation.

- A blood clot is eliminated through two processes: **clot retraction** and **thrombolysis**.

- Platelets have a cytoskeleton made of actin and myosin proteins that cause platelet contraction and squeezes serum out of a clot. This makes the clot smaller and dryer.

- Thrombolysis begins with degradation of the fibrin network that cements a clot: 1) endothelial cells release an enzyme, **tissue plasminogen activator** or **tPA**; 2) inactive protein **plasminogen** circulates in the bloodstream. This protein creates chemical bonds with fibrin. Within few days after clot formation, it becomes saturated with plasminogen molecules bound to fibrin. The tPA released by endothelial cells transforms inactive plasminogen in an active enzyme **plasmin**; 3) plasmin degrades both fibrin and fibrinogen. Broken fibrin does not hold the clot; it falls apart and dissociates from the endothelium. Clot components are moved out by blood flow.

- The endothelium and liver produce **anticoagulants**: **antithrombin III**, **heparan sulfate**, and **protein C**. Antithrombin III binds and deactivate factor Xa and thrombin. It inhibits already existing and prevents formation of new thrombin molecules. Heparan sulfate stimulates antithrombin III activity. Protein C degrades factors Va and VIIIa.

- An inability to control blood clot formation is termed a **clotting disorder**. Clotting disorders are classified as 1) **bleeding disorders** and 2) **hypercoagulation disorders**. Bleeding disorders increase blood loss and are caused by deficiency of clotting proteins: 1) **hemophilia A**, by a shortage of factor VIII; 2) **hemophilia B**, by low factor IX. An inappropriate clot formation is called **thrombosis**. A **thrombus** obstructs blood flow and can cause an ischemic effect.

- Blood type refers to the presence of glycoproteins on the red blood cell surface that are important for self-recognition and known as **antigens**. Blood plasma of some species may contain **antibodies** that create chemical bonds with antigens, a process called **agglutination**.

- Dogs have eight blood groups, called **dog erythrocyte antigen (DEA) system**. A presence of antigen is termed positive and called negative when it is absent. The immune system of DEA-negative dogs recognizes DEA positive as a foreign substance and attacks it. Dogs do not have antibodies, and there is no risk at the first transfusion. Antibodies form within five to seven days of the first transfusion, and a second transfusion after five days can cause severe consequences if the blood is not matched.

- Cats have an **AB** blood group system. Their blood type is a simple dominant trait, where A is dominant over B. Cats have three blood groups: **A**, **B**, and **AB**. Group A has A/A or A/B genotype and is the most common blood type of domestic cats. Group B has only B/B genotype and is common in Devon rex, Persian, British shorthair, Somali, Himalayan, and Birman breeds. Rarely do cats have AB group. Cats with blood type A have antibody B in their blood plasma. Cats with blood type B have A antibody in their blood plasma. Cats with blood type AB have no antibodies. Antibody A reacts only on antigen A, and antibody B agglutinates only with antigen B. Group A cats have a low amount of anti-B antibodies, and giving group A cats type B blood will cause destruction of red blood cells and a mild transfusion reaction. Group B cats have high amount of anti-A antibodies, and giving group B cats type A blood can result in a potentially fatal transfusion reaction. Type AB cats can receive AB or A blood.

- Antibodies can be transmitted in milk, and kittens with type A blood can have a fatal reaction (**neonatal isoerythrolysis**) when they drink the milk of a type B queen.

CHECK YOUR KNOWLEDGE

LEVEL 1. CHECK YOUR RECALL

1. What percentage of the blood is composed of plasma?
   A. 75 percent
   B. 65 percent
   C. 15 percent
   D. 55 percent
   E. 45 percent

2. Normal blood pH should fall between:
   A. 7.35 and 7.45
   B. 7.15 and 7.25
   C. 6.95 and 7.15
   D. 7.65 and 7.85
   E. 5.45 and 5.55

3. The most abundant component of plasma is:
   A. Ions
   B. Proteins
   C. Water
   D. Gases
   E. Glucose

4. Which plasma protein forms blood colloid osmotic pressure?
   A. Transport proteins
   B. Antibodies
   C. Fibrinogen
   D. Albumin
   E. Collagen

5. Which statement best describes red blood cells?
   A. Red blood cells have a nucleus and most organelles.
   B. Red blood cells live about ten days.
   C. Red blood cells form antibodies to fight antigens.
   D. Red blood cells possess a protein known as hemoglobin.
   E. Red blood cells may leave the blood flow and move into body tissues.

6. The function of red blood cells is to:
    A. Stop blood loss from an injured blood vessel
    B. Transport oxygen and carbon dioxide
    C. Transport nutrients to the body's cells and tissues
    D. Phagocytize bacteria
    E. All of the above

7. What organ serves as a control center for the regulation of erythropoiesis?
    A. Kidney
    B. Duodenum
    C. Spleen
    D. Pancreas
    E. Heart

8. Which organ traps older erythrocytes so they will be removed from circulation?
    A. Pancreas
    B. Gallbladder
    C. Spleen
    D. Heart
    E. Stomach

9. The process of red blood cell production is known as:
    A. Polycythemia
    B. Erythropoiesis
    C. Erythropenia
    D. Erythrocytosis
    E. Erythroblastosis

10. Which of the following might trigger erythropoiesis?
    A. Decreased tissue demand for oxygen
    B. An increased number of RBCs
    C. Moving to a lower altitude
    D. Increase of blood oxygen above the norm
    E. Blood oxygen levels fall below normal

11. The percentage by volume of red blood cells in a blood sample is called:
    A. Red blood cell count (RBCC)
    B. White blood cell count (WBCC)
    C. Differential white blood cell count (DIFF)
    D. Hematocrit (HCT)

12. The biconcave cells in blood that have no nuclei when they are mature are:
    A. Neutrophils
    B. Basophils
    C. Erythrocytes
    D. Lymphocytes
    E. Eosinocytes

13. Lymphocytes play major role in:
    A. Production of histamine
    B. Immunity
    C. Creation of a blood clot
    D. Moderate allergic reaction
    E. Oxygen transport

14. Erythrocytes are derived from _____ stem cells, whereas lymphocytes are from _____.
    A. megakaryoblast; proerythroblast
    B. proerythroblast; myeloblast
    C. myeloblast; lymphoblast
    D. lymphoblast; megakaryoblast
    E. proerythroblast; lymphoblast

15. Oxygen attaches to _____, and carbon dioxide attaches to _____ in hemoglobin.
    A. Ca^{2+}; Fe^{2+}
    B. Fe^{2+}; $-NH_2$
    C. $-NH_2$; Ca^{2+}
    D. Ca^{2+}; $-NH_2$
    E. $-NH_2$; Fe^{2+}

16. The extrinsic pathway is triggered by _____, whereas the intrinsic pathway is triggered by _____.
    A. tissue factor; factor XII
    B. prothrombin; factor X
    C. factor I; factor V
    D. factor X and Ca^{2+}; tissue factor
    E. fibrinogen; fibrin

17. True or false: Cat blood type is defined by AB antigen system.
18. True or false: Prostacyclin promotes platelet adhesion and plug formation.
19. True or false: Albumins are fibrous proteins responsible for blood clot formation.

20. Match the term with its description:

_____ DEA	a. Converts plasminogen in plasmin
_____ Embolus	b. Coagulation cascade triggered by factor XII
_____ tPA	c. Blood accumulated in tissue
_____ Intrinsic pathway	d. Hormone that regulates platelet production
_____ Hemorrhage	e. Lymphocyte that directly attacks pathogens
_____ Thrombopoietin	f. Piece of thrombus moving in bloodstream
_____ NK cell	g. Dog antigen system

LEVEL 2. CHECK YOUR UNDERSTANDING

1. A dog's blood test demonstrates a higher-than-normal neutrophil count. This suggests that the dog may have what condition?

2. Cirrhosis of the liver often reduces production of albumin. How it can this effect the organism's well-being?

LEVEL 3. APPLY YOUR KNOWLEDGE TO REAL LIFE

1. Aspirin **irreversibly blocks** platelet receptor proteins responsible for plug formation. Why does aspirin intake have to be stopped at least five days before surgery procedure?

2. Warfarin is a drug that primarily disrupts the extrinsic coagulation pathway. Why does warfarin disrupt the entire coagulation cascade?

Chapter 18

The Lymphatic System and Immunity

LEARNING OBJECTIVES

The lymphatic system has two principal functions: 1) transporting and housing lymphocytes and other immune cells that help the immune system defend against potentially harmful objects, and 2) aiding the cardiovascular system in recovering fluids that can accumulate in tissues and returning it into the bloodstream. Thus, the lymphatic system serves to defend an organism from pathogens and helps the cardiovascular system maintain fluid balance, blood volume, and blood pressure.

In this chapter you will learn about the following:

1. The anatomy of the lymphatic system and lymphatic organs.

2. The mechanisms of fluid recovery and movement along the lymphatic vessels.

3. The role of the lymphatic system in immunity.

4. Innate immunity.

5. Adaptive immunity.

INTRODUCTION

The lymphatic system is a partner with the circulatory system. It has two principal components: lymphatic vessels and lymphatic tissue. The fluid that circulates inside lymphatic vessels is called **lymph**. The lymphatic system has two important functions: 1) helping the cardiovascular system in maintaining fluid balance and transporting some special substances, such as lipids; and 2) housing critical elements of the immune system, which protect an organism against harmful substances and pathogenic agents.

18.1 The Lymphatic System

Role of the Lymphatic System

The lymphatic system does not have its own unique function, but it provides critical support to other body systems, without which normal functioning of these systems will be impossible. Its two significant functions are: 1) The lymphatic system helps the cardiovascular system by recovering excess of interstitial fluid and returning it into the bloodstream, which is critical to maintaining fluid balance, blood volume, and blood pressure; 2) the lymphatic system harbors lymphocytes and other elements of the immune system, which serve to defend organism against pathogens and potentially harmful substances; 3) absorption and initial transportation of dietary fat. The lymphatic system is composed of lymphatic vessels and lymphatic tissues.

Anatomy of Lymphatic Vessels and Recovery of Interstitial Fluids

Lymphatic vessels are blind-ended tubes that pick up an interstitial fluid and return it to the cardio-vascular circulation. Lymphatic vessels begin in the tissues with tiny **lymphatic capillaries**. Lymphatic capillaries form microscopic network interspersed throughout the areolar connective tissue surrounded blood capillary beds (fig. 18.1). They are found in all tissues except red bone marrow, the central nervous system, and avascular tissues, such as epithelium and tendons. Special lymphatic capillaries called **lacteals** occupy centers of villi in walls of the small intestine, where they serve for absorption of a dietary fat. Recent studies have found lymph vessels in dural venous sinuses that drain blood away from the brain.

The blind-ended lymphatic capillaries can transport lymph only away from tissue. Like in blood capillaries, their walls are composed of endothelial cells. However, lymphatic capillaries are typically larger in diameter than blood capillaries and have no basement membrane. Endothelial cells that form lymphatic

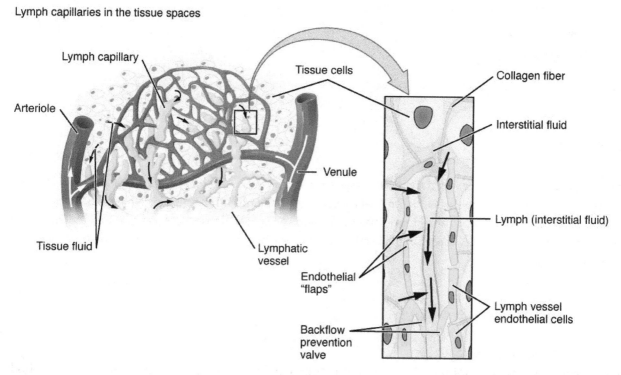

FIGURE 18.1   Network of Lymphatic Capillaries in the Tissue.

capillary wall are not tightly joined and overlap, like shingles. Their membrane is anchored by **anchoring filaments**, with the surrounding elastic fibers of the extracellular skeleton. The main molecular component of anchoring filaments is glycoprotein **fibrillin**. This structural organization of lymph capillary walls allows endothelial cells to rotate around the axis created by anchoring filaments and act as one-way flaps that permit interstitial fluid to enter the lymphatic capillary, but prevent its backward flow (fig. 18.2).

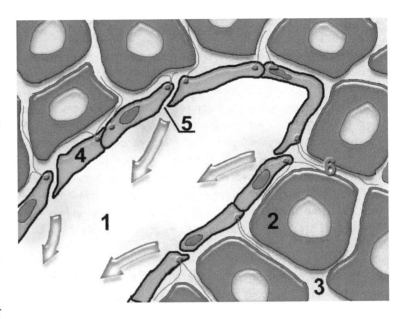

FIGURE 18.2   Structural Organization of Lymphatic Capillary. 1. Lymph; 2. Surrounding Tissue Cells; 3. Interstitial Fluid; 4. Endothelial Cell; 5. Open Pore between Endothelial Cells; 6. Anchoring Filaments.

Pressure within the arterioles of the blood arises from three sources: 1) blood hydrostatic pressure, 2) blood colloid osmotic pressure, and 3) hydrostatic pressure of interstitial fluid around blood vessels. Hydrostatic pressure is a force exerted by blood on capillary walls. Blood hydrostatic pressure is a major force that drives blood plasma to leave the capillary. Colloid osmotic pressure is a difference between blood plasma and interstitial fluid osmotic pressure. Because blood plasma contains high concentration of plasma proteins, its osmotic pressure is much higher than the osmotic pressure of the surrounding interstitial fluid. Thus, colloid osmotic pressure in healthy organisms seeps fluids back inside capillaries. At the arteriole end capillaries' hydrostatic pressure is usually higher than osmotic pressure. As a result, fluid exits capillaries and fills surrounding tissues. At the venule side capillary hydrostatic pressure dissipates and osmotic pressure becomes dominant. The net inward pressure recovers almost 90 percent of the fluid that left blood. The remaining 10 percent forms interstitial fluid. Further accumulation of this fluid causes the tissue to swell, a condition known as **edema**. In a healthy organism edema does not occur because excess of the interstitial fluid is picked up by the lymphatic capillaries. Accumulation of extracellular fluid increases its hydrostatic pressure, which presses on endothelial cells in lymphatic capillaries and forces these cells to rotate and open flaps through which fluid enters the lymphatic capillary. The lymph volume inside lymphatic capillary grows and its pressure on the endothelial cells increases. When hydrostatic pressure of the lymph overcomes pressure of interstitial fluid, cells are forced to return to the initial position and close passages and lymph becomes trapped within the lymphatic capillary. From here lymph has only one way to move—into a network of increasingly larger vessels that create a continuous chain of lymphatic vessels. Lymphatic vessels drain into **lymphatic trunks**, and then **lymphatic ducts**, which carry lymph into the cardiovascular blood flow.

Lymphatic vessels are structurally similar to small veins. Usually, superficial lymphatic vessels are associated with the superficial veins, whereas deep lymphatic vessels are located close to deep arteries and veins. The wall of a lymphatic vessel has three layers or tunics: the tunica intima, or endothelium; The tunica media; and the tunica externa, or adventitia. Endothelial cells in the tunica intima are folded and form valves within the lumen. There is not a special organ which can force lymph movement, and valves prevent its backward flow. These valves are especially numerous in vessels were lymph has to move against gravity; in the legs, for example. The functional unit of a lymph vessel is called a **lymphangion**, which is the segment between two valves. The tunica media of the lymph vessel contains smooth muscles, and because of that, lymphangion is contractile. The tension of smooth muscles in the lymphangion wall depends on the ratio of its length to its radius. It can act either like a contractile chamber propelling the fluid ahead, or as a resistance vessel tending to stop the lymph in its place and prevent lymph back flow (fig. 18.3). Beside valves, the lymphatic system relies on other mechanisms that move lymph inside vessels: 1) Contraction of surrounding skeletal muscles in limbs and respiratory pump in the torso (see chapter 17, page 501); 2) rhythmic contraction of smooth muscles within the vessel's wall; and 3) pulsatile movement of blood in the nearby arteries.

Lymphatic trunks collect lymph from lymphatic vessels. In human, for example, there are four pairs of lymphatic trunks on both sides of the body: 1) jugular trunks that collect lymph from head and neck; 2) subclavian trunks that drain lymph from the upper limbs, breasts, and superficial thoracic wall; 3) bronchomediastinal trunks, which drain deep thoracic structures; 4) lumbar trunks that collect lymph from the lower limbs, abdominopelvic wall, and pelvis; and 5) a single interstitial trunk, which collects lymph from most abdominal organs.

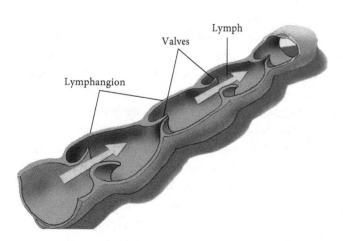

FIGURE 18.3   Lymphatic Vessel.

The largest lymphatic vessels are called **lymphatic ducts**. Lymphatic ducts collect lymph from lymphatic trunks. There are two lymphatic ducts in mammals. The **right lymphatic duct** receives lymph from the lymphatic trunks on the upper right side of the body and drains it into the bloodstream in subclavian vein near its fusion with right internal jugular vein. The **thoracic duct** is shorter; it extends from the diaphragm to the junction of the left subclavian vein with left internal jugular vein. Thoracic duct drains lymph from the thoracic tissues on the left side (fig. 18.4).

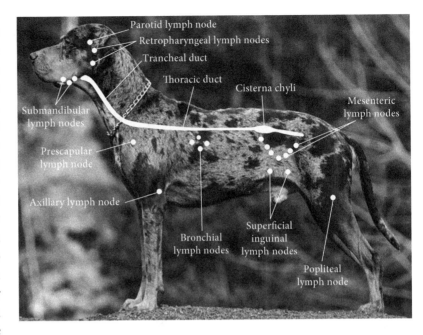

FIGURE 18.4   The Lymphatic System of the Dog.

CHECK YOUR UNDERSTANDING

- List the main functions of the lymphatic system.

- What are the major differences between lymphatic and blood capillaries?

- Describe the mechanism that assists in the return of fluids into the blood circulation.

Lymphoid Tissues and Organs

The second component of the lymphatic system is lymphatic tissue organized in lymphatic organs. The main type of lymphatic tissue is **reticular connective tissue** (see chapter 4, page 106). The principal characteristic of this tissue is reticulin fibers in the matrix, which creates a web-like network. This fibrous network creates a frame of lymphatic organs and traps pathogen agents. Several cell types constitute formed elements of the lymphatic tissue, including 1) **leukocytes** (see chapter 17, page 496), 2) **dendritic cells** (see chapter 5, page 138), and 3) **reticular cells**. Leukocytes include macrophages, T cells, and B cells. Dendritic cells are immune cells with spiny projections that looks like neuron dendrites. There are several types of dendritic cells of different origin. Some dendritic cells are produced in the red bone marrow, and the others are from connective tissue. A reticular cell is a type of fibroblast that produces collagen type III and makes from it web-like reticular fibers. Reticular cells provide a structural framework for most lymphoid organs. They are found in many tissues, including the spleen, lymph nodes, and lymph nodules.

Lymphatic tissue is organized in lymphatic organs that are classified in two groups: **primary** and **secondary lymphatic structures**.

Primary (or **central**) lymphoid tissues are also referred to as primary lymphoid organs. They are responsible for lymphopoiesis (see chapter 17, page 501) and lymphocyte development. The primary lymphoid tissues include:

1. **Red bone marrow.** In some primates, bone marrow acts as a primary lymphoid organ; in other species it can also be a secondary lymphoid tissue.

2. **The bursa of Fabricius.** The bursa of Fabricius is a primary lymphoid organ in birds. It is a round out-pouching on the posterior-dorsal wall of the cloaca called **proctodeum**. The bursa consists of a number of lymphoid lobules and folds surrounding the lumen. The lumen is lined with a thin layer of stratified squamous epithelium and opens into the proctodeum. Every lobule is stratified into three layers: the outermost cortex, medulla, and lymphocytes supported by epithelial cells at the center. In six weeks chicken bursa reaches its maximum size. After that, it slowly regresses (involutes), and in an adult bird, only a small remnant remains. In 1956 Bruce Glick found that removal of the bursa of Fabricius in newly hatched chicks severely impaired the ability of the adult birds to produce antibodies. Timothy S. Chang continued to study chickens he obtained from Glick and demonstrated that they failed to produce antibody in response to an immunization with staphylococcus bacteria; the two scientists realized that the bursa is necessary for antibody production. Later, it was found that these are white blood cells named B lymphocytes or B cells, where *B* is an abbreviation of "bursa." The bursa is involved in the development and maturation of B cells that produce antibodies. Lymphoid precursor cells migrate into the developing bursa during the first few weeks of bird embryo development.

3. **The thymus.** The thymus plays a key role in the maturation of immature T lymphocytes called **prothymocytes** into mature T cells. In juvenile animals the thymus produces significant numbers of new T cells, but with aging this production decreases and thymus T cell population is maintained by multiplication of already mature T cells. The thymus develops from the left and right third pharyngeal pouches and extends caudally until it fuses with the pericardium. Then the thymus follows the heart, when the latter migrates into the thoracic cavity. At this point the thymus has a Y shape, and this shape persists in neonatal ruminants. Lateral arms of the gland are called **thymus lobes**, which are connected by a bridge known as an **isthmus**. In horses the isthmus is lost and leaves two separate lobes, while in carnivores only the thoracic part (isthmus) persists and the cranial portion (lobes) regresses. During development T lymphocytes' precursor cells (CFU-L cells) from the red bone marrow migrate to the thymus and concentrate around the thymus, producing a dense cortex. Eventually, they give rise to the inner medulla. Endodermal reticular cells in the medulla are arranged in concentric structures and form the structures known as **Hassall's corpuscles**. These concentric corpuscles are composed of a central mass, consisting of one or more granular cells, and of a capsule formed by epithelioid cells. A thin connective tissue membrane surrounds the thymus and forms its capsule. Trabeculae from capsule connective tissue extend inside the thymus and divide its internal space into compartments called **lobules**.

The connective tissues house blood vessels, efferent lymphatic vessels, and nerves. The thymus cortex is dense and consists of rapidly dividing **thymocytes**. A network of **epithelioreticular cells** support developing thymocytes. There are six types of epithelioreticular cells. Types I–III are found in the cortex and types IV–VI in the medulla. Type VI forms Hassall's corpuscles. The medulla has nondividing, more mature

T cells with dendritic cells at the corticomedullary junction. The blood-thymus barrier protects T lymphocytes from exposure to antigens in the blood. It is formed in the capillaries by a continuous endothelium with occluding junctions surrounded by connective tissue and then surrounded by a second layer formed from the processes of epithelioreticular cells (type I). The blood-thymus barrier also has macrophages surrounded capillaries and engulf any antigenic substances that penetrate the barrier (figs. 18.5 and 18.6).

1. **The fetal liver.** As embryological development progresses during pregnancy hematopoiesis shifts from the yolk sac to the fetal liver. The liver becomes the main hematopoietic organ in the developing fetus. Erythropoiesis is the dominant process that takes place in the fetal liver, but some leukopoiesis also occurs. That is why the fetal liver can be considered a primary lymphoid organ.

Secondary (or **peripheral**) lymphoid tissues provide a site for immune responses and houses populations of mature T cells, B cells, macrophages, and dendritic cells. The secondary lymphoid tissues include:

Lymph nodes. The lymph nodes are round or bean-shaped bodies with an outer **cortex** and inner **medulla**. Node structure includes **follicles, paracortical zones, medullary cords**, and **sinuses**. Lymph nodes are connected to lymphatic vessels. Afferent vessels enter the node on its convex side, and efferent vessels exit on the concave side (**hilum**). The nodes are surrounded by a fibrous capsule that extends inside the node interior as trabeculae. Below the capsule are the subcapsular sinuses. Reticular fibers and reticular cells form a fine network, which provides a frame for attachment of other cells. The cortex contains round groups of B cells called **follicles**

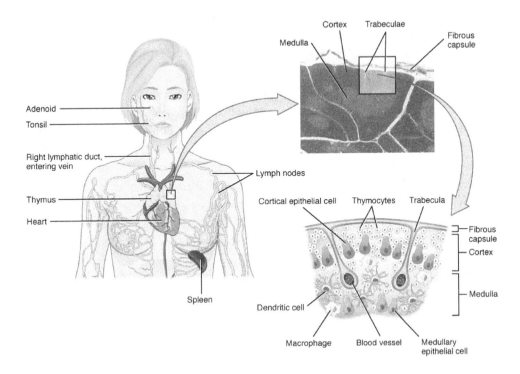

FIGURE 18.5   Human Thymus.

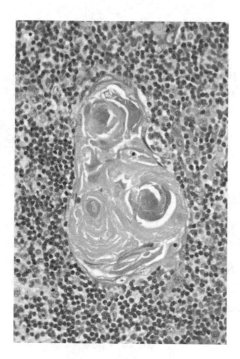

FIGURE 18.6   Hassall's Corpuscles.

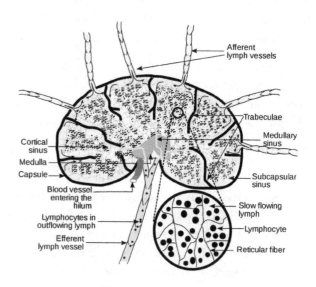

FIGURE 18.7   Schematic Diagram of Lymph Node.

in its outer region. Every follicle is surrounded by a layer of T cells and some amount of dendritic cells called **paracortex**. B cells, plasma cells, and some macrophages in medulla are organized into **medullary cords**. Between medullary cords is the medullary sinus lined with endothelial cells and macrophages. Lymph from afferent vessels passes through sinuses, where it is filtered by macrophages and antigens, and leaves the lymph node via efferent vessel. Lymph nodes have two types of follicles: **primary** and **secondary**. Primary follicles contain activated B cells differentiated into plasma B cells or **plasmablasts**, and memory B cells or **lymphoblasts**. Secondary follicles are sites of B cells proliferation and have three layers: 1. Central dark zone contains dividing B cell precursors called **centroblasts**; 2. **Basal zone**, where B cells express surface immunoglobulin and expose them to the follicular dendritic cells. This zone is characterized by a high rate of apoptosis (programmed death) among B cells. Those B cells that survive negative selection migrate to the apical zone; 3. **Apical zone** (also called **mantle zone**) contains cells programmed to become B memory (lymphoblasts) or plasma cells (plasmablasts). **High endothelial venules** (**HEV**) are composed of cuboidal and columnar epithelium. They are the major route for lymphocytes to enter the lymph node. HEV contain a large number of aquaporin channels allowing for a large uptake of water, which in turn drives lymph flow through the cortex. This fluid is then returned to the bloodstream. The walls of venules are impregnated with selectins, receptor proteins for B and T lymphocytes primed with antigens. Selectins bind to antigens on the plasma membrane of circulating lymphocytes and help them leave the bloodstream and enter the lymphatic tissue (fig. 18.7).

The structure of lymph nodes in pigs, dolphins, hippopotamuses, and rhinoceroses is different from other mammals. Most follicles in lymph nodes of these animals are found deep in the paracortex. The paracortex is surrounded by loose medullary tissue. Afferent lymphatic vessels enter at the hilum.

As a rule, lymph nodes are organized in clusters. Lymph moves from node to node, where it is filtered and cleaned from pathogens and toxins. During infection, some lymph nodes become swollen and tender to the touch. These enlarged nodes are a sign that lymphocytes are multiplied to fight infection. Swollen superficial lymph nodes in the neck and axilla often can be palpated (fig. 18.8).

Spleen. The spleen is the largest lymphatic organ. It is located in the left upper quadrant of the abdomen, posterior to the diagram, dorsolateral to the stomach, and adjacent to ribs 9–11. The spleen has convex and rounded dorsolateral (also called **diaphragmatic**) surface; and concave ventromedial or **visceral surface**. **Splenic artery**, **splenic vein**, and nerves enter and exit spleen through the opening in visceral surface called **hilum**. The spleen serves as a blood filter. A connective tissue capsule surrounds the spleen. Its extensions termed **trabeculae** project inside the spleen. Trabeculae subdivide the spleen into compartments called **white pulp** and **red pulp**. At the center of white pulp is a **central artery**, surrounded by circles of T cells, B cells, and macrophages. Red pulp is composed of erythrocytes, platelets, macrophages, and B cells. The reticular connective tissue forms structures called **splenic cords**. A network of porous capillaries with discontinuous basal lamina (see chapter 16, page 466) called **splenic cords** are part of red pulp. The porous discontinuous capillaries allow red blood cells and platelets leave the bloodstream, fill lacunae called **sinusoids**, and return back to bloodstream through small venules that lead into the splenic vein. Red pulp serves as a blood reservoir, including a storage of erythrocytes and platelets (fig. 18.9).

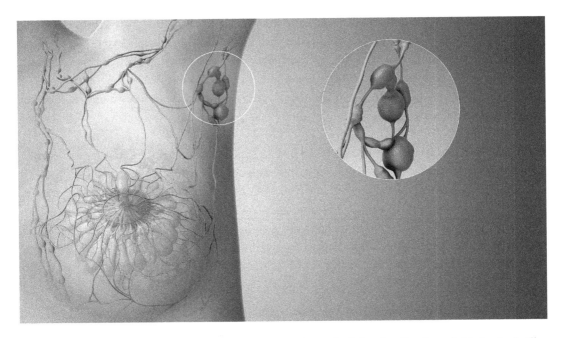

FIGURE 18.8   Clusters of Lymph Nodes in Human Torso. Red Are Swollen Lymph Nodes in Axilla.

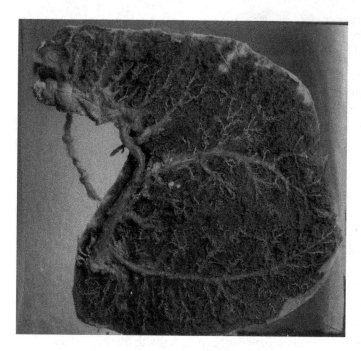

FIGURE 18.9   Structure of Donkey Spleen.

Blood, which enters the spleen via the splenic artery, moves into central arteries in white pulp. Here the incoming blood is examined on presence of pathogens. From central arteries blood flows into the sinusoids in red pulp. Macrophages in the sinusoids phagocytize bacteria, foreign materials, as well as both old and defective erythrocytes and platelets. In general, the pathway of blood flow in the spleen is: **splenic artery → central artery → splenic sinusoid → venule → splenic vein**.

The spleen serves several functions: 1) phagocytosis of bacteria and other foreign substances; 2) phagocytosis of old and defective erythrocytes and platelets; 3) reservoir and storage site of erythrocytes and platelets. Besides that, during the fetal development the spleen engages in the hematopoietic function. After birth, the hematopoiesis concentrates in red bone marrow. However, spleen hematopoiesis remains possible and can be reactivated under some medical conditions called **extramedullary hematopoiesis**.

Tonsils. Tonsils have no completed connective tissue capsule. They are located in the pharynx and oral cavity. The **pharyngeal tonsil** is in the posterior wall of the nasopharynx. The enlarged pharyngeal tonsil condition is known as **adenoids**. **Palatine tonsils** are in the dorsolateral surfaces of the oral cavity. **Lingual tonsils** are located along the dorsal one-third of the tongue. Tonsils protect the organism against foreign substances that try to invade with air, water, and food via the nose and mouth (fig. 18.10).

Mucosal associated lymphoid tissue (MALT). MALT includes many different organs associated with the mucosa lamina propria and are scattered along gastrointestinal, respiratory, urinary, and reproductive organs. The lymphatic cells in MALT help defend against foreign substances that come in contact with mucosal membranes. MALT is nonencapsulated lymphoid tissue. Strategically, MALT is located to intercept pathogens before they enter the body. Depending on the location, they are classified into 1) **GALT**, or gut associated lymphoid tissue; 2) **BALT**, or branchial associated lymphoid tissue; 3) **CALT**, or conjunctiva associated lymphoid tissue; and 4) **VALT**, or vulvo-vaginal associated lymphoid tissue.

GALT include **appendix/caecal pouch**, **Peyer's patches**, and mucosa in the large intestine and rectum. Lymphatic tissue in the appendix develops during early life and reaches maximum size at early adulthood. Some regression (involution) occurs as the animal is aging, but some amount of tissue retains throughout life. The

(a) Locations of the tonsils

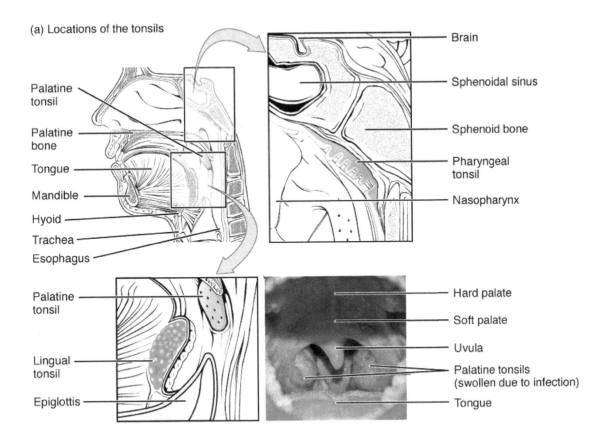

Palatine tonsil

Palatine bone

Tongue

Mandible

Hyoid

Trachea

Esophagus

Brain

Sphenoidal sinus

Sphenoid bone

Pharyngeal tonsil

Nasopharynx

Palatine tonsil

Lingual tonsil

Epiglottis

Hard palate

Soft palate

Uvula

Palatine tonsils (swollen due to infection)

Tongue

(b) Histology of palatine tonsil

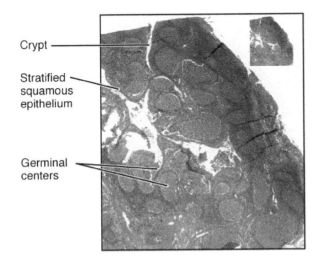

Crypt

Stratified squamous epithelium

Germinal centers

FIGURE 18.10 Human Tonsils.

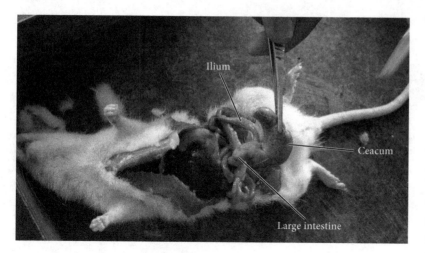

FIGURE 18.11   Rat Caecum.

appendix is a pouch of the caeca at the ileocolic junction. The appendix opens inside caeca on one side and is blind closed on the other. The lamina propria of the appendix have a number of lymphatic nodules with lymphocytes. The mammalian appendix corresponds to the birds' bursa of Fabricius and, consequently, has functions associated with maturation and differentiation of B lymphocytes. In rabbits the appendix is a primary lymphoid organ, whereas in other mammals it is a secondary lymphoid organ (fig. 18.11).

Peyer's patches are lymphoid tissues found in the wall of the small intestine. In many species (cattle, sheep, pigs, horses, dogs, and rabbits), they act as a primary lymphoid tissue.

In cattle, sheep, pigs, horses, and dogs, over 8 percent of the patches are found in the ileum, where they form a continuous structure. They develop to their maximum before birth, and during the adulthood they regress to detectable structures. The rest of the patches are found in the jejunum and are represented there by patches of lymphatic tissue isolated from each other, where they last throughout the adult life. In rabbits and rodents the patches are randomly located along both the ileum and jejunum and persist throughout life (fig. 18.12).

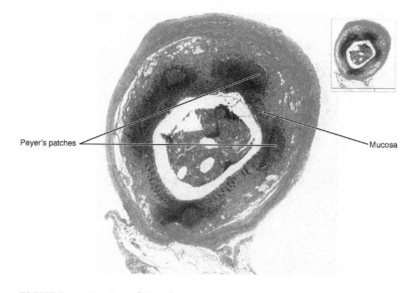

FIGURE 18.12   Peyer's Patches.

Peyer's patches in the small intestine may be found by the lack of villi covering. The patches are composed of B cells covered by a specialized **follicle associated epithelium (FAE)**, which consists of **enterocytes** and **M (microfold** or **multifold) cells**. M cells transport antigens from the intestinal lumen to the lymphocytes. Their free surface is folded and exposed inside the intestines. Membrane of these folds carry receptors for exogenous antigens. Receptors on the M cell surface bind with antigens, take them up from the intestine via endocytosis, and transport them to the extracellular space on their basal surface, where the antigen is processed by antigen presenting cells. Peyer's patches have a similar role to that of the avian bursa in maturing and differentiation immature B lymphocytes. Presentation of antigen activates B lymphocytes, which begin to synthesize IgA for this antigen. In ruminants and pigs. Peyer's patches in the ileum have a primary lymphoid function, while those in the jejunum are secondary lymphoid tissue.

Bronchial associated lymphoid tissue (BALT) is located at the bronchial bifurcations under nonciliated epithelium. BALT, like Peyer's patches, is covered by M cells that recognize and transport antigens captured by mucous membrane from the inhaled air and present them to B lymphocytes.

CHECK YOUR UNDERSTANDING

- What is the principal difference between primary and secondary lymphatic organs?
- How are the two types of T lymphocytes arranged in the thymus cortex and medulla?

- What is the function of lymph nodes?
- Describe the main types and functions of MALT.

18.2 Overview of the Immune System

The immune system serves to protect organisms from pathogenic agents. The immune system does not have its own organs. It consists of many different types of cells, proteins, and structures spread across the body. Together, they create three lines of defense against pathogens:

1. The first line of defense is created by cutaneous and mucous membranes that act as a physical barrier, which blocks the entry of pathogens into the body.
2. The second line of defense consists of the responses of the cells and extracellular matrix chemicals to create an inhospitable environment to pathogens. Together with the first line, the second line of defense constitutes innate immunity.
3. The third line of defense consists of a highly selective responses of the immune system on particular pathogen agents, which constitutes an **adaptive immunity**.

An **infectious agent** is any organism that may cause damage or death to the host. Collectively, infectious agents are called **pathogens**. The five major categories of pathogens that may cause disease are bacteria, viruses, fungi, protozoans, and multicellular parasites.

Bacteria are microscopic prokaryotic organism. Bacteria are fundamentally different from multicellular organisms. They have no nucleus. A single DNA molecule of prokaryotes has a ring shape; the plasma membrane is enclosed in a cell wall, formed by complex carbohydrates linked with peptides. Some bacteria have an external sticky polysaccharide capsule, which protects bacteria from the host's immune system and increases their **virulence**. Additionally, bacteria can release enzymes or toxins that cause severe damage to host cells.

Viruses are not cells. They are much smaller than bacteria. Their "body" is composed of viral DNA or RNA enclosed in a protein capsid, or shell. Some viruses also have capsid covered by a membrane. Viruses do not have their own metabolic mechanism for development and reproduction and can do it only by using the biochemical machinery of the host cell. Thus, they are **obligatory parasites**, which cannot survive without a host.

Fungi are multicellular eukaryotic organisms. Fungi have a cell wall external to their plasma membrane. Here belong different forms of molds, yeasts, and fungi that produce spores. Fungal diseases are called **mycoses**.

Protozoans are microscopic, unicellular eukaryotic organisms that lack a cell wall. An example of protozoan disease is malaria caused by a plasmodium. Multicellular parasites include worms and arthropods.

Prions are fragments of abnormal proteins that cannot be destructed by animal enzymes and can be transmitted from organism to organism. Prions can cause damage to nervous tissue. The example of a prion-caused infection is mad cow disease or Variant Creutzfeldt-Jakob disease.

CHECK YOUR UNDERSTANDING

- Which pathogen must enter a cell to reproduce?

- What elements constitute innate immunity?

Types of Immunity: Innate Immunity and Adaptive Immunity

Immunity is classified according to the means by which it responds to pathogen agents. The first two lines of defense are formed by physical and chemical barriers that develop together with the organism and have the same mechanisms that deal with all pathogens. These mechanisms are inbuilt in body organization and cannot be changed. That is why they collectively constitute **nonspecific** or **innate immunity**. The innate immune system consists of cells and chemicals that create physical and chemical body barriers, spread in body tissues, or circulate with blood. They guarantee an immediate response to a pathogen invasion.

The **adaptive** or **specific immunity** is characterized by a selective specific response to unique glycoprotein markers called **antigens**. Antigens are present on the surface of all cells and most biological molecules and serve for their recognition. Adaptive immunity requires time for its development and responds slower than innate immunity. This response has to be initiated by the presence of a particular antigen. That is why adaptive immunity is also called **acquired immunity**. Adaptive immunity has a capacity termed **immunological memory**. This memory guarantees a fast and effective response to exposure to the same already familiar antigen. The innate immunity has no such capacity and will response the same way as before (fig. 18.13).

Both types of immunity function together, and one does not act independent from the other. The final response of an organism to a pathogen is a highly integrated series of events within all parts of the immune system. The dysfunction of one component of the immune system can cause catastrophic consequences to the entire system.

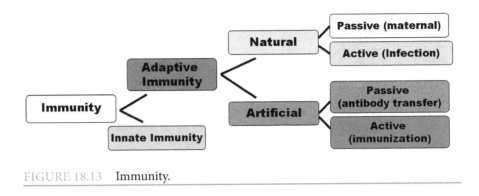

FIGURE 18.13   Immunity.

CHECK YOUR UNDERSTANDING

- What are the three lines of defense?

- Which immunity type has immunological memory?

Brief Characteristics of Innate Immunity

The first line of defense is the body's surface, provided by skin, mucous membranes, and their secretions. Altogether they form a continuous physical **surface barrier**, which blocks entry of potential pathogens inside the body. The importance of surface barriers becomes obvious when these barriers are compromised by wounds, burns, or chemical trauma. Every wound immediately becomes a window for different types of infectious agents.

Stratified keratinized epithelium and irregular dense connective tissue of the skin are resistant to mechanical stress. Dry hydrophobic keratin is not a proper media for most bacteria and fungi to grow and multiply. Keratinized epithelium is too hard to pass through towards the more sensitive body regions. Gelatinous polysaccharide—hyaluronic acid—in areolar tissue of the dermis slows down the entry of pathogenic microorganisms. Numerous exocrine glands in the skin, such as sweat, sebaceous, and ceruminous glands, release oily secretions with acidic pH that prevents growth of most pathogenic organisms that are evolutionarily adapted to alkaline blood and other body fluids. Tears and sweat contain antimicrobial lysozyme, defensins, and dermcidin.

Mucous membranes line all passages that have external openings, such as respiratory, gastrointestinal, and urogenital tracts. Mucous membranes have no keratin, but mucus produced by numerous goblet cells can trap and discourage pathogen invasion. Besides its high viscosity, mucus contains a number of antimicrobial substances, such as lysozyme, defensins, and immunoglobulins (IgA). Mucous membranes of the gastrointestinal tract, especially the stomach, also secrete digestive juices, which destroy and digest most pathogens. The viscous saliva has alkaline pH and contains antimicrobial lysozyme and IgA. The pH between the mouth and stomach changes dramatically from lightly alkaline to highly acidic, which does not give most microorganisms a chance to adapt. The very high acidity in the stomach may kill almost all invaders. Only very high specialized pathogens, such as *Helicobacter pylori*, can withstand the acidity of gastric juice. The respiratory tract is lined with ciliated pseudostratified (respiratory) epithelium (see chapter 4, page 104), whose cilia sweep mucus with trapped microbes out of the air passages (fig. 18.14).

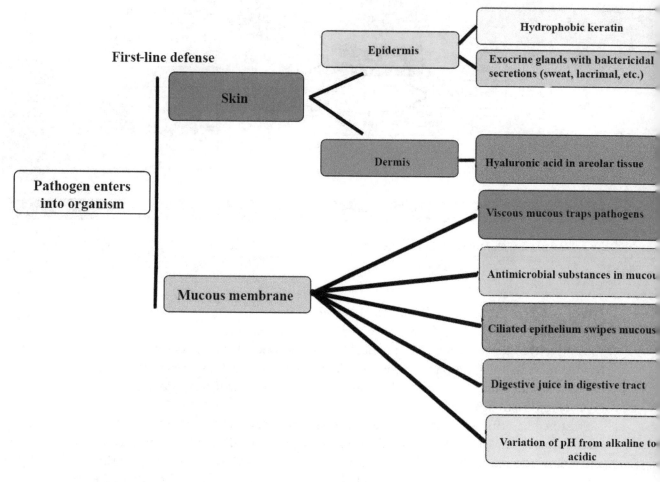

FIGURE 18.14   The First-Line Barrier of the Innate Immune System.

Diverse microflora normally populate a healthy organism. This microflora is called **commensal microflora**. It is found in all types of covering membranes. Nonpathogenic microorganisms of commensal flora protect their territory and prevent growth of other potentially pathogenic microorganisms. The real role of the normal microflora in an organisms' well-being is just beginning to be understood.

Surface barriers create a very strong defense line but cannot guarantee an absolute protection. Pathogens that pass through this barrier face the next line of defense. The second line of the innate immune system includes 1) cellular responses, 2) defensive chemicals, and 3) physiological processes that include inflammation, fever, diarrhea, and so on.

Microbes have molecular structures called **motifs** that they have in common. These molecular structures may be on the microbe surface or inside it. Innate immune cells carry **pattern recognition receptors** on their plasma membrane that recognize and bind with these molecular motifs. Physical contact of innate immune cells with motifs triggers an active immune response. The cellular component of the innate immune system includes four groups of cells identified by the defensive mechanisms they use against pathogens: 1) phagocytic cells, 2) inflammatory chemical-secreting cells, 3) apoptosis initiating cells, and 4) eosinophils.

Phagocytic cells include neutrophils, macrophages, and dendritic cells. They catch, engulf, and digest foreign substances and bodies. Phagocytosis of bacteria and viruses within neutrophils and macrophages is facilitated by the production of reactive oxygen-containing molecules, such as nitric oxide, hydrogen peroxide, and superoxide. The release of these molecules generates a so-called **respiratory burst** that depletes oxygen and kills aerobic microorganisms. Most microbes that enter the body are phagocytized by these cells. However, participation of neutrophils in phagocytosis is fatal for them. Dead neutrophils become the major component of the pus produced during some infections. Macrophages and dendritic cells, in opposite to neutrophils, continue

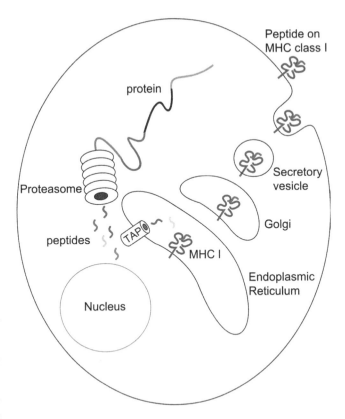

FIGURE 18.15   Major Histocompatibility Complex Class I Processing.

to function after phagocytosis pathogenic microorganisms. They serve in the process called **antigen presentation**. Fragments of phagocytized microbe are exposed in the special structures called **major histocompatibility complex I (MHC I)** on the plasma membrane of these cells for T lymphocytes, which activates them (fig. 18.15).

Basophils and mast cells secrete chemicals that generate inflammatory reaction. These cells release histamine and heparin. The first chemical causes vasodilation and increases capillaries' permeability. Heparin is an anticoagulant (see chapter 17, page 499). Basophils also secrete chemicals that attract other immune cells, such as neutrophils and macrophages.

Apoptosis is a programmed cellular suicide. Natural killer (NK) cells residing within secondary lymphatic structures directly attack unwanted cells. For that quality they are called **cytotoxic lymphocytes**. Attacking NK cells release a number of cytotoxic chemicals. **Perforin** makes holes in plasma membrane of attacked cell. **Granzymes** are enzymes that enter via the pore made by perforin unwanted cell interior and trigger its apoptosis. NK cells constantly patrol body tissues in search of unhealthy cells. The process is referred to as **immune surveillance**. NK cells eliminate cells already infected by virus or bacteria, but are most effective in destruction of tumor cells and transplanted tissues (fig. 18.16).

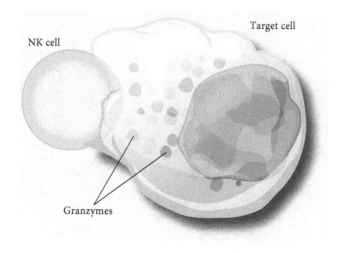

FIGURE 18.16   NK Cell Injects Granzymes in Target Cell.

Eosinophils are granulocytes, which targets are multicellular parasites, such as tapeworms (see chapter 17, page 499). Mechanisms of destruction include degranulation and release of enzymes and other substances lethal to the parasite. Eosinophils also release proteins that form a transmembrane pore to destroy cells of the multicellular organism (fig. 18.17).

Interferons (IFNs) are a special category of proteins called **cytokines**. A virus-infected cell produces and releases into surrounding space two types of interferons: **INF-α** and **INF-β**, which serve as signaling molecules that inform other nearby still uninfected cells about close presence of virus. All cells in the body have receptors to these interferons and, when **INF-α** and **INF-β** produced by infected cells bind to them, the transduction cascade of chemical reactions triggers in receiving cell production of special enzymes called **restriction factors**. Restriction factors cut down and destroy viral nucleic acids. Thus, the cell that receives signal from interferons becomes protected, and when a virus tries to invade it, it degrades viral hereditary molecules and prevents further spread of infection. In addition to that, **INF-α** and **INF-β** attract and stimulate NK cells to attack virus-infected cells that secrete these interferons and destroy them through apoptosis. In their turn NK cells also release **INF-γ** that mobilizes macrophages to aid NK cells in destruction of virus-infected cells (fig. 18.18).

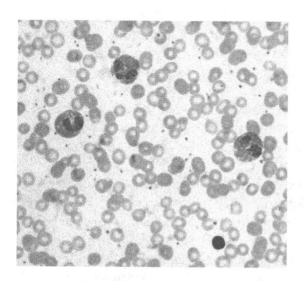

FIGURE 18.17   Eosinophils.

Tumor necrosis factor (TNF) is a cytokine that induces necrosis of tumor cells. Necrosis is a premature cell death caused by factors external to the cell or tissue, such as infection, toxins, or trauma which result in the unregulated digestion of cell components. Apoptosis, in opposite to necrosis, is a naturally programmed physiological process of cell death. TNF is secreted primarily by activated macrophages in response to certain bacteria and other pathogens. TNF attracts phagocytes to the area of infection, increases their activity, and stimulates phagocytes to release other cytokines. A severe infection can cause massive production of TNF, which may result in the potentially fatal condition of **septic shock**.

Another big group of 36 cytokines is called **interleukins**. Interleukins stimulate production of neutrophils, mobilize NK cells, trigger production of interferons, and activate T cells.

Many cytokines generate flu-like symptoms, including fever, chills, and aches. Cytokines have been actively studied for their possible therapeutic use in conditions such as persistent viral infections and certain cancers.

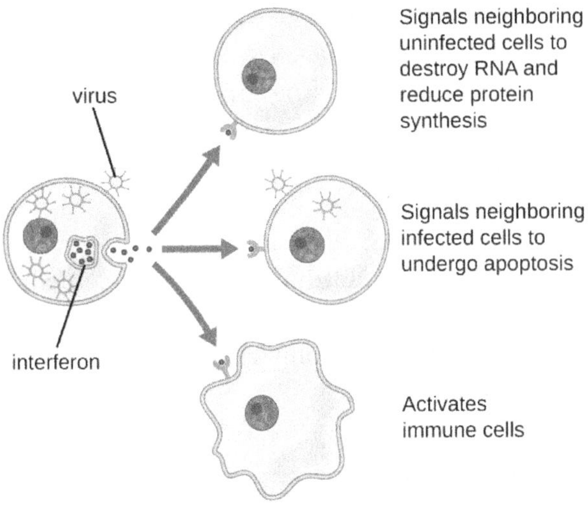

The complement system is a group of more than 20 plasma proteins produced by the liver. Their inactive form is released into the bloodstream, where they circulate until they become activated via two cascade reactions called the **classical** and **alternative pathways**. The classical pathway begins when inactive complement proteins bind to antibodies bound to antigen. The alternative pathway begins with cleavage of an inactive complement protein called **C3** into the active form **C3b**. This can also occur when inactive complement proteins encounter foreign cells such as bacteria. The two pathways converge when active C3b protein cleaves the inactive protein C5 and converts it into an active C5b. Activated complement proteins initiate the next processes (fig. 18.19):

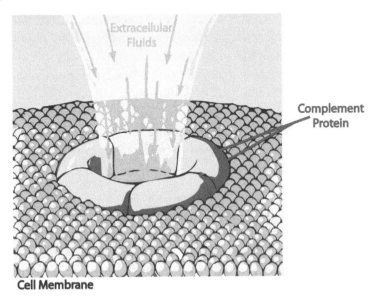

FIGURE 18.18 Interferon Signaling.

Signals neighboring uninfected cells to destroy RNA and reduce protein synthesis

Signals neighboring infected cells to undergo apoptosis

Activates immune cells

virus

interferon

1. **Cytolysis.** Some complement proteins are able to **lyse** the plasma membrane of pathogens, leading to their destruction. This process is mediated by C5b, which binds to the surface of the pathogen and provides a docking site for several other activated complement proteins. Together these complement proteins form a structure collectively known as a **membrane attack complex**, or **MAC**, which inserts into the plasma membrane of the target cell and create pore in it. Hydrolytic enzymes enter the cell through this pore and lyse it.

2. **Inflammation.** Inflammation is a nonspecific response to a cellular injury. Several complement proteins enhance this response by triggering basophils and mast cells to release histamine and heparin that mediate inflammation.

Extracellular Fluids

Complement Protein

Cell Membrane

FIGURE 18.19 Membrane Attack Complex.

3. **Neutralization of viruses.** C3b and components of the membrane attack complex bind to certain viruses and neutralize them physically block them from infecting host cells.

4. **Opsonization.** The complement protein binds to bacteria or other cell surfaces. This protein plays the role of a marker. Attached to a pathogen, the complement protein makes this pathogen "visible" to other immune cells. Phagocytes recognize complement proteins and attack pathogenic organisms. The protein is called **opsonin**. Besides that, opsonization immobilizes pathogenic organism.

5. **Clearance of immune complex.** C3b also binds to immune complexes (complexes created by bound antigens and antibodies) and stimulates their phagocytosis. This action cleans circulation from immune complexes, which is critical to preventing them from lodging in different tissues around the body.

CHECK YOUR UNDERSTANDING

- Which structures create a surface barrier?

- What is a membrane attack complex, and how does it work against pathogens?

- Describe the role of interferons in an immune reaction.

- What mechanisms activate the complement system?

Inflammation

Cellular injury triggers a series of events termed **inflammatory response**. The damaged cell releases inflammatory mediators that cause local changes in the damaged tissue. Inflammatory mediators attract phagocytes to the area and clean up damaged tissue. The inflammatory mediators include histamine, serotonin, cytokines, a peptide called **bradykinin**, a group of local signaling molecules collectively termed **prostaglandins**, and **leukotrienes**. Basophils and mast cells also produce some additional amount of inflammatory mediators. Inflammatory mediators increase blood influx to the affected area and its leaking into the surrounding tissues. Three symptoms of any inflammation include redness, swelling, and pain are known as **cardinal signs of inflammation**. These symptoms are results of the following processes:

1. **Vasodilation of arterioles.** Inflammatory mediators such as histamine and bradykinin are potent vasodilators, and their release increases blood flow to injured tissues. This causes injured area becomes congested with blood, a condition termed **hyperemia**. Hyperemia is responsible for the redness and heat that accompany inflammation.

2. **Increase of capillary permeability.** The structure of most capillaries prevents them from leaking. Inflammatory mediators increase the permeability of local capillaries. This allows protein-rich fluid to exit the blood vessels and accumulate in the surrounding tissues. The proteins in the fluid

include clotting proteins such as fibrinogen, complement proteins, and proteins needed for tissue repair. Tissue becomes congested with blood and swells.

3. **Pain.** Many of the inflammatory mediators, particularly bradykinin and prostaglandins, trigger action potentials in the peripheral processes of sensory neurons.

4. **Chemotaxis.** The final effect of inflammatory mediators is the recruitment of leukocytes to the damaged area via a process known as **chemotaxis**. Inflammatory mediators attract and activate a number of leukocytes, particularly macrophages and neutrophils.

The second component of the inflammatory response deals with the phagocytes that ingest pathogens and cellular debris.

1. **Local macrophages are activated.** Within minutes of a cellular injury, macrophages already present in the area enlarge and begin to phagocytize pathogens and damaged cells.

2. **Neutrophils migrate by chemotaxis to the damaged tissue and phagocytize bacteria and cellular debris.** Neutrophils migrate from the blood to the damaged tissue. Inflammatory mediators and activated complement proteins attract neutrophils and enable them to leave the blood and enter the tissue. The inflammatory mediators make the capillary endothelium in the damaged area "sticky," and the neutrophils adhere to the capillary wall, a process called margination. The inflammatory mediators also increase capillary permeability. So, neutrophils can squeeze between endothelial cells and enter the damaged tissue. This process is termed **diapedesis** (fig. 18.20).

3. **Monocytes migrate to the tissue by chemotaxis and become macrophages, which phagocytize pathogens and cellular debris.** The next group of cells to be attracted to the area by

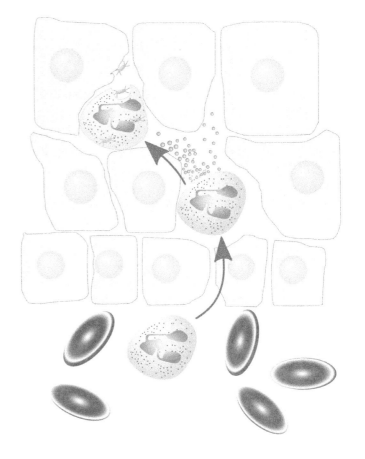

FIGURE 18.20   Extravascular Migration of Neutrophils.

chemotaxis is the circulating monocytes. Monocytes exit the blood the same way as neutrophils. In the damaged tissue, monocytes enlarge and mature into macrophages. This process is much slower than mobilization of neutrophils. However, monocytes live longer and are more aggressive than neutrophils.

4. **Leukocytosis is a process of producing new leukocytes that takes place in the red bone marrow.** Cytokines produced by the activated phagocytes act on cells of the red bone marrow to increase the production of neutrophils and monocytes over the next few days. This leads to an elevated number of circulating leukocytes or leukocytosis.

CHECK YOUR UNDERSTANDING

- What are inflammatory mediators, and what do they do?

- What is role of phagocytes in the inflammatory response?

- What is inflammation, and what are its main signs?

Fever

Fever is an innate immune system general response to cellular injury. This response is initiated by chemicals collectively known as **pyrogens**. Pyrogens are released from damaged cells or some bacteria. Neurons in the hypothalamus' body temperature control center have receptors sensitive to pyrogens. The receptor-pyrogen complex resets the thermoregulation center to a higher-than-normal temperature range. At that point, the hypothalamus is programmed to maintain a higher body temperature level and interprets normal temperature as low. That is why fever is often accompanied by feeling cold and experiencing chills. The hypothalamus elevates body temperature to a new higher level. For that, the hypothalamus uses different mechanisms; for example, shivering: uncontrollable muscle activity that generates heat in the body.

Medications that reduce an inflammation-mediated fever are called **antipyretics**. Most antipyretics work in the same way as anti-inflammatories. They inhibit formation of prostaglandins. Aspirin and ibuprofen, which are used as anti-inflammatory medicine, are also antipyretics.

CHECK YOUR UNDERSTANDING

- Which part of the brain controls body temperature?

- What causes the elevation of body temperature?

- Explain why a patient can have a fever during a heart attack.

Adaptive Immunity: Cell-Mediated Immunity and Antibody-Mediated Immunity

Adaptive immune response is initiated by entrance of foreign antigen. It works through two different, but tightly associated, mechanisms: 1. **cell-mediated immunity**, and 2. **antibody-mediated immunity**, also called **humoral immunity**. Both are performed by lymphocytes. For that, lymphocytes have to make contact with an antigen. This contact causes a lymphocyte to proliferate and differentiate. Emerged new lymphocytes create a group of specialized immune cells that can respond only to a particular antigen. This group of lymphocytes is called a **clone**.

CHECK YOUR UNDERSTANDING

- What is the difference between cell-mediated and anti-body-mediated immunity?

- What is a clone?

Cell-Mediated Immunity

Cell-mediated immunity functions through different classes of T cells. T cells originate from lymphoid line cells in the red bone marrow. Soon, they leave the bone marrow and migrate to the thymus. Here, they undergo **gene rearrangements** that lead to a huge variety of genetically distinct T cells. There are millions of different clones in the immune system, but only a few cells of each clone exist in the body at any given time. T cells have receptor molecules called corereceptors, which facilitate T cell physical interaction with a cell presenting antigen. The most important category of core-receptors is the CD molecules. T lymphocytes are divided in two principal groups in accordance with the type of CD core-receptors: **helper T cells (T_H)**, also called **CD4 cells**, and **cytotoxic T cells (T_C)**, also known as **CD8 cells**. These cells respond to cells infected by viruses, bacteria, cancer, and foreign cells, such as transplanted tissues. **Helper T lymphocytes (T_H)** initiate cell-mediated and humoral immune reactions, activate NK cells; that is, enhance innate immunity. **Cytotoxic T lymphocytes (T_C)** release chemicals that kill pathogen cells (fig. 18.21).

Additional types of T lymphocytes include: 1. **memory T lymphocytes** (both T_C and T_H). Memory T cells serve to "preserve" memory about certain infection in order to be able rapidly develop immune response in case of repeated invasion;

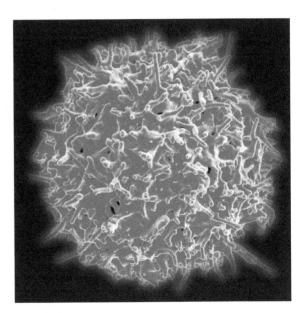

FIGURE 18.21   Healthy Human T Lymphocyte. Electron Microscope Image.

2. **regulatory T lymphocytes (T$_{regs}$)** suppress immune response and prevent development of allergic and autoimmune reactions.

To perform their function, T lymphocytes have to be able to recognize an antigen of interest. T cell acquire their antigen recognition through the process termed **antigen presentation**. There are several cell types that present antigen to T lymphocytes, termed **antigen-presenting cell (APC)**. APC includes dendritic cells, macrophages, and B cells.

Antigen presentation begins from attachment of antigen to a special transmembrane proteins called **major histocompatibility complex (MHC)**. There are two primary categories of MHC molecules: **MHC class I** and **MHC class II**. All cells are able to present antigen with MHC class I molecules, but only APCs display antigen with both MHC classes.

MHC class I are glycoproteins. They are genetically determined and are unique to every organism. MHC class I are continuously synthesized by the rough endoplasmic reticulum (RER), inserted into the ER, shipped within and modified by the endomembrane system. Finally, they incorporate into the plasma membrane and display peptide fragments of **endogenous proteins** ("self" proteins of the cell). This process is called **endogenous pathway**. In the endogenous pathway, peptide fragments in the cell randomly bind with the MHC class I molecules. These peptide fragments in uninfected, healthy cells are simply partially degraded proteins of the cell and are considered "self." Consequently, in uninfected, healthy cells, MHC class I molecules are displaying only self-antigens on their surface. These self-antigens are ignored or tolerated by the T lymphocytes.

However, if the cell is infected, the antigens presented are foreign antigens. Proteins of an intracellular infectious agent are cleaved by a proteasome into peptide fragments of 3 to 15 amino acids; these degraded peptide fragments of the infectious agent are considered "nonself." The peptide fragments of the infectious agent that are in the cytosol are shipped into the RER, where the peptide fragments combine with MHC class I molecules, within the RER. Through the endomembrane system, the MHC class I molecules with bound foreign antigen are shipped to the plasma membrane, where they are displayed at the cell surface.

The **MHC class II** molecule is a glycoprotein continuously synthesized by the rough endoplasmic reticulum, modified by the endomembrane system, and then embedded within the plasma membrane. However, antigens are presented with MHC molecules only after an APC (macrophage and dendritic cell) first engulfs **exogenous antigens**. The process involving proteins that originate outside a host cell is referred to as the **exogenous pathway**. In the exogenous pathway, the microbe is engulfed by the APC through phagocytosis. The phagosome with a foreign antigen merges with a lysosome. Enzymes of the lysosome digest the microbe into peptide fragments. The vesicle containing peptide fragments (antigens) then merges with vesicles containing newly synthesized MHC class II molecules. The peptide fragments bind with the MHC class II molecules. The MHC class II-antigen complex incorporates into the APC plasma membrane and displays exogenous antigen outside the cell membrane. The **helper T cells** recognize the antigen as a signal to step up their actions (fig. 18.23). A similar effect has display of antigen with MHC class I molecules. However, this display of foreign antigen with MHC class I molecule provides the means of communicating specifically with **cytotoxic T cells** only. In both cases, the communication between T lymphocyte and exogenous antigen causes T cell activation (fig. 18.22).

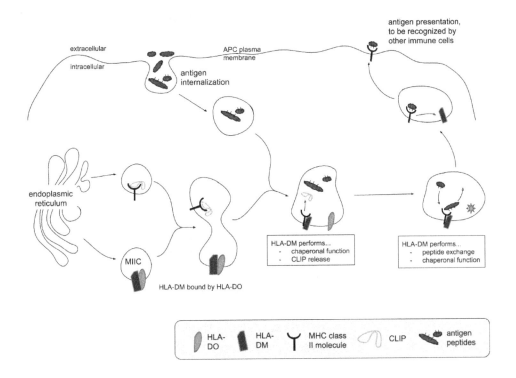

FIGURE 18.22   Antigen Presentation by the MHC Class II Molecule in APC.

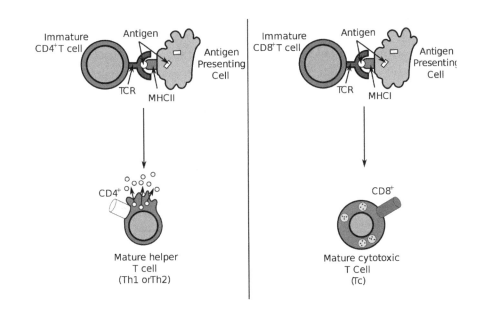

FIGURE 18.23   Antigen Presentation by MHC Class I Activates T$_C$ Cells, Whereas Antigen Presentation by MHC Class II Activates T$_H$ Cells.

CHECK YOUR UNDERSTANDING

- What is the role of helper T cells in acquired immunity?

- What do cytotoxic T lymphocytes do?

- Explain the role of antigen presenting cells.

- What is the difference between the functioning of MHC class I and MHC class II molecules?

T Lymphocyte Formation, Selection, and Activation

Millions of immature T lymphocytes, called **thymocytes**, migrate to the thymus. In —thymus they transform into the mature T lymphocytes and become **immunocompetent**. They get a unique receptor called **T cell receptor**, or **TCR**. This receptor is responsible for recognition of antigen fragments and binding to both class I and class II MHC molecules. Each lymphocyte has a unique TCR. In the thymus, the TCR of each lymphocyte is examined on its ability to bind with exogenous antigen presented by the MHC molecule, but ignores all MHC molecules associated with self-antigens. This process of TCR testing is called **thymic selection**. The thymic selection proceeds in two steps:

1. **Positive selection.** Positive selection occurs within the outer cortex of the thymus. The TCR embedded in the plasma membrane of a T lymphocyte must be able to recognize and bind an MHC molecule. Thymic epithelial cells have MHC molecules in their plasma membrane. Those thymocytes that can bind with the MHC of thymic epithelial cells are survive. The thymocytes that do not recognize the MHC molecules are destroyed. The selection of T lymphocytes that are able to bind with MHC molecules suggests the name of this process as a **positive selection**. Selected T lymphocytes migrate into the medulla, where they come through the next step, called **negative selection**.

2. **Negative selection.** In the medulla, lymphocytes are tested by thymic dendritic cells that present their self-antigens with MHC class I and II molecules. This selection is called negative because those T lymphocytes that bind with presented within the MHC molecule are destroyed. Only those T lymphocytes that disregard self-antigens and bind with foreign antigens stay alive. Through the negative selection, lymphocytes learn to "ignore" self-antigens and react only on foreign antigens, the quality termed **self-tolerance**. Development of self-tolerant T cells in primary lymphatic organs collectively called **central tolerance**.

Thymocytes that survive both positive and negative selections can bind an MHC molecule and recognize foreign antigen, but ignore self-antigens. Only approximately 2 percent of the originally formed thymocytes survive both selection processes; the remaining 98 percent are eliminated in the thymus by apoptosis.

The final step in T lymphocyte selection is a **differentiation** of each thymocyte into either a helper T lymphocyte (CD4 cell) by the selective loss of the CD8 protein, or a cytotoxic T lymphocyte (CD8 cell) by the selective loss of CD4 protein. After differentiation, two primary types of T lymphocytes become **naive immunocompetent** cells. Helper T lymphocytes also are called **CD4+** and cytotoxic T lymphocytes—**CD8+**.

The naive immunocompetent lymphocytes migrate from the thymus to secondary lymphatic organs and populate them (fig. 18.24).

To exercise their immune responsibilities, T lymphocytes have to be activated. Lymphocytes activation begins with recognition and physical contact between lymphocyte and antigen. The binding of lymphocyte with antigen triggers a cascade of chemical reactions leading to the lymphocyte's mitotic divisions and differentiation into a clone of identical cells with the same TCRs that match that specific antigen. This clone-forming process in response to a specific antigen is called **clonal selection**.

The first contact between an antigen and a lymphocyte is called an **antigen challenge**. It takes place in secondary lymphatic structures. The antigen challenge has many different forms, depending on the entry pathway of the antigen. Antigen in the blood is transported to the spleen; antigen that invades through the skin is engulfed and transported by epidermal dendritic cells to a lymph node; and antigen that enters through the mucous membrane of the respiratory, gastrointestinal, urinary, or reproductive tract comes into contact with the tonsils or MALT.

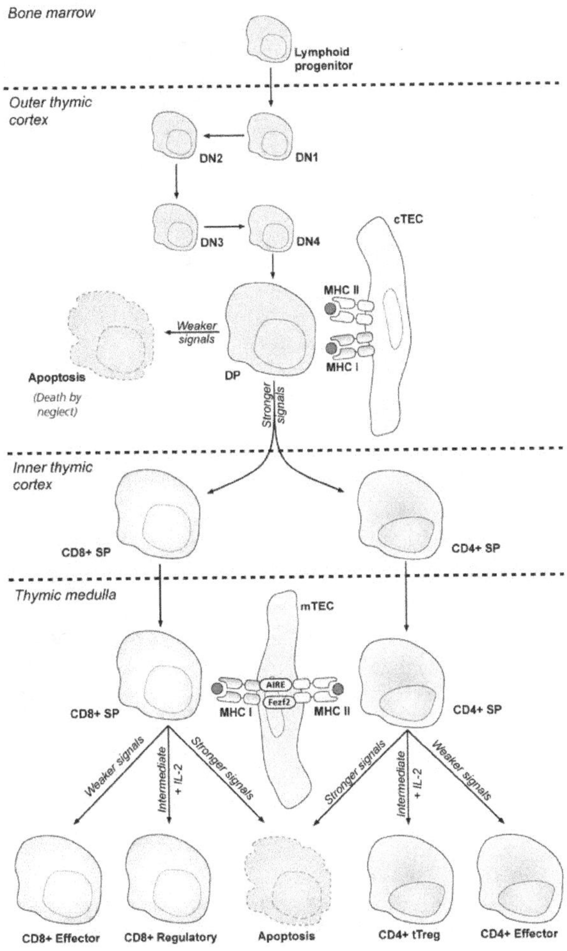

The lymphocyte TCR connection with the peptide fragment presented with an MHC class II molecule of the APC constitutes the **first signal** in activation process. This interaction is stabilized by the CD4 molecule in the helper T cell binding to other regions of

FIGURE 18.24 Thymic Selection.

the MHC class II molecule. If the TCR does not recognize the presented antigen, it disengages from the APC. If it does recognize the antigen, contact between the two cells lasts several hours.

The **second signal** takes place when other receptors of the APC interact with receptors of the helper T lymphocyte. Ultimately, helper T cells are induced to synthesize and release the cytokine interleukin 2 (IL-2), which occurs within about 24 hours. IL-2 acts as an autocrine hormone to further stimulation of the helper T cell from which it was released. On this step T lymphocytes divide in two groups. Some of activated T lymphocytes become dedicated producers of IL-2, whereas another small group develops in **memory helper T cells**. The role of memory cells is to preserve "memory" of infectious antigen and be available in the future if specific antigen again invades organism. The lack of the second signal is thought to result in formation of helper T lymphocytes become regulatory T lymphocytes (T_{Treg}) (fig. 18.24).

A simple activation of naive CD8$^+$ T cells requires the interaction with professional APCs, mainly with matured dendritic cells. To generate long-lasting memory T lymphocytes and to allow repetitive

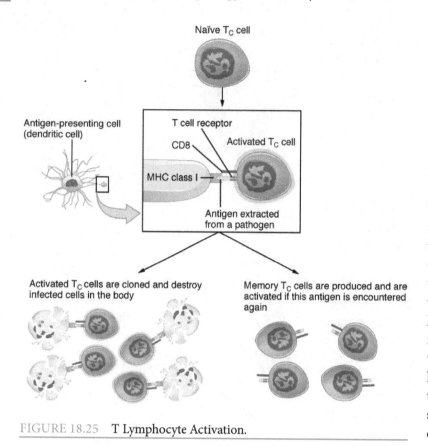

FIGURE 18.25   T Lymphocyte Activation.

stimulation of cytotoxic T cells, dendritic cells have to interact with both, activated CD4+ helper T cells and CD8+ T cells. During this process, the CD4+ helper T cells "license" the dendritic cells to give a potent activating signal to the naive CD8+ T cells. In most cases, activation is dependent on TCR recognition of antigen. An alternative pathways include activation of cytotoxic T cells by other CD8 T cells. An activated T_C cell undergoes clonal expansion with the help of the cytokine interleukin-2 (IL-2). This increases the number of cells specific for the target antigen. These cells then leave the lymphatic organ and travel throughout the body in search of antigen-positive somatic cells.

CHECK YOUR UNDERSTANDING

- What is the difference between thymocytes and immunocompetent T lymphocytes?

- What is the difference between positive and negative selection?

- What does "central tolerance" mean?

- What is the difference between the development of helper and cytotoxic T cells?

Effects of T Cells

The primary function of cytotoxic T cells is direct destruction of pathogen cells that carry foreign antigens bound to MHC class I molecules. Their ability to interact with MHC class I molecules means that they can detect abnormalities in any cell type with a nucleus, which is critical for the detection of cancer cells, foreign cells, and cells infected with intracellular pathogens such as viruses and bacteria. T_C cells are activated in the same way as T_H cells, with the addition that they require IL-2 from T_H cells in order to be completely activated. This mechanism protects organism from abnormal T_C cell activation.

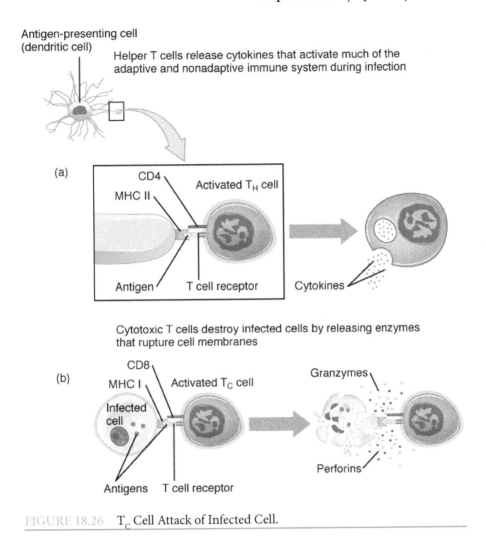

FIGURE 18.26 T_C Cell Attack of Infected Cell.

An activated T_C cell searches and binds with target cell. Connection with target antigen triggers release of protein called **perforin**. Perforin forms pores in, or perforates, the target cell's plasma membrane. After that, T_C cell releases enzymes that can now enter the target cell cytosol. These enzymes catalyze reactions that degrade target cell proteins and eventually lead to its DNA fragmentation and cellular death. T_C cells also bind to proteins on the plasma membrane of the target cell and initiate its programmed death—apoptosis. When the target cell begins to degrade, the T_C cell detaches and leaves it for search of another target cell (fig. 18.26).

Helper T cells have no phagocytic or cytotoxic abilities. Their function in an immune response consists of synthesis and release of **cytokines**. Cytokines activate and enhance various components of the immune system. Cytokine **interleukin-3** stimulates macrophages' phagocytic activity. It also causes macrophages to produce an **interleukine-12**, which stimulates T_H cells to generate more interleukine-3. Cytokine **interleukine-2** (IL-2) is needed for activation of T_C cells. In the absence of T_H cells and IL-2, most T_C cells fail to activate and become unresponsive to the antigen. IL-2 also stimulates the T_C cells' proliferation.

VETERINARY APPLICATION

Feline immunodeficiency virus (FIV) is a lentivirus that affects cats worldwide. From 2.5 percent to 4.4 percent of cats worldwide are infected with FIV. FIV is closely related to human immunodeficiency virus (HIV). FIV is the only nonprimate lentivirus to cause an AIDS-like syndrome, but FIV is not typically fatal for cats, as they can live relatively healthily as carriers and transmitters of the disease for many years.

FIV was discovered in 1986 by Dr. Niels Pedersen at the UC Davis School of Veterinary Medicine. He studied a colony of cats that had a high level of opportunistic infections and degenerative conditions and was originally called feline T lymphotropic virus (FTLV). Since that time, it has been found in domestic cat populations worldwide. FIV can compromise the cat's immune system. FIV infects many cell types in its host, including CD4+ and CD8+ T lymphocytes, B lymphocytes, and macrophages. FIV can be tolerated well by cats but can eventually lead to debilitation of the immune system in its feline hosts by the infection and exhaustion of T-helper (CD4+) cells. The primary mode of FIV transmission is via deep bite wounds, where the infected cat's saliva enters the other cat's tissues. FIV may also be transmitted from pregnant females to their offspring in utero; however, this vertical transmission is considered to be relatively rare based on the small number of FIV-infected kittens and adolescents.

The development of an effective vaccine against FIV is difficult because of the high number and variations of the virus strains. A dual-subtype vaccine for FIV released in 2002 called Fel-O-Vax made it possible to immunize cats against some FIV strains. In 2006 a new treatment aid was developed, termed Lymphocyte T-Cell Immunomodulator, manufactured by T-Cyte Therapeutics, Inc. Lymphocyte T-Cell Immunomodulator is a potent stimulator of CD-4 cell's production of IL-2.

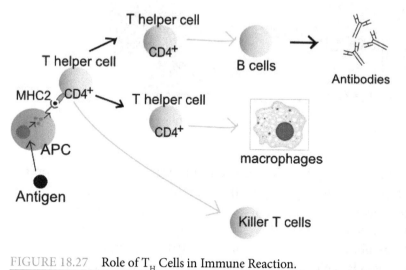

T_H cells directly bind to B cells and stimulate them to proliferate and differentiate. They also secrete various interleukins that stimulate B cells proliferation and increase antibody production. T_H cells are required for normal function of all components of the immune system, including innate, antibody mediated, and cell mediated immunity. Because of that, failure of T_H cells to function leads to failure of the entire immune system (fig. 18.27).

FIGURE 18.27   Role of T_H Cells in Immune Reaction.

CHECK YOUR UNDERSTANDING

- What are the main functions of T_C cells?
- What are the main functions of T_H cells?

- How do T_C cells fight infectious cells?

Antibody-Mediated Immunity

The naive immunocompetent B lymphocytes are also activated by a specific antigen in secondary lymphatic structures. As with T lymphocytes, two signals are required. However, B lymphocytes do not require antigen to be presented by other nonlymphocyte cells. B lymphocytes can recognize and respond to antigens by themselves. For that, B lymphocyte has a transmembrane receptor protein called **B cell receptor**, or **BCR**. BCR is an immunoglobulin located on the outer surface of the cell.

The **first signal** occurs when an antigen binds to the BCR, and the antigen cross-links BCRs. The stimulated B lymphocyte engulfs, processes, and presents the antigen to the helper T lymphocyte that recognizes that antigen. The **second signal** occurs when an activated helper T lymphocyte releases the IL-4, which stimulates the B lymphocyte.

Activation of B lymphocytes causes them to proliferate and differentiate. Most of the activated B lymphocytes differentiate into **plasma cells** that produce antibodies, and the remainder become **memory B lymphocytes** that can be activated upon reexposure to the same antigen. Memory B lymphocytes differ from plasma cells in some respects: 1) the memory B lymphocytes retain their BCRs, and 2) the memory B lymphocytes have a much longer life span (months to years) than plasma cells.

The antibody-mediated immune response has three basic phases. The first phase involves a B cell clone all cells of which recognize one specific antigen. Contact with this antigen triggers B cell to undergo changes and start secreting antibodies. The second phase begins when the antibody level in the blood rises dramatically. Antibodies, also known as **immunoglobulins** or **gamma globulins**, are active components of antibody-mediated immunity (fig. 18.28).

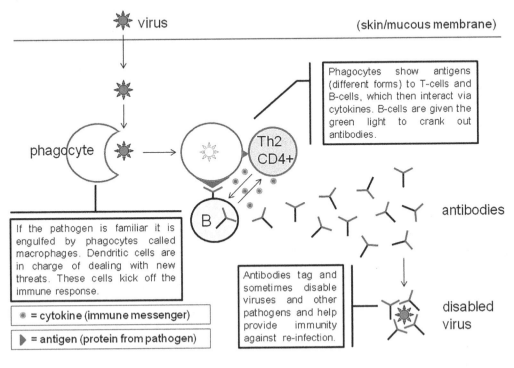

FIGURE 18.28   Humoral Immune Reaction.

- What do plasma cells do?
- What is the role of memory B cells?

B Lymphocyte Formation, Selection, and Activation

B cells develop from hematopoietic stem cells (HSCs) in the red bone marrow. HSCs give rise to the lymphoid cell line. From here, B cells' development proceeds through two selective processes. **Positive selection** occurs through antigen-independent signaling involving the pre-BCR and the BCR. At this step, the B cell receptor has to bind with presented antigen. If BCR do not bind to their ligand, B cells do not receive support and cease to further development. **Negative selection** occurs through the binding of self-antigen with the BCR. If the BCR binds to self-antigen, the B cell faces one of four options: 1) clonal deletion, 2) receptor editing, 3) anergy, or 4) ignorance. **Clonal deletion** means that all B cells that belong to the clone and do not pass negative selection are programmed to apoptosis. **Receptor editing** occurs during the B cells' maturation. It is a process of change of the antigen structure, in order to rescue B cells from programmed cell death (apoptosis). It is thought that 20 to 50 percent of all peripheral naive B cells have undergone receptor editing. **Anergy** describes a procedures that lead to inability of B cell to respond to antigen or B cell deactivation. Negative selection results in development of **central tolerance** expressed in inability of the mature B cells to bind with self-antigens present in the bone marrow. To complete development, immature B cells, called **transitional B cells**, migrate from the red bone marrow into the spleen, where they differentiate into mature but naive B cells.

B cell activation takes place in the secondary lymphoid organs, such as the spleen and lymph nodes. The activation begins when the B cell binds to an antigen via its BCR. B cell activation is enhanced through the activity of a surface receptor CD21 in complex with surface proteins CD19 and CD 81 (all three are collectively known as the **B cell coreceptor complex**). This process can proceed with help of T lymphocytes, called **T cell-dependent antigens (TD)**, or without T lymphocytes' help, called **T cell-independent antigens (TI)**.

Antigens that activate B cells with the help of T cells include foreign proteins. B cell response to these antigens takes many days. TD antigens have higher affinity and are more functionally versatile than that generated through T cell-independent antigens. Once a BCR binds a TD antigen, the antigen is phagocytized by the B cell through receptor-mediated endocytosis, degraded, and, finally, presented to helper T cell through the MHC class II complex. When the T_H recognizes and binds MHC-II-TD antigen it expresses the surface protein CD40L and cytokines IL-4 and IL-21. CD40L binds with B cell receptor CD 40. Cytokines bind with B cell cytokine receptors. Altogether they trigger B cell multiplication and activation. Activated B cells participate in a two-step differentiation process that yields short-lived B cells called **plasmablasts** for immediate protection and long-lived plasmablasts or memory B cells. Plasmablasts produce early, weak antibodies mostly of class IgM. The long-lived plasmablasts secrete large amounts of antibody and either stay within the spleen and lymph nodes, but most often migrate to the red bone marrow.

Antigens that activate B cells without T_H cells include foreign polysaccharides and unmethylated CpG DNA. B cell responses to these antigens is rapid, but has lower affinity and is less functionally versatile than generated through T cell-dependent activation. The process results in development of short-lived plasmablasts that produce early, weak antibodies mostly of class IgM, but also some populations of long-lived plasma cells.

Some memory B cells can be activated without T cell help, such as certain virus-specific memory B cells, but others need T cell help. Upon antigen binding, the memory B cell takes up the antigen through receptor-mediated endocytosis, degrades it, and presents it to T cells as peptide pieces in complex with MHC-II molecules on the cell membrane. Memory T helper (T_H) cells recognize and bind these MHC-II-peptide complexes through their TCR. Following TCR-MHC-II-peptide binding and the relay of other signals from the memory T_H cell, the memory B cell is activated and differentiates either into plasmablasts.

CHECK YOUR UNDERSTANDING

- How is a B cell activated?

- What does the term *clonal deletion* mean?

- What is the difference between the two ways of B cell activation?

Antibodies and Their Effects

The science that studies antibodies and their effects is called **serology**. The basic subunit of an every antibody is a **Y**-shaped molecule formed from four peptide chains: two **heavy (H)** and two **light (L) chains**. Every chain has two regions or motifs: **constant (C)** and **variable (V) regions**. Constant regions are relatively similar among all antibodies. Variable regions are unique sequences of amino acids responsible for antigen recognition and binding. An antibody has **V** regions at the tips of the two arms of the molecule, so the basic antibody subunit has two **antigen-binding sites**—one on each arm (fig. 18.29).

A single antibody subunit, called a **monomer**, can be combined with other subunits to form a larger structure of two monomers called **dimer** or five monomers, called **pentamer**. Five classes of antibodies are grouped in accordance to the structure of their **C regions**. Each antibody is named with the two-letter abbreviation Ig. The following capital letter designates immunoglobulin to one of these five classes: **IgG, IgA, IgM, IgE,** and **IgD**.

1. **IgG** are the most common antibodies. They account about 75 to 80 percent of the serum antibodies. It consists of a single subunit. IgG is the only antibody able to cross placenta and enter into the fetal circulation during pregnancy. In primates this immunoglobulin is responsible for Rh reaction of the Rh- female on the Rh+ fetus during the second pregnancy.

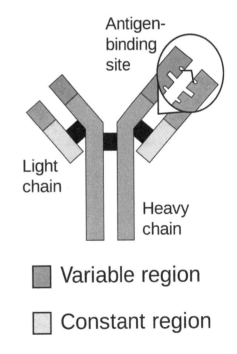

Antigen-binding site

Light chain

Heavy chain

■ Variable region

□ Constant region

FIGURE 18.29   Antibody Structure.

2. **IgA** is usually a dimer, made of two Y-shaped subunits and having four antigen-binding sites. IgA was found in skin secretions, mucous membranes, and such exocrine glands as lacrimal (tears), salivary, sweat, and lactiferous (milk).

3. **IgM** is the largest pentamer antibodies. Its five subunits are arranged in a star pattern and has 10 antigen-binding sites. IgM is generally the first antibody secreted by plasma cells on pathogen invasion. IgM also can be a part of the B cell plasma membrane, where it functions as a B cell receptor (BCR).

4. **IgE** is a single-subunit antibody, presented in very low amounts in body fluids. IgE binds to two types of antigen: 1) antigens associated with parasites, such as tapeworms or pathogens, and 2) allergens linked with inflammatory reactions. IgE binds to mast cells in mucous membranes, and when they come into contact with their specific antigens, they trigger mast cells to release the content of their granules, a process called **degranulation**. Mast cell granules contain inflammatory mediators such as histamine that initiate a local inflammatory response.

5. **IgD** is the only antibody not secreted by B cells. It has only one subunit located on the B cell surface and acts as an antigen receptor that helps activate B cells in a similar manner to IgM.

The basic effects of antibodies include:

1. **Agglutination and precipitation.** Antibodies can bind to more than one antigen on different cells. This creates a clump of cells that are cross-linked by their attachment to antibodies. The clumping of cells is known as **agglutination**. Similar to agglutination is the process called **precipitation**, which involves soluble antigens instead of whole cells. Both agglutination and precipitation allow these antigen-antibody complexes to precipitate out of body fluids and therefore make the complexes easier for phagocytes to ingest. IgM is the most potent agglutinating and precipitating antibody as a result of its ten antigen-binding sites.

2. **Opsonization.** Opsonization involves complement proteins coating the pathogen and activating phagocytes. IgG antibodies are also opsonins able to coat pathogens and bind and activate phagocytes, which greatly enhances phagocytosis.

3. **Neutralization.** Bacterial toxins, viral proteins, and animal venoms are molecules with specific components that are harmful. Antibodies bind to these components, as well as certain viruses and bacteria, and prevent them from interacting with cells. This renders the toxin inactive, which is known as **neutralization**. Most neutralizing antibodies are of either the IgG or the IgA class.

4. **Complement activation.** Several antibodies, particularly IgM and IgG, bind and activate the complement proteins of innate immunity. When several antibodies bind a single cell, their complement binding sites are exposed. This allows complement to activate and lyse the foreign cell with its membrane attack complex. This effect is particularly important in defense against cellular pathogens such as bacteria (fig. 18.30).

5. **Stimulation of inflammation.** The antibody IgE directly triggers inflammation by initiating the release of inflammatory mediators from mast cells and basophils. Antibodies also trigger inflammation indirectly through their activation of complement.

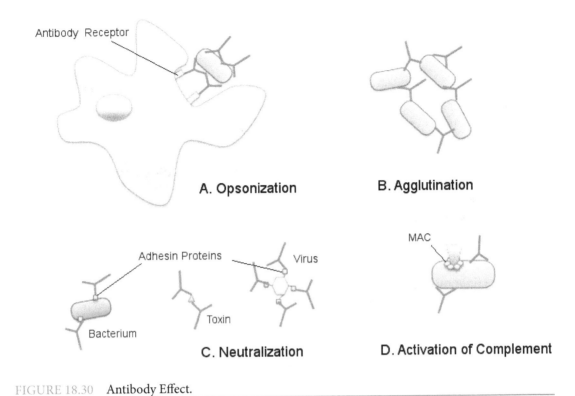

Antibody Receptor

A. Opsonization

B. Agglutination

Adhesin Proteins

Virus

Toxin

Bacterium

C. Neutralization

MAC

D. Activation of Complement

FIGURE 18.30   Antibody Effect.

CHECK YOUR UNDERSTANDING

- Describe the five classes of antibodies.
- Describe the five principal functions of antibodies.

- What is the role of the variable region of an immunoglobulin molecule?

CHAPTER SUMMARY

- Functions of the lymphatic system include: 1) to help the cardiovascular system by recovering excess interstitial fluid and returning it back to bloodstream; 2) to harbor cells of the immune system; 3) to absorb and transport dietary fat. The lymphatic system contains lymphatic vessels and lymphatic tissues. A fluid within lymphatic vessels is called **lymph**.

- Lymphatic capillaries form a network interspersed throughout the areolar tissue that surrounds capillary beds. **Lacteals** are lymphatic capillaries at the centers of villi in walls of small intestine where they serve for absorption of dietary fat.

- Endothelial cells in lymphatic capillary are not tightly joined, overlap and are bound by **anchoring filaments** to elastic fibers in extracellular skeleton. This structural organization allows endothelial cells to rotate and act as a one-way flaps that permit interstitial fluid to enter lymphatic capillary but prevent its exit.

- Wall of lymphatic vessel has three layers or tunics: the intima, media, and externa. The tunica intima form valves inside the lumen, which are especially numerous in vessels were lymph moves against gravity. Lymph movement is also facilitated by 1) contraction of surrounding skeletal muscles and respiratory pump in torso; 2) rhythmic contraction of smooth muscles within the vessel's wall; and 3) pulsatile movement of blood in nearby arteries.

- The main type of lymphatic tissue is **reticular connective tissue** composed of **leukocytes, dendritic cells**, and **reticular cells**. Leukocytes include macrophages, T cells, and B cells. Dendritic cells are several cell types with spiny projections. Reticular cell is a fibroblast that produce collagen type III. They form structural framework of lymphoid organs.

- There are two groups of lymphoid organs: **primary** and **secondary lymphatic structures**.

- Primary or **central** organs are responsible for lymphopoiesis and lymphocyte maturation. They include 1) **red bone marrow**; 2) **bursa of Fabricius**—a primary lymphoid organ in birds involved in development and maturation of B cells; 3) the **thymus**, which has a key role in maturation of T cells; and 4) the **fetal liver**, which is a main hematopoietic organ in an embryo.

- Secondary or **peripheral** lymphoid organs are sites of immune responses populated by T cells, B cells, macrophages, and dendritic cells. They include 1) the **lymph nodes**; 2) the **spleen**; 3) the **tonsils**; and 4) the **mucosal associated lymphoid tissue (MALT)**.

- Lymph nodes have round or bean-shaped bodies with outer **cortex** and inner **medulla**. Afferent lymphatic vessels enter the node on convex side and efferent vessels exit on the concave side (**hilum**). Fibrous capsule around the node extends inside and forms trabeculae. Below the capsule is a subcapsular sinus. Cortex contains groups of B cells called **follicles**. Every follicle is surrounded by a layer of T and dendritic cells called **paracortex**. B cells, plasma cells, and macrophages in medulla are organized in **medullary cords**. Between medullary cords is a medullary sinus lined by endothelial cells and macrophages. Lymph from afferent vessels passes through sinuses, where it filtered by macrophages, and leaves the node via efferent vessel. Lymph nodes have two follicle types: **primary** and **secondary**. Primary follicles contain plasma B cells or **plasmoblasts**, and memory B cells or **lymphoblasts**. Secondary follicles are sites of B cell proliferation and have three layers: 1) a central dark zone contains B cell precursors called **centroblasts**; 2) a **basal zone** where B cells express surface Ig and are exposed to follicular dendritic cells; and 3) an **apical** or **mantle zone**, which is programmed to become memory or plasma B cells.

- The spleen is the largest lymphatic organ. Folds of splenic capsule called **trabeculae** project inside the spleen and subdivide it into compartments called **white** and **red pulps**. White pulp has a **central artery** surrounded by circles of T cells, B cells, and macrophages. Red pulp consists of erythrocytes, platelets, macrophages, and B cells. It is a blood reservoir. Cells in the red pulp are located in reticular connective tissue organized in **splenic cords**. Red blood cells from capillaries fill lacunae called **sinusoids** and return back to bloodstream through small venules that lead to splenic vein. White pulp surveys blood for pathogens. From central arteries blood enters sinusoids in red pulp. Macrophages in sinusoids phagocytize bacteria, foreign materials, as well as old erythrocytes and platelets. In a fetus, the spleen is engaged in hematopoiesis.

- The tonsils are located in the pharynx and oral cavity, including pharyngeal, palatine, and lingual tonsils.

- MALT unites organs in mucosa of gastrointestinal, respiratory, urinary, and reproductive organs. It includes 1) **GALT**, or gut associated lymphoid tissue; 2) **BALT**, or branchial associated lymphoid tissue; 3) **CALT**, or lymphoid tissue in conjunctiva; and 4) **VALT**, or vulvo-vaginal lymphoid tissue.

- GALT includes the **appendix/caecal pouch**, **Peyer's patches**, large intestine, and rectum mucosa. The appendix is a pouch of caeca. The mammalian appendix is a site of maturation and differentiation of B cells. In rabbits the appendix is a primary lymphoid organ, whereas in other mammals it is a secondary lymphoid organ. Peyer's patches are located in the wall of the small intestine. In cattle, sheep, pigs, horses, dogs, and rabbits, they act as a primary lymphoid tissue over 8 percent of which are found in ileum. Patches are composed of B cells covered by **follicle associated epithelium (FAE)** composed of **enterocytes** and **M (microfold** or **multifold) cells**. M cells pick up antigens from digested food and present them to B cells. Antigen presentation commits B cells to synthesize IgA. BALT, CALT, and VALT lymphoid tissues have similar organization.

- The immune system consists of cells, proteins, and structures organized in three defense lines: 1) The first line is created by cutaneous and mucous membranes acting as a physical barrier, which blocks pathogens entry; 2) The second line is created by chemicals that kill pathogens; 3) The third line consists of selective responses on particular pathogen agents or **adaptive immunity**. First two lines of defense constitute **nonspecific** or **innate immunity**. **Adaptive** or **specific immunity** is a specific response to unique **antigens** on pathogen cell surface. Adaptive immunity has to be initiated and need a time for development. It has a capacity termed **immunological memory**.

- Body surface—skin, mucous membranes, and their secretions—makes the first line of defense. Altogether they form continuous physical barriers that block pathogen entry.

- The second line includes 1) cellular responses; 2) chemicals: interferons and complement system; and 3) physiological responses: inflammation, fever, and diarrhea.

- Microbes have characteristic molecular structures called **motifs**. These motifs are signals to innate immune cells that have **pattern recognition receptors** on their plasma membrane. Physical contact between immune cell and motif triggers immune response. The innate immune system has four cell groups: 1) phagocytes, 2) inflammatory chemical-secreting cells, 3) apoptosis initiating cells, and 4) eosinophils.

- Phagocytes include neutrophils, macrophages, and dendritic cells. Phagocytosis is enforced by production of reactive oxygen-containing molecules that generate a **respiratory burst**. The respiratory burst depletes oxygen and kills aerobic microorganisms. Phagocytes expose fragments of phagocytized microbe in structures called **major histocompatibility complex I (MHC I)** on plasma membrane. This process is called **antigen presentation**.

- Basophils and mast cells release histamine and heparin. Histamine causes vasodilation and increases capillaries permeability. Heparin is an anticoagulant. Together they cause inflammation. Basophils also releases substances that attract other immune cells.

- Apoptosis is a programmed cellular death. Natural killer (NK) cells or **cytotoxic lymphocytes** eliminate infected, cancer, and transplanted cells by chemicals: 1) **perforins** make whole in plasma membrane, 2) **granzymes** enter cell and trigger its apoptosis.

- Eosinophils attack multicellular parasites with enzymes that are lethal to them.

- **Interferons (IFNs)** are proteins—**cytokines**. A virus-infected cell releases **INF-α** and **INF-β** that inform nearby uninfected cells about the close presence of a virus. All cells in the body have receptors to these interferons and react on them by production of **restriction factors**—enzymes that destroy viral DNA or RNA. Interferons stimulate NK cells to attack virus-infected cells. NK cells release **INF-γ** that stimulates macrophages to attack virus-infected cells.

- **Tumor necrosis factor (TNF)** is a cytokine that induces necrosis of tumor cells. It is secreted by activated macrophages in response to certain pathogens. TNF attracts phagocytes to the infected area and stimulates them to release other cytokines. Massive production of TNF may cause a potentially fatal condition called **septic shock**.

- Interleukins are a group of 36 cytokines. Interleukins stimulate production of neutrophils, activate NK and T cells, and trigger production of interferons.

- The **complement system** is a group of more than 20 plasma proteins produced by the liver. Their inactive form is released into the bloodstream and circulates until become activated via two cascade reactions: **classical** and **alternative pathways**. The complement system generates 1) **cytolysis**, a lysis of pathogen plasma membrane with help of a **membrane attack complex** (**MAC**) that makes pore in pathogen plasma membrane; 2) **inflammation**, a response to cellular injury. Several complement proteins stimulate basophils and mast cells to release inflammatory chemicals; 3) **virus neutralization**, a blocking of virus by C3b and components of membrane attack complex; 4) **opsonization**, an attaching of protein opsonin to pathogen surface and marking it for attack of phagocytes; and 5) **clearance of immune complex**, a phagocytosis of antigen-antibody complex by attaching C3b protein.

- **Inflammatory response** is executed by inflammatory mediators: histamine, serotonin, cytokines, **bradykinin**, **prostaglandins**, and **leukotrienes**. They attract phagocytes and increase blood influx to affected area.

- There are two mechanisms of adaptive immunity: 1) **cell-mediated immunity** and 2) **antibody-mediated**, also called **humoral immunity**.

- Cell-mediated immunity is executed by T cells. There are millions of different T cell clones, but only a few cells of each clone exist in the body at any given time. T cells have receptors, called core-receptors, responsible for T cell physical interaction with presented antigen. The most important core-receptors are CD molecules. T lymphocytes are divided in 2 groups according type of CD core-receptors: **helper T cells (T_H)** or **CD4 cells**, and **cytotoxic T cells (T_C)** or **CD8 cells**. T_H initiate cell-mediated and humoral immune reactions and activate NK cells. T_C release chemicals that kill pathogen. T lymphocytes also include: 1) **memory T cells** (both T_C and T_H), which are responsible for rapid development of immune response to repeated infection; and 2) **regulatory T lymphocytes (T_{regs})**, which suppress immune response.

- Antigen recognition by T cell begins with **antigen presentation**. Cell that presents antigen (dendritic cell, macrophage, or B cell) is termed **antigen-presenting cell (APC)**. At first exogenous antigen is attached to a transmembrane protein called **major histocompatibility complex (MHC)**. There are two categories of MHCs: **MHC class I** and **MHC class II**. All cells have MHC class I molecules, but only APCs have both classes.

- MHC class I are glycoproteins. They are continuously synthesized by cells and incorporated into their plasma membrane. Proteins of an infectious agent are cleaved in fragments of 3–15 amino acids. These fragments are shipped to the RER, where they combine with MHC class I molecules. The endomembrane system ships this complex to plasma membrane, where it is displayed at the cell surface. This display activates cytotoxic T cells.

- **MHC class II** molecule is also a glycoprotein continuously produced by the rough endoplasmic reticulum, modified by the endomembrane system, and then embedded within the plasma membrane. MHC class II molecules present antigen only by APC after a phagocytosis of **exogenous antigens**.

- Lymphocytes are produced in red bone marrow and migrate to thymus, where they become **immunocompetent** T cells. Millions immature T cells, called **thymocytes**, get a unique **T cell receptor (TCR)** that recognizes antigens bound to MHC.

- Each TCR is tested on its ability to bind with MHC and presented foreign antigen complex. This process is called **thymic selection**. It has two steps: 1) **positive selection** occurs within the thymus cortex. TCR must recognize and bind an MHC molecule. Thymocytes that does not pass this test are destroyed. Survived T cells migrate to medulla; 2) in medulla T cells pass through **negative selection** Dendritic cells present their self-antigens with MHC class I and II molecules. T cells that bind with self-antigens are destroyed. Finally, only T cells that bind with foreign antigens, but not self-ones, survive. This is called **central tolerance**.

- The final step in T cell development is **differentiation**, when each thymocyte becomes either a helper T (CD4) or cytotoxic T (CD8) cell. This **naive immunocompetent** T cells leave thymus and migrate to secondary lymphatic organs.

- Activation of naive immunocompetent T cells includes physical contact between lymphocyte and exogenous antigen and following proliferation into a clone of identical cells with the same TCR. This process is called **clonal selection**.

- The first contact between antigen and T cell is called **antigen challenge**. It proceeds through two signals. The first signal T cell receives during a direct physical contact with MHC class II molecule. The second signal requires interaction among other receptors of the APC and helper T cell. Ultimately, helper T cell is induced to produce cytokine interleukin 2 (IL-2), which occurs within 24 hours. IL-2 acts as an autocrine signal. T cells are activated and proliferate to form clones of T_H cells. Some **activated T lymphocytes** continue to produce IL-2; the others become **memory helper T cells** available for future encounters with this particular antigen.

- Activation of naive CD8$^+$ T cells requires an interaction with APC. For that dendritic cell has to interact with both, activated CD4$^+$ helper T cell and CD8$^+$ cytotoxic T cell. During this interaction, CD4$^+$ helper T cell "licenses" the dendritic cell to give an activating signal to the naive CD8$^+$ T cell. The activated T_C cell undergoes clonal expansion with the help of IL-2 and a number of cells sensitive for target antigen increases.

- Cytotoxic T cells directly attack and destroy pathogen cells. Their ability to interact with MHC class I molecules means they can detect abnormalities in any cell type: cancer cells, foreign cells, and cells infected by intracellular pathogens. T_C cells are activated the same way as T_H cells with addition of IL-2 from T_H cells to be fully activated.

- An activated T_C cell binds to target cell and releases a protein **perforin**. Perforin makes pores in the plasma membrane of target cell. After that, T_C cell releases enzymes that enter the target cell cytosol, degrade target cell proteins, destroy DNA, and cause cell death. T_C cells also initiate target cell apoptosis. After target cell death, T_C cells leave it in search of another one.

- Helper T cells release **cytokines** that activate various components of the immune system. **Interleukin-3** stimulates macrophages' phagocytic activity and increases production of **interleukine-12**, which stimulates T_H cells to produce even more interleukine-3. T_H cells also secrete IL-2, which is required to activate T_C cells. T_H cells are required for normal functioning of all components of the immune system, including innate, antibody mediated, and cell mediated immunity. Disfunction of T_H cells leads to failure of the entire immune system.

- Naive immunocompetent B cells are activated in secondary lymphatic organs. Two signals are required. The **first signal** occurs when antigen binds and cross-links B cell receptors (BCR). B cell phagocytizes and presents the antigen to a T_H cell that recognizes it. The **second signal** occurs when an activated T_H cell releases an IL-4 that stimulates B cell to produce antibodies.

- Most of activated B cells become **plasma cells** that produce antibodies; some become **memory B cells** that become active upon second exposure of the same antigen. B_M cells 1) retain their BCRs and 2) have a long (months to years) life span.

- The antibody-mediated immune response proceeds in three phases: 1) recognition of specific antigen by a B cell clone, which triggers antibodies' secretion of **immunoglobulins** or **gamma globulins**; 2) dramatic increase of antibodies' level; and 3) involvement of **B_M cells**.

- **Positive selection** of B cells occurs through antigen-independent signaling. If BCR does not bind to its ligand, B cell is ceased to develop. **Negative selection** includes binding of BCR with self-antigen. If BCR binds to it, B cell faces the following options: 1) clonal deletion, 2) receptor editing, 3) anergy, or 4) ignorance.

- B cells are activated in the spleen and lymph nodes. For that, B cells bind to antigen with the help of surface proteins CD21, CD19, and CD81 (all three constitute BCR).

- An antibody is a Y-shaped molecule formed by four peptide chains: two **heavy (H)** and two **light (L)**. Every chain has two regions: **constant (C)** and **variable (V)**. Constant regions are relatively similar among all antibodies. Variable regions are unique and responsible for antigen recognition. An antibody has two V-shaped **antigen-binding sites**.

- A single antibody subunit, called a **monomer**, can be combined with other subunits to form a larger structure. There are five classes of antibodies according structure of **C region**: **IgG, IgA, IgM, IgE**, and **IgD**.

- Antibodies have a number of functions: 1) they bind antigens and clump cells together; this process is called **agglutination**; 2) opsonization is a coating of pathogen surface that involves complement proteins; 3) they bind bacterial toxins, viral proteins, animal venoms, and deactivate or **neutralize** them; 4) IgM and IgG activate complement proteins; 5) IgE initiates release of inflammatory mediators.

CHECK YOUR KNOWLEDGE

LEVEL 1. CHECK YOUR RECALL

1. Which of the following is **not** a function of the lymphatic system?
   A. Absorption of dietary fat
   B. Oxygen transportation
   C. Regulation of interstitial fluid volume
   D. Immune surveillance of body fluids
   E. Housing lymphocytes and macrophages

2. Which of the following make up the first line of the immune system?
   A. Skin and mucous membranes
   B. T and B lymphocytes
   C. Interferons, cytokines, and complement system
   D. Macrophages and dendritic cells
   E. Inflammation and fever

3. Which of the following functions are performed by complement system proteins?
   A. Lysis
   B. Opsonization
   C. Clearance of immune complexes
   D. Inflammation
   E. All of the above

4. An activated B cell differentiates into:
   A. Cytotoxic cell
   B. Plasma cell
   C. Memory cell
   D. B and C only
   E. All of the above

5. What type of cells have MHC class I molecules?
   A. Antigen presenting cells only
   B. B cells only
   C. T cells only
   D. All nucleated cell
   E. All of the above

6. Which of the following is **not** a function of T_H cells?
   A. Stimulation of macrophages
   B. Activation of T_C cells
   C. Stimulation of plasma cells
   D. Stimulation of memory cells
   E. Stimulation of clonal selection

7. Which of the following conditions leads to inflammation?
   A. Vasodilation of arterioles
   B. Release of pyrogens
   C. B cell activation by exogenous antigens
   D. Plasma cells releasing antibodies
   E. Agglutination and precipitation of pathogenic agents

8. All of the following are phagocytes **except**:
   A. Neutrophils
   B. Cytotoxic T lymphocytes
   C. Macrophages
   D. Dendritic cells
   E. Microglia

9. T_c cells produce _____, whereas plasma cells produce _____.
   A. interferon; immunoglobulins
   B. immunoglobulins; granzymes
   C. granzymes; immunoglobulins
   D. immunoglobulins; interferon
   E. interferon; granzymes

10. MHC class I are presented by _____, whereas MHC class II are presented by _____.
    A. all nucleated cells; macrophages only
    B. macrophages only; antigen presenting cells only
    C. antigen presenting cells and B lymphocytes; all nucleated cells
    D. B lymphocytes; all nucleated cells
    E. all nucleated cells; antigen presenting cells and B lymphocytes

11. Lymph nodes filter _____, whereas the spleen filters _____.
    A. blood; lymph
    B. lymph; blood
    C. lymph and blood; blood
    D. lymph; lymph and blood
    E. both filter lymph and blood

12. True or false: Nonspecific immunity is also called adaptive immunity.
13. True or false: Neutrophils may generate an oxygen burst.
14. True or false: NK cells kill cancerous cells by apoptosis.
15. True or false: Interferon is a complement system protein.
16. Match the term with its description:

    _____ Helper T cell   a. Major histocompatibility complex of professional APC
    _____ Clone   b. Programmed cell death
    _____ Cytotoxic T cell   c. A genetically identical group of cells
    _____ Membrane attack complex d. CD8 cell directly attacks and kills pathogen cells
    _____ Apoptosis   e. Active complement that forms transmembrane channel
    _____ Necrosis   f. CD4 cell that stimulates B cells produce antibodies
    _____ MHC class II   g. Chemicals that cause fever
    _____ Pyrogens   h. Injury that causes premature cell death

LEVEL 2. CHECK YOUR UNDERSTANDING

1. The blood test of your dog shows a greatly elevated neutrophil count. What does this tell you about your dog's condition?

2. You are walking in the park with your dog. The dog finds a nest of ground wasps. The dog tries to play with a wasp, but the wasp stings the dog in the nose. Immediately the dog's nose becomes swollen, red, and in pain. Describe what has happened with your dog's nose.

3. In chapter 17, you learned about neonatal isoerythrolysis that may develop if blood type A kittens drink milk from a type B mother. Explain why kittens may develop such a severe reaction to their mother's milk.

LEVEL 3. APPLY YOUR KNOWLEDGE TO REAL LIFE

1. Diabetic type I is an autoimmune disease. It is caused by an abnormal reaction of the immune system on pancreatic β cells that produce insulin. Which malfunction of immune system causes such an abnormal reaction?

Chapter 19

The Digestive System

LEARNING OBJECTIVES

The digestive system serves to transform a meal into fuel for the body. Organs of the digestive system ingest food, digest it, and absorb nutrients. The principal structure of the digestive system is the alimentary canal, which includes the mouth, pharynx, esophagus, stomach, and intestines. The alimentary canal is supported by a set of accessory organs that help process food physically and chemically. In this chapter you will find a description of the anatomy and physiology of the digestive system. It is expected that after reading the chapter, you will be able to answer the following questions:

1. What are the major parts of the mammalian alimentary canal, and how are they structurally organized?

2. What accessory organs form the digestive system, and what role in digestion does each organ have?

3. What mechanisms control and regulate digestion?

4. What effect does feeding strategy have on the structural organization of the digestive system?

5. How are different nutrients absorbed, and what are essential nutrients?

INTRODUCTION

Digestion is a breakdown of large insoluble pieces of food into small water-soluble nutrient molecules and their absorption into the blood for further distribution among body cells. Two major processes break the food down in the digestive system: mechanical and chemical digestions. The term *mechanical digestion* refers to the physical breakdown of large pieces of food into smaller particles that can subsequently be accessed by digestive enzymes. In *chemical digestion*, enzymes break food into progressively smaller molecules, which the body can use. In vertebrates, nutrients, as a rule, are absorbed in the small intestine.

19.1 Overview of the Digestive System

The digestive system takes many forms. Its structural organization and functioning influence body shape and feeding behavior and vice versa. Digestion takes place in the gastrointestinal tract. The process begins in the mouth with the mechanical processing of food with the teeth and tongue, and the accompanying secretion of saliva containing digestive enzymes. In the mouth, food is formed into a bolus by the mechanical mastication and swallowed into the esophagus, through which it enters the stomach. In the stomach gastric enzymes continue to break down the food. This action is combined with the churning movements of the stomach wall. The partially digested food enters the duodenum as a thick semiliquid **chyme**. In the small intestine, with the help of bile and pancreatic and intestinal juices, digestion comes to its end. The epithelial lining of the small intestines absorbs nutrients. In the large intestine food moves slower, gut flora ferments indigestible food remnants and supplies the organism with some essential nutrients, such as vitamins. The colon serves to absorb water and form waste material into feces for defecation via the rectum and anus.

Most parts and organs of the digestive system are inside the abdominal cavity. They are covered by a common set of serous membranes and supported by blood vessels and nerves. The serous membrane that covers the digestive tract in the abdomen is known as the **peritoneal membrane** or **peritoneum** (see chapter 5, page 135). Like other serous membranes, it has two folds: one that occupies an external position and is attached to the walls of the abdominal cavity is called the **parietal peritoneum**, and the other fold that occupies an inner position and is attached to the internal organs is called the **visceral peritoneum**, or **serosa**.

Organs located entirely within the peritoneal cavity are termed **intraperitoneal**, whereas organs located outside the peritoneum are known as **retroperitoneal**. The peritoneum that wraps around the intestine and holds it is called a **mesentery**. The mesenteries support and bind organs, hold them in place, and form their shape. Mesenteries also house blood vessels, nerves, and lymphatic vessels, anchoring them to their position. The mesentery that holds the large intestine is called the **mesocolon**. The most prominent mesentery that covers the abdominal cavity like an apron from the ventral side is called **greater omentum**. The greater omentum consists of four layers. It extends from the base of the stomach to the pelvis (fig. 19.1).

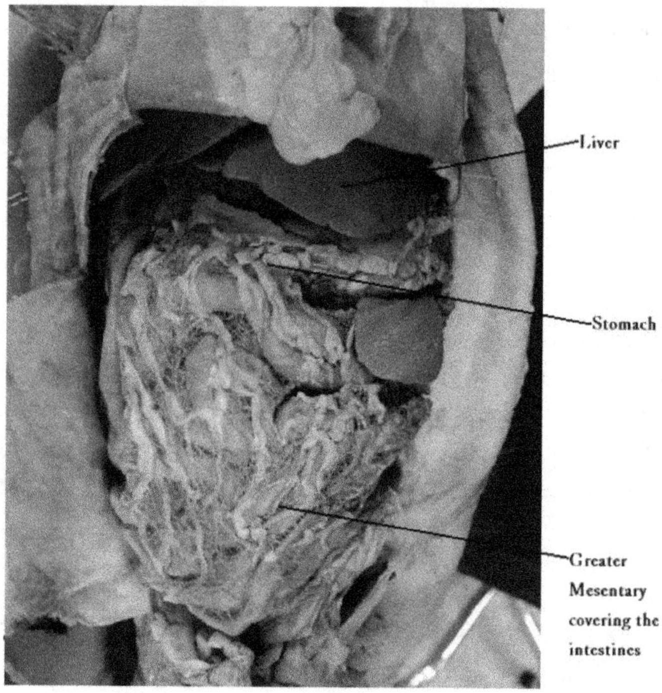

Blood vessels that deliver and drain blood to and from the digestive organs collectively are called **splanchnic circulation**. Three branches of abdominal aorta supply digestive organs with blood: **celiac trunk** (its branch is called the **gastric artery**), **superior mesenteric**, and **inferior mesenteric arteries**. The veins that drain the digestive tract inside the abdominal cavity are organized into a set of veins known as the **hepatic portal vein system**. The hepatic portal veins transport blood to the liver, where blood is filtered and examined for presence of pathogens and toxins. From the liver, blood is drained into the **hepatic veins**, which empty into the posterior vena cava.

Digestive organs are supplied with very extensively developed and complexly organized nerves of the autonomic

FIGURE 19.1   Greater Omentum; Monogastric Stomach.

nervous system in three main clusters: the **celiac plexus**, **superior mesenteric plexus**, and **inferior mesenteric plexus**. The neurons of the ANS and ENS are involved in multiple digestive reflex arcs. The sensory component of the reflex arcs is provided by receptors located in the walls of the alimentary canal organs. These receptors respond to stimuli such as stretching, pH, and presence of certain chemicals in digested food. The motor reaction on the received stimuli include peristalsis and glandular secretion.

CHECK YOUR UNDERSTANDING

- Where is the greater omentum located?

- What is a mesocolon?

- Which blood vessels constitute splanchnic circulation?

Digestive System Functions

Digestion is a multistage process. It starts with ingestion of raw materials, most often other organisms, and usually involves mechanical and chemical processing of the ingested food. In general, digestion proceeds in four steps:

1. Ingestion: placing food into the mouth.
2. Mechanical and chemical breakdown: mastication and the mixing of the resulting bolus with water, acids, bile, and enzymes to break complex materials into simple molecules termed nutrients.
3. Absorption: transport of nutrients from the lumen of an alimentary canal to the circulatory and lymphatic capillaries through diffusion and active transport.
4. Egestion (excretion): Expelling of undigested materials from the body by defecation.

In mammals, preparation for digestion begins with the cephalic phase, in which saliva is produced in the mouth and digestive enzymes are produced in the stomach. Mechanical and chemical digestion begin in the mouth, where food is chewed and mixed with saliva. The stomach continues to break food down mechanically and chemically through churning and mixing with both acids and enzymes. The major part of digestion takes place in the small intestine. The large intestine primarily serves as a site for fermentation of indigestible materials by gut bacteria and for resorption of water from remaining undigested substances before excretion.

CHECK YOUR UNDERSTANDING

- What processes are involved in digestion?

- What is absorption?

Histology of the Digestive System

The walls of the alimentary canal follow the same general tissue pattern of other hollow organs. Most regions of the alimentary canal have four tissue layers or tunics: the **mucosa**, **submucosa**, **muscularis externa**, and **serosa** or **adventitia**.

Mucosa is an innermost layer that lines the space inside the alimentary canal called **lumen**. Mucosa has three layers. First is a layer of epithelium facing the lumen; cells that form this layer are called **enterocytes**. Following this is a thin layer of loose connective tissue called the **lamina propria**. The deepest layer in mucosa is made of two layers of smooth muscle collectively known as the **muscularis mucosae**. A simple columnar epithelium lines the stomach and the small and large intestines. Columnar epithelium has high protective properties. Its goblet cells secrete an alkaline mucus (see chapter 4, page 106). This mucus coats the epithelium and protects it and the underlying tissues from ingested food and chemicals secreted by digestive glands. The mucosa also houses regenerative epithelial cells that have a high rate of mitosis. These cells replace damaged and dead cells of mucosa. The lamina propria houses blood and lymphatic vessels, glands, and mucosa associated lymphoid tissue (MALT) (see chapter 18, page 536). The fibers of smooth muscles in muscularis mucosae are arranged in two directions. The inner smooth muscle layer has a circular arrangement, and the outer layer has a longitudinal arrangement. This organization of smooth muscles in the wall of the digestive tract generates wavy contraction of the alimentary canal that propels food forward.

Submucosa is composed of irregular dense connective tissue with blood and lymphatic vessels and submucosal glands. Submucosa houses a part of the enteric nervous tissue called **submucosal** or **Meissner's plexus**. This plexus mostly serves to control secretion of glands and regulation of blood flow.

Muscularis externa is a thick muscular layer composed of smooth muscle in most of the alimentary canal. Smooth muscles in this layer are organized in two layers in the same way as in muscularis mucosae. The contractions of smooth muscles in this layer are controlled by an extensive group of motor neurons called **myenteric** or **Auerbach's plexus**.

The serosa or **adventitia** is an outermost membranous layer. The serosa corresponds with the visceral peritoneum. It is composed of a simple squamous epithelium and areolar connective tissue. The adventitia is an external membrane that corresponds parietal peritoneum. It is composed of irregular dense connective tissue. The serosa and adventitia anchor digestive organs to surrounding structures (fig. 19.2).

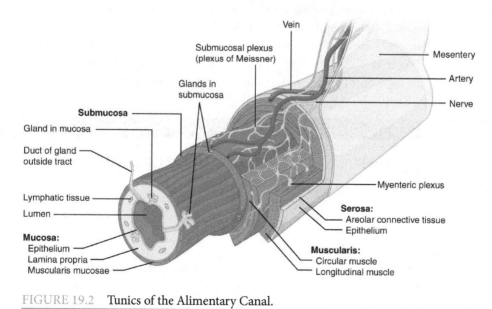

FIGURE 19.2   Tunics of the Alimentary Canal.

CHECK YOUR UNDERSTANDING

- List and describe the four tunics that make up the wall of the alimentary canal.

- Where in the wall of the GI tract is the myenteric plexus located, and what is its function?

- What is the structure and role of the adventitia?

19.2 From Oral Cavity to Stomach

Oral Cavity: Teeth, Tongue, Salivary Glands

The mouth is an entry point for food. It is the first part of the upper gastrointestinal tract and is equipped with several structures that initiate digestion. Accessory organs of the oral cavity include salivary glands, teeth, and tongue. The teeth divide the mouth in two regions: the **vestibule** and the **oral cavity proper**. The vestibule is the area between the teeth, lips, and cheeks. This area is lined with squamous nonkeratinized epithelium called **gum** or **gingiva**. The oral cavity proper is located behind the teeth. Most of the oral cavity is lined with a mucous membrane, which produces a lubricating mucus. Mucus is secreted either by surface cells or by glands. The mucous membrane in the mouth continues as the thin mucosa that lines the bases of the teeth. The main component of mucus is a viscous clear glycoprotein called **mucin**. A thin layer of smooth muscles underlines the mucous membrane and gives it its great elasticity. It covers the inside of the cheeks, inner surfaces of the lips, and floor of the mouth.

The roof of the mouth is termed the palate. The palate separates the oral cavity from the nasal cavity. The anterior part of palate is formed by premaxilla, maxilla, and palate bones and is called the **hard palate**. The posterior portion of the palate does not contain bone and is made of muscle and connective tissue. This part of palate is called the **soft palate** (fig. 19.3). The

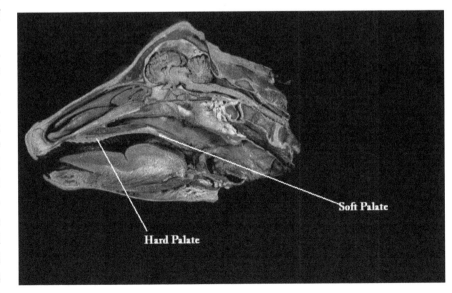

FIGURE 19.3   Hard Palate and Soft Palate.

surface of the hard palate helps to masticate food and keeps the nasal passage clear. The soft palate ends at the **uvula**.

Teeth are complex structures made of **dentin** covered by the **enamel**. Enamel is the hardest tissue in the body, composed of calcium hydroxyapatite crystals with a small inclusion of collagen fibers that bind crystals together. In mammals, cells that secrete enamel degrade after the tooth erupts. As a result, the organism is unable to repair enamel damage, and teeth deteriorate with aging. Enamel forms a tooth portion that is visible above the gum, termed **crown**. The part of the tooth hidden within the alveolus is called the **root**. Externally, the root is composed of a mineralized bonelike tissue called **cementum**. The inner body of the tooth consists of **dentin**, composed of about 70 percent calcium hydroxyapatite crystals. Dentin is the second-hardest tissue in the mammalian body. The inner surface of dentin is lined by specialized cells called **odontoblasts**. Odontoblasts persists throughout the animal's life and continuously generate new dentin. A loose connective tissue called **pulp** fills the space at the center of the tooth called the **pulp cavity**. Pulp contains blood vessels and nerves that nurture and innervate internal tissues of the tooth. The pulp cavity extends into the root via the **root canal** (fig. 19.4). Teeth have different shapes. Some are designed to tear, whereas others are designed to chew food. The teeth are named after the role they play in mastication: incisors are used for cutting or biting off pieces of food; canines are used for tearing; premolars and molars are used for chewing and grinding. Teeth sit in bony sockets known as **alveoli**. **Periodontal ligaments** hold them and prevent their displacement. The periodontal ligament consists of collagen fibers that on one side are intertwined with collagen inside the cementum, and on the other side with collagen from the denture's bone matrix. Mastication of food with the help of saliva and mucus results in formation of a soft bolus, which then can be swallowed to make its way to the stomach. The digestive enzymes and bactericide chemicals in saliva keep teeth clean and healthy.

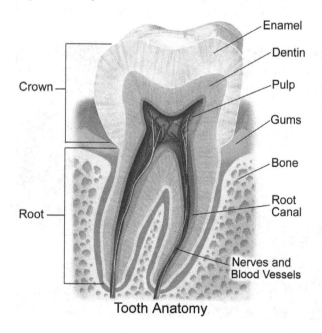

Tooth Anatomy

FIGURE 19.4   Tooth Anatomy.

Mastication or chewing is a mechanical breakdown of the ingested food characteristic of mammals. The mastication reduces a large chunk of food into small bolus particles. A small moist bolus is easy to swallow. These small boluses have bigger surface area for attack of digestive enzymes. Mastication strongly depends on the food's physical properties. Soft but sinewy foods, such as muscles and skin, are best cut up by the blades of specialized canine (carnassial) teeth of carnivores. Fibrous food, like grass or leaves, are best broken down by grinding. The molar teeth of ungulates, subungulates, and rodents are corrugated on their working surface.

There are three pairs of main **salivary glands** and between 800 and 1,000 minor salivary glands. Altogether, they serve the digestive process, and also play an important role in the maintenance of dental health and mouth lubrication. The salivary glands are exocrine glands that secrete **saliva** in the mouth via ducts. Saliva is a composite fluid that consists of water and electrolytes, such as sodium, potassium, and chloride. Mucus also constitutes a major saliva component. Saliva moisturizes the oral cavity, dissolves food, lubricates, and cleans the oral cavity. It protects the organism from pathogens and functions in mechanical and chemical digestions. It has the following components:

1. **Salivary amylase** is an enzyme that hydrolyses polysaccharides into the smaller saccharide molecules and first of all transforms starch into maltose.
2. **Lingual lipase** is an enzyme that catalyzes the hydrolysis of lipids (fats).
3. **Bicarbonate ions** (HCO_3^-) neutralize acids released from the food and regurgitated from the stomach.
4. **Lysozyme** is an enzyme that catalyzes the perforation (making holes) in bacterial plasma membranes and thus helps destroy them.
5. **Immunoglobulins A (IgA)** bind specific antigens on the pathogen's surface and mediate their destruction.

The secretory cells of the salivary glands are called **acinar** cells. Two types of acinar cells are **serous** and **mucous cells**. The secretions of serous cells are involved in digestion and contain a water-based fluid with enzymes and other supporting digestion components. As a rule, they release their secretions during or after eating. The mucous cells secrete mucus that keeps the oral cavity moist. These cells produce their secretions continuously. There are three main and numerous minor salivary glands. The largest of these are the **parotid glands**—their secretion is mostly serous. A pair of salivary glands underneath the jaw is called the **submandibular glands**. These glands produce both serous fluid and mucus. About 70 percent of the oral cavity saliva is produced by these glands. The **sublingual glands** are located underneath the tongue, and their secretion is mostly mucous with a small percentage of saliva (fig. 19.5).

Within the oral mucosa, tongue, palates, and floor of the mouth are the minor salivary glands. They mostly secrete mucus. There are other glands on the surface of the tongue that encircle bases of taste buds on the dorsal side of the tongue, and these also produce lingual lipase. These glands are termed **Von Ebner's glands**. These glands secrete histamine.

Saliva moistens and softens food, and along with the chewing action of the teeth, transforms the food into a smooth soft bolus. Salivary amylase initiates digestion of the starch, breaking it down into maltose and dextrose. About 30 percent of starch is digested in the mouth by the salivary amylase. Other food molecules that initiate digestion in the mouth are lipids. Lingual lipase triggers this process, which later is accomplished in the small intestine by the

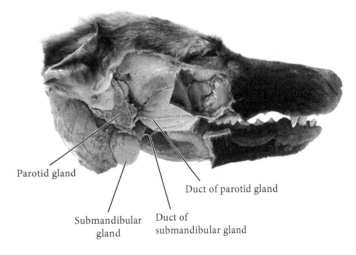

Parotid gland

Duct of parotid gland

Submandibular gland

Duct of submandibular gland

FIGURE 19.5 Dog Salivary Glands.

pancreatic lipase. The presence of salivary lipase is of prime importance in a neonatal whose pancreatic lipase has yet to be developed.

Saliva also contains a glycoprotein called **haptocorrin**. The haptocorrin firmly binds vitamin B$_{12}$ and safely transports it through the acidic content of the stomach. In the duodenum, pancreatic enzymes break down the chemical bond between glycoprotein and B$_{12}$, and free the vitamin, which then binds with intrinsic factor.

Most birds, particularly those feeding in water, lack oral glands. However, some passerine birds use oral mucus secretions to glue together materials composing their nests. Salivation primarily is controlled by the parasympathetic nervous system via a reflex arc. The reflex response is initiated by sensory stimuli such as the smell and taste of food. The sensory input passes to **salivatory nuclei** in the ponce. There are two salivatory nuclei in pons: the **superior salivatory nucleus**, and the **inferior salivatory nucleus**, which house motor neurons that innervate the salivary glands. The superior salivatory nucleus via the facial nerve (CN VII) controls the submandibular and sublingual glands. The inferior salivatory nucleus gives rise to the glossopharyngeal nerve (CN IX), which innervates the parotid gland.

The tongue is a fleshy and muscular sensory organ, covered by the stratified squamous epithelium. The skeletal muscles make it main inner body mass. Taste buds (see chapter 13, page 356) are the source of sensory information about food. If the taste is agreeable, the tongue will go into action, manipulating the food in the mouth, which stimulates the secretion of saliva from the salivary glands. The tongue is attached to the floor of the mouth by a ligamentous band called the **frenulum**. Frenulum guarantees tongue mobility for the food manipulation. The manipulations are controlled by the action of several muscles and limited in its external range by the stretch of the frenulum. The tongue has two sets of skeletal muscles: four **intrinsic muscles** that originate inside the tongue and are involved in formation of tongue's shape; and four **extrinsic muscles** attached to the mandible, hyoid, and temporal bones. These muscles are involved in tongue movement.

CHECK YOUR UNDERSTANDING

- What structures form the superior wall of the oral cavity?

- What structures hold a tooth in the bone socket? What are they made off?

- What components of saliva have a digestive function?

- Why is saliva important for tooth health?

Pharynx

The pharynx or throat sits posterior to the nasal and oral cavities. It is divided into three regions: superior **nasopharynx**, middle **oropharynx**, and posterior **laryngopharynx** (fig. 19.6). The nasopharynx is a passage for air only, whereas the last two are parts of both the respiratory and digestive systems. Like the oral cavity, the oropharynx and laryngopharynx are lined with stratified squamous epithelium. The oropharynx harbors palatine and lingual tonsils. The pharynx is a passage for food and air. Swallowing, or **deglutition**, begins with a forceful movement of the food bolus from the mouth into the pharynx and from there to the esophagus. The pharynx is surrounded by three pairs of skeletal muscles: the **upper**, middle, and **lower pharyngeal constrictor muscles**. Constriction of these muscles pushes the food bolus towards the esophagus.

The **epiglottis** is a spoon-shaped structure of the larynx made of elastic cartilage. It is covered with a mucous membrane and carries taste buds on its lingual surface, which faces into the mouth. The epiglottis guards the entrance into the **glottis**, the opening between vocal cords. During swallowing, the epiglottis folds and closes the entrance into the larynx. This maneuver prevents food from going into the trachea and directs it to the esophagus.

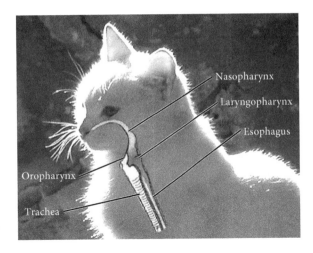

FIGURE 19.6　Cat Pharynx.

CHECK YOUR UNDERSTANDING

- Which regions of the pharynx are parts of the digestive system?

- What is the primary digestive function of the pharynx?

Esophagus

The esophagus transports the food bolus from the pharynx to the stomach. It is a soft muscular tube that can be easily distended to accommodate a large food bolus. The esophagus does not participate in mechanical or chemical digestion. In some vertebrates, the esophageal mucosa is covered by a ciliated epithelium that controls the flow of lubricating mucus around the food. The ciliated epithelium may also help gather small meal crumbs and move them to the stomach. In most cases, the mucosa of the esophagus is a stratified epithelium. It may be keratinized in animals that eat rough or abrasive food. In vertebrates that swallow large quantities of food at once, the esophagus serves as a site of temporary storage. Anteriorly, the esophagus is coated by skeletal muscles. At its posterior region the skeletal muscles are replaced by smooth muscle.

At the junction of the pharynx and esophagus, the circle of external muscles forms the **upper esophageal sphincter** that controls the bolus entering into the esophagus. On the opposite side, a **lower esophageal sphincter** guards movement of the bolus into the stomach and prevents reflux of gastric juice from stomach to the esophagus. Combination of skeletal and smooth muscles surrounded esophagus propels food bolus by wavelike contractions termed **peristalsis**.

Birds have no teeth and swallow the food in big chunks. Their esophagus expands into a baglike structure called **crop** (fig. 19.7). Crop is

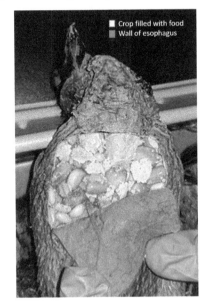

FIGURE 19.7　Crop of Fowl.

used as a temporary food storage before it will be proceeded further along the digestive tract or regurgitated as a meal for nestlings. In pigeons, the crop secretes a nutritional fluid called "milk." Parents feed their nestlings with this milk for several days after hatching. The bird's esophagus joins the thin-walled glandular section of the stomach called **proventriculus** connected to the posterior gizzard. The proventriculus secretes gastric juice to help digest the bolus, and the gizzard, together with selected pieces of hard grit and pebbles, grinds large food into smaller pieces. In mammals, the esophagus usually lacks a crop, and the stomach shows no tendency to form a gizzard. In some cetaceans, the stomach or esophagus may expand into a pouch that apparently serves, like an avian crop, to store food temporarily, although some gastric digestion may begin as well in this pouch.

CHECK YOUR UNDERSTANDING

- What is the primary function of the esophagus?

- What is the crop's function?

- What is the role of the upper and lower esophageal sphincters?

19.3   Stomach

The esophagus passes the diaphragm through the **esophageal hiatus** and delivers the bolus to the stomach: an expanded region of the alimentary canal. Animals that intake large amounts of food on an irregular basis, such as many carnivores, have stomachs that serve as a storage. Such food storage, probably, has been an initial function of the stomach, when early vertebrates evolved from suspension feeding to feeding on larger chunks of food. Hydrochloric acid, produced by the stomach, may have functioned to retard food putrefaction by bacteria, thus preserving it until digestion was underway. In most vertebrates, the stomach performs an expanded role. Some absorption of water, salts, and vitamins occurs in the stomach, but predominantly it serves to churn and mix food mechanically and add digestive chemicals collectively called **gastric juice**. Gastric juice includes some enzymes and mucus but is primarily composed of hydrochloric acid released from the mucosal wall of the stomach.

Gross Anatomy

The stomach sits right beneath the diaphragm in the left upper quadrant of the abdominal cavity. It is a curved elongated balloon. Its lateral border is long and is called the **greater curvature**. The internal medial side is shorter and is termed the **lesser curvature**. There are four anatomic regions in the stomach: the **cardia, fundus, body,** and **pylorus**. The pylorus has two parts: a wide **pyloric antrum** and a progressively narrowing **pyloric canal**. It empties into the first part of the small intestine, called the **duodenum**. The **pyloric sphincter** separates the stomach and duodenum and controls passage of acidic chyme into the small intestine. Internally, the stomach wall is folded and forms ridges called **rugae**. Rugae allow the stomach to expand when it receives a big meal (fig. 19.8).

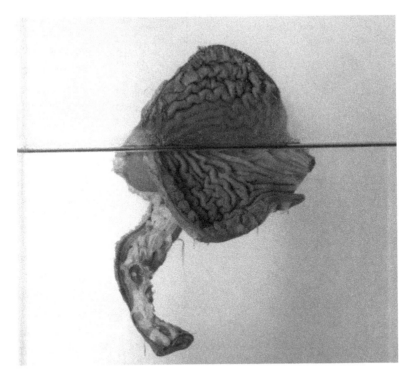

FIGURE 19.8   Longitudinal Section Through a Dog Stomach.

CHECK YOUR UNDERSTANDING

- What are the primary functions of the stomach?

- Which major parts constitute the stomach?

- What is the role of rugae?

- What is the function of the pyloric sphincter?

Histology and Function

In general, the stomach wall has the same main tunics as the other parts of the alimentary canal: mucosa, submucosa, muscularis externa, and adventitia. The muscular tunic of the stomach is thick, strong, and has three layers of smooth muscles. The external and middle layers, like in other regions of the alimentary canal have circular and longitudinal orientation of the muscle fibers, whereas muscle cells of the internal layer are oriented oblique and spiral around stomach wall. The oblique layer of smooth muscle adds to peristaltic movement characteristic to all parts of the digestive tract **churning** motions that toss and mix food with gastric juice, forming a liquid substance called **chyme**.

There are two types of gastric mucosa: the **glandular** and **nonglandular epithelium**. The stomach's glandular epithelium is characterized by the presence of **gastric glands**. Gastric glands are located in deep **gastric pits**. The lining between gastric pits is made of columnar cells with numerous goblet cells.

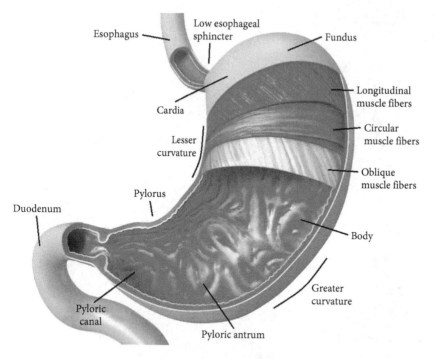

FIGURE 19.9   Anatomy of the Human Stomach.

Both secrete a thick mucus that covers and protects the stomach wall from its own highly acidic secretions. The gastric glands are branched tubular glands. The gastric glands are distributed over three regions of the stomach—the cardia, fundus, and pylorus. The cardia is a very narrow region found only in mammals. It forms the transition zone between the esophagus and the stomach. Its gastric glands are termed **cardiac glands**. These glands are composed predominantly of mucus-secreting cells. The fundus is usually the largest region of the stomach. It contains most important gastric glands called **fundic glands**. Mucous cells are present in fundic glands, but in addition to them, these glands have numerous **parietal cells** and **chief cells**. The parietal cells produce hydrochloric acid. HCl is important component of **gastric juice** necessary for activation of proteolytic enzymes produced by chief cells (fig. 19.10). In addition, parietal cells secrete **intrinsic factor**, a chemical needed for absorption of vitamin B_{12} in the small intestine. The chief cells secrete several proteolytic enzymes, particularly **pepsinogen**, a precursor of the active enzyme **pepsin**. In the lumen of the stomach, pepsinogen mixes with the hydrochloric acid and converts into pepsin. Some vertebrates have **oxyntopeptic cells** that produce both HCl and pepsinogen. The wall of the pylorus is mostly composed of mucous cells, which form distinct gastric glands called **pyloric glands**. The mucus of pyloric glands helps neutralize the acidic chyme as it moves towards the intestine. Thus, most of the chemical and mechanical processes of gastric digestion occur in the fundus. The cardia and pylorus add mucus. Smooth muscle bands in their walls act as sphincters to prevent the retrograde transfer of food.

In addition to the exocrine secretions, gastric glands produce hormones. **Enteroendocrine cells** that produce hormones are located at the bottom of the gastric glands (fig. 19.9). **G cells**, for example, secrete hormone **gastrin**, which stimulates exocrine cells of the gastric glands to increase their secretions.

The stomach of some vertebrates also has region of nonglandular epithelium. In some herbivores, the nonglandular region may develop from the base of the esophagus. In other species, such as rodents, loss of gastric glands in the mucosa creates a stomach region with nonglandular epithelium in which smooth muscle contractions churn and mix food with gastric juice. In rodents, this nonglandular epithelium often is keratinized, which helps them process rough foods such as seeds, grasses, and chitin of insect exoskeletons.

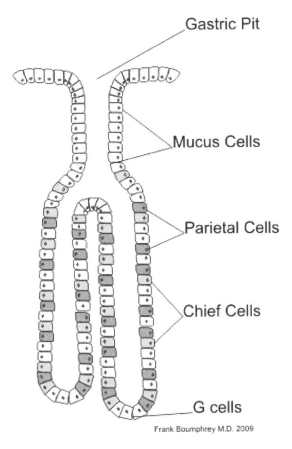

Gastric Pit

Mucus Cells

Parietal Cells

Chief Cells

G cells

Frank Boumphrey M.D. 2009

FIGURE 19.10   Gastric Gland.

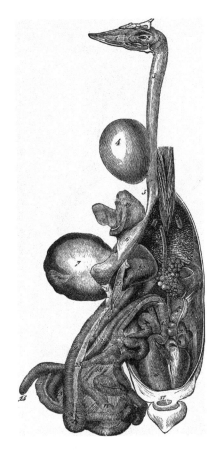

FIGURE 19.11   Gizzard and Proventriculus.

Crocodiles and alligators have a **gizzard**. The gizzard is a region of the stomach with thick strong musculature that grinds food against ingested hard objects, usually small stones deliberately chosen and swallowed into the stomach. The thin-walled glandular region of the crocodilian stomach lies in front of the gizzard. This region is rich with gastric glands that produce gastric juices. The gizzard is well developed in birds, especially in those that feed on seeds. The muscular wall of gizzard tosses the swallowed stones against the bolus and grinds it into smaller pieces. Eventually, more gritty stones are swallowed to replace those ground up along with the food. The gizzard is especially important in animals that process plant materials with tough cellulose walls (fig. 19.11).

In ruminants, the stomach is highly specialized. It has four chambers, although the first three—the **rumen**, **reticulum**, and **omasum**—arise from the esophagus and only the fourth—the **abomasum**—is a real stomach. The large rumen, which gives its name to these mammals, receives the food after it is clipped by teeth and swallowed. The reticulum is a small accessory chamber with a honeycombed texture. Like the first two chambers, the omasum is lined with esophageal epithelium. It is folded into overlapping leaves. The three types of mucosa characteristic to the mammalian stomach (cardia, fundus, and pylorus) are found only in the abomasum. Camels also have stomach similar to that of ruminants, even though they lack the omasum. Their stomach has three chambers: rumen, reticulum, and abomasum (fig. 19.12).

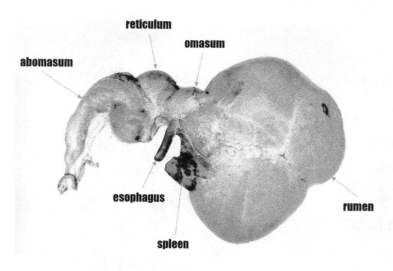

FIGURE 19.12   Ruminant Stomach.

When a ruminant feeds, food initially collects in the rumen. The rumen is thin walled and lined with numerous projecting papillae that increase its absorptive surface. It serves as a large holding and fermentation vat. Processed in rumen food regurgitated back into the mouth, remasticated, and swallowed again. The process is repeated until there has been thorough mechanical breakdown of plant material and chemical attack on cellulose.

Rumination involves complicated waves of contraction that sweep through the rumen and that are synchronized with remastication and with passage of food along the digestive tract. Initially, ruminant animals clip plant material, mix it with saliva, roll it into bolus, and swallow into the rumen. Cycles of contraction pass through the rumen and reticulum to circulate and mix the ingested food with microorganisms. In grazers, this mixing also results in physical separation of coarse and fine food particles. Small particles sink into the fluid that accumulates ventrally within the rumen. Large, undigested plant fibers float on top of this fluid. Methane gas that forms during fermentation collects above this fluid and plant fiber.

The regurgitation proceeds in three steps. First, the ruminant contracts its diaphragm as if taking a breath but keeps the glottis closed. This produces a negative pressure in the thorax around the esophagus. Second, the gastroesophageal sphincter is relaxed, and digesta are aspirated from the rumen into the esophagus. Third, peristaltic contractions sweep the digesta up the esophagus into the mouth, so the animal can rechew the undigested plant material. The process of regurgitation and remastication is termed **ruminating**. The ruminating repeats until most of the food material is broken down mechanically. The amount of time an animal spends ruminating depends proportionately on the fiber content of the food. In grazing cattle, this may occupy up to eight hours per day and involve rumination of each bolus 40–50 times. The reticulum contracts to move digested food between itself and the rumen.

The omasum operates like a two-phase pump to transfer digesta from the reticulum to the abomasum. First, relaxation of the muscular walls of the omasum aspirates fluid and fine particles from the reticulum into the lumen of the omasum. Second, the omasum contracts to force this digesta into the abomasum. The abomasum is the fundic part of the stomach in which further digestion occurs before chyme passes to the intestines.

In animals that feed on fibrous plants, the combination of remastication and fermentation is very efficient. In cattle, organic acids produced in the rumen alone make up 70 percent of their total energy requirements. Eventually, rechewed food travels through the reticulum into the omasum. The omasum absorbs volatile fatty acids, ammonia, and water. At the same time, omasum separates the fermenting contents of the rumen and reticulum from the highly acidic content of the abomasum. The omasum moves smaller food particles into the abomasum, the true stomach, in which enzymatic and acidic hydrolysis takes place. Finally, chyme enters the intestine.

In the suckling ruminant neonate, the abomasum and intestine digest milk, so fermentation in the rumen is unnecessary. Milk bypasses the rumen of a neonate through a **reticular groove** that reflexively closes when the neonate swallows milk. Thus, milk passes directly from the esophagus to the abomasum via the reticular groove.

Foregut fomentation has arisen independently in groups other than ruminants, such as leaf-eating sloths, langur monkeys, elephants, hippopotamuses, and many rodents. The stomach of these animals is similar to that of ruminants. Marsupials, wallabies, wombats, and kangaroos depend on microbial fermentation in a specialized region of the stomach to digest plants on which they feed. Kangaroos, for example, have two stomach chambers: the **sacciform** and the **tubiform**. The sack-like front chamber contains bacteria, fungi, and protozoa that begin the fermentation process. Food may remain in the sacciform stomach for many hours for fermentation. Much like a cow chewing cud, the kangaroo may spit up bits of undigested food to be chewed and then swallowed again. As food ferments, it passes into the kangaroo's second stomach chamber, where acids and enzymes finish digestion.

The stomach does not create a surface for substances absorption. Its main roles in food processing include digestion of protein molecules, formation of chyme, and its propulsion to the small intestine. Pepsin in the stomach lumen initiates chemical digestion of proteins. Churning movements facilitate this process by mechanically mixing food with gastric juice. When the churning is completed, the peristaltic movements propel chyme into duodenum via the pyloric sphincter. All these actions are tightly controlled by endocrine and nervous systems.

A group of special pacemaker cells known as **interstitial cells of Cajal** in the stomach wall has the ability to build a membrane potential and then, when the membrane potential reaches some threshold level, spontaneously depolarize with around four times per minute. This rhythmic change of the membrane potential in the Cajal cells generates the basic rhythm of muscular contraction. Pacemaker cells are bound with other smooth muscle cells in the stomach wall via gap junctions and trigger rhythmic contractions in the muscular layer. These basic contractions are modified by both nervous reflexes and hormones.

Control over gastric secretion is organized in three phases: **cephalic**, **gastric**, and **intestinal**. The cephalic phase is based on the **cephalic reflex**. The cephalic reflex is initiated by the smell, sight or taste of the food. It develops before or at the beginning of eating. Nerve impulses from special sense organs are transferred to the hypothalamus and from here to the medulla oblongata. The parasympathetic nucleus of the vagus nerve (CN X) sends nerve impulses to the stomach. The vagal stimulation increases muscular contractions in the stomach wall and triggers secretion of gastric juice.

The gastric phase begins when the bolus enters the stomach. This phase is controlled by both nervous signals via the gastric reflex and endocrine G cells in the gastric glands. The food bolus presses on the stomach wall and distends it. Baroreceptors in the stomach wall monitor its tension; together with chemoreceptors that sense the presence of food, they trigger release of gastric juice. At the same time, enteroendocrine cells in gastric glands release gastrin in the bloodstream. When gastrin returns back to the stomach, it increases the strength of muscle contraction and stimulates production of HCl by the parietal cells. Gastrin also forces the pyloric sphincter to contract more strongly, which prevents premature movement of chyme into the small intestine.

The intestinal phase is initiated by the entrance of the chyme into the duodenum. It is also regulated by the nervous and endocrine systems. The nervous system responds on the presence of the chyme in the small intestine by the **intestine reflex**. Intestine reflex develops on the change of pH, which normally is alkaline. The entrance of an acidic chyme from the stomach dramatically changes pH in the duodenum on acidic. The sensory impulses from the small intestine cause decrease nerve impulses to the medulla oblongata and, as a result, inhibit vagal stimulation of the stomach. The enteroendocrine cells in the duodenum release two principal hormones: **cholecystokinin (CCK)** and **secretin**. The cholecystokinin is released at the response to chemoreceptors sensitive to presence of fats. CCK decreases stomach movements and inhibits gastric emptying. It stimulates the acinar cells of the pancreas to release pancreatic enzymes that catalyze the digestion of fat, protein, and carbohydrates. CCK also stimulates production of hepatic bile, and initiates the gallbladder contractions, which result in the release of the bile into the duodenum. Besides that, CCK mediates satiety by acting on the CCK receptors in the satiety center of the hypothalamus. The secretin is released in response to the presence of the acidic chyme in the duodenum. Secretin inhibits secretion of gastric juice and gastrin. It also stimulates the production of bicarbonate (HCO_3^-) by pancreas. The bicarbonate ions bind with H^+ and neutralize acidic chyme. Besides that, secretin stimulates liver to produce more bile.

CHECK YOUR UNDERSTANDING

- What is the function of the oblique muscular layer in the stomach wall?

- What are the primary cell types of the gastric gland, and what does each type do?

- What is the role of gastric motility?

- What mechanism controls the stomach emptying into the duodenum?

19.4   Small Intestine

The small intestine (also called **small bowel**) serves to finish food digestion and nutrient absorption. It is divided into three continuous regions: the **duodenum, jejunum**, and **ileum**. The small intestine is associated with accessory organs such as the liver and pancreas. These organs produce bile and pancreatic juice for complete digestion of all major types of macromolecules: carbohydrates, proteins, lipids, and nucleic acids. The jejunum and ileum are best delineated in mammals on the basis of histological features of their mucosal wall. Such distinct regions are absent or less well defined in other vertebrates. The **ileocecal vale** is a sphincter between the ileum of the small intestine and the cecum of the large intestine. This valve regulates the movement of chyme into the large intestine.

Gross Anatomy

The small intestine is a long, coiled tube. Three structures serve to increase the total surface of the small intestine wall: **circular folds** or **plicae circulares**, **villi**, and **microvilli**. Plicae circulares are macroscopic ring folds of the mucosa and submucosa. They are most numerous in duodenum and jejunum, and less abundant in ileum. The **villi** are small projections of mucosa only. The free surface of mucosa epithelial cells facing the lumen carry numerous **microvilli**, perhaps up to several thousand per cell. Both microscopic and macroscopic structures increase surface area. The numerous villi on the epithelial lining of the intestine increase 10- to 20-fold the area available for absorption. The microvilli, in their turn, contribute to a 100-fold overall increase in surface area. A free surface of apical cells also harbors digestive enzymes, which are bound to it. The intestinal mucosa also has **intestinal glands** that secrete enzymes and hormones (fig. 19.13).

The mammalian small intestine has three distinctive regions: the **duodenum, jejunum** (fig. 19.14), and **ileum**. The duodenum receives chyme from the stomach and exocrine secretions primary from the liver and pancreas. The mammalian small intestine is coiled and usually has distinctive histological differences

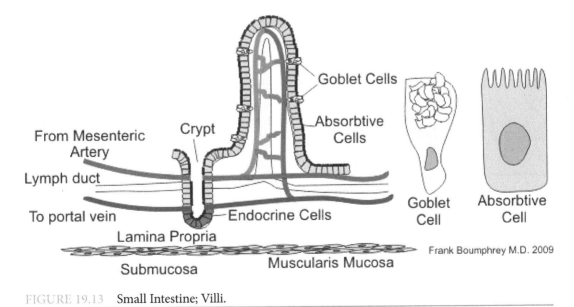

FIGURE 19.13   Small Intestine; Villi.

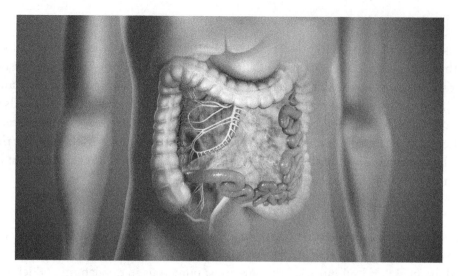

FIGURE 19.14   Jejunum and Mesenteries.

among duodenum, jejunum, and ileum. Birds have no jejunum. Their long, coiled small intestine consists of a duodenum and ileum only.

CHECK YOUR UNDERSTANDING

- Why is the internal surface of the small intestine arranged into progressively smaller folds?

- What is the role of the brush border?

- How does motility of the small intestine differ along the small intestine, and why?

Histology and Function

Absorption of food begins in the stomach. Water, salts, and simple sugars often cross the mucosa and are absorbed in blood capillaries. However, the end products of digestion are mostly absorbed in the intestine. The rate of absorption strongly depends on the area available and time which nutrients spent in the alimentary canal. In herbivores, the intestines usually are quite long, and their intestinal ceca extended. These modifications increase absorption surface and prolong the time food travel through the intestines. Many vertebrates are able to move food inside the digestive tract in both directions. A retrograde peristalsis prolongs the time digesta spend in the digestive tract. In birds, retrograde peristalsis forces intestinal contents back into the gizzard. It especially characteristic of birds that feed on fruits with a waxy coating of saturated fats.

A villus is a small fingerlike projection of the simple columnar epithelium and lamina propria of the mucosa. Villi are larger and more numerous in the jejunum. Each villus contains a capillary network that receives blood from an arteriole and drains it into venule. A blind ended lymphatic capillary called **lacteal** occupies the center of the villus. Capillaries receive absorbed through the small intestine wall water soluble nutrients and transport them across the circulatory system. However, lipids are not water soluble and cannot be directly absorbed into the bloodstream. They are absorbed into the lacteals and transported through the lymphatic vessels.

Microvilli are microscopic extensions on the free surface of apical mucosa cells. They form a continuous field with a velvet-like surface called a **brush border** (fig. 19.15). The brush border holds various enzymes between microvilli. These enzymes complete the chemical digestion of most nutrients just before absorption. Collectively, these enzymes are called **brush border enzymes**. Located in close proximity or even embedded within the plasma membrane are the proteins that transport nutrients.

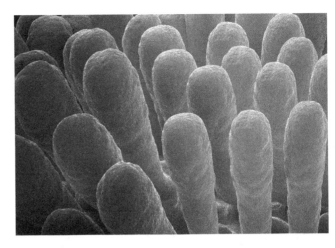

FIGURE 19.15   Brush Border.

The intestinal glands located between the villi are structurally similar to the gastric glands. These glands produce secretions. Three cell types produce **intestinal juice** and fourth type of cell secretes hormones into the blood.

1. **Goblet cells** produce mucus. Mucus lubricates and protects the intestinal cells. The number of these cells continuously increases from the duodenum to the ileum. This increase correlates with the increased proportion of undigested materials that remain in the intestinal lumen.
2. Special glands that are found only in submucosa on proximal duodenum called **duodenal submucosal** or **Brunner glands** produce a viscous, alkaline mucus that protects the duodenum from the acidic chyme entering from the stomach.
3. **Unicellular gland cells** synthesize enzyme **enteropeptidase**. Enteropeptidase converts **trypsinogen** (**zymogen**) into its active form, **trypsin**, which triggers a cascade of activation reactions of pancreatic digestive enzymes.
4. **Enteroendocrine cells** secrete hormones such as CCK and secretin.

Smooth muscle contraction within the small intestine wall has three functions: 1) mixing chyme with accessory gland secretions, 2) moving the chyme against the brush border, 3) propelling the content towards the large intestine. There are three levels of control of small intestine movements: local, nervous, and endocrine.

At the **early interstitial phase**, the chyme from the stomach is thoroughly mixed with intestinal juice and accessory gland secretions for fast and effective digestion. This process is termed **segmentation**. Muscular contractions are generated by the **pacemaker cells** (interstitial cells of Cajal). They generate waves of changes in plasma membrane potential, which via the gap junctions between adjacent smooth muscle cells travel along the small intestine muscular layer. This establishes a basic rhythm of smooth muscles contraction, which is a primary cause of the food segmentation. This type of movements prevails in the duodenum and proximal part of the jejunum.

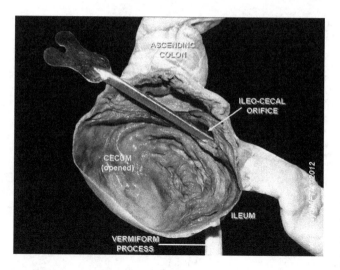

FIGURE 19.16   Ileocecal Valve.

At the **late intestinal phase**, movements of the intestinal wall become more wavelike. It helps propel indigestible materials along the small intestine towards the large intestine. This type of movement is called **peristalsis**. Peristalsis is characteristic of the ileum. When the food reaches this part of the small intestine, the major portion of valuable nutrients are already released from the food and absorbed. The peristalsis removes remaining materials from the organism. The peristalsis is enforced by a hormone **motilin** produced in the duodenum. A peristaltic wave of muscle contractions squeezes the content and moves it towards the large intestine. This moving wave of contraction is called the **migrating motility complex**.

The small intestine is separated from the large intestine by the **ileocecal valve** (fig. 19.16). Most of the time the ileocecal valve is closed and opens only for a short period to allow chyme to enter the cecum. The opening of the ileocecal valve is under control of the **gastroileal reflex**. The gastroileal reflex arc includes the vagus nerve and centers in the medulla oblongata. The reflex is stimulated by presence of food in the stomach and gastric peristalsis. Initiation of the reflex causes peristalsis in the ileum and the opening of the ileocecal valve, resulting in emptying the contents of the ileum into the large intestine.

CHECK YOUR UNDERSTANDING

- What are the hormones secreted by duodenal enteroendocrine cells?

- What role in digestion does cholecystokinin play?

- What role does the gastroileal reflex play?

- What is the function of the enteropeptidase?

19.5   Large Intestine

The large intestine is also called the **large bowel**. It is a relatively wide tube. Most nutrients are processed and absorbed in the small intestine. Thus, when the chyme reaches the large intestine, it has almost no nutrients to be absorbed, and the large intestine is preoccupied with other functions. First of all, the large intestine absorbs water and returns it to the body fluids. It also absorbs some electrolytes (primarily sodium and chloride). The large intestine harbors rich symbiotic microflora. Microflora ferments remaining from the food materials. By-products of its metabolism microflora produce some chemicals essential to the host organism, such as vitamins B and K, which then are absorbed in the large intestine. The remaining fecal materials are formed into feces, which later are removed from the body through defecation.

Gross Anatomy

The large intestine is a tube connecting the small intestine to the **cloaca** or **anus**. In most mammals it contains three distinct parts: a **cecum**, **colon**, and **rectum**. The cecum is a blind ended outgrowth at the junction of the small and large intestines. In many mammals, the large intestine forms a large, gentle loop called the **colon**. The large intestine often straightens near its end, forming a distinctive terminal portion before exiting. If this terminal section also receives products of the urinary and/or reproductive systems, it is called the **cloaca**. The external opening of the cloaca is called a **vent**. If the external exit only receives products from the alimentary canal, it is called a **rectum** and its opening is termed **anus**. The rectum narrows into the **anal canal**. A smooth muscle sphincter within the muscular layer of the anal canal controls the release of feces from the digestive tract (fig. 19.17).

The large intestine is often long, although not as long as the small intestine. The passage from the last segment of the small intestine—the ileum—and large intestine—the cecum—is guarded by a valve called

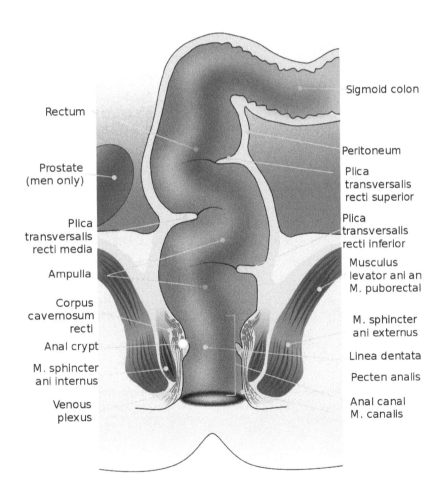

FIGURE 19.17   Human Rectum and Anus.

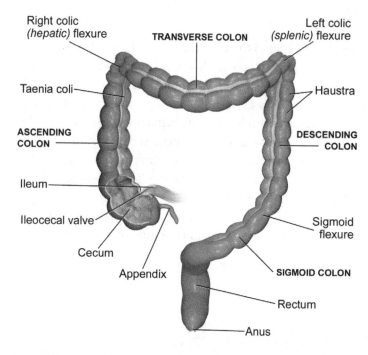

Right colic (hepatic) flexure
TRANSVERSE COLON
Left colic (splenic) flexure
Taenia coli
Haustra
ASCENDING COLON
DESCENDING COLON
Ileum
Ileocecal valve
Sigmoid flexure
Cecum
Appendix
SIGMOID COLON
Rectum
Anus

FIGURE 19.18   Human Large Intestine.

the **ileocecal valve**. In herbivores, a cecum is usually present at the junction between the large and small intestine. In humans, this much reduced cecum is called the appendix, or more specially the **vermiform appendix**. In monotremes and a few marsupials, the large intestine terminates in the cloaca. In eutherian mammals, it opens directly to the outside through the anal sphincter. In many herbivores, digestion of plant cellulose is enhanced by a cecum. The cecum houses microorganisms effective in cellulose digestion. Many species have several ceca that sprout from the intestine near the ileocecal junction.

The rectum is a muscular tube that easily expands to accumulate feces. Three thick transverse folds of the rectum, called **rectal valves**, retain fecal materials. The internal lining of the anal canal has thin longitudinal ridges called **anal columns**. Small depressions between anal columns are called **anal sinuses**. Cells at the bottoms of the anal sinuses produce mucus and release it, when feces pass anal canal. At the base of the anal canal there are two sphincters: a smooth muscle **internal anal sphincter** and a skeletal muscle **external anal sphincter**.

Three anatomic structures are specific to the large intestine: the **teniae coli**, **haustra**, and **epiploic appendages**. The teniae coli are thin longitudinal bundles of smooth muscles. The haustra are sacs that partition the large intestine into short fragments. The epiploic appendages, also called **omental appendages**, are fat lobules on the external surface of the haustra (fig. 19.18).

CHECK YOUR UNDERSTANDING

- What are the primary functions of the large intestine?

- What is the difference between the rectum and cloaca?

- How do the internal and external sphincters differ?

- What are the teniae coli?

Histology and Function

The mucosa of the large intestine is lined by a simple columnar epithelium with numerous goblet cells. The large intestine mucosa has no villi. Its wall is smooth, goblet cells are organized in **intestinal glands**, and numerous lymphatic nodules and lymphatic cells are scattered on its surface (fig. 19.19). The muscular

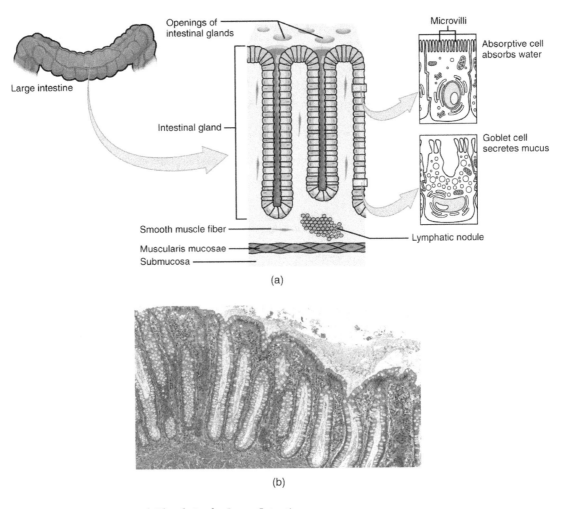

(a)

(b)

FIGURE 19.19   Intestinal Glands in the Large Intestine.

layer of the cecum and colon has two layers, but its outer longitudinal layer is discontinuous and does not completely surround the colon and cecum. These longitudinal smooth muscles form the teniae coli.

Rabbits, hares, many rodents, and even gorillas eat their feces, a behavior termed **coprophagy**. Usually, eaten feces come only from the cecum, but not from the main intestine. The cecum is emptied in the early morning, and only these droppings are consumed. Within the alimentary canal, there is also a selection process at the ileocecal junction. Liquids and fine particles are diverted into the cecum for extended fermentation, and coarse fibers are excluded. Thus, the coarse fiber that bypasses the cecum is not reingested, and only a small percentage of the digesta from the cecum is consumed a second time. Coprophagy allows reingestion, an additional opportunity for the full length of the alimentary canal to capture the products of fermentation, such as vitamins (K and all B vitamins), amino acids, and volatile fatty acids. If normal coprophagy is prevented, the animal requires vitamin supplements to remain healthy. Growing neonates of the marsupial koala from Australia eat feces during the transition from the milk food and leaves eating. The koala mother feeds her own droppings to the six-month-old neonate to begin the process of weaning it from milk to feces to eucalyptus leaves.

Microbial digestion of cellulose centered in the intestine is called **hindgut fermentation**. Extensive elongation of the intestine and large ceca extends the volume available for fermentation. Rabbits, pigs, horses, and koalas are examples of hindgut fermenters, as are herbivorous and omnivorous birds.

VETERINARY APPLICATION

Colonic impaction is intractable constipation that can occur in all species, including dogs and cats. There are hardened feces in the colon and a delayed or failed passage of fecal matter. The slower transit time allows more salt and water to be reabsorbed, leaving drier feces in the colon, which are more difficult to pass. Peristalsis may increase initially but is then significantly reduced or even absent due to **chronic distension**. Chronic cases may progress to **obstipation**, the feces become so hard and dry that defecation is no longer possible and ultimately there is secondary degeneration of the colonic musculature.

There are numerous causes of the disease, including: dietary, mechanical obstruction, colonic weakness, and problems with defecation. Symptoms of the disease include presence of firm fecal material in the colon on abdominal palpation. Digital rectal examination shows hardened fecal balls; there also may be an anal sac disease or perineal hernia.

The treatment depends on the severity and duration of the condition. Dehydrated patients should receive **IV fluid therapy**, with correction of any concurrent electrolyte and acid-base abnormalities. A warm water **enema** can be used to soften and allow the impaction to pass. **Laxatives** such as emollient laxatives (docusate sodium), stimulant laxatives (bisacodyl), saline laxatives and disaccharide laxatives (lactulose) are also beneficial. Surgical removal of feces under general anesthesia is necessary in severe cases where enemas and laxatives fail. A colectomy is required in cases of obstipation or recurrent cases.

The odor from feces can alert a predator to the presence of vulnerable young. Among many herbivores that hide from predators, the young animal does not pass feces until it is licked by its mother. Licking stimulates elimination of feces, which the mother eats so that feces do not collect at sites where young hide and leave a telltale odor. Many young birds bundle their feces. As feces move into the cloaca, its walls secrete a mucous bag that holds the digested food. Parents carry off these bundles of dirty feces, both contributing to a good housekeeping and removing any smelly feces that might attract the attention of a predator.

The activity of the large intestine is regulated by two major reflexes: **gastrocolic** and **defecation reflexes**. The gastrocolic reflex is initiated by stomach distention. It increases the peristaltic movements of the colon consisting of giant migrating contractions or mass movements, in response to stretch in the stomach and by-products of digestion in the small intestine. Thus, this reflex is responsible for the urge to defecate following a meal. The defecation reflex is triggered by accumulation of feces, which stretches the rectum. The stretch of the rectum stimulates one of two main defecation reflexes; **myenteric** or **parasympathetic**. The **myenteric defecation reflex** is responsible for increasing peristalsis and propelling stool toward the rectum. This eventually signals the internal anal sphincter to relax and reduce sphincter constriction. The **parasympathetic defecation reflex** proceeds through parasympathetic nerves from the sacral region of the spinal cord.

- What tissue lines the internal wall of the large intestine?

- What is the role of the gastrocolic reflex?

- How is the myenteric defecation reflex different from the parasympathetic defecation reflex?

Microflora of the Large Intestine and Its Role in Normal Physiology

Gut flora, or **gut microbiota**, or **gastrointestinal microbiota** is the complex community of microorganisms that live in the alimentary canal. The relationship between the host organism and its gut flora can be identified as a mutualistic or mutually beneficial relationship. Some microorganisms, for example, benefit by fermenting dietary fibers into fatty acids, such as acetic acid and butyric acid. Intestinal flora synthesizes vitamin B and K, metabolize bile acids and sterols. The short-chain fatty acids and other compounds they produce function like hormones, and the gut flora itself appears to function like an endocrine organ. Recent studies show that imbalance of the gut flora causes an inflammatory and autoimmune condition in the host organism.

In both foregut and hindgut fermenters, microorganisms of the digestive tract release enzymes that digest the plant cellulose. However, the physiological advantages of such fermentation differ between foregut and hindgut fermenters. At first glance, it might seem that foregut fermenters—such as ruminants, camels, kangaroos, and wallabies—enjoy all the advantages when it comes to efficient digestion. First, fermentation takes place in the anterior part of the alimentary canal, yielding end products of digestion early in the digestive process so they are ready for uptake next in the intestine. Second, the ruminant system allows rechewing and more complete mechanical breakdown of the cell walls. By shuttling food between the mouth and rumen via the esophagus, the ruminant can keep grinding away at plant fibers. The distant ceca of intestinal fermenters make such shuttling impossible. Third, the ruminant system turns much of the nitrogen, which in most vertebrates is a waste product, into a resource. This is particularly useful in ruminants that consume low-protein diets. Initially, the ruminant system converts nitrogen into waste products, such as ammonia and urea. Nitrogen in the form of ammonia is a by-product of fermentation of protein in the rumen. Microorganisms take up ammonia, combine it with organic carbon compounds, and use it to make their own cell proteins as they proliferate. Periodically, the rumen contracts, flushing these microorganisms into the abomasum and intestine, where, like any food, the microorganisms themselves are digested and their high-quality proteins are absorbed.

Foregut fermenters are also able to turn urea, another waste product, into a resource. For example, a camel fed nearly protein-free foods excretes almost no urea in its urine. Urea certainly forms during metabolism, but it reenters the rumen, partly by direct transfer across the rumen wall and partly in the camel's saliva. In the rumen, urea is broken down into carbon dioxide and ammonia.

Thus, foregut fermentation is especially efficient at extracting the most nutrients, even from food of poor quality. Ruminant animals have been especially successful in habitats where the forage is scarce, fibrous, and poor for at least part of the year, such as in alpine regions (goats), deserts (camels), and harsh winter areas (bison). Further, the action of fermentation in foregut animals early in the passage of digesta destroys or neutralizes potential plant toxins.

Hindgut fermentation has some advantages. For the hindgut fermenter, the bolus passes through the major absorptive regions of the alimentary canal before reaching the principal sites of fermentation, usually the ceca. Thanks to that, soluble nutrients such as carbohydrates, glucose, and proteins can be safely absorbed before they become fermented.

The foregut fermentation is thorough, and it is also slow. To ferment fibrous plants, food must occupy the rumen for extended cellulose processing. Where forage is abundant, the hindgut fermenter can move large quantities of food through the digestive tract, process the most easily digestible component of the forage, excrete the low-quality component, and replace low-quality food with fresh forage. Horses are hindgut fermenters. They depend on a high food intake and rapid transit to meet their nutritional needs. In addition, coprophagy allows rabbits and some rodents to reingest feces containing fermentation products produced on the first pass through the digestive tract. This gives these hindgut fermenters a second chance to extract some of the undigested material.

CHECK YOUR UNDERSTANDING

- What kind of relation exists between the host organism and its gut microflora?

- What is the difference between foregut fermenters and hindgut fermenters?

- What type of essential nutrients do microflora provide host organisms?

- What is the meaning of the coprophagy in hindgut fermenters?

Cloaca

The cloaca is a common chamber that receives products from the intestines and urogenital tracts. In some fishes and most mammals, the cloaca is absent. Instead, the intestine opens to the outside through the anus, which is a separate opening from that of the urogenital system.

Birds reproduce using their cloaca; this occurs during a cloacal kiss in most birds. Birds that mate using this method touch their cloacae together to transfer sperm from the male to the female (fig. 19.20).

Most mammals have no cloaca. Even in those that have one, the cloaca is partially subdivided into separate regions for the anus and urethra. Only monotremes (platypus), marsupial moles, and some small placental mammals, such as golden moles, tenrecs, and shrews have a true cloaca.

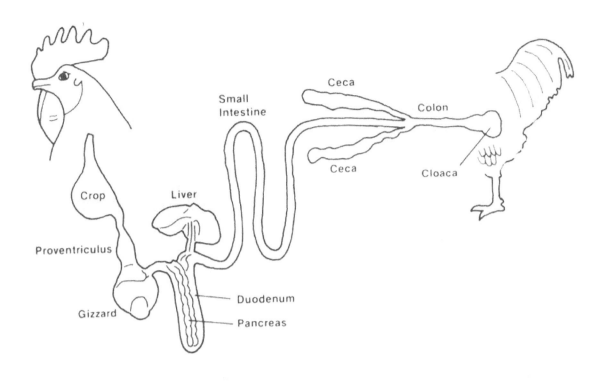

FIGURE 19.20   Bird Digestive System.

- What tracts open into the cloaca?
- Name animals that have a cloaca.

19.6   Accessory Organs

Pancreas

The pancreas (fig. 19.21) has both exocrine and endocrine glands organized into a single organ located near duodenum (see chapter 14, page 392). Exocrine cells known as **acinar cells** produce pancreatic juice with digestive enzymes and bicarbonate ions. In mammals, the pancreas usually has a wide head that occupies space made by the curved duodenum. Cuboidal secretory epithelial acinar cells are organized in saclike structures called **acini**. Each acinus empties its secretion via the small ducts into the **main** or **accessory pancreatic ducts**.

Secretions of acinar cells and cells that line the pancreatic ducts form **pancreatic juice**. The pancreatic juice is an alkaline watery solution of HCO_3^- and mixture of digestive enzymes, including 1) **pancreatic amylase** to digest carbohydrates; 2) **pancreatic lipase** to digest triglycerides; 3) **trypsinogen**,

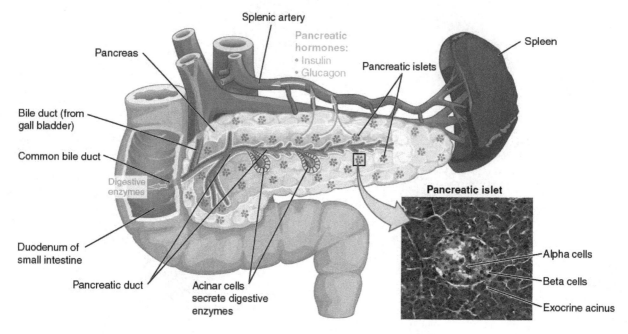

FIGURE 19.21   Sheep Pancreas. R—Right Lobe of Pancreas; B—Body; L—Left Lobe of Pancreas.

chymotrypsinogen, procarboxypeptidase—inactive forms of proteolytic enzymes to digest proteins; and 4) nucleases to digest nucleic acids.

CHECK YOUR UNDERSTANDING

- What cells produce pancreatic juice?
- What chemicals constitute pancreatic juice?
- How do CCK and secretin affect pancreatic secretion?

Liver and Gallbladder: Their Anatomy and Function

The liver has a wide variety of roles. Early in fetal life, the liver is directly involved in the production of red blood cells. In an adult organism, it is the site of old red blood cells' destruction and storage of iron released from the hemoglobin. It removes toxins from the blood. Hepatocytes secrete bile and release it into the duodenum to **emulsify** fats (break big clumps of fat down to small droplets). Carbohydrates, proteins, and fats are stored and metabolized in the liver.

The liver is covered by a connective tissue capsule. At one side this capsule has opening called the **porta hepatis**. The organ consists of several lobes and supported by two ligaments. The **falciform ligament** separates right and left lobes. The **round ligament** or **ligamentum teres** is a remnant of the fetal umbilical vein.

The liver is one of the most heavily vascularized organs of the body, being supplied with arterial blood via the **hepatic artery**, a branch of the celiac trunk. The **hepatic vein** drains blood from liver directly to the posterior vena cava. The liver also receives blood from the **hepatic portal vein**. The hepatic portal vein collects blood rich with nutrients from the intestines and spleen and delivers absorbed products to the liver. Blood circulation through the liver can be presented in following scheme:

IN	OUT
Portal vein and hepatic artery → interlobular vessels → portal vessels →	→ Central vein → sublobular vein → hepatic veins → posterior vena cava

At the gross level, the vertebrate liver is bulky and situated within the rib cage, conforming to the available shape of the body cavity. In snakes, it is long and narrow within the tubular body cavity. Although details differ, the microscopic structure of the liver basically remains the same throughout vertebrates. It is composed of sheets of hepatocytes separated by blood sinuses, through which courses venous blood returning from the intestines and arterial blood from the hepatic artery.

The connective tissue of the liver capsule makes deep folds that branch throughout the organ and form **septa** that partition the liver into thousands of microscopic polyhedral **hepatic lobules**. The hepatic lobule is constructed of liver cells called **hepatocytes**. A set of vessels, which consists of bile ductule, micro-scopic branches of portal vein and hepatic artery, called **portal triad** occupy peripheral areas of each lobule. The center of every lobule is occupied by a **central vein**. Central veins drain lobules and via the numerous hepatic veins empty into the posterior vena cava (fig. 19.22). Between the portal triads and the central vein are hepatocytes, organized into columns separated by spaces filled with blood, known as **hepatic sinusoids**.

Cells in the liver receive blood from two sources: the hepatic artery and hepatic portal vein. The hepatic artery supplies the liver with oxygenated blood, whereas the hepatic portal vein transports deoxygenated but nutrient-rich blood from capillaries in the GI tract, spleen, and pancreas. Both types of vessels deliver their blood to each sinusoid inside the hepatic lobule. There, blood is processed by the hepatocytes and then drained into the central vein. In hepatic

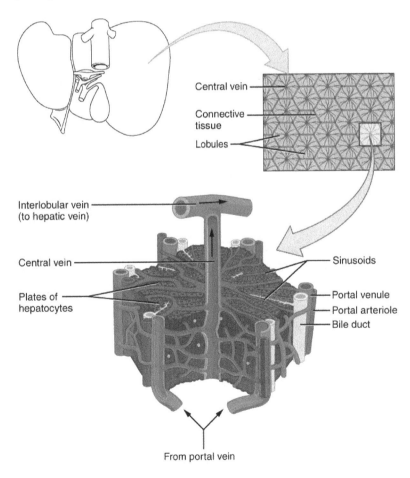

FIGURE 19.22   Hepatic Lobule.

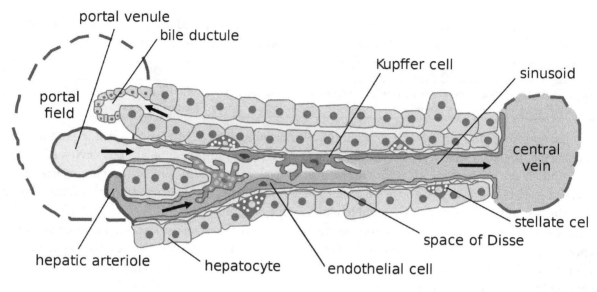

FIGURE 19.23   Segment of Hepatic Lobule.

sinusoids, nutrients and oxygen from the blood are absorbed into the hepatocytes. Special sedentary macrophages called **stellate** or **Kupffer cells** line walls of sinusoids. They thoroughly examine blood for presence of pathogens and toxins and phagocytize them.

The exocrine product of the liver is bile, which is delivered to the intestine, where it serves to emulsify fats. Bile is a fluid containing mostly water, bicarbonate ions (HCO_3^-), bile salts, bile pigments (**bilirubin**), cholesterol, lecithin, and mucin. Bile is produced by the hepatocytes. Hepatocytes release the bile into the **bile canaliculi**, a tiny tube that drains into the bile ductules of the portal triads (fig. 19.23). Bile within the bile ductules flows into the progressively larger bile ducts, until it enters the hepatic duct.

The system of ducts known as a **biliary apparatus** transports bile from the liver and gallbladder. The biliary apparatus is a network of ducts that include the right and left hepatic ducts. The merge of these ducts forms **common hepatic duct**. The gallbladder does not produce bile. It is just a temporary bile storage site. Bile enters and leaves the gallbladder through the **cystic duct**. The fusion of the cystic duct with common bile duct creates a **common bile duct** that empties into the **hepatopancreatic ampulla**. The hepatopancreatic ampulla is an enlarged chamber that receives bile from the common bile duct and secretions of the pancreas from the **main pancreatic duct** (fig. 19.24). It opens inside the duodenum via the **hepatopancreatic sphincter**. Most of the time, the sphincter is closed, but duodenal hormone CCK relaxes smooth muscles of the sphincter and opens it. Thus, the sphincter opens only when the acidic chyme from the stomach enters into the duodenum.

Bile has the following functions: 1) bicarbonate in the bile neutralizes acidic chyme from the stomach; 2) bile salts and lecithin emulsify fat molecules and make them accessible to lipases; and 3) elimination of the waste by-product of erythrocyte destruction—bilirubin.

The gallbladder is a sack organ that serves for temporary bile storage. Its wall contains three tunics: an inner tunic is mucosa, a middle tunic is muscularis, and an external tunic is serosa. At the gallbladder junction with the cystic duct, there is a sphincter valve that controls bile flow.

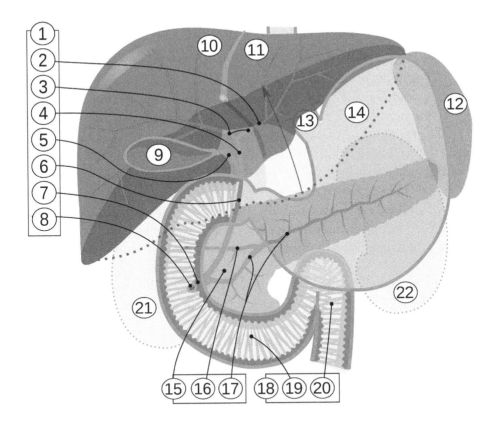

FIGURE 19.24   Biliary Apparatus. 1) Bile Ducts; 2) Intrahepatic Bile Ducts; 3) Left and Right Hepatic Ducts; 4) Common Hepatic Bile Duct; 5) Cystic Duct; 6) Common Bile Duct; 7) Hepatopancreatic Sphincter; 8) Duodenal Papilla; 9) Gallbladder; 10–11) Right and Left Lobes of Liver; 12) Spleen; 13) Esophagus; 14) Stomach; 15) Pancreas; 16) Accessory Pancreatic Duct; 17) Main Pancreatic Duct; 18) Small Intestine; 19) Duodenum; 20) Jejunum; 20–21) Right and Left Kidneys.

In most vertebrates, bile is stored in the **gallbladder** and released in sufficient quantities when chyme enters the intestine. The gallbladder is absent in most birds and some mammals. For example, among ungulates, the gallbladder is absent in cervids but present in bovids.

CHECK YOUR UNDERSTANDING

- What is a portal triad?

- What triggers bile release?

- What components constitute bile, and what is their role in digestion?

- What is the function of the stellate cells?

19.7   Nutrients and Metabolism

Nutrients: Water, Carbohydrates, Proteins, Lipids, Vitamins, and Minerals

Nutrients are small organic molecules that result from food digestion. Among nutrients are those molecules which organism can manufacture by itself, such as glucose or certain amino acids. These nutrients are called dispensable or nonessential nutrients. Nutrients necessary for normal functioning that cannot be synthesized by the organism and can be obtained only from food are called **indispensable** or **essential**. Depending on the amount of a nutrient needed for a normal healthy life, they are divided into two groups: macronutrients and micronutrients. Macronutrients include chemical elements consumed in large quantities, such as carbon, hydrogen, nitrogen, oxygen, phosphorus, and sulfur; chemical compounds consumed in large quantities, which provide bulk energy: carbohydrates, proteins, and fats. Micronutrients support metabolism. They include dietary minerals such as copper and iron, as well as vitamins.

Water is absorbed across the epithelial lining of the small and large intestines into the blood capillaries by osmosis.

The main sites of carbohydrate digestion are the oral cavity and small intestine. Starch digestion begins in the oral cavity by the enzyme **salivary amylase** and ends in the small intestine with the help of pancreatic amylase and other enzymes secreted by the intestinal glands. Complete carbohydrate breakdown to monosaccharides is accomplished by brush border enzymes embedded within the epithelial lining of the small intestine. These enzymes include **dextrinase**, **glucoamylase**, and **maltase**. The digestion of lactose into glucose and galactose is performed by **lactase**. **Sucrase** digests sucrose to glucose and fructose. The released monosaccharides glucose, fructose, and galactose are absorbed into the blood. All venous blood from the small intestine is transported through the hepatic portal vein to the liver, where fructose and galactose is converted into glucose.

Amino acids are the structural components of proteins in all plants, animals, and fungi. Amino acids are considered either **indispensable (essential)** or **dispensable (nonessential)**. Essential amino acids are those that are required preformed in the diet as the animal either lacks the metabolic pathway to synthesize the given amino acid or is unable to make sufficient quantities for growth and normal functioning. Nonessential amino acids are those that can be produced endogenously from available nitrogen and carbon sources. Dogs and cats, for example, have a requirement for ten amino acids: methionine, lysine, phenylalanine, arginine, histidine, threonine, tryptophan, leucine, isoleucine, and valine.

Proteins digestion begins in the stomach by pepsin and ends in the small intestine. Proteolytic enzymes are produced in inactive form and activated in the lumen of the alimentary canal. In small intestine works enzymes produced by the pancreas and intestinal glands. Trypsin and chymotrypsin break the bonds between specific amino acids within the protein to produce smaller strands of amino acids. Carboxypeptidase is restricted to breaking the bond only between an amino acid on the carboxyl end and the remaining protein. The brush border enzyme **dipeptidase** breaks the final bond between the two amino acids of a dipeptide so that both may be absorbed. The brush border enzyme **aminopeptidase** generate free amino acids from the amino end of peptides.

Saliva contains lingual lipase. Thus, digestion of lipids begins in the mouth. However, lingual lipase is active only in an alkaline environment and becomes inactive in a highly acidic stomach. A new step of lipids chemical digestion takes place in the small intestine. Pancreatic lipase digests each triglyceride into a monoglyceride and two free fatty acids. Lipids are hydrophobic and tend to self-organize in big masses, when they surround by body fluids. That is why, large lipid droplets, first of all, have to be mechanically broken into smaller droplets, so the pancreatic lipase can digest the fat molecules. This separation of large fat droplets into small is called **emulsification**, which is executed by **bile salts**. Bile salts are amphipathic molecules with that are hydrophobic on one side and hydrophilic on the other. Bile salts combined with water and fat molecules will automatically turn with their hydrophilic sides towards water molecules and their hydrophobic side towards the fat molecules. This orientation of bile salt molecules will lead to the formation of **micelle**. Thus, bile function in digestion is emulsification of fat molecules and makes them accessible to lipases (fig. 19.25).

Digested triglycerides and cholesterol are absorbed into the columnar epithelial cells in small intestine. Here monoglycerides and fatty acids are reorganized into new triglycerides. These triglycerides and cholesterol are rapped into the protein capsule form **chylomicron**. The Golgi apparatus packages chylomicrons into secretory vesicles. Vesicles with chylomicrons merge with the plasma membrane of epithelial cells to release chylomicrons by exocytosis. Chylomicrons are too large to pass through blood capillary walls, but they can enter the lacteals, the lymphatic capillaries (fig. 19.26).

Nucleic acids are digested by pancreatic enzymes **nucleases** in small intestine. The breakdown of nucleic acids is accomplished by the brush border enzymes including **phosphatase** and **nucleosidase**. The phosphatase breaks the bond between phosphate and the rest of the nucleotide. The nucleosidase breaks the bond between the sugar and the nitrogenous base of the nucleotide, releasing the sugar and nitrogenous base.

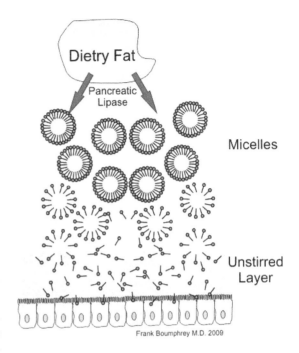

FIGURE 19.25   Bile and Chemical Digestion of Lipids.

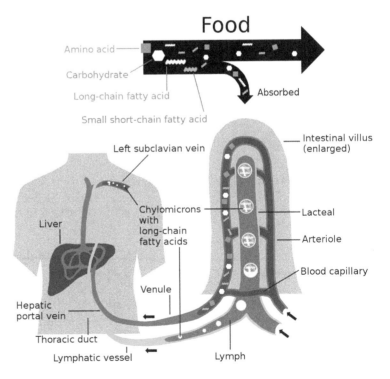

FIGURE 19.26   Absorption of Nutrients in Small Intestine.

Electrolytes are absorbed in the small intestine. Iron is an unusual element. Its absorption is controlled by the hormone **hepcidin**. The hormone is produced by the liver and is released in response to iron levels. Hepcidin inhibits the transport protein **ferroportin** located in the epithelial membrane of the GI tract. The hormone production decreases in accordance to the decrease of iron level. The decrease of hepcidin secretion decreases its inhibitory effect on ferroportin and allows an increase in iron transportation.

Vitamins are organic molecules divided in two principal groups: **fat-soluble** and **water-soluble**. Fat soluble vitamins (A, D, E, and K) are absorbed from the small intestine lumen into epithelial cells together with lipids within micelles. Thus, fat-soluble vitamins for their absorption need dietary fats. Water-soluble vitamins (B and C) are absorbed through various transport mechanisms: simple diffusion and active transport. Vitamin B_{12} is a large molecule and is transported through the receptor-mediated endocytosis. The process requires **intrinsic factor** released from the parietal cells in the stomach.

CHECK YOUR UNDERSTANDING

- Which nutrients are called essential?

- Where does nucleic acid digestion occur?

- What are the roles of bile and chylomicrons in lipid digestion?

- Explain why proteolytic enzymes need to be activated for protein digestion.

CHAPTER SUMMARY

- Organs of the digestive system are covered by a serous membrane called **peritoneal membrane** or **peritoneum** that has two folds: **parietal** and **visceral peritoneum**, or **serosa**.

- Blood vessels that serve digestive organs create **splanchnic circulation** (**gastric**, **superior mesenteric**, **inferior mesenteric arteries** and **hepatic portal vein system**).

- Actions of digestive organs are controlled by enteric nervous system (ENS) organized in three plexuses: **celiac**, **superior mesenteric**, and **inferior mesenteric**.

- Digestion proceeds in four steps: 1) ingestion; 2) mechanical and chemical breakdown; 3) absorption; and 4) egestion or excretion.

- Most regions of alimentary canal have four layers or tunics: **mucosa**, **submucosa**, **muscularis externa**, and **serosa** or **adventitia**.

- **Mucosa** is a three-layered innermost tunic: 1) epithelium that faces the lumen, 2) a thin layer of loose connective tissue called **lamina propria**, and 3) smooth muscles called **muscularis mucosae**. The stomach and the small and large intestines are lined by simple columnar epithelium with goblet cells that secrete mucus. Lamina propria houses blood and lymphatic vessels, glands, and MALT. Smooth muscles in muscularis mucosae are arranged in 1) an inner layer that has a circular arrangement and 2) an outer layer that has a longitudinal arrangement.

- **Submucosa** is composed of irregular dense connective tissue with blood and lymphatic vessels and submucosal glands. Submucosa houses **submucosal** or **Meissner's plexus** of ENS. This plexus controls secretion of glands and regulates blood flow.

- **Muscularis externa** is composed of smooth muscles organized in two layers. Contractions of muscles are controlled by motor neurons in the **myenteric** or **Auerbach's plexus**.

- The **serosa** is an outermost layer composed of irregular dense connective tissue.

- The mouth accommodates salivary glands, teeth, and tongue. It has two regions: the **vestibule** and **oral cavity proper**. The vestibule is an area between the teeth, lips, and cheeks. It is lined by squamous nonkeratinized epithelium called **gum** or **gingiva**. The oral cavity proper is behind teeth. It is lined by a mucous membrane.

- Teeth are made of **dentin** covered by **enamel**. Enamel is composed of calcium hydroxyapatite crystals with inclusion of organic component, mostly collagen. Enamel forms a **crown**. Part of the tooth inside alveolus is called **root**. It is composed of a mineralized tissue called **cementum**. Inside, tooth consists of **dentin**, about 70 percent of which is calcium hydroxyapatite. **Odontoblasts** are cells that continuously produce dentin. The center of the tooth is filled by a loose connective tissue called **pulp**. The center of the tooth filled by pulp is called the **pulp cavity**. Pulp cavity extends into the root via a **root canal**. **Periodontal ligaments** anchor teeth and prevent their displacement.

- Saliva consists of water, electrolytes, and mucus. It moisturizes the oral cavity, dissolves food, lubricates, and cleans the oral cavity, and along with teeth action, transforms food into a bolus. **Salivary amylase** is an enzyme that hydrolyses polysaccharides. Saliva accounts for 30 percent of starch digestion. **Lingual lipase** hydrolyses fats. **Bicarbonate ions** (HCO_3^-) neutralize acids. **Lysozyme** and **IgA** protect from pathogenic microorganisms. A glycoprotein **haptocorrin** binds vitamin B_{12} and carries it safely through acidic stomach to the duodenum.

- Salivary glands are exocrine glands. They are made of **serous** and **mucous** acinar cells. Serous cells secrete watery fluid with enzymes and other digestion components. Mucous cells secrete mucus. Three major salivary glands are: **parotid**, **submandibular glands**, and **sublingual**.

- The tongue is composed of skeletal muscles. It is attached to the mouth floor by a ligamentous band called the **frenulum**. There are two sets of tongue muscles: 1) four **intrinsic muscles** originate inside the tongue and form its shape; and 2) four **extrinsic muscles** that are attached to mandible, hyoid, and temporal bones and are involved in tongue movement.

- The throat or pharynx is posterior to the nasal and oral cavities. It has three parts: superior **nasopharynx**, middle **oropharynx**, and posterior **laryngopharynx**. Swallowing or **deglutition** triggers by a forceful movement of the food bolus. The pharynx is surrounded by three pairs of skeletal muscles: **upper**, **middle**, and **lower pharyngeal constrictor muscles**. They propel food bolus towards the esophagus.

- The **epiglottis** is a spoon-shaped elastic cartilage in the larynx. It is covered with a mucous membrane. The epiglottis guards the entrance into the **glottis**: an opening between the vocal cords.

- Between the pharynx and esophagus there is a circle of external muscles called the **upper esophageal sphincter**. A **lower esophageal sphincter** guards the bolus entrance into the stomach. A combination of skeletal and smooth muscles surrounding the esophagus propels food bolus by wavelike contractions termed **peristalsis**.

- Birds have an esophagus expanded into a **crop**. A crop is a temporary food storage site. In pigeons, it secretes a nutritional fluid called "milk" for feeding chickens. The stomach of birds has two parts: 1) a thin-walled glandular section called the **proventriculus** and 2) the posterior muscular section called the gizzard. The proventriculus secretes gastric juice to help digest the bolus, and the gizzard, together with selected pieces of hard grit and pebbles, grinds food.

- The stomach is an enlarged part of the digestive tract. It has five regions: the **cardia, fundus, body, pyloric antrum**, and **pylorus**. The pylorus empties into the first part of the small intestine, called the **duodenum**. A **pyloric sphincter** controls passage of acidic chyme. Internally, the stomach wall has folds called **rugae**.

- The stomach muscular tunic has three layers of smooth muscles. The external and middle layers have a circular and longitudinal orientation of muscle fibers. Muscles in the internal layer have an oblique orientation and spiral around the stomach. The oblique layer adds to peristaltic movement **churning** motions that toss and mix food with gastric juice.

- Gastric mucosa can be **glandular** or **nonglandular**. Nonglandular epithelium often is keratinized. It processes rough food: seeds, grasses, and chitin of insect exoskeletons. Glandular epithelium has **gastric glands** in **gastric pits**. The space between gastric pits is lined by columnar cells with goblet cells. Both secrete a thick mucus that protects stomach wall from its own acidic secretions. Gastric glands are distributed over the cardia, fundus, and pylorus. The cardia is a narrow region found only in mammals. It marks the transition between the esophagus and stomach. Its glands are termed **cardiac glands**. They mostly secrete mucus. **Fundic glands** have **parietal** and **chief cells**. The parietal cells produce hydrochloric acid and **intrinsic factor**, a chemical needed for absorption of vitamin B_{12}. The chief cells secrete **pepsinogen**, a precursor of **pepsin**. These secretions form **gastric juice**. **Pyloric glands** release mucus that neutralize acidic chyme as it moves towards the small intestine.

- Ruminants have four chambers. The first three—**rumen, reticulum**, and **omasum**—arise from the esophagus and only the fourth—**abomasum**—is a real stomach. The large rumen receives the food. The reticulum is a small accessory chamber with a honeycombed wall texture. The omasum is lined with esophageal epithelium, although it is folded into overlapping leaves. The three types of mucosa distinctive of the mammalian stomach are found only in the abomasum.

- The process of regurgitation and remastication is termed **ruminating**. It repeats until most of the material is broken down mechanically. In grazing cattle, this may take up to eight hours per day and repeats 40–50 times.

- The omasum operates as a two-phase pump to push a food bolus from the reticulum to the abomasum.

- In a suckling ruminant neonate, the abomasum and intestine digest milk. Milk bypasses the rumen via the **reticular groove** and moves directly from the esophagus to the abomasum.

- A group of cells known as **interstitial cells of Cajal** in the stomach wall has the ability to generate muscular contractions. These cells are bound with other smooth muscle cells by gap junctions and trigger rhythmic contractions.

- Gastric secretion has three phases: **cephalic, gastric**, and **intestinal**. The cephalic phase is based on **cephalic reflex** initiated by food smell, sight or taste. The gastric phase begins when bolus enters stomach. It is controlled by nervous signals via the gastric reflex and endocrine G cells in gastric glands. The intestinal phase is initiated by an entrance of chyme into the duodenum. Presence of acidic chyme in duodenum triggers an **intestine reflex**. Sensory impulses from duodenum inhibit vagal stimulation of the stomach. Enteroendocrine cells in the duodenum release hormones **cholecystokinin (CCK)** and **secretin**. CCK decreases stomach movements, stimulates pancreas release pancreatic enzymes, production of bile, and emptying of the gallbladder. CCK mediates satiety by acting on CCK receptors in hypothalamic satiety center. Secretin inhibits secretion of gastric juice and gastrin. It also stimulates production of HCO_3^- by pancreas. HCO_3^- binds H^+ and neutralizes acidic chyme.

- The small intestine or **small bowel** is a part of the **lower gastrointestinal tract**. It serves to finish food digestion and nutrients absorption. It has three regions: the **duodenum**, **jejunum**, and **ileum**. The **ileocecal vale** separates the ileum and cecum.

- The total surface of the small intestine is large because of **circular folds** or **plicae circulares**, **villi**, and **microvilli**. Plicae circulares are macroscopic ring folds of mucosa and submucosa. They are most numerous in duodenum and jejunum. The **villi** are mucosal projections. Mucosa cells carries **microvilli**.

- Villus contains a capillary network and lymphatic capillary called **lacteal**. Capillaries receive absorbed water-soluble nutrients. Lymph in lacteal transports lipids.

- Microvilli form a **brush border** that increases absorptive surface and accumulates enzymes between microvilli called **brush border enzymes**.

- The intestinal glands located between the villi structurally similar to the gastric glands. These glands produce **intestinal juice** and hormones.

- **Duodenal submucosal** or **Brunner glands** in proximal part of duodenal submucosa produce a viscous alkaline mucus that protects duodenum from the acidic chyme.

- **Unicellular gland cells** synthesize enzyme **enteropeptidase** that converts **trypsinogen (zymogen)** into active **trypsin**. Active trypsin activates other pancreatic enzymes.

- Smooth muscle contraction within the small intestine wall functions to 1) mix chyme with accessory gland secretions, 2) move chyme against the brush border, and 3) propel intestine content towards the large intestine. Peristalsis is initiated by a hormone **motilin** produced in duodenum. Peristaltic wave of muscles contraction squeezes content and moves it towards the large intestine. The moving wave of contraction is called **migrating motility complex**.

- **Ileocecal valve** opens only for a short time to allow chyme enter the cecum. This opening is controlled by the **gastroileal reflex**.

- Large intestine or **large bowl** absorbs water and electrolytes. It houses symbiotic microflora that digests remaining materials and produces some essential chemicals, including vitamins B and K.

- Large intestine has three distinct parts: **cecum**, **colon**, and **rectum** ended by **cloaca** or **anus**. Cecum is a pouch at the junction of small and large intestines. In many mammals, large intestine forms a large, gentle loop called **colon**. The straight part of large intestine near its end is called **rectum** and its opening is termed **anus**. If this terminal section also receives products of the urinary and/or reproductive systems, it is called **cloaca** and its opening is called **vent**.

- Folds called **rectal valves** help rectum to retain feces. Internal lining of the anal canal has thin longitudinal ridges called **anal columns** and depressions between them—**anal sinuses**. Cells at the bottom of anal sinuses produce mucus and release it, when feces pass anal canal. At the base of the anal canal there are two sphincters: **internal** and **external anal sphincters**.

- Rabbits, hares, rodents, and gorillas eat their feces: a habit termed **coprophagy**. Coprophagy is an additional opportunity to capture products of fermentation: vitamins K and all B, amino acids, and volatile fatty acids.

- Intestinal microbial digestion of cellulose is called **hindgut fermentation**.

- Large intestine activity is regulated by: **gastrocolic** and **defecation reflexes**. The gastrocolic reflex is initiated by stomach distention. The defecation reflex is triggered by accumulation of feces in rectum. Stretch of the rectum stimulates one of two defecation reflexes: **myenteric** or **parasympathetic**.

- **Gut flora (gut microbiota** or **gastrointestinal microbiota)** is a community of microorganisms that live in the alimentary canal. The relationship between the host organism and its gut flora can be identified as a mutually beneficial.

- Pancreatic secretory acinar cells are organized in structures called **acini**. Each acinus release secretion in a small duct, which empties into the **main** or **accessory pancreatic ducts**. Pancreatic juice is an alkaline watery solution of HCO_3^- and digestive enzymes, including 1) **pancreatic amylase** to digest carbohydrates; 2) **pancreatic lipase** to digest triglycerides; 3) **trypsinogen, chymotrypsinogen, procarboxypeptidase**—inactive forms of proteolytic enzymes to digest proteins; and 4) **nucleases** to digest nucleic acids.

- The liver removes toxins from the blood, secretes bile, and stores and metabolizes carbohydrates, proteins, and fats. It is covered by a capsule, one side of which has an opening called the **porta hepatis**. The organ consists of several lobes and is supported by 1) the **falciform ligament**, which separates the right and left lobes; and 2) the **round ligament** or **ligamentum teres**, which is a remnant of the fetal umbilical vein.

- The liver is supplied with arterial blood via the **hepatic artery**. It also receives blood from the **hepatic portal vein** that collects nutrient-rich blood from the intestines and spleen. The **hepatic vein** drains blood from the liver to the posterior vena cava.

- The tissue of the liver capsule makes folds that divide the liver interior in **septa** that partition it into thousands of microscopic polyhedral **hepatic lobules**. Bile ductule, microscopic branches of portal vein, and hepatic artery form **portal triad** that occupy peripheral position of the lobule. At center of the lobule is a **central vein**. Central veins drain lobules. Between the portal triads and central vein are hepatocytes, organized in columns separated by spaces filled with blood called **hepatic sinusoids**. In hepatic sinusoids nutrients and oxygen from the blood are absorbed into hepatocytes. Macrophages called **stellate** or **Kupffer cells** line walls of sinusoids. They examine blood for pathogens and toxins and phagocytize them.

- Bile serves to emulsify fats. It contains water, HCO_3^-, bile salts, bile pigments, cholesterol, lecithin, and mucin. Hepatocytes release bile into the **bile canaliculi**, a tiny tube that drains into the bile ductules of the portal triads. Within the ductules bile flows into the progressively larger bile ducts until it enters the hepatic duct.

- The **biliary apparatus** includes right and left hepatic ducts, which merge in the **common hepatic duct**. Bile enters and leaves the gallbladder through the **cystic duct**. The fusion of the cystic duct with common bile duct creates **common bile duct** that empties into the **hepatopancreatic ampulla**. The hepatopancreatic ampulla opens inside the duodenum via the **hepatopancreatic sphincter**. Bile: 1) neutralizes acidic chyme; 2) bile salts and lecithin emulsify fat molecules and make them accessible to lipases. The gallbladder serves as a temporary bile storage site. It is absent in most birds and some mammals.

- Molecules released from digested food are called **nutrients**. Nutrients that organism can produce are called **dispensable** or **nonessential nutrients**. Nutrients that organism cannot produce are called **indispensable** or **essential**. Depending the amount of nutrient needed for a healthy life, they are divided into **macronutrients** and **micronutrients**.

- Water is absorbed across the epithelial lining of the small and large intestines by osmosis.

- Carbohydrate digestion begins in the oral cavity by salivary amylase and ends in the small intestine by pancreatic amylase and enzymes of intestinal glands. Complete carbohydrate breakdown is accomplished by brush border enzymes within epithelial lining of small intestine, including **dextrinase**, **glucoamylase**, and **maltase**. The digestion of lactose into glucose and galactose performed by **lactase**. **Sucrase** digests sucrose to glucose and fructose. In the liver fructose and galactose are converted in glucose.

- Dogs and cats have ten essential amino acids: methionine, lysine, phenylalanine, arginine, histidine, threonine, tryptophan, leucine, isoleucine, and valine.

- Digestion of proteins begins in the stomach by pepsin and ends in the small intestine. Trypsin and chymotrypsin break the bonds between specific amino acids within protein. Carboxypeptidase cuts bonds at amino acid carboxyl side. The brush border enzyme **dipeptidase** breaks dipeptides and **aminopeptidase** cuts peptides at amino ends.

- Triglycerides and cholesterol are absorbed by columnar epithelial cells in small intestine. Here monoglycerides and fatty acids are reassembled into new triglycerides and covered by protein capsule called **chylomicron**. Chylomicrons enter lacteals.

- Nucleic acids are digested by pancreatic enzymes **nucleases** in the duodenum. Their breakdown is accomplished by the brush border enzymes **phosphatase** and **nucleosidase**.

- Electrolytes are absorbed in small intestine. Absorption of iron is controlled by the hormone **hepcidin** produced by the liver.

- Vitamins are organic molecules divided in two groups: **fat-soluble** and **water-soluble**. Fat-soluble vitamins (A, D, E, and K) are absorbed together with lipids. Water-soluble vitamins (B and C) are absorbed through various transport mechanisms. Vitamin B_{12} is transported via receptor-mediated endocytosis with the help of **intrinsic factor**.

CHECK YOUR KNOWLEDGE

LEVEL 1. CHECK YOUR RECALL

1. Required molecules that animals cannot synthesize are called:
    A. Essential nutrients
    B. Enzymes
    C. Proteins
    D. Carbohydrates

2. The liver functions to:
   A. Synthesize glucose from noncarbohydrates
   B. Store vitamin D
   C. Destroy damaged red blood cells
   D. Produce bile from cholesterol
   E. All of the above

3. The parietal cells of gastric glands secrete:
   A. Mucus
   B. Pepsinogen
   C. Hydrochloric acid
   D. Pepsin
   E. Gastrin

4. Bile is composed of:
   A. Water
   B. Electrolytes
   C. Bile salts
   D. Cholesterol
   E. All of the above

5. The sphincter muscle located between the small intestine and the large intestine is called:
   A. Pyloric
   B. Low esophageal
   C. Hepatopancreatic
   D. Internal anal
   E. Ileocecal

6. What component of bile has a digestive function?
   A. Bile salts
   B. Bile pigments
   C. Cholesterol
   D. Electrolytes
   E. Water

7. In mammals, how and where are carbohydrates digested?
   A. By lipase in the small intestine
   B. By pepsin and HCl in the stomach
   C. By aquaporins in the large intestine
   D. By amylases in the mouth and small intestine
   E. By nucleases in the stomach

8. One of the major functions of the large intestine is to:
   A. Secrete digestive enzymes
   B. Reabsorb water from chyme
   C. Regulate the release of bile
   D. Break down hemoglobin
   E. Absorb amino acids and fats

9. An example of a digestive specialization is seen in:
   A. The long intestine and enlarged cecum of herbivores
   B. The incisors being the dominant teeth in wolves
   C. Canine teeth being the dominant teeth in deer
   D. Salivary lipase being made by human
   E. Enlarged cecum of cats

10. The crop is a modification of the _____, whereas the gizzard is a part of bird's _____.
    A. stomach; small intestine
    B. esophagus; stomach
    C. small intestine; colon
    D. esophagus; small intestine
    E. stomach; colon

11. Pancreatic juice contains:
    A. HCO_3^- and digestive enzymes
    B. Bile
    C. Bile and digestive enzymes
    D. Hormone gastrin
    E. HCO_3^- and bile

12. The _____ of the stomach secrete _____.
    A. chief cells; gastrin
    B. parietal cells; HCl
    C. parietal cells; pepsinogen
    D. chief cells; HCl
    E. chief cells; pepsinogen

13. The most common movement in the duodenum is _____, whereas in the ileum it is _____.
    A. churning; peristalsis
    B. peristalsis; segmentation
    C. segmentation; churning
    D. churning; segmentation
    E. segmentation; peristalsis

14. _____ increases gastric secretion, whereas _____ inhibits it.
    A. Secretin; gastrin
    B. Gastrin; intrinsic factor
    C. Gastrin; CCK
    D. CCK; gastrin
    E. Secretin; CCK

15. True or false: Bile is transported through the lacteals.
16. True or false: Digestion of proteins begins in the oral cavity.
17. True or false: Cholecystokinin (CCK) is produced by the duodenal mucosa.
18. Match the term with its description:

    _____ Acinar cell   a. Initiate peristalsis
    _____ Chief cell   b. Inhibit production of gastric juice and gastrin
    _____ Parietal cell   c. Stimulate gastric juice production
    _____ Motilin   d. Exocrine cell that produces pancreatic juice
    _____ Hepatocyte   e. Produce pepsinogen
    _____ Intrinsic factor   f. Produce bile
    _____ Secretin   g. Produce HCl
    _____ Gastrin   h. Facilitate absorption of vitamin B_{12} in the ileum

LEVEL 2. CHECK YOUR UNDERSTANDING

1. Why can the release of intrinsic factor be considered the only essential function of the stomach in meat-eating animals?
2. Often manufacturers advertise dietary supplements that contain digestive enzymes needed for proper food digestion. Do you think that these supplements are likely to be useful? Explain your answer.
3. General anesthesia eliminates the swallowing reflex, but it does not eliminate the ability to vomit. Why must patients not eat or drink anything for at least 12 hours prior to undergoing surgery?

LEVEL 3. APPLY YOUR KNOWLEDGE TO REAL LIFE

1. Research shows that a dry mouth is correlated with dental problems, such as cavities. What are the possible reasons for that?
2. The disease cystic fibrosis is characterized by an excess production of highly thick, sticky mucus, which can block the pancreatic duct. What digestive problems are characteristic of cystic fibrosis?

Chapter 20

The Respiratory System

LEARNING OBJECTIVES

Oxygen is a unique chemical element. It is the second-most electronegative element in the periodic table after fluorine. An electronegative element tends to create chemical bonds with most elements by taking or pulling onto itself their electrons. The reactions with oxygen are commonly called oxidation reactions, and they are accompanied by a release of a substantial amount of energy. This energy may be utilized in multiple ways for vital organism needs. That is why organisms that use oxygen and oxygenation reactions as a foundation for metabolic processes get an evolutionary advantage and are the most prosperous on earth. There are organisms that get energy from other recourses then oxidative-reduction reactions, but all of them are not effective. The amount of energy harvested via oxidation reactions is incomparably larger than via other reactions; for example, fermentation. The respiratory system includes organs that participate in taking in oxygen, absorbing it into body fluids, and expelling by-products of oxygen metabolism, which otherwise will accumulate up to toxic levels. Upon completion of this chapter, you should be able to do the following:

1. Describe the structural organization of the respiratory system.
2. Describe the passageways of oxygen and carbon dioxide in the body.
3. Explain the role of environmental factors in respiration.
4. Describe the mechanisms underlining regulation of respiration and gas exchange.

INTRODUCTION

The respiratory system serves in exchanges of gases between an organism and the environment. In terrestrial animals, gas exchange takes place in the lungs. It occurs in millions of small air sacs called **alveoli** in mammals and reptiles, and in **parabronchi** of birds. These microscopic air sacs bring the air into close contact with the blood. A system of airways, or hollow tubes, of which the largest is the **trachea** connects alveoli with external environment. The trachea branches in the middle of the chest into the two main **bronchi**. These enter the lungs where they branch into progressively narrower secondary and tertiary bronchi that branch into numerous smaller tubes, the bronchioles. In birds the bronchioles are ended by **parabronchi**. It is the bronchioles that generally open into the microscopic alveoli in mammals. Air is pumped into the alveoli or parabronchi by the process of breathing, which involves the respiratory muscles.

Gases move between alveoli and blood by passive diffusion. The rate of passive diffusion between an organism and its environment depends on surface area, distance, and resistance. The relation between diffusion rate and surface area is direct: the greater the available surface area, the higher the rate of diffusion. The distance has a negative effect on gas diffusion. The greater the distance, the longer it will take for molecules to reach their destination. Thick tissues slow diffusion, and thin barriers aid the process. The resistance to diffusion by the tissue barrier can be demonstrated by the example of skin. The moist skin of amphibians facilitates gas transfer. In contrast to that, the skin of most mammals is cornified, thick, and makes exchange of gases impossible.

The respiratory and circulatory systems are functionally coupled in the process of **respiration**. Respiration is divided in two sequential and dependent steps. ***External respiration*** refers to gas exchange between the environment and blood via the respiratory surface. ***Internal respiration*** refers to gas exchange between the blood and the deep body tissues.

During external respiration, gases diffuse between the environment and the organism—oxygen enters, carbon dioxide departs. **Ventilation**, or breathing, is the active process of moving the respiratory medium, water or air, across the exchange surface. Stopping of the respiratory medium movement causes **apnea**, or breath holding. Pumping of blood through an organ via capillaries is termed **perfusion**. The **respiratory organs** specialize in ventilation to deliver oxygen and remove carbon dioxide.

Structurally, the respiratory system is organized in two regions: the **upper respiratory tract** and **lower respiratory tract**. The upper respiratory tract includes the nose, nasal cavity, and pharynx. The larynx, trachea, bronchi, bronchioles, respiratory bronchioles, alveolar ducts, and alveoli are components of the lower respiratory tract.

Functionally, the respiratory system organs are divided in two groups. The first group is responsible for transporting air, but does not participate in gas exchange. This group includes air passageways from the nose to the terminal bronchioles, altogether called the **conducting zone**. The second group of structures is responsible for gas exchange. It is called the **respiratory zone**. The respiratory zone consists of respiratory bronchioles, alveoli ducts, and alveoli.

CHECK YOUR UNDERSTANDING

- What are external and internal respirations?

- What structures compose the upper respiratory tract?

- What structures compose the conducting zone?

- What three structures compose the respiratory zone?

20.1   Anatomy of the Respiratory System

Nose and Nasal Cavity

The respiratory system begins with **nares**, or **nostrils**. The nostrils have an outer ring made of cartilage (the **alar cartilage**), which serves to hold them open during inhalation. A small pocket within nares, called the **nasal diverticulum**, filters debris with the help of the hairs lining the inner nostril. The nasal cavity contains the nasolacrimal duct, which drains tears from the eyes.

The nasal passages contain nasal conchae on both sides. Nasal conchae make air passages through the nasal cavity longer and increase the surface area to which the air is exposed. They are covered by a nonkeratinized mucous membrane with numerous goblet cells, mucous glands, and blood vessels in the

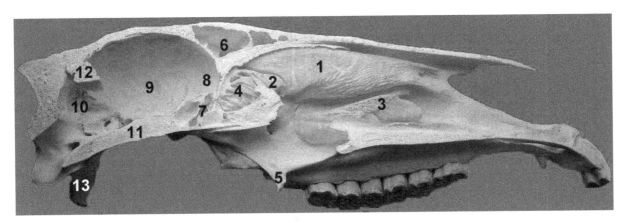

FIGURE 20.1   Horse Skull: 1. Superior (Dorsal) Nasal Concha; 2. Medial Nasal Concha; 3. Ventral (Inferior) Nasal Concha; 4. Ethmoid Bone; 5. Pterygoid Bone; 6. Frontal Bone; 7. Sphenoid Sinus; 8. Fossa Cranii Rostralis; 9. Fossa Cranii Media; 10. Fossa Cranii Caudalis; 11. Porus Acusticus Internus; 12. Tentorium Cerebelli Osseum; 13. Processus Paracondylaris.

lamina propria. The close contact of the inhaled air with walls of the nasal cavity prepares it to enter the lungs. Air is cleaned of contaminants such as dust particles and microorganisms, moisturized by mucus vapor, and warmed up by blood flow close to the surface. The sinuses within the skull are able to drain through the nasal passage. The nasal passage joins to the larynx via the pharynx. The pharynx includes the nasopharynx, which protects the entrance to the auditory tubes; the oropharynx, which contains tonsillar tissue; and the laryngopharynx (fig. 20.1).

Parallel to the main nasal passages there is a complex system of paranasal sinuses—spaces within head bones filled by air and connected with the respiratory tract (fig. 20.2). They serve to reduce the weight of the head and consist of the following types of sinuses:

1. **Frontal sinuses** are located within frontal bones between eyes. There are two, one on each side, divided by a bony septum. They are open inside the nasal conchae, forming the **conchofrontal sinuses**. Drainage into the nasal passages is via the caudal maxillary sinus.

2. **Maxillary sinuses** are spaces within the maxilla, above the tooth roots. Each is divided into two compartments: the **rostral maxillary sinus** in front, and the **caudal maxillary sinus** behind. They do not communicate. In addition, each of *these* is subdivided into a medial (inside) and lateral (outside) component, by an incomplete bone wall that carries the infraorbital canal containing nerves and blood vessels. The close proximity to the tooth roots means that as the teeth erupt with age, the maxillary sinuses become larger.

3. **Sphenopalatine sinuses** are small pouches medial (inside) to the caudal maxillary sinus.

A flap of tissue called the **soft palate** blocks off the pharynx from the oral cavity. It prevents food inhaling. A horse, for example, cannot breathe through the mouth when it is in respiratory distress. It can breathe only through the nostrils. For this same reason, horses also cannot pant as a method of thermoregulation. The horse has a unique part of the respiratory system called the **guttural pouch**, which is thought to equalize air pressure across the tympanic membrane. The guttural pouch is present only in nonruminant ungulates:

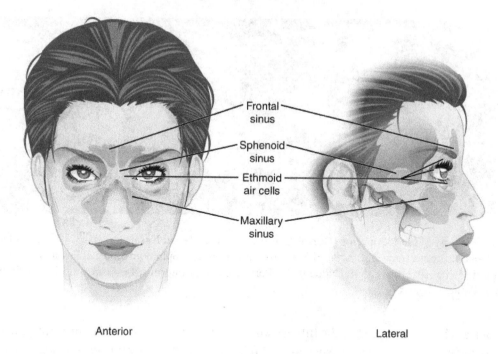

Anterior

Lateral

FIGURE 20.2   Sinuses in Human Skull.

horses, tapirs, rhinoceros, and some small mammals including hyraxes (dassies), certain bats, and a South American mouse. The guttural pouches are paired ventral diverticulae of the eustachian (auditory) tubes, formed by mucosal lining of the tube through a relatively long ventral slit in the supporting cartilages. The auditory tube connects the nasal cavity and middle ear, and the diverticulum dilates to form pouches, which can have a capacity of 300 to 500 ml in the domestic horse. The pouches are normally filled with air. Laterally the guttural pouch is covered by the pterygoid muscles, parotid, and mandibular glands. The floor lies mainly on the pharynx and beginning of the esophagus. The medial retropharyngeal lymph node lies between the pharynx and ventral wall of the pouches. The pouch has a very thin wall lined by respiratory epithelium. The mucus of the epithelium drains into the pharynx when the horse is grazing. The pouch is drained through the slit-like pharyngeal openings of the eustachian tube in the lateral wall of the nasopharynx. The connection opens when the horse swallows, and grazing normally provides drainage.

The function of guttural pouches is largely unknown; however, there are two hypotheses:

1. It may influence internal carotid artery blood pressure. Air pressure varies with the phase and forcefulness of respiration, and the artery in the mucosal fold is exposed sufficiently to be affected.
2. The cerebral blood-cooling mechanism operates at times of physical stress/exercise, when core body temperature is raised. Vigorous respiration, cool air in guttural pouches, and the exposed artery all lead to cooling of the blood.

The vomeronasal organ is also known as the **olfactory organ**, or **Jacobson's organ**. It is an olfactory sense organ that is found in most animals. It is positioned at the base of the nasal cavity, within the roof of the mouth, and is separated into two parts by the nasal septum. It is situated close to the vomer and nasal bones; hence the name vomeronasal organ. It is contained within a bony capsule which opens into the base of the nasal cavity, and is lined with olfactory mucosa. The vomeronasal organ contains sensory chemoreceptors, and is involved in the first processing step of the accessory olfactory system (see Chapter 13, pages 355–356). The vomeronasal organ carries information via the **olfactory nerve** (CN I), which travels through the cribriform plate, to the accessory olfactory bulb (the vomeronasal bulb), and then to the hypothalamus. The sensory receptors are found on the medial inner surface of the vomeronasal organ. The lateral inner surface is covered with sensory cilia. Basal cells are also found in this region. The dorsal and ventral inner surfaces of the vomeronasal organ comprise the vomeronasal glands, which function to fill the organ with fluid.

The function of the vomeronasal organ is carried out by the sensory chemoreceptors. They can detect specific chemical compounds, including pheromones. As the information that is picked up by the vomeronasal organ is sent to the accessory olfactory bulb and then the hypothalamus, as opposed to the olfactory bulb and then the cerebral cortex; this may explain why some specific chemical compounds within scents may induce aggressive or mating behavior. It can also be used in kin recognition (e.g., lambs by their dam).

CHECK YOUR UNDERSTANDING

- What is the function of nasal conchae?
- What are the major functions of the nasal cavity?
- What is the function of the vomeronasal organ?

VETERINARY APPLICATION

Feline upper respiratory infection (URI) is the common term for a respiratory infection caused by viral or bacterial agents. The most common viruses that cause upper respiratory infections in cats are feline herpesvirus *type 1* (also known as feline viral rhinotracheitis or FVR) and feline calicivirus (FCV). Herpesvirus and calicivirus are responsible for approximately 90 percent of all feline URIs. The typical URI involves the nose and throat, causing symptoms such as sneezing, nasal congestion, conjunctivitis, and discharges from the nose or eyes. The discharges may be clear or purulent (cloudy containing pus). A cat may develop ulcers in the mouth. In severe cases, the cat may have difficulty breathing. Usually, a URI in cats lasts seven to ten days.

A URI in cats is highly contagious. An infected cat will shed contagious particles in saliva or secretions from the nose or eyes. Susceptible cats can get an infection by direct contact with another infected cat or by environmental exposure to objects that have been contaminated with infectious secretions such as food and water bowls, litter boxes, toys, and bedding. Usually, a cat gets an infection by direct contact since the viruses and bacteria can only survive for a short period of time in the environment, and they are readily destroyed by proper disinfection procedures. It is estimated that herpesvirus can survive less than 18 hours outside the host's body, while calicivirus may live up to ten days. Dilute bleach solution will destroy both viruses, but calicivirus will withstand washing with bleach-free laundry detergents. An incubation period is 2 to 10 days before developing symptoms. The disease typically lasts 7 to 21 days, depending on the particular agent, with 7 to 10 days being the average duration of illness.

A cat that catches FVR (herpesvirus) becomes a chronic carrier. In some cats that carry FVR, stress (surgery, other illnesses, age, boarding, etc.) may cause virus reactivation. With calicivirus, about half of the cats that are infected will become carriers of disease. In some of these cats, the carrier state may only last for a few months, but in a small percentage of cats the carrier state may persist for life. These persistent carriers are usually free of symptoms but serve as a constant source of virus to susceptible cats.

Pharynx

The **pharynx** (plural: **pharynges**) is the part of the throat behind the mouth and nasal cavity and above the esophagus and larynx. In mammals and birds, the pharynx is part of both the digestive and respiratory systems. The pharynx lies immediately behind the nasal cavity. It is conventionally divided into three sections: the nasopharynx, oropharynx, and laryngopharynx.

The nasopharynx encloses the space between the internal nares and the soft palate, and lies above the oral cavity. The adenoids, also known as the pharyngeal tonsils, are lymphoid tissue structures located in the dorsal wall of the nasopharynx. Waldever's tonsillar ring is an annular arrangement of lymphoid tissue in both the nasopharynx and oropharynx. The nasopharynx is lined by respiratory epithelium. The auditory tube connects the middle ear to the pharynx. It opens into the nasopharynx at the pharyngeal opening of the auditory tube. The opening and closing of the auditory tube equalize the air pressure between the middle ear and atmosphere.

CHECK YOUR UNDERSTANDING

- What is the function of the pharynx?
- What is the role of the tonsillar ring?

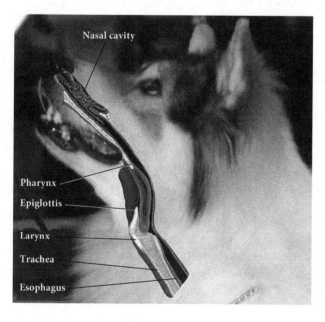

FIGURE 20.3   Dog Pharynx.

Oropharynx

The oropharynx lies behind the oral cavity, extending from the uvula to the level of the hyoid bone. Anteriorly, it opens into the mouth. The anterior wall consists of the base of the tongue. The lateral wall is made up of the tonsil, tonsillar fossa, and tonsillar pillars; the superior wall consists of the inferior surface of the soft palate and the uvula. Epiglottis closes over the glottis when food is swallowed to prevent aspiration. The oropharynx is lined by nonkeratinized squamous stratified epithelium (fig. 20.3).

Laryngopharynx

The laryngopharynx, also known as the **hypopharynx**, is the caudal part of the pharynx. Posteriorly, it opens into the esophagus. It lies inferior to the epiglottis and extends to the location where this common pathway diverges into the respiratory (larynx) and digestive (esophagus) pathways. The esophagus conducts food and fluids to the stomach; air enters the larynx anteriorly. During swallowing, food has the "right of way," and air passage is temporarily closed. The laryngopharynx includes three major sites: the pyriform sinus, postcricoid area, and the posterior pharyngeal wall. Like the oropharynx, the laryngopharynx serves as a passageway for food and air and is lined with a stratified squamous epithelium. It is innervated by the pharyngeal plexus. The vascular supply to the laryngopharynx includes the superior thyroid artery, the lingual artery, and the ascending pharyngeal artery. The primary neural supply is from both the vagus and glossopharyngeal nerves. These nerves are responsible for the ear-cough reflex in which stimulation of the ear canal causes coughing.

CHECK YOUR UNDERSTANDING

- Which tissues line three areas of the pharynx?

- Which nerves serve to trigger the swallowing and coughing reflexes?

Larynx

From the laryngopharynx, inhaled air moves into the **larynx**. This short tube lies anterior to the esophagus and extends from about the third to the sixth cervical vertebra. The larynx keeps food and liquids out of the rest of the respiratory tract and, as its common name implies, it houses the vocal cords, which are involved in sound production.

Superior to the vocal cords, the larynx is lined with a stratified squamous nonkeratinized epithelium that is continuous with that of the laryngopharynx. This prevents the larynx surface from abrasion due to contact with food. Inferior to the vocal cords, the epithelium changes to a pseudostratified ciliated columnar epithelium, which also presents in the nasal cavity and the nasopharynx. Because this epithelium is tightly associated with the respiratory tubular organs, it is also called the **respiratory epithelium**. The cilia in the larynx propel mucus and debris upward and out.

The flexible framework for the larynx is made of nine pieces of cartilage. The cartilage framework is supported by muscles that attach larynx to other structures of the neck and by muscles within the larynx itself. The three largest cartilages are unpaired, whereas the other six occur as three pairs of smaller cartilages.

The three unpaired cartilages are the **thyroid cartilage**, the **epiglottis**, and the **cricoid cartilage**. The thyroid cartilage is the largest piece of the larynx. It forms the anterior and superior walls and is attached superiorly to the hyoid bone and inferiorly to the cricoid cartilage by a fibrous membrane (fig. 20.4).

Posterior to the thyroid cartilage there is a spoon-shaped elastic cartilage called the **epiglottis**. The base of the epiglottis is attached to the posterior wall of the thyroid cartilage, and its superior edge stands above the larynx. Normally, the epiglottis's superior edge stands upright to allow air to enter the larynx via an opening called **glottis**. During swallowing, the larynx is elevated by surrounding muscles, so that the epiglottis covers the glottis, preventing food and liquids from entering the larynx. The tongue also pushes the epiglottis down during swallowing, helping to keep the larynx sealed off. The third piece of unpaired cartilage is the cricoid cartilage. It is located inferior to the thyroid cartilage with which it is bound by the **cricothyroid ligament** (fig. 20.5).

The three pairs of cartilages in the larynx are:

1. **Arytenoid cartilages** are triangular structures involved in sound production. They are attached to the **vocal folds** and the intrinsic muscles of the larynx.

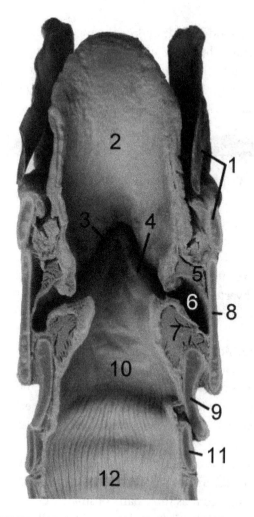

FIGURE 20.4   Larynx of a Horse. 1. Hyoid Bone; 2. Epiglottis; 3. Vestibular Fold (False Vocal Fold/Cord—Plica Vestibularis); 4. Vocal Fold (True Volcal Cord—Plica Vocalis); 5. Musculus Ventricularis; 6. Ventricle of Larynx (Ventriculus Laryngis); 7. Musculus Vocalis; 8. Thyroid Cartilage; 9. Cricoid Cartilage; 10. Cavum Infraglotticum; 11. First Cartilage Ring of Trachea; 12. Trachea.

2. **Corniculate cartilages** are small cap-shaped cartilages. These cartilages are also associated with vocal folds.
3. **Cuneiform cartilages** are located in the lateral wall of the larynx. They support the epiglottis.

The thyroid, the cricoid, and most parts of the arytenoid cartilages are made of hyaline cartilage. The epiglottis, corniculate, and cuneiform cartilages consist of elastic cartilage. The larynx is lined by mucosa which forms folds projected inside the lumen. These folds anteriorly are attached to the thyroid cartilage and posteriorly to the arytenoid cartilage. The superior pair of folds, termed **vestibular folds**. The opening between the vestibular folds is called the **rima vestibuli**. The second folds are called **true vocal cords**. At the core of these folds there are bands of elastic tissue called **vocal ligaments**. These cords got their name in recognition of the fact that they can vibrate and produce sound when air passes through them. Vocal cords are avascular and because of that have a distinctive white color. The opening between folds is called the **rima glottis**. The rima glottis and vocal cords together form the **glottis** (fig. 20.6).

Skeletal muscles compose part of the larynx wall and are classified as either extrinsic or intrinsic muscles. The **extrinsic muscles** attach to the thyroid cartilage on one end and extend either superiorly to the hyoid bone or inferiorly to the sternum. These muscles elevate the larynx during swallowing. The **intrinsic muscles** are located within the larynx and attach to arytenoid and corniculate cartilages. Contraction of these muscles causes pivot of the arytenoid cartilages. Rotating arytenoid cartilages pull on the vocal cords and change the size of the rima glottis, make it more or less open. This maneuver functions in two ways: it closes the larynx during swallowing (evolutionarily, it is probably a primary function of this structure) and participates in sound production. The air passing through the rima glottis causes vibration of the vocal cords. In horses, the two plates of the thyroid cartilage are fused incompletely, forming a rostral notch, which is a good site for surgical entry into the larynx. The **thyroarytenoid muscle** is divided into two parts. the **rostral** and **caudal vocalis**, which are situated within the vocal folds and vestibular folds. The **cuneiform processes** are attached to the epiglottis.

Dogs also have the **thyroarytenoid muscle** divided into two parts, and the **rostral** and **caudal vocal cords**, which are situated within the vocal folds and vestibular folds. Feline species have thick vocal folds. Purring occurs due to vibration of the vocal folds (and of the diaphragm) by rapid twitching of the laryngeal muscles. They have very sensitive mucosa, making intubation tricky. The **thyroid cartilage** in ruminants is completely ventral. It has a narrow rima glottis, which makes intubation difficult. The larynx is close to the median **retropharyngeal lymph node**, so enlargement of the lymph nodes may compress the larynx as well as the pharynx (fig. 20.6).

There are no vocal folds in avian species. Birds produce sound in the syrinx (fig. 20.7). The larynx is on the hyoid apparatus. There are paired arytenoids, one constrictor and one dilator muscle only. Birds have no epiglottis. The syrinx is located at the caudal end of the trachea, at the beginning of the primary bronchi and is surrounded by an air sac. Tracheal cartilages of the syrinx are complete and sturdy, whereas bronchial cartilages are incomplete. The syrinx is

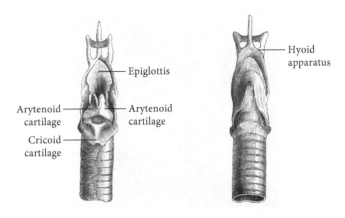

FIGURE 20.5   Horse Larynx.

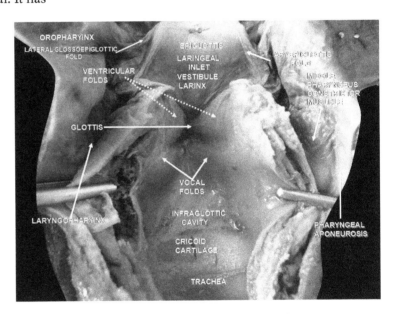

FIGURE 20.6   Human Vestibular and Vocal Cords.

composed of ossified cartilages, vibrating membranes, and muscles. A paired **sternotrachealis muscle** pulls the trachea towards the syrinx. The shape and size of the syrinx varies between species. The lateral and medial walls of the primary bronchi are membranous and flutter, which produces sound on expiration. An increased pressure in the clavicular air sac causes the tympanic membrane of the syrinx to be forced into the lumen and vibrate. Tension of the membranes is controlled by the **tracheolateral muscles**. Each half of the syrinx can function independently, allowing two different notes to be produced at the same time. **Drakes and cobs** (male swans) have an enlarged osseous bulla on the left side of the syrinx which acts as a resonator. **Songbirds** have a complex set of syringeal muscles. Sexual dimorphism occurs in songbirds, with the males of the species usually producing a more complex birdsong, which directly relates

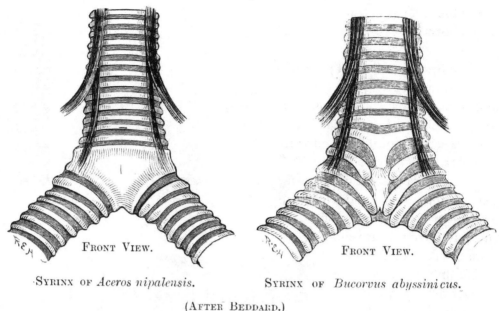

FRONT VIEW.

SYRINX OF *Aceros nipalensis.*

FRONT VIEW.

SYRINX OF *Bucorvus abyssinicus.*

(AFTER BEDDARD.)

FIGURE 20.7   Syrinx.

to the size of the area of the brain responsible for song. **Parrots** have a thick tongue which allows them to make sounds similar to humans. Sound travels from the syrinx and is modified in the throat, tongue, and mouth in parrots.

CHECK YOUR UNDERSTANDING

- What are the three unpaired cartilages in the larynx?

- What are the differences between the vocal and vestibular folds?

- What is the difference between sounds' production in mammals and birds?

Trachea

The trachea is an open (patent) tube between the larynx and bronchi. It is located in the mediastinum of the thoracic cavity. The ventral and lateral walls of the trachea are supported by C-shaped rings of hyaline cartilage called **tracheal cartilages** (fig. 20.8). Tracheal cartilages are connected each other by sheets of elastic connective tissue called **anular ligaments**. The dorsal ends of tracheal cartilage rings are open and connected by the **trachealis muscles** and elastic ligamentous membrane. The C-shape of tracheal cartilages guarantee that trachea will remain open at all time. The trachealis muscles adjust tracheal airflow to the organism's needs. Their contraction and relaxation control the diameter of the trachea and

Anatomy of the Trachea

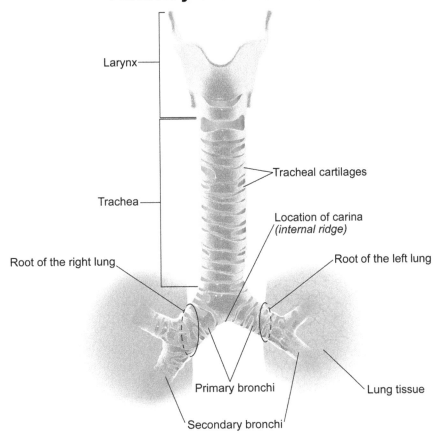

Larynx

Tracheal cartilages

Trachea

Location of carina
(internal ridge)

Root of the right lung

Root of the left lung

Primary bronchi

Lung tissue

Secondary bronchi

FIGURE 20.8   Trachea General View.

affect lung ventilation. Ability to distend the trachea's diameter is also very important for movement of a big bolus along the esophagus, when an animal swallows a substantial chunk of food. Fast contraction of trachealis muscles leading to rapid reduction of the tracheal diameter causes coughing and expulsion of air and material dislodged in the respiratory passages.

An internal ridge of mucosa-covered cartilage called the **carina** is located at the area where the trachea splits into two main (primary) bronchi. The carina has sensory receptors that are sensitive to touch with foreign materials and able to induce a forceful cough.

Walls of the trachea are made of 1) mucosa, which is composed of a pseudostratified ciliated columnar epithelium with goblet cells and lamina propria; 2) submucosa with large blood vessels, nerve endings, serous, mucous glands, and lymphatic tissue; 3) tracheal cartilage; and 4) the adventitia, composed of elastic connective tissue. The movement of cilia in the mucosal epithelium propels mucus laden with dust,

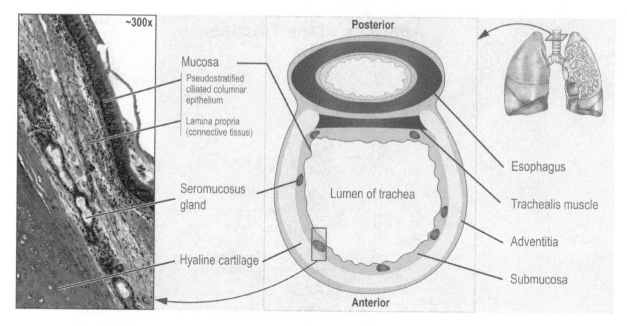

FIGURE 20.9   Cross Section through Trachea.

microbes, and other particles toward the larynx and pharynx, where it may be swallowed into the stomach and digested or expelled out of the respiratory passage (fig. 20.9).

CHECK YOUR UNDERSTANDING

- What is the function of the C-shaped tracheal cartilages?

- What is the function of trachealis muscles and elastic ligaments that complete each tracheal cartilage ring posteriorly?

- What is the function of the carina?

Bronchial Tree

The **bronchial tree** is a highly branched system of air-conducting passages that originates at the main bronchi and progressively branches into narrower tubes that diverge throughout the lungs before ending in the **alveoli**. The trachea bifurcates at the levels of the fourth to sixth intercostal space, approximately halfway between the thoracic inlet and the diaphragm. It divides into two **principle bronchi**, also called **main** or **primary bronchi**—tubes that conduct air into the lungs. The right main bronchus is shorter, wider, and branches at almost a right angle to the trachea. The left main bronchus is longer and separates from the trachea at other than right angle. That is why the right bronchus more often is lodged with foreign particles and prone to infection. The main bronchus, together with pulmonary blood vessels, lymph vessels, and nerves, enters the lung via an opening at the medial surface of lung's capsule called the **hilum**.

Each main bronchus branches into **lobar** or **secondary bronchi**. Each lobar bronchus is associated only with one lobe of the lung. Because the left and right lungs have a different number of lobes, there are also a different number of lobar bronchi on the left and right sides. Humans have three lobar bronchioles on the right side and only two on the left; dogs have four right lobar bronchi and two left bronchi. Lobar bronchi have a smaller diameter than main bronchi. They further divide into **segmental bronchi** that serve a division of the lung called a **bronchopulmonary segment**. The bronchial tree continues to divide into numerous smaller bronchi. The bronchial tree ends by small **bronchioles**, which are ended by **terminal bronchioles**. Terminal bronchioles are the last segments of the conducting zone. They lead into **respiratory bronchioles**, the first elements of the respiratory zone.

The bronchi and bronchioles are part of the **conduction zone** of the respiratory system, allowing the passage of air from the external environment into the lungs where gaseous exchange can take place. Some of the bronchioles have alveoli scattered along their length, and thus form part of the **respiratory zone**, the site for gaseous exchange. Between species the diameter of the bronchi and bronchioles vary greatly and more significantly than the variations in trachea. The number of bronchial tree divisions also varies by species—small mammals such as mice may have only 4 or 5 generations, whereas large animals may have 12 or more generations.

The histology of the **bronchi** is similar to that of the trachea. The lumen of the bronchus is lined by a pseudostratified epithelium, including goblet cells, and serous cells. Beneath the narrow layer of connective tissue under the epithelium lie well-developed spiral bands of smooth muscle. Thus, bronchi, like a trachea, are able to trap airborne microorganisms into the mucus coverage and then remove them through the rhythmic beating of the cilia.

The bronchioles have no cartilage rings but have well developed muscular walls to enclose the lumen. The epithelium is reduced to cuboidal that has no cilia on the free cell surface. Normally, the bronchiole lining has no goblet cells or mucus-secreting glands; but it has numerous lymphoid nodules beneath the epithelial layer. These monitor incoming air on the presence foreign particles and pathogens. The cuboidal epithelium has no cilia or mucus-producing cells, and all responsibility for cleaning incoming air of airborne pathogens relies on lymphatic tissues.

The **respiratory bronchioles** have few alveoli scattered along the length. The entrance into the alveoli is guarded by a simple squamous epithelium and bundles of smooth muscles. Smooth muscles control alveoli ventilation and simple squamous epithelium allows gases to diffuse between airflow and blood flow (fig. 20.10).

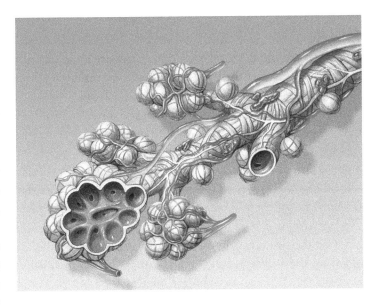

FIGURE 20.10   Bronchial Tree and Alveoli.

CHECK YOUR UNDERSTANDING

- What are the structural differences between bronchi and bronchioles?

- Which are the last segments of the conduction zone, and which are the first structures of the respiratory zone?

- What are the structures in bronchioles that protect an organism from airborne infection?

Lungs

The lungs are the site for gas exchange and are situated within the thoracic cavity. They occupy approximately 5 percent of the body's volume in mammals when relaxed, and their elastic nature allows them to expand and contract during the inhalation and exhalation.

Evolutionarily, the lungs are homologs to the fish **swim bladder**, an internal gas-filled organ that contributes to the ability of most bony fish to control their buoyancy. Together with the larynx and trachea, lungs develop from ventral pockets of the esophagus. This process is not completed at the time of parturition, and the lungs of a fetus are not functional. The left and right lungs lie within their pleural sac and are only attached by their roots, to the mediastinum, so they are fairly free within the thoracic cavity. The right lung is always larger than the left, due to the position of the heart. The apex of the lungs is their cranial point.

Each lung is placed within a separate layer of membrane, thus there are two pleural sacs. The space between the two sacs is known as the mediastinum, and is almost in the midline of the thorax. The pleura covering the surface of the lung is known as the **pulmonary pleura** or **visceral pleura**. This becomes continuous with the **mediastinal pleura**, as it wraps around the lung. The **diaphragmatic and costal pleura** are continuous with the mediastinal pleura. Together, these three membranes form the **parietal pleura** (fig. 20.11).

Between the parietal and visceral pleura is the **intrapleural space**, or **pleural cavity**. The cavity contains a small amount of serous fluid. Watery serous fluid generates adhesion, through the water molecules' surface tension, between the membranous fold and holds them firmly, allowing smooth movement between the lung and chest wall, and between individual lobes of the lungs. Thus, the pleural membrane guarantees coordinated movements of the lungs and the walls of the thoracic cavity during the respiratory cycle. Pulled by a surface-tension force between the parietal and visceral pleura, the lungs passively follow the movements of the diaphragm and ribs. The left and right pleural sacs are not connected, and injury (for example, puncture) of one pleural membrane does not affect the functioning of the other.

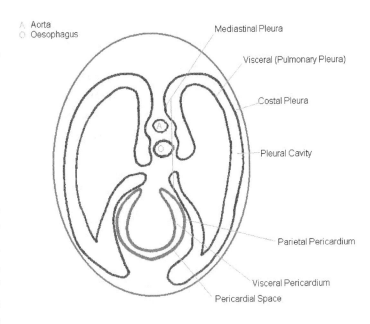

FIGURE 20.11   Schema of Pleural Membranes.

The **pericardial space**, containing the heart, separates the two membranes. Cranially, the costal and mediastinal pleura adjoin to form a "dome" of pleura which extends to the thoracic inlet. This is known as the **cupulae pleurae**. This region is only protected by soft tissue and, thus, is vulnerable to injury. Within the pleural sac encasing the right lung, there is a fold which encases the vena cava. It is known as the **plica venae cavae**.

Blood supply to the pleural membranes is provided by the **bronchial** and **pulmonary arteries**. The parietal pleura is innervated by the intercostal nerves, with the mediastinal and diaphragmatic pleura also innervated by the phrenic nerve. The visceral pleura is innervated by the vagus nerve and sympathetic fibers. It is insensitive to pain stimuli.

In **cattle**, the mediastinum is a tough membrane, in contrast to **horses**, **dogs**, and **cats**, where it is thin and delicate. **Birds** do not have a pleural cavity as avian lungs do not have the capacity to inflate.

In most mammals, the lungs are divided into lobes by the bronchial tree: 1) the **left lung** is divided into the **cranial** and **caudal lobes**; and 2) the **right lung** is partitioned into the **cranial**, **caudal**, **middle**, and **accessory** lobes. The cranial lobe is further divided by an external fissure (fig. 20.12).

The bulk of the lungs consists of bronchi, blood vessels, and connective tissue. The terminal bronchioles have alveoli scattered along their length and are continued by alveolar ducts, alveolar sacs, and finally alveoli. Openings to individual alveoli are guarded by smooth muscle. These are rotunda-like areas on the end of each alveolar ducts which are usually organized in clusters.

Alveoli are minute, polygonal chambers, whose diameter changes with the inspiration and expiration and varies by species. The wall of the alveoli is extremely thin, consisting of two irregular layers of epithelial sheets, "sandwiching" a network of capillaries. Thus, the blood-gas barrier at the

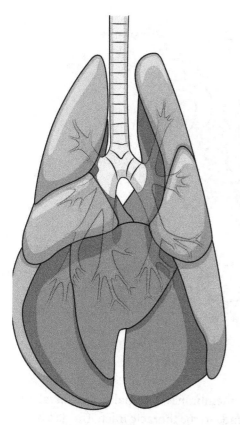

FIGURE 20.12   Inflated Left Dog Lung.

thinnest portions is a tripartite structure consisting of the pulmonary capillary endothelium, a common basal lamina and the alveolar epithelium. This structure is ideal for gas exchange. The alveolar interstitial space is filled with connective tissue fibers and cells, which include collagen and elastin fibers.

Respiratory bronchioles typically are composed of a simple cuboidal epithelium, whereas both the alveolar ducts and alveoli are composed of a simple squamous epithelium. Alveoli are tightly attached and press each other. The optimal configuration of tightly packed soft bubbles resembles a hexagonal tiling of the plane. Thus, alveolus in cross section actually looks more like bees' honeycombs than circular. Small openings in the alveoli walls, called **alveolar pores**, occur between some adjacent alveoli. These openings provide a collateral ventilation of alveoli. Pulmonary capillaries surround each alveolus to facilitate gas exchange between the alveolus and blood within the pulmonary capillaries. The **intraventricular septum** contains elastic fibers that contribute to the ability of the lungs to stretch during inspiration and recoil during expiration.

The cells in alveoli are called **pneumocytes**. There are two types of pneumocytes:

1. **Type I** pneumocytes are simple squamous epithelium cells with a flattened central nucleus that protrudes into the alveolar lumen. These cells constitute about 95 percent of the alveolar surface. These simple squamous cells are the primary cells that form **alveolar epithelium** of the respiratory membrane.
2. **Type II** pneumocytes, or **septal cells**, are round to pyramidal-shaped cells found among the type I pneumocytes. They have a larger centrally placed nucleus with a prominent nucleolus and a slightly vacuolated, foamy, basophilic cytoplasm. Septal cells secrete an oily fluid called **pulmonary surfactant**. This fluid prevents an alveoli collapse.

Alveoli are moist inside. Their surface tension is high. It makes alveoli prone to collapse and to stay collapsed. Surfactant secreted by alveolar type II cells coats the inner alveolar surface. When an alveolus is going to collapse, which occurs with each expiration, the pulmonary surfactant molecules become more tightly packed together and collectively tend to oppose the collapse of the alveolus.

There is a third type of cells in the alveoli—**alveolar macrophages**, also called **dust cells**. They are leukocytes that can have a fixed location or wonder within alveolus. Both types survey lungs for presence of pathogens and engulf microorganisms and organic contaminants inside the alveoli (fig. 20.13).

The thin barrier that oxygen and carbon dioxide have to trespass is called the **respiratory membrane**. It consists of two cellular layers of simple squamous epithelial cells and basement membrane between them.

This layer on the alveolar side is created by the type I pneumocytes and endothelial cells on the capillary side. Oxygen diffuses from the alveolus across the respiratory membrane into the pulmonary capillary blood. Carbon dioxide diffuses from the blood within the pulmonary capillary into alveoli (fig. 20.14).

The main function of lungs is gas exchange. The **pulmonary arteries** follow the bronchi, while the **pulmonary veins** sometimes run separately. **Bronchial arteries** from the aorta supply the bronchi, and **bronchial veins** may drain this blood to the right atrium via the **azygous vein**. More often the blood from the bronchi drains directly to the left atrium.

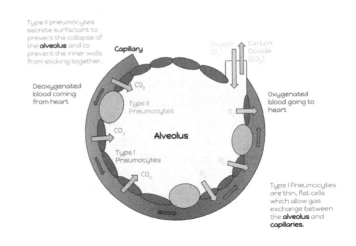

FIGURE 20.13   Alveolus.

The **pulmonary plexus** within the mediastinum supplies lungs with nerves. The pulmonary plexus consists of sympathetic fibers largely from the **stellate ganglion**, and parasympathetic fibers from the vagus nerve. Lymph drains to the **tracheobronchial** and **mediastinal** lymph nodes.

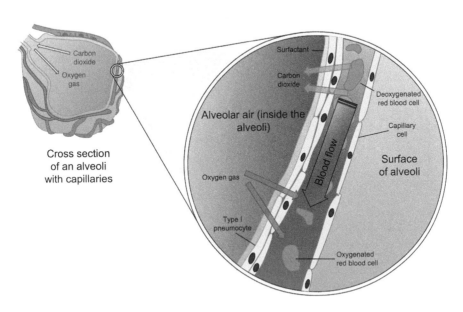

FIGURE 20.14   Respiratory Membrane and Gas Diffusion.

The lungs of a horse have no lobes. In comparison to this, the lungs of ruminants and pigs are obviously lobed. The fissures between the lobes (**interlobar fissures**) are deeper in the dog and cat lung compared to other species.

The diaphragm is a dome-shaped musculotendinous sheet separating the thoracic and abdominal cavities. It is convex on its cranial surface. In the neutral position between full inspiration and full expiration, the most cranial part of the diaphragm is in line with the sixth rib. The muscular part of the diaphragm is peripheral, surrounding the central tendinous area. The muscular part has sections which arise from the xiphoid process of the sternum, vertebral column and caudal ribs.

The diaphragm has three openings (fig. 20.15):

1. **Aortic hiatus** is the most dorsal opening; it contains the aorta, azygous vein, and thoracic duct.
2. **Esophageal hiatus** contains the esophagus, dorsal, and ventral vagal trunks.
3. **Caval foramen** lies within the central tendinous region of the diaphragm and contains the caudal vena cava. This opening does not allow movement. Here the diaphragm is fused with the vena cava wall.

During inspiration, the diaphragm contracts and increases the volume of the thoracic cavity. It causes the decrease of thoracic pressure that pulls air in. The diaphragm relaxation leads to elastic recoil and

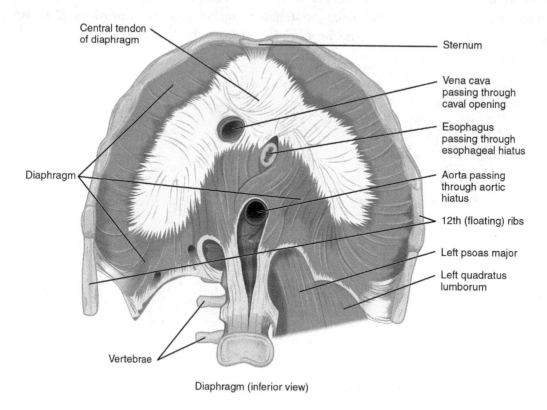

Diaphragm (inferior view)

FIGURE 20.15   Diaphragm, Caudal View.

expelling air from lungs. The **phrenic nerve** that springs from the cervical plexus regulates rhythm and strength of diaphragm contractions.

Because of the shorter thorax, the diaphragm is steeper in the **ruminant** compared to the **horse**. **Avian** species do not possess a diaphragm. Air moves in and out of their lungs via air sacs.

CHECK YOUR UNDERSTANDING

- What structures make up the respiratory membrane?

- What is the function of serous fluid 1) within the pleural cavity, and 2) within alveoli?

- What prevents alveoli from collapsing at the end of exhalation?

- Why is the pressure in the pleural cavity normally lower than the pressure in the lungs? What is the function of this difference in pressure?

20.2   Physiology of Respiration

Pulmonary Ventilation

Respiration is a general term for the exchange of respiratory gases (oxygen and carbon dioxide) between the atmosphere and the systemic cells of the body. It is organized into four continuous and simultaneously occurring processes:

1. **Pulmonary ventilation** is a movement of respiratory gases between the atmosphere and the alveoli of the lungs.
2. **Alveolar gas exchange** (also known as an **external respiration**) is an exchange of respiratory gases between the alveoli and the blood in the pulmonary capillaries.
3. **Gas transportation** is a transport of respiratory gases within the blood between the lungs and systemic cells of the body.
4. **Systemic gas exchange** (also known as an **internal respiration**) is an exchange of respiratory gases between the blood in the systemic capillaries and systemic cells of the body.

The respiration events are organized in eight steps:

1. Air containing oxygen is inhaled into the alveoli during the inspiratory phase of pulmonary ventilation.
2. Oxygen diffuses from alveoli into the blood in pulmonary capillaries during alveolar gas exchange.
3. Oxygen is transported within the blood from the lungs to systemic cells of the body.
4. Oxygen diffuses from the blood within systemic capillaries into the systemic cells during systemic gas exchange.
5. Carbon dioxide diffuses from systemic cells into the blood within systemic capillaries during systemic gas exchange.
6. Carbon dioxide is transported within blood to the lungs.

7. Carbon dioxide diffuses from the blood within the pulmonary capillaries into the alveoli during alveolar gas exchange.
8. Air containing carbon dioxide is then exhaled from the alveoli into the atmosphere during the expiratory phase of pulmonary ventilation.

Pulmonary ventilation is a movement of air into and out of the lungs. Air moves from high pressure to low pressure with the rate of flow being proportional to the pressure difference. As environmental pressure is generally constant, the respiratory system must change its internal pressure to maintain airflow. The lungs are not fixed to the thoracic wall, but follow the movements of the thoracic cavity hold in tight touch by the surface tension of serous fluid covered pleural cavity. Pulmonary ventilation has two phases: **inspiration**, or inhalation of the outside air into the lungs, and **expiration**, or exhalation that expels air from the lungs.

Air is a complex mixture of gases and water molecules. The movement of these molecules follows the basic physical principle of pressure gradient. The gas pressure in lungs varies with change of the total size of the lungs or with change of the temperature of the gas. The variation of the gas pressure by changing the volume of the container is described by **Boyle's law**. The law states that at the constant temperature and constant number of gas molecules, the pressure and volume of a gas are related inversely. The increase of the container's volume causes a decrease of the gas pressure, and vice versa. Robert Boyle formulated this law in the 17th century in a simple formula: $P_1 V_1 = P_2 V_2$, where P is a gas pressure and V is its volume. The dependence of gas pressure on the temperature is described by **Charles's law**. It was discovered by Jacques Charles in 1787. The law states that, for a given mass of an ideal gas at constant pressure, the volume is directly proportional to its absolute temperature: $V = kT$, where T is an absolute temperature of the gas and k is a non-zero constant. Gay-Lussac combined Boyle's and Charles's laws and created the generalized gas law. He concluded that there is a constant relationship among gas pressure, temperature, and volume: $PV/T = \text{constant}$.

The pulmonary ventilation in reptiles, mammals, and birds is based on Boyle's law, and involves volume changes in the thoracic cavity and lungs that generates development of pressure gradient between external air and that inside the lungs. This gradient, in turn, causes air to move into or out of the lungs. During inspiration, the pressure within the pleural cavity drops below that outside of the body. This is achieved by increasing the lung volume by the inspiratory muscles. The diaphragm contracts, causing the dome to flatten and move caudally. The external intercostal muscles contract and pull the ribs causing their rotation and movement of the medial sternum forward. Because the ribs are bow shaped, this rotation results in outward cranial expansion of the thoracic cage around lungs. Together, these maneuvers increase total volume and the air pressure inside lungs drops. This mechanism of lung ventilation is called **negative ventilation**. It is negative because the air is pushed inside the lungs by creation of lower-than-outside pressure. A set of anatomic structures that generate low air pressure inside lungs is called **aspiration pump**. The lungs are located within the pump so that the force required to ventilate them is applied directly. This pump consists of rib cage and a diaphragm. The diaphragm, like a plunger, alters the pressure on the lungs to favor entry or exit of air. Intercostal muscles between ribs, the transverse abdominis muscles, serratus, and rectus abdominis aid in lung ventilation.

During expiration, the pressure within the pleural cavity increases to greater than that of the external environment, in order to expel air from the lungs. This is achieved by decreasing the lung volume, and is brought about by relaxation of inspiratory muscles. The dome of the diaphragm is pushed back by the intrathoracic pressure and the ribs recoil back to their original position.

During active exhalation, internal intercostal muscles slant in the opposite direction of the relaxed external intercostals and pull the ribs back. Relaxation of the diaphragm causes it to recoil and resume its arched, dome shape. Rib retraction and diaphragm relaxation decrease chest volume, forcing air from lungs. Elastic energy stored in the lungs and gravity acting to fold or collapse the rib cage may aid exhalation.

During quiet breathing, only inhalator muscles are at work. At such times, exhalation muscles may not contract, and compression of the rib cage results from elastic recoil and gravitational forces only. There also is a coupling of breath cycles with body movement cycles so that both are synchronized. When the animal is at rest, the diaphragm is the principal component in mammalian lung ventilation. During locomotion the rib cage may receive ground reaction forces through the forelimbs that slightly change its shape. The abdominal viscera at that time is free to move within the body cavity and slide forward and backward in synchrony with the rhythm of the limbs' oscillation. In this situation, the abdominal viscera act as a piston: first pressing anteriorly on the lungs and then moving posteriorly and decreasing pressure in the thoracic cage. A running mammal takes advantage of this rhythmic movements of the viscera, expelling air when the viscera press against the thorax and inhaling when they move posteriorly.

CHECK YOUR UNDERSTANDING

- What forces drive the movement of gases during breathing?

- What structures constitute the respiratory pump?

Factors That Influence Pulmonary Ventilation

Three factors have a strong impact on pulmonary ventilation: resistance of airways to airflow, alveolar surface tension, and pulmonary compliance.

Airway resistance is a cumulative effect of different factors that oppose to airflow. It is defined as the ratio of driving pressure to the rate of airflow: $R = \Delta P/V$, where R is resistance, ΔP is an air pressure gradient, and V is a rate of airflow. Resistance to flow in the airways depends on whether the flow is laminar or turbulent, on the diameter and length of the airway, and on the viscosity of the gas. Thus, varying these factors, an organism may change airway resistance and by that the rate of pulmonary ventilation.

The most variable and easily controlled way to adjust airway resistance is to alter the pressure gradient. Aspiration pump may increase or decrease number of muscles that participate in drawing air into the lungs and strength of their contraction. It alters the total volume of thoracic cage during inhalation and exhalation, and the gradient of air pressure between lungs and air outside of the body. Neural and hormonal control over contraction of the aspiratory pump have a principal role in this process. Body motion is also very important. Walking, running, and especially jumping may significantly affect pressure gradient. As a rule, airway resistance dramatically decreases during running or jumping.

The diameter of the airways is controlled by the smooth muscles of the trachea, bronchi, and bronchioles. Constriction of the smooth muscles in bronchi and bronchioles is called **bronchoconstriction** and their relaxation is **bronchodilation**. The bronchodilation increases diameter of the bronchioles and lows airway resistance. The sympathetic motor neurons release norepinephrine that causes smooth muscles in bronchioles to relax. Stress reaction leads to release a significant amount of norepinephrine and epinephrine from adrenal glands. It also decreases resistance to airflow. Irritants and some pollutants in the air can trigger bronchoconstriction and decrease airflow to lungs through the parasympathetic nervous system.

The **alveolar surface tension** is a strength with which molecules in surface film of a liquid attract each other. This attraction holds molecules together and minimizes surface area. Water is a polar covalent molecule (see chapter 2, page 33). The presence of oppositely charged atoms in water molecule results in attraction between positive hydrogens and negative oxygen and formation of weak chemical bonds called hydrogen bonds. The cells of the alveoli are coated by a serous fluid film composed mostly of water. When alveoli surface decreases during exhalation, water molecules come closer and hydrogen bonds between them become stronger. The increase of hydrogen bonds' strength increases surface tension. If this process is not opposed, alveoli may collapse. The collapse of alveoli caused by the surface tension is known as **atelectasis**. Thus, surface tension in alveoli resists inflation of lungs and decreases pulmonary ventilation.

The complete collapse of lungs during exhalation is prevented by a **pulmonary surfactant**. Pulmonary surfactant is a lipoprotein complex formed by type II alveolar cells. The proteins and lipids that make up the surfactant have both hydrophilic and hydrophobic regions. By adsorbing to the air-water interface of alveoli, with hydrophilic head groups in the water and the hydrophobic tails facing towards the air. They disrupt hydrogen bonds between water molecules, reduce surface tension, and prevent collapse of alveoli.

The term **pulmonary compliance** refers to the ability of the lungs and the chest wall to stretch. The pulmonary compliance is determined by three main factors: 1) **alveolar surface tension**; 2) **distensibility of elastic tissue in the lungs**; 3) **ability of the chest wall to move**.

Factors that influence pulmonary compliance may dramatically change ventilation efficiency. Thus, decrease of a surfactant production results in increase of the alveolar surface tension and decrease their ability to inflate during inspiration. The set of bones in the sternum is connected by cartilages, which make the sternum moveable and increase the size of the thoracic cage for inhalation. With age, these cartilages tend to ossify and become rigid and immovable. This change results in a significant decrease of pulmonary compliance.

CHECK YOUR UNDERSTANDING

- What are the main factors that determine airway resistance?

- What creates surface tension?

- How does surfactant influence surface tension?

- What factors influence pulmonary compliance?

Pulmonary Volumes and Capacities

The state of the respiratory system is very important for the health of the organism. Measuring the volume of inhaled and exhaled air provide important information about the health of the respiratory organs and their ability adjust their activity to the organism's needs. These characteristics are species specific. Next respiratory volumes and capacities are of clinical primary interest:

1. **Respiratory rate (RR)** is the number of inhalation and exhalation cycles per minute.
2. **Tidal volume (TV)** is the amount of air inspired or expired during a quiet ventilation at rest.

3. **Minute volume** is the total volume of air inhaled or exhaled in a minute of quiet resting ventilation. This volume can be calculated by multiplying TV and RR: $\mathbf{MV = TV \times RR}$.

4. **Inspiratory reserve volume (IRV)** is the amount of air that can be forcefully inhaled on the top of the TV. This volume characterizes the ability of the respiratory system to adjust ventilation to meet the need of maximal body activity or stress.

5. **Expiratory reserve volume (ERV)** is the amount of air which an organism can forcefully exhale after a normal tidal expiration.

6. The **inspiratory pulmonary capacity** is the total amount of air that an organism can inhale with all its strength. It is a combination of TV and IRV: $\mathbf{IPC = TV + IRV}$.

7. **Vital capacity** is the total amount of air that an organism can exchange forcefully. It is the sum of TV, IRV, and ERV: $\mathbf{VC = TV + IRV + ERV}$.

8. The multiple measurements of respiratory volumes and capacities show that normally IRV always is larger than ERV in all mammals. This difference exists because even after the most forceful exhalation, some amount of the air remains in lungs. The volume of this remaining air is called **residual volume (RV)**. Residual air remains inside lungs due to the intrapleural pressure and outward recoil of the chest wall, which prevents lungs from collapsing.

9. **Total lung capacity** is the total amount of exchangeable and nonexchangeable air in the lungs. It is calculated as: $\mathbf{TLC = IRV + TV + ERX + RV}$ (fig. 20.16).

10. Respiratory windpipes only conduct airflow. Together they constitute the **conduction zone** of the respiratory system. The air in the conducting zone cannot exchange its gases with blood. The total

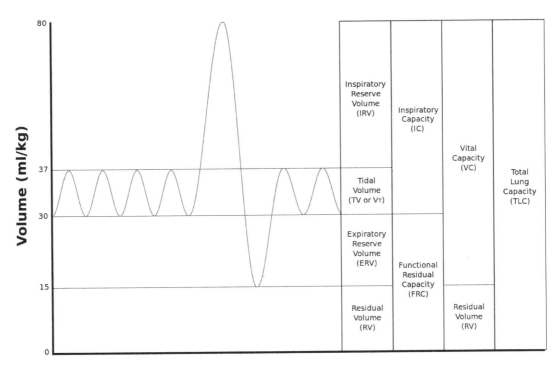

FIGURE 20.16   Pulmonary Volumes and Capacities.

volume of air in the conduction zone depends on the anatomy of the respiratory system, which suggests its name: **anatomic dead space**.

11. **Physiologic dead space** in a healthy organism is equal to the anatomic dead space. However, if pathologic process develops in the lungs, some alveoli continue to be ventilated, but gas exchange (perfusion) in them decreases or is absent. The total volume of alveoli where ventilation remains but perfusion is reduced is called **alveoli dead space**. Thus, physiologic dead space is the sum of anatomic and alveoli dead spaces: **PhDS = AnDS + AlDS**.

CHECK YOUR UNDERSTANDING

- What is a tidal volume?

- Why may vital capacity increase in a trained animal?

- What may cause physiological dead space to be larger than anatomic dead space?

20.3 Gas Exchange

Gas exchange proceeds in two steps: 1) **pulmonary** or **alveolar gas exchange**, and 2) **tissue gas exchange**. The first one takes place in the alveoli and consists of the movement of gases across the respiratory membrane: oxygen diffuses from alveolar space into the blood, whereas carbon dioxide diffuses in the opposite direction—from blood into the alveolar space. The second process consists of gas exchanges between blood flow and tissues of the body.

Air is a mixture of many different gases, including oxygen, nitrogen, carbon dioxide, vapored water, and others. Together, they create air pressure. All gases in the air contribute in formation of the air pressure. Their contribution is described by **Dalton's law of partial pressure**. The law states that each gas in a mixture of gases exerts its own pressure, called **partial pressure**, proportional to its percentage in gaseous mixture, so the total pressure of all gases is equal the sum of their partial pressures. The air usually contains 78 percent of nitrogen and 21 percent of oxygen, whereas carbon dioxide constitutes less than 1 percent. If the air pressure on the sea level varies around 760 mm Hg, then the partial pressure of oxygen is $P_{O2} = 760 \times 0.21 = 160$ mm Hg, and nitrogen is $P_{N2} = 760 \times 0.78 = 593$ mm Hg.

Gases move from a place where their concentration is high to areas where their concentration is lower. Because concentration of gases directly correlates with their partial pressure, one can state that **every gas moves from a place with high partial pressure to a place where its partial pressure is low**. The higher the gradient of partial pressure, the faster gas moves.

Alveoli are covered inside by a tiny film made of water and surfactant. To diffuse across the respiratory membrane, gases have to be dissolved in water. The ability of gas to dissolve in water is called **solubility**. The degree at which gases dissolve in water is described by **Henry's law**, which states that gas dissolves in water proportional of its partial pressure and its solubility. This law explains behavior of gases during the pulmonary gas exchange. For example, partial pressure of nitrogen in the air is high, but its solubility in water is very low. That is why there is much less nitrogen present in a blood then oxygen, which partial pressure much lower than nitrogen, but its solubility is significantly higher. Carbon dioxide has a very low partial pressure, compare with the previous two gases, but its solubility is much higher than other gases and it is always present in the blood in some amount.

CHECK YOUR UNDERSTANDING

- What two processes constitute gas exchange?

- What is gas partial pressure, and how does it relate to atmospheric pressure?

Alveolar Gas Exchange

During the alveolar gas exchange, oxygen diffuses from the air in alveoli, where its partial pressure is always higher, into the blood, and carbon dioxide diffuses in the opposite direction for the same reason. Blood comes to the lungs from the ventricle, which collects deoxygenated but carbon dioxide–rich blood that returns after traveling through the systemic circuit. The oxygen partial pressure in the deoxygenated blood varies around 40 mm Hg, whereas its partial pressure in the inhaled air is about 104 mm Hg. This gradient drives oxygen to the blood. It takes only about a quarter of a second for oxygen to reach equilibrium.

The partial pressure of carbon dioxide in blood is around 45 mm Hg and in exhaled air 40 mm Hg. The difference, compared with oxygen, is not so big, but because of the much higher solubility (CO_2 solubility is 20 times higher than that of O_2), it does not need high partial pressure gradient and diffuses very rapidly across the respiratory membrane.

Avian lungs are relatively compact, with a bird's lungs being approximately 50 percent as large as the lungs of a mammal of similar size. The lungs are unlobed and do not expand. Birds do not have a pleural cavity as the lungs do not expand, and thus the membranes are not necessary. One **primary bronchus** from the trachea enters each lung, narrowing as it travels through, and communicates with the **abdominal air sac**. This bronchus gives off branches as it travels through the lung, known as **secondary bronchi**. Each of these gives off a further 400 to 500 **parabronchi**, in the walls of which gaseous exchange takes place.

Birds have no diaphragm. Their thoracic and abdominal cavities are continuous. The bird has a number of thin walled, easily distensible **air sacs** which can extend to approximately ten times the volume of the lungs. They are present within body cavities, and extend inside some bones, where they replace bone marrow. This reduces the weight of the bone, as they become filled with air. The air sacs create unidirectional flow of air to maximize oxygen extraction and reduce heat production during flight. A chicken has eight air sacs: 1) the **cervical** sac extends within the cervical and thoracic vertebrae; 2) the **clavicular** sac lies within the thoracic inlet, surrounding the heart, and within the humerus in the forelimb; 3) two **cranial thoracic** sacs are located ventral to the lungs; 4) two **caudal thoracic** sacs are located between the body wall and the thoracic air sacs; and 5) two **abdominal** are the largest air sacs and fill the posterior-dorsal region of the abdomen near the small and large intestines, kidneys, and reproductive organs. In addition, these air sacs utilize space within the acetabulum and synsacrum.

The cervical, clavicular, and cranial thoracic air sacs form the **cranial functional group**. The caudal thoracic and abdominal air sacs form the **caudal functional group**. The air sacs have a vital role in ventilation, but do not have the capacity for gaseous exchange. Thus, they are a part of the avian conduction zone.

Ventilation in birds is strikingly different from that of mammals in that air flows through the lungs in the same direction during both inspiration and expiration. In addition, both inhalation and exhalation are active processes, requiring muscle contraction.

During **inspiration**, the ribs are drawn forwards and the sternum lowered, and the caudal air sacs receives fresh air. At the same time, the cranial air sacs receive air which was inhaled at the previous inhalation and now is expelled from the lungs. This air has lost much of its oxygen.

During **expiration**, the sternum is drawn caudal and dorsal. The air sacs are compressed. Air from the caudal air sac passes through the lungs, while the air in the cranial air sac is exhaled via the trachea. Thus, oxygenated air passes through the lungs two times: first time during inspiration and the second during expiration.

Avian gas exchange takes place not in alveoli, as in mammals, but within **air capillaries** which are extensions of the parabronchial lumen.

CHECK YOUR UNDERSTANDING

- What causes oxygen and carbon dioxide to move across the respiratory membrane?

- What structures are responsible for exchange of gases in birds?

Factors Affecting Pulmonary Gas Exchange

Three factors have a major impact on the rate of pulmonary gas exchange: 1) the size of the surface area of the respiratory membrane, 2) the thickness of the respiratory membrane, and 3) the degree of matching air and blood flows.

The surface area of the respiratory membrane has to be large enough that every erythrocyte in the capillaries associated with alveoli can get a contact with the respiratory surface. Factors that decrease the surface area of the respiratory membrane decrease the efficiency of pulmonary gas exchange. For example, the disease **emphysema** is characterized by destruction of the alveolar walls, which reduces the surface area of the respiratory membrane to as little as one-fifth of normal. This reduction results in severely impaired pulmonary gas exchange, leading to **hypoxemia**, or low blood oxygen level, and **hypercapnia**, or high blood carbon level.

Normally, the respiratory membrane is very thin, having only two squamous epithelial cells and a basement membrane between them. Anything that increases the thickness of the respiratory membrane, such as inflammation, increases the time needed for gas diffusion.

In effective respiration the amount of oxygen available for gas exchange in alveoli has to match the amount of blood able to pick up oxygen for transportation. This relationship is known as **ventilation-perfusion matching** or **coupling**. Ventilation matches perfusion via two mechanisms:

1. Changes in alveolar ventilation lead to changes in perfusion, so blood flow is directed to areas with the most oxygen. When an alveolus is insufficiently ventilated, the oxygen partial pressure (P_{O2}) of the air within that alveolus drops. The pulmonary arteriole serving that alveolus constricts and decreases blood flow. When the P_{O2} rises, the pulmonary arteriole dilates and increases blood flow.

Thus, low alveolar P_{O_2} causes pulmonary arterioles to constrict, and high alveolar P_{O_2} causes them to dilate. These responses by the arterioles redirect blood flow to the alveoli with the greatest P_{O_2}, maximizing the efficiency of pulmonary gas exchange.

2. Changes in the efficiency of perfusion lead to changes in the amount of ventilation, so airflow is directed to areas with the most blood flow. When the pulmonary capillaries bring blood with less carbon dioxide to the alveoli, lowering carbon dioxide partial pressure (P_{CO_2}), the bronchiole constricts. Conversely, when pulmonary capillaries bring more carbon dioxide to the alveoli, raising P_{CO_2}, the bronchioles dilate. Therefore, high arteriolar P_{CO_2} causes bronchioles to dilate, and low arteriolar P_{CO_2} causes them to constrict. These responses by the bronchioles allow the lungs to ventilate the areas that have the greatest blood flow, so that gas exchange takes place efficiently.

These two processes combine to ensure a close match of pulmonary ventilation and pulmonary capillary perfusion. Success of this coupling is represented by the **ventilation/perfusion (V/Q) ratio**. Ideally, the V/Q ratio has to be 1.0, but in all known mammals, from mice to giraffes, it is lower because of the effect of gravity on pulmonary blood flow.

CHECK YOUR UNDERSTANDING

- What is the relation between respiratory membrane surface area and gas exchange?

- What is the relation between respiratory membrane thickness and gas exchange?

- How does the alveoli perfusion influence gas exchange?

Tissue Gas Exchange

The exchange of oxygen and carbon dioxide between the blood and tissues is called **tissue gas exchange**. In tissue gas exchange, oxygen moves from the blood in the systemic capillaries into tissue. The main driving force of tissue gas exchange is a gas partial pressure gradient. The cells constantly consume oxygen in cellular respiration, and for this reason, the P_{O_2} in the tissues is always low, averaging about 40 mm Hg. P_{O_2} in the systemic capillaries is comparatively high, measuring about 100 mm Hg. Thus, the pressure gradient facilitates rapid exchange of oxygen between the capillaries and the tissues. The pressure gradient functions in the reverse direction for carbon dioxide. The tissues produce large quantities of carbon dioxide as a waste product of cellular respiration, so the P_{CO_2} in the tissues is relatively high, whereas P_{CO_2} in the blood is low. This pressure gradient, combined with carbon dioxide's high solubility in water, facilitates its rapid transport into systemic capillaries.

Factors Affecting Tissue Gas Exchange

Factors that influence gas exchange in tissues include:

1. **The surface area available for gas exchange.** Capillaries form web-like capillary beds. The capillary bed increases the surface area available for tissue gas exchange and makes the process more efficient.

2. **The distance over which diffusion must occur.** Gases move by diffusion, which is fairly slow process. Cells that are too distant from capillaries do not receive adequate oxygen and die.
3. **The perfusion of the tissue.** Tissue gas exchange is most efficient when tissues are adequately supplied with blood via the capillaries. Inadequate perfusion can lead to damage and death of a tissue.

- Why is P_{O2} in tissues always lower than in blood?

- Why is P_{CO2} in tissue always higher than in blood?

- How will P_{O2} and P_{CO2} change if the perfusion of the tissue decreases?

- Rapidly metabolizing tissues generate a large amount of CO_2. How does this affect O_2 transport?

20.4   Gas Transportation

Gas transportation is the movement of respiratory gases within the blood between the lungs and systemic cells. Two main gases are of primary interest: oxygen and carbon dioxide. They are transported separately and do not directly influence each other's transportation.

Oxygen Transport

Oxygen is transported within blood from the alveoli through pulmonary veins of the pulmonary circulation to the left atrium of the heart. After that the oxygenated blood enters systemic circuit via the left ventricle and aorta. In capillaries oxygen diffuses into the interstitial fluid where it is picked up by systemic cells. Transportation of oxygen is based on its solubility and the presence of oxygen binding molecules of hemoglobin. It means, that oxygen partially transported being dissolved in blood plasma, but the most portion is bound with hemoglobin. Only 2 percent of oxygen is dissolved in the blood plasma, and remain 98 percent is transported within erythrocytes. A hemoglobin that carries oxygen molecules is called **oxyhemoglobin**. The hemoglobin without oxygen is termed **deoxyhemoglobin**.

Hemoglobin is a protein found in erythrocytes. It consists of four polypeptide chains, each containing a **heme group**. Heme group has one atom of iron (Fe^{2+}) that can bind with one molecule of oxygen. Thus, each molecule of hemoglobin can carry maximum 4 molecules of oxygen (see chapter 17, page 492). The process of binding hemoglobin molecule with O_2 is termed **loading**, and release of O_2 is called **unloading**.

During loading, oxygen from alveoli binds to hemoglobin in the pulmonary capillaries. When all four heme groups in the hemoglobin bind with four oxygen molecules, this hemoglobin is called **fully saturated**. When hemoglobin carries three or less oxygen molecules, it is called **partially saturated**.

The fully saturated hemoglobin travels with blood from lungs to the left atrium of the heart via four pulmonary veins and from here oxygenated blood is injected into the systemic circuit. In the body tissues hemoglobin releases its oxygen cargo. Poorly oxygenated blood then returns to the right atrium of the heart, ready to go to the pulmonary circuit again.

The ability of hemoglobin to load and unload oxygen depends on two factors: 1) the gradient of the oxygen partial pressure, and 2) the strength of chemical bonds between hemoglobin and oxygen. The ability of hemoglobin to bind and hold oxygen molecules is termed **affinity**. The percentage of Hb bound to oxygen is called the **percent saturation of Hb**. One of the main determinants of the percent saturation of Hb is the P_{O_2} of the blood and tissues. A high P_{O_2} favors hemoglobin loading, because more O_2 molecules are available.

The oxygen binding capacity of hemoglobin is between 1.36 and 1.40 ml O_2 per gram of hemoglobin. It increases the total blood oxygen carrying capacity seventyfold, compared to carry it solely as a dissolved gas with oxygen solubility only 0.03 ml O_2 per liter at arterial P_{O_2} is about 100 mm Hg.

Under normal conditions at rest, the hemoglobin that leaves the lungs is about 98 to 99 percent saturated with oxygen, achieving an oxygen delivery between 950 and 1150 ml/min to the body. In a healthy adult at rest, oxygen consumption is approximately 200 to 250 ml/min, and deoxygenated blood returning to the lungs is still roughly 75 percent (70 to 78 percent) saturated. Increased oxygen consumption during sustained physical activity reduces the oxygen saturation of venous blood, which can drop below 15 percent. The increased breath rate and blood flow compensate it and continue to maintain oxygen saturation in arterial blood at 95 percent level or less under these conditions. Sustained hypoxia (oxygenation less than 90 percent), is dangerous to health, and severe hypoxia (saturations less than 30 percent) may be rapidly fatal.

A fetus receives oxygen via the placenta. Its oxygen pressure is low (about 21 percent of the level found in an adult's lungs), so fetuses produce another form of hemoglobin (hemoglobin F) with a much higher affinity for oxygen to function under these conditions.

CHECK YOUR UNDERSTANDING

- How is oxygen transported in the blood?

- What factors affect hemoglobin O_2 loading and unloading?

Carbone Dioxide Transport

Cells typically produce about 200 mL/min of carbon dioxide as a waste product during cellular respiration. Carbon dioxide is transported from systemic cells within deoxygenated blood through veins of the systemic circulation to the right side of the heart, then pumped into the pulmonary trunk and pulmonary arteries to enter pulmonary capillaries. Carbon dioxide then diffuses from the blood within pulmonary capillaries into the alveoli.

Carbon dioxide has three means of being transported in the blood from the systemic cells to the alveoli: 1) CO_2 dissolved within plasma, 2) CO_2 attached to the globin portion of hemoglobin, and 3) as bicarbonate (HCO_3^-) dissolved within blood plasma. Due to high solubility of carbon dioxide (0.57) and small partial pressure gradient for CO_2, approximately 7 percent of carbon dioxide is transported to the alveoli as a dissolved gas within the blood plasma. Hemoglobin is capable of transporting about 23 percent of the CO_2 as a carbaminohemoglobin compound. The CO_2 is attached to amine groups ($-NH_2$) in the globin protein: $CO_2 + Hb \leftrightarrow HbCO_2$ **(carbaminohemoglobin)** (fig. 20.17).

The remaining 70 percent of the CO_2 diffuses into erythrocytes and combines with water to form bicarbonate (HCO_3^-) and H^+: $CO_2 + H_2O \leftrightarrow H_2CO_3 \leftrightarrow H^+ + HCO_3^-$. HCO_3^- then diffuses into the blood

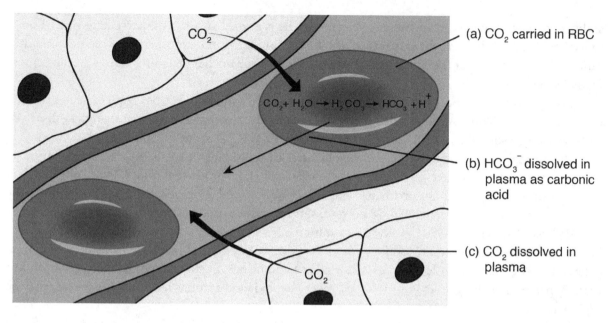

(a) CO_2 carried in RBC

$$CO_2 + H_2O \rightarrow H_2CO_3 \rightarrow HCO_3^- + H^+$$

(b) HCO_3^- dissolved in plasma as carbonic acid

(c) CO_2 dissolved in plasma

FIGURE 20.17   Carbon Dioxide Transport.

plasma. Thus, the largest percentage of carbon dioxide is carried from systemic cells to the lungs in plasma as dissolved HCO_3^-. Carbon dioxide is regenerated when blood moves through pulmonary capillaries and this process is reversed.

The P_{CO2} within the blood is normally lower than in systemic cells. The partial pressure gradient forces CO_2 to diffuse from the systemic cells into the capillary blood. In blood CO_2 is converted by the enzyme **carbonic anhydrase** into HCO_3^-. This conversion keeps P_{CO2} inside the systemic capillaries low at all times and stimulates diffusion of more CO_2 from systemic cells. The hydrogen ions that result from dissociation of carbonic acid are bound with hemoglobin, which acts as a buffer to resist change of blood pH. Because bicarbonate ions have a negative charge, the influx of negative charged ions into the blood plasma could create serious problems, but it is balanced by movement of also negatively charged chloride ions in the opposite direction—from plasma into the erythrocytes. This phenomenon is termed **chloride shift**. Chloride shift maintains a stable electric charge of blood plasma and by that holds pH homeostasis.

In lungs the P_{CO2} in pulmonary capillaries is higher than in alveoli, and the gradient of partial pressure favors CO_2 to diffuse from blood into the alveoli. In lungs the P_{O2} increases and P_{CO2} falls down. These changes trigger the release of hydrogen ions from hemoglobin. Concentration of H^+ in erythrocyte cytoplasm rises, and the equilibrium of reaction between water and carbon dioxide shifts toward the release of CO_2 and water. Bicarbonate and hydrogen ions react and produce CO_2 and H_2O. The decrease of HCO_3^- inside the erythrocyte reverses chloride-bicarbonate shift in the opposite direction; that is, bicarbonate moves inside the erythrocyte, whereas chloride moves out. This keeps P_{CO2} inside erythrocytes high comparatively to the blood plasma and facilitates continuous diffusion of CO_2 from erythrocytes. At the same time, this conversion keeps the concentration of the blood plasma carbon dioxide higher than in alveoli, allowing it to continue to diffuse into alveoli.

CHECK YOUR UNDERSTANDING

- What is the main transport mechanism of CO_2?

- What is the function of carbonic anhydrase in CO_2 transport?

- What will happen if Cl⁻ transport across erythrocytes' membrane is blocked?

20.5 Control of Respiration

Carbonic acid–bicarbonate conversion is a very important part of the blood buffer system. Under normal conditions, the pH of the blood varies very little. The change is small because the hydrogen ions bind with buffers such as bicarbonate ions to form carbonic acid, which acts as a weak acid. When the blood pH increases and the level of hydrogen ions drops too low, hydrogen ions are released from the carbonic acid to yield bicarbonate ions, which in this situation act as a weak base.

The major force that determines the amount of carbonic acid in the blood is the partial pressure gradient of CO_2. This gradient also depends on 1) the rate and depth of ventilation and 2) the rate at which carbon dioxide is generated by metabolic reactions in the cells. Thus, the pattern of ventilation has a dramatic impact on the concentration of H⁺ and, thus, pH of the blood. Two main processes have this profound effect on the blood pH: **hyperventilation** and **hypoventilation**.

Hyperventilation is an abnormally high rate and/or depth of breath. In general, hyperventilation increases the amount of carbon dioxide that is expired and decreases the blood P_{CO_2}. As a result, less carbonic acid is formed, less hydrogen ions are released, and the pH of the blood increases; that is, becomes basic more than normal. This condition is called **alkalosis**. When an organism chronically hyperventilates, the relative lack of carbon dioxide leads to development of a condition called **hypocapnia**. Hyperventilation also increases P_{O_2} in the blood.

Hypoventilation results from a decrease in the rate and/or depth of ventilation. It causes retention of CO_2 and increase of its partial pressure in the blood. As a result, more carbonic acid is formed and more hydrogen ions are released. The excess of hydrogen ions above the norm causes decrease of blood pH or its **acidosis**. The chronic hypoventilation leads to development of condition called **hypercapnia**. Hypoventilation also decreases the arterial P_{O_2}, called **hypoxemia**.

CHECK YOUR UNDERSTANDING

- Why does hyperventilation cause alkalosis?

- What is the relation between CO_2 level in the blood and acidosis?

Neural Control of Ventilation

Eupnea is a restful unlabored breathing. Breathing is controlled by the brain stem, particularly the medulla oblongata. The collection of neurons that generate the basic rhythm of eupnea spring from breathing centers called the **respiratory rhythm generator (RRG)**. There are two RRGs, known as the **ventral respiratory group (VRG)** and **dorsal respiratory group (DRG)**.

The nuclei of the DRG occupy the posterior medulla oblongata. These neurons form an elongated mass that extends most of the length of the dorsal medulla. They are located near the central canal of the spinal cord, just behind the ventral group. The nuclei contain the inspiratory neurons that send signals to the **phrenic nerve**, which generates contractions of the diaphragm and **intercostal nerves** that control contractions of external intercostal muscles. The DRG has the most fundamental role in initiating inspiration. It sets and maintains the basic rhythm of respiration. Most neurons of the DRG are located in the nucleus of the **solitary tract**. Other important neurons are found in the adjacent areas, including the **reticular formation** of the medulla. The solitary nucleus is the endpoint for sensory information from the pontine respiratory group, and from two cranial nerves: the glossopharyngeal and vagus.

The VRG consists of nuclei located in the anterior and lateral regions of the medulla oblongata. They contain both inspiratory and expiratory neurons. Inspiratory neurons send signals that eventually trigger action potentials in the **phrenic** and **intercostal nerves**. In quiet, restful breathing, the ventral respiratory group of neurons are inactive. They become active in forceful breathing. The VRG sends inhibitory commands to the **apneustic center**.

The second main center that contains neurons serving to maintain the eupnea is the **pontine respiratory group (PRG)**. The PRG includes the **pneumotaxic** and **apneustic centers**. The pneumotaxic center is located in the upper part of the pons. This center controls both the rate and the pattern of breathing. The pneumotaxic center is considered an antagonist to the apneustic center. The pneumotaxic center is responsible for limiting inspiration. It limits the burst of action potentials in the phrenic nerve, which results in decreasing of the tidal volume and regulates the respiratory rate. The pneumotaxic center regulates the amount of air that can be taken into the body with each breath. The dorsal respiratory group has rhythmic bursts of activity that are constant in duration and interval. When a faster rate of breathing is needed, the pneumotaxic center signals the dorsal respiratory group to speed up. When longer breaths are needed, the bursts of activity are elongated. All the information that the body uses to help respiration is collected in the pneumotaxic center. An injury of this center causes an increase in respiration depth and a decrease in respiratory rate.

The apneustic center of the lower pons appears to promote inhalation by constant stimulation of the neurons in the medulla oblongata. The apneustic center sends signals to the dorsal group in the medulla to delay the switching off. It controls the intensity of breathing, giving positive impulses to the neurons involved with inhalation. The apneustic center is inhibited by pulmonary stretch receptors and also by the pneumotaxic center. It also discharges an inhibitory impulse to the pneumotaxic center (fig. 20.18).

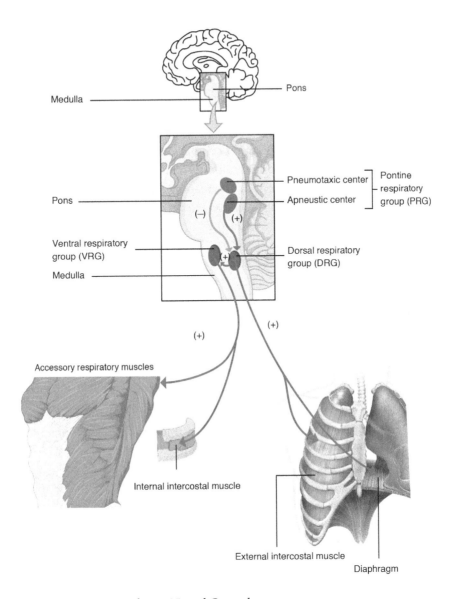

Medulla

Pons

Pneumotaxic center ⎤ Pontine
⎥ respiratory
Apneustic center ⎦ group (PRG)

Pons

(−) (+)

Ventral respiratory
group (VRG)

Dorsal respiratory
group (DRG)

Medulla

(+)

(+)

(+)

Accessory respiratory muscles

Internal intercostal muscle

External intercostal muscle

Diaphragm

FIGURE 20.18   Ventilation Neural Control.

CHECK YOUR UNDERSTANDING

- Which brain area generates the basic respiratory rhythm?

- What nerves have a major influence on ventilation?

- What is the function of the ventral respiratory group?

Chemical Control of Ventilation

Chemical regulation of breathing is part of the involuntary (autonomic) control of breathing. This mechanism is part of the body's homeostasis to maintain an appropriate balance and concentration of CO_2, O_2, HCO_2^-, and pH and is based on negative feedback loops that ensure the organism's respiratory needs. These feedback loops are initiated by receptors that gathering chemical information on the current levels of oxygen, carbon dioxide, and pH. There are two types of chemoreceptors that strongly monitor level of these parameters in the blood: **central** and **peripheral chemoreceptors**.

Central chemoreceptors are located in the medullary reticular formation. The central chemoreceptors are responsible for approximately 80 percent of the response to CO_2 concentration. These receptors generate the most powerful stimuli that induce alterations in ventilation. They respond to concentration of P_{CO2} in the cerebrospinal fluid, but not to P_{O2}. CO_2 diffuses across the blood-brain barrier from blood to cerebrospinal fluid (CSF), while H^+ and HCO_3^- are unable to. As the blood CO_2 readily passes the blood-brain barrier into the CSF, it will react with H_2O to make H_2CO_3 that dissociates into HCO_3^- and H^+: $CO_2 + H_2O \rightarrow HCO_3^- + H^+$. An increase in H^+ concentration stimulates the chemoreceptor neurons in the reticular formation of the medulla oblongata. They relay this information to the DRG, which, in its turn, sends signals to the VRG. In response, the VRG changes the rate and depth of ventilation, which leads to a decrease in CO_2 level in CSF. Decrease of the carbon dioxide level returns the pH to the norm.

Peripheral chemoreceptors are located in the carotid arteries and aorta and are called **carotid** and **aortic bodies** respectively. They are made of neuroepithelial cells that contact with glossopharyngeal (CN IX) and vagus (CN X) sensory nerve terminals. They respond to changes in P_{O2}, P_{CO2}, and pH. The peripheral chemoreceptors are responsible for about 20 percent of the response to an increase in P_{CO2}. But they are most sensitive to the oxygen concentration in the blood. When the concentration of O_2 drops below 70 mm Hg (the norm is 100 mm Hg), they close their K^+ channels and open Ca^{2+} channels. This causes an increase in initiation of dopamine impulses to the DRG. The DRG relays these impulses to the VRG and the last triggers an increase in the rate and depth of ventilation.

CHECK YOUR UNDERSTANDING

- Where are the central chemoreceptors located?
- What do center chemoreceptors detect?

- Where are the peripheral chemoreceptors located, and what do they detect?

CHAPTER SUMMARY

- The respiratory system serves in exchanges of gases between an organism and the environment. It occurs in millions of small air sacs called **alveoli** in mammals and reptiles, and in **atria** of birds.

- Respiration proceeds in two steps: 1) **external respiration** refers to gas exchange between environment and blood via a respiratory surface; 2) **internal respiration** refers to gas exchange between blood and body tissues.

- **Ventilation** is an active process of moving the respiratory medium (water or air) across the exchange surface. Arrest of the respiratory medium movement causes **apnea**. Movement of blood through an organ via capillaries is termed **perfusion**.

- The respiratory system has two regions: the **upper respiratory tract** and **lower respiratory tract**. The upper respiratory tract includes the nose, nasal cavity, and pharynx. The larynx, trachea, bronchi, bronchioles, and alveoli belong to the lower respiratory tract.

- Respiratory organs that transport air but do not participate in gas exchange are called the **conducting zone**. Structures that serve in gas exchange are called the **respiratory zone**. The respiratory zone consists of respiratory bronchioles, alveoli ducts, and alveoli.

- The respiratory system opens by **nares** or **nostrils**. A small pocket within nares, called **nasal diverticulum**, filters debris. The nasal cavity has a nasolacrimal duct that drains tears from eyes.

- Nasal conchae increase surface area to which the air is exposed and are covered by a nonkeratinized mucous membrane with goblet cells, mucous glands, and blood vessels.

- A complex system of paranasal sinuses consists of spaces within skull bones filled by air. They include 1) **frontal sinuses** are within frontal bones; 2) **maxillary sinuses** are spaces within the maxilla, above the tooth roots; and 3) **sphenopalatine sinuses**.

- The **soft palate** blocks off the pharynx from oral cavity.

- The vomeronasal organ, also known as the **olfactory** or **Jacobson's organ**, is found in most animals. It is located at the base of nasal cavity and is divided in two parts by the nasal septum.

- The **pharynx** is a part of the throat between the nasal cavity and larynx. In mammals and birds, it is part of both the digestive and respiratory systems. It is subdivided in the naso-, oro-, and laryngopharynx.

- The larynx keeps food and liquids out of the respiratory tract and houses the vocal cords. It consists of nine cartilages: 1) three unpaired cartilages are **thyroid cartilage, epiglottis,** and **cricoid cartilage**; and 2) six paired cartilages called **arytenoid cartilages** are attached to the **vocal folds** and larynx intrinsic muscles; **corniculate cartilages** are also associated with vocal folds; **cuneiform cartilages** support the epiglottis.

- The larynx is lined by mucosa that forms folds projected inside the lumen. The superior pair of folds is termed **vestibular folds**. The opening between them is called the **rima vestibuli**. The second folds are called **true vocal cords**. At the core of these folds there are bands of elastic tissue called **vocal ligaments**. These cords can produce sound. The opening between them is called the **rima glottis**. The rima glottis and vocal cords together form the **glottis**.

- Skeletal muscles of the larynx are organized in two groups: 1) **extrinsic muscles** elevate the larynx during swallowing, and 2) **intrinsic muscles** pivot arytenoid cartilages, pull vocal cords, and change the size of the rima glottis. This maneuver closes the larynx during swallowing and participates in sound production.

- Birds produce sound in a syrinx. It is located between the trachea and primary bronchi, and is surrounded by air sacs. It is composed of ossified cartilages, vibrating membranes, and muscles.

- The trachea is located in the mediastinum between the larynx and bronchi. Ventral and lateral walls of the trachea are supported by C-shaped rings of **tracheal cartilages**. Cartilages are connected to each other by sheets of elastic connective tissue called **anular ligaments**. The dorsal ends of tracheal cartilage rings are open and connected by the **trachealis muscles** and elastic ligamentous membrane. This structural organization guarantees that trachea will remain open at all times. Tracheal muscle contraction controls the trachea's diameter and the lungs' ventilation.

- The **carina** is located in the area where the trachea splits into the main bronchi. It has sensory receptors that are sensitive to touch with foreign materials and are able to induce a forceful cough.

- Walls of the trachea are made of: 1) mucosa composed of a pseudostratified ciliated columnar epithelium with goblet cells and lamina propria; 2) submucosa with large blood vessels, nerve endings, serous, mucous glands, and lymphatic tissue; 3) tracheal cartilage; and 4) the adventitia, composed of elastic connective tissue. The movement of cilia in the mucosal epithelium propels mucus laden with dust, microbes, and other particles toward the pharynx, where it is swallowed into the stomach and digested or expelled out of the respiratory passages.

- The **Bronchial tree** is a branched system of air-conducting passages ended in **alveoli**. It begins by two **principle bronchi**, also called **main** or **primary bronchi**. The right main bronchus is shorter, wider, and branches at almost right angle to trachea. Main bronchi, together with pulmonary blood vessels, lymph vessels, and nerves, enter the lung via an opening at the medial surface of lung capsule called the **hilum**.

- The main bronchus branches into the **lobar** or **secondary bronchi**. Because left and right lungs have a different number of lobes, there are a different number of lobar bronchi that are divided in **segmental bronchi**. The bronchial tree ends by **bronchioles** terminated with **terminal bronchioles**, the last segments of the conducting zone. They lead to **respiratory bronchioles**, the first elements of the respiratory zone.

- The lumen of the bronchus is lined by a pseudostratified epithelium, containing goblet and serous cells. Beneath the narrow layer of connective tissue under the epithelium lie well-developed spiral bands of smooth muscle. Bronchi trap airborne particles and remove them by cilia.

- Entrance to the alveoli is guarded by bundles of smooth muscles that control alveoli ventilation.

- Each lung is placed within a separate layer of membrane. Thus, there are two pleural sacs. The pleura has two folds: the **pulmonary pleura** or **visceral pleura** and **parietal pleura**. Serous fluid that fills the pleural cavity creates adhesion between folds, allowing smooth movement of the lungs.

- Blood supply to the pleural membranes is provided by **bronchial** and **pulmonary arteries**. The parietal pleura is innervated by intercostal nerves. The mediastinal and diaphragmatic pleura also are innervated by the phrenic nerve, and the visceral pleura is innervated by the vagus nerve and sympathetic fibers.

- In most mammals, the lungs are divided into lobes: 1) the **left lung** is divided into the **cranial** and **caudal lobes**; and 2) the **right lung** is partitioned into the **cranial**, **caudal**, **middle**, and **accessory lobes**.

- Alveoli are minute, polygonal chambers. Their walls consist of two layers of epithelial sheets, "sandwiching" a network of capillaries: the blood-gas barrier consists of capillary endothelium, basal lamina, and alveolar epithelium. Small openings in alveoli walls called **alveolar pores** between adjacent alveoli provide their collateral ventilation. Pulmonary capillaries surround each alveolus. The **intraventricular septum** has elastic fibers that guarantee lung elasticity.

- Cells in alveoli are called **pneumocytes**. There are two types of pneumocytes: 1. **type I** pneumocytes are squamous epithelium cells. They constitute about 95 percent of alveolar surface and form respiratory membrane; 2. **type II** pneumocytes or **septal cells** are round to pyramidal cells. They secrete an oily fluid called **pulmonary surfactant** that prevents alveoli collapse.

- The internal surface is moist, causing a high surface tension, which makes alveoli prone to collapse. An oily surfactant coats the alveolar surface. Pulmonary surfactant opposes collapse of the alveolus. A third type of alveoli cells is called **alveolar macrophages** or **dust cells**. They are leukocytes that survey the lungs for the presence of pathogens.

- The diaphragm is a dome-shaped musculotendinous sheet separating the thoracic and abdominal cavities. It is convex on its cranial surface. It has the following openings: 1) the **aortic hiatus** is the most dorsal opening, containing the aorta, azygous vein, and thoracic lymphatic duct; 2) the **esophageal hiatus** contains the esophagus, dorsal and ventral vagal trunks; and 3) the **caval foramen** lies within the diaphragm central tendinous region and contains caudal vena cava.

- Because of the shorter thorax, the diaphragm is steeper in the **ruminant** compared to the **horse**. **Avian** species do not possess a diaphragm.

- **Respiration** is a general term for the exchange of respiratory gases. It consists of continuous and simultaneous processes: 1) **pulmonary ventilation** is a movement of respiratory gases between the atmosphere and the alveoli of lungs; 2) **alveolar gas exchange** or **external respiration** is an exchange of gases between alveoli and blood; 3) **gas transportation** is movement of gases within the blood; 4) **systemic gas exchange** or **internal respiration** is an exchange of respiratory gases between blood and cells of the body.

- **Pulmonary ventilation** is air movement in and out of lungs. Air flows from an area with high pressure to a place with low pressure. Rate of the flow is proportional to the pressure difference. Pulmonary ventilation has two steps: **inspiration**, or inhalation, and **expiration**, or exhalation.

- Gas pressure follows **Boyle's law**, which states that at constant temperature its pressure and volume are related inversely: **P1V1 = P2V2**, where P is a gas pressure and V is its volume. During inspiration, lung volume increases by inspiratory muscles and the air pressure inside lungs drops. The force that sucks air into lungs is called the **aspiration pump**. Lungs are located within this pump that consists of a rib cage and diaphragm.

- Relaxation of inspiratory muscles decreases lung volume and increases pressure within the pleural cavity, which results in expiration.

- Three factors affect pulmonary ventilation: **resistance of airways to airflow**, **alveolar surface tension**, and **pulmonary compliance**.

- **Airway resistance** is a cumulative effect of different factors that causes friction opposing to airflow. It depends on diameter and length of the airway, and gas viscosity.

- Diameter of airways is controlled by smooth muscles of trachea, bronchi, and bronchioles. Constriction of muscles in bronchi and bronchioles is called **bronchoconstriction**, and their relaxation is **bronchodilation**. The bronchodilation lows airway resistance.

- **Alveolar surface tension** holds water molecules together and minimizes surface area. When alveoli surface decreases during exhalation, water molecules come closer and force of their attraction increases. This attraction generates a high amount of surface tension that can collapse alveoli—the phenomenon known as **atelectasis**. Surface tension works against inflation of lungs and decreases pulmonary ventilation. **Pulmonary surfactant** reduces surface tension by disruption of hydrogen bonds between water molecules and prevents collapse of lungs.

- **Pulmonary compliance** is an ability of lungs to stretch. It is determined by 1) degree of alveolar surface tension, which resists to lungs stretch; 2) distensibility of elastic tissue in the lungs that is determined by an ability of tissues to stretch; and 3) ability of the chest to expend that depends on quality of joints, bones, and cartilages in thoracic cage.

- **Respiratory rate (RR)** is the number of respiratory cycles per minute.

- **Tidal volume (TV)** is the amount of air inspired or expired during quiet ventilation at rest.

- **Minute volume** is the total volume of air inhaled or exhaled in a minute of quiet resting ventilation. This volume can be calculated by multiplying TV and RR: **MV = TV × RR.**

- **Inspiratory reserve volume (IRV)** is the amount of air that can be forcefully inhaled on the top of TV. This volume characterizes the ability of the respiratory system to adjust ventilation to meet maximal body activity.

- **Expiratory reserve volume (ERV)** is the amount of air that an organism can forcefully exhale after a normal tidal expiration.

- The **inspiratory pulmonary capacity** is the total amount of air that an organism can exhale with all its strength. It is a combination of TV and IRV: **IPC = TV + IRV**.

- **Vital capacity** is the total amount of air that an organism can exchange forcefully. It is a sum of TV, IRV, and ERV: **VC = TV + IRV + ERV**.

- The volume of air that remains after exhalation is called **residual volume (RV)**. RV remains inside lungs due to intrapleural pressure and recoil of the chest wall that prevents lungs from collapsing.

- Combination of ERV and RV is known as **functional residual capacity: FRC = ERV + RV**.

- **Total lung capacity** is the total amount of exchangeable and nonexchangeable air in the lungs.

- The air in the conducting zone that does not exchange in alveoli is called **anatomic dead space**.

- Gases' contribution in air pressure is described by **Dalton's law of partial pressure**, which states that each gas in a mixture exerts pressure, called **partial pressure**, proportional to its percentage. Total air pressure is the sum of partial pressures of all gases. The air usually contains 78 percent N_2, 21 percent O_2, and 1 percent CO_2. Air pressure at sea level is around 760 mm of Hg. At this condition, the O_2 partial pressure is $P_{O2} = 760 \times 0.21 = 160$ mm Hg; $P_{N2} = 760 \times 0.78 = 593$ mm Hg; and $P_{CO2} = 760 \times 0.01 = 7.6$ mm Hg.

- Avian lungs are compact. Their lungs are approximately 50 percent as large as lungs of a similar-sized mammal. Birds do not have a pleural cavity as the lungs do not expand. One **primary bronchus** from the trachea enters each lung, travels through, and communicates with an **abdominal air sac**. This bronchus branches as it travels through the lung in **secondary bronchi**. Each of these gives off 400 to 500 **parabronchi** serving for gas exchange. Birds have no diaphragm. Birds have thin distensible **air sacs**, which extend ten times the volume of lungs. Air sacs create airflow in one direction that maximize oxygen extraction and reduce heat production during flight. A chicken has eight air sacs: 1) **cervical**; 2) **clavicular**; 3) two **cranial thoracic**; 4) two **caudal thoracic**; and 5) two **abdominal**.

- The pulmonary gas exchange rate depends on 1) surface size of respiratory membrane, 2) thickness of respiratory membrane, and 3) correlation between air and blood flows.

- In effective respiration, the amount of air matches blood perfusion. This relationship is known as **ventilation-perfusion matching** or **coupling**. Change in alveolar ventilation causes change in perfusion and blood flow is directed to areas where there is more oxygen. At the same time, perfusion affects ventilation, and airflow is directed to areas with highest blood flow.

- Gas exchange in tissues depends on 1) surface area available for gas exchange, 2) distance over which diffusion must occur, and 3) perfusion of the tissue.

- Two percent of O_2 travels inside blood plasma and 98 percent is transported by erythrocytes. Hemoglobin with O_2 is called **oxyhemoglobin**. Hemoglobin without O_2 is termed **deoxyhemoglobin**.

- Hemoglobin consists of four polypeptide chains containing **heme group**. Heme group is responsible for carrying oxygen. One heme group can carry one molecule of oxygen. The process of binding hemoglobin with O_2 is termed **loading**, and its release is called **unloading**.

- When all four hemes are bound with four O_2, the hemoglobin is called **fully saturated**. Hemoglobin with three or fewer oxygen molecules is called **partially saturated**.

- The ability of hemoglobin to load and unload oxygen depends on 1) gradient of P_{O_2}, and 2) strength with which hemoglobin binds with O_2 or its **affinity**. The percentage of Hb bound to oxygen is called the **percent saturation of Hb**.

- Active cells produce about 200 mL/min of CO_2 waste product. It is transported 1) dissolved within plasma, 2) attached to the hemoglobin, and 3) as bicarbonate (HCO_3^-) dissolved within blood plasma. Due to both the high solubility of carbon dioxide (0.57) and its small partial pressure gradient, about 7 percent of CO_2 is transported to alveoli as a dissolved within blood. Hemoglobin transports about 23 percent of CO_2 as a carbaminohemoglobin.

- Seventy percent of CO_2 diffuses in erythrocytes and combines with water to form bicarbonate (HCO_3^-) and H^+: $$CO_2 + H_2O \leftrightarrow H_2CO_3 \leftrightarrow H^+ + HCO_3^-.$$ HCO_3^- then diffuses in blood plasma. In lungs CO_2 is regenerated and exhaled with air.

- P_{CO_2} within the blood is normally lower that in systemic cells. Partial pressure gradient forces CO_2 to diffuse from systemic cells in blood where it is converted by enzyme **carbonic anhydrase** in HCO_3^-. This conversion keeps P_{CO_2} inside systemic capillaries low at all times. H^+ from carbonic acid binds with hemoglobin, which resist change of blood pH. HCO_3^- is balanced by movement of Cl^- in opposite direction. This phenomenon is termed **chloride shift**. Chloride shift maintains stable electric charge of blood plasma and pH homeostasis.

- In alveoli, the gradient of partial pressure favors CO_2 to diffuse from blood inside alveoli. Depletion of CO_2 in blood stimulates HCO_3^- to leave erythrocytes and diffuse in blood. The carbonic anhydrase converts HCO_3^- in CO_2.

- **Hyperventilation** is an abnormally high rate and/or depth of breathing. It decreases blood P_{CO_2}. As a result, pH of the blood increases: a condition called **alkalosis**. Chronic hyperventilation leads to development of **hypocapnia**.

- **Hypoventilation** is an abnormally low rate and/or depth of ventilation. It increases the carbonic acid level in blood. Increase of blood H^+ level above the norm decreases blood pH. Low pH condition is called **acidosis**. Chronic hypoventilation leads to **hypercapnia**. It also decreases arterial P_{O_2}, a condition called **hypoxemia**.

- **Eupnea** is a restful breathing. The basic rhythm of eupnea is generated by the breathing centers called the **respiratory rhythm generator (RRG)**. The medulla oblongata has two RRG: **ventral respiratory group** and **dorsal respiratory group**.

- The dorsal respiratory group (**DRG**) is in the posterior medulla oblongata. It contains inspiratory neurons that send signals via **phrenic nerve** to diaphragm and **intercostal nerves** to external intercostal muscles. DRG initiates inspiration, sets and maintains basic respiratory rhythm.

- The ventral respiratory group (**VRG**) is located in anterior and lateral parts of the medulla oblongata. It contains both inspiratory and expiratory neurons. Inspiratory neurons send signals to the **phrenic nerve** and **intercostal nerves**. In quiet, restful breathing, it is inactive. The VRG is active in forceful breathing and sends inhibitory impulses to the **apneustic center**.

- The **pontine respiratory group (PRG)** includes **pneumotaxic and apneustic centers**. The pneumotaxic center is located in the upper part of pons. It controls rate and pattern of breathing, and regulates the amount of inhaled air. When a faster breathing is needed, the pneumotaxic center signals the dorsal respiratory group to speed up.

- Apneustic center in lower pons promotes inhalation. It controls intensity of breathing, giving positive impulses to the neurons involved with inhalation. The apneustic center is inhibited by pulmonary stretch receptors and also by the pneumotaxic center.

- There are two types of chemoreceptors that monitor a change in blood level of O_2, CO_2, and pH: **central** and **peripheral chemoreceptors**.

- Central chemoreceptors are located in the medullary reticular formation. They monitor P_{CO_2} in cerebrospinal fluid and send sensory signals to DRG.

- Peripheral chemoreceptors are located in carotid arteries and aorta, and are called **carotid** and **aortic bodies**. They contact with the glossopharyngeal and vagus nerves and are sensitive to O_2.

CHECK YOUR KNOWLEDGE

LEVEL 1. CHECK YOUR RECALL

1. What is the function of the cilia in the trachea and bronchi?
    A. Movement of air into and out of the lungs
    B. Increase the surface area for gas exchange
    C. Vibrate when air rushes past them to produce sounds
    D. Sweep mucus with the airborne particles trapped in it

2. In a mixture of gases, the pressure created by each gas is called:
    A. Partial pressure
    B. Special pressure
    C. Differential pressure
    D. Particular pressure

3. Minute ventilation is:
    A. Tidal volume multiplied by breathing rate
    B. Amount of air inhaled and exhaled in one respiratory cycle
    C. Air volume that remains in respiratory organs at all times
    D. Amount of air that may be forcefully exhaled
    E. Total amount of air that may be inhaled

4. The respiratory rhythmicity group is a group of neurons in:
    A. Pons
    B. Medulla oblongata
    C. Dorsal and ventral respiratory groups
    D. A and C only
    E. B and C only

5. Oxygen and carbon dioxide are exchanged in the lungs by:
    A. Active transport
    B. Diffusion
    C. Filtration
    D. Osmosis

6. Physiological dead space is:
    A. The air that enters the respiratory tract but fails to reach alveoli
    B. The air that remains in the lungs all the time
    C. The air in alveoli, which fails to participate in the gas exchange
    D. The combination of the anatomical and alveolar dead spaces
    E. The difference between total lung capacity and vital capacity

7. Carotid bodies are:
    A.   Stretch receptors that react to stretching of the diaphragm
    B.   Stretch receptors in the aortic wall, which monitor blood pressure
    C.   Stretch receptors that react on the stretch of the intercostal muscles
    D.   Chemoreceptors in carotid arteries that monitor sodium concentration in the blood
    E.   Chemoreceptors in carotid arteries that monitor oxygen concentration in the blood

8. The detergent-like substance that keeps the alveoli from collapsing between breaths because it reduces the surface tension of the water film in the alveoli is called:
    A.   Lecithin
    B.   Bile
    C.   Surfactant
    D.   Reluctant

9. A pleural cavity is a:
    A.   Space between ribs
    B.   Space inside lungs
    C.   Space between lungs and ribs
    D.   Space between parietal and visceral pleurae
    E.   Space between pleural membrane and walls of thoracic cavity

10. One inspiration plus the following expiration constitute a:
    A.   Respiratory volume
    B.   Respiratory cycle
    C.   Breathing rate
    D.   Internal respiration
    E.   External respiration

11. The alveolar ventilation rate is:
    A.   The amount of air that moves into the respiratory passages each minute
    B.   The frequency of ventilation
    C.   The air that reaches the alveoli and is available for gas exchange in a minute
    D.   The air that remains in the alveoli at all times

12. The trachea can be described as:
    A.   Lined with a ciliated mucous membrane
    B.   Including C-shaped cartilage semi-rings
    C.   An air passageway
    D.   All of the above

13. The force responsible for normal expiration is supplied by the:
    A. Diaphragm
    B. External intercostal muscles
    C. Elastic recoil of tissues and surface tension
    D. Contraction of smooth muscles in air passages
    E. Pressure of abdominal organs on lungs

14. The amount of air that enters or leaves the lungs during a restful respiratory cycle is called:
    A. Tidal volume
    B. Residual volume
    C. Vital capacity
    D. Total lung capacity
    E. Inspiratory reserve volume

15. The first event in inspiration is:
    A. The sternocleidomastoid muscle contracts.
    B. The diaphragm moves downward and the external intercostals muscles contract.
    C. Atmospheric pressure forces air into the respiratory tract.
    D. Intra-alveolar pressure is decreased.
    E. The lungs become inflated.

16. O_2 will diffuse from blood to tissue faster in response to which of the following conditions?
    A. An increase in the P_{O_2} of the tissue
    B. A decrease in the P_{O_2} of the tissue
    C. An increase in the thickness of the capillary wall
    D. A decrease in the surface area of the capillary

17. The walls of the alveoli are composed of:
    A. Ciliated columnar epithelium
    B. Simple squamous epithelium
    C. Stratified squamous epithelium
    D. Loose connective tissue
    E. Elastic connective tissue

18. Gas exchange takes place in:
    A. Alveoli
    B. Primary bronchi
    C. Lobar bronchi
    D. Alveolar ducts
    E. Intralobular bronchioles

19. Anatomic dead space is the volume of air that:
    A. Enters the respiratory tract, but fails to reach the alveoli
    B. Doesn't exchanges because of the nonfunctioning of lung's regions
    C. Remains in the lungs all the time
    D. Is a combination of expiratory and residual volumes

20. Central chemoreceptors monitor _____, whereas peripheral chemoreceptors monitor _____.
    A. CO_2 in blood; O_2 in cerebrospinal fluid
    B. CO_2 in blood; CO_2 in cerebrospinal fluid
    C. CO_2 in cerebrospinal fluid; O_2 in blood
    D. O_2 in cerebrospinal fluid; CO_2 in blood
    E. O_2 in blood; O_2 in cerebrospinal fluid

21. True or false: The respiratory membrane consists of pseudostratified epithelium.
22. True or false: The increase of alveolar surface tension increases pulmonary compliance.
23. True or false: Vital capacity is the total amount of exchangeable air.
24. True or false: Chronic hyperventilation leads to development of alkalosis.
25. Match the term with its description:

    _____ Respiratory mucosa   a. Extended from the posterior nares to the uvula
    _____ Nasopharynx   b. Unicellular gland that secrete mucus
    _____ Paranasal sinuses   c. Pseudostratified ciliated columnar epithelium
    _____ Goblet cell   d. Hollow cavities inside bones connected to nasal cavity
    _____ Pulmonary surfactant   e. Alveoli collapse
    _____ Tidal volume   f. Lipoproteinous complex that decreases surface tension
    _____ Atelectasis   g. Amount of air inhaled or exhaled at rest

LEVEL 2. CHECK YOUR UNDERSTANDING

1. How does hypoventilation affect pH of the blood?
2. How does fever (elevated body temperature) affect unloading of oxygen from hemoglobin?
3. Why does a punctured lung collapse?

LEVEL 3. APPLY YOUR KNOWLEDGE TO REAL LIFE

1. A dog was hit by a car. You find that the dog is breathing erratically. What injury does the dog have that must be addressed first?
2. Prolonged vomiting can result in loss of hydrogen ions from the blood and, as a result, development of alkalosis. Would you expect a patient with this condition to hyperventilate or hypoventilate?

Chapter 21

The Urinary System

LEARNING OBJECTIVES

Evolutionarily, the primary function of the urinary system is elimination of wastes and potentially toxic substances from an organism. The urinary system of seawater vertebrates concentrates mostly on this process. Life in an aquatic environment normally does not face the risk of dehydration. This challenge is only faced by life in freshwater. Freshwater with its very low osmotic pressure tends to suck solutes such as sodium, potassium, and calcium from the body fluids; high osmotic pressure of body fluids attracts water to move inside the body. Thus, freshwater organisms additionally have to control their water and solute balance. Terrestrial animals have to develop a mechanism that preserves water inside the body, prevents dehydration, maintains solute balance, and maintains blood pressure. The urinary system takes responsibility for all these vital functions. The system includes the kidneys that filtrate blood and remove wastes from it, the ureters that transport waste products to the urinary bladder, and the urethra that excretes urine collecting in the bladder through a process termed micturition.

In this chapter, you will find information on the anatomy and physiology of the urinary system. After reading it, you will be able to describe:

1. What organs constitute the urinary system.

2. The anatomy and histology of the urinary system organs.

3. What processes constitute the formation of urine.

4. How the urinary system maintains homeostasis of body fluids.

5. The mechanisms that control urinary system functioning.

INTRODUCTION

The urinary system is composed of the pairs of kidneys and ureters, and single urinary bladder and urethra. The kidneys filter blood to remove metabolic wastes and toxins. This action is crucial for maintaining a stable chemical composition of body fluids and blood electrolyte balance, pH, and pressure. Waste compounds form **urine**. Urine is transported along the tubular **ureters** to the **urinary bladder** and eliminated via the **urethra**. Organs that transport, store, and remove urine from the body constitute the **urinary tract**.

Mammalian kidneys, as a rule, are bean shaped and have brown color. They occupy a **retroperitoneal** position, meaning they are located dorsal to the peritoneal membrane on the back side of the abdominal wall. The locations of both kidneys

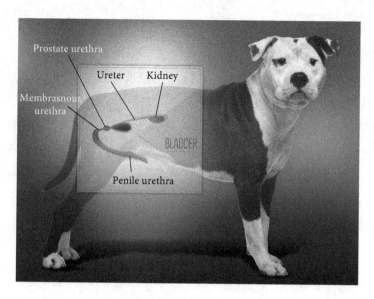

Prostate urethra

Ureter   Kidney

Membrasnous
urethra

BLADDER

Penile urethra

FIGURE 21.1   Male Dog Urinary System.

are not exactly symmetric. As a rule, the left kidney has little bit more cranial position than the right one. From the dorsal side the kidneys are protected by the vertebral column and partially by the ribs. They receive blood supply from the abdominal aorta though the short **renal artery**. Cleaned blood leaves the kidney through the **renal vein**, which empties into the posterior vena cava. The adrenal glands sit on the cranial surface of the kidneys. They receive blood through the suprarenal arteries, which may be a branch of the renal arteries or may directly spring from the abdominal aorta.

Ureters collect urine from the kidneys and deliver it for storage to the urinary bladder. Ureters are soft collapsible tubes between the dorsal wall of the abdominal cavity and peritoneal membrane. Thus, like kidneys, they occupy a retroperitoneal position. The urinary bladder is a muscular sac on the floor (posterior portion) of the pelvic cavity. It has two input openings for the urine that enters from the ureters and one output opening for the urethra (fig. 21.1). The urethra conducts urine from the urinary bladder out of the body through the opening known as the **urethral orifice**.

CHECK YOUR UNDERSTANDING

- What organs constitute the urinary tract?

- What are the blood vessels that serve to deliver blood to and take blood away from the kidneys?

Role of the Urinary System in Homeostasis

The kidney are key players in whole-body homeostasis. They regulate acid-base balance, concentration of electrolytes, total volume of extracellular fluid, and blood pressure. Various hormones coordinate their performance, including aldosterone, antidiuretic hormone, and atrial natriuretic peptide.

The kidneys excrete a variety of waste products produced by an organism. These include the nitrogenous wastes urea, from protein catabolism, and uric acid, from nucleic acid metabolism. The ability of mammals and some birds to concentrate wastes into a volume of urine much smaller than the volume of blood from which the wastes were extracted depends on an elaborate countercurrent multiplication mechanism. These functions that are critical for an organism may be categorized as:

1. **Elimination of metabolic wastes**. The kidneys filter blood, remove wastes, and from these wastes form urine, which then eliminates from the body.

2. **Maintenance of homeostasis of body fluids and electrolyte balance**. The kidneys maintain a stable solute concentration and, by that, blood colloid osmotic pressure. They control sodium, potassium, and calcium blood levels through their retention in the blood or excretion with urine.

3. **Regulation of pH of body fluids.** The kidneys have a primary role in regulation of acid-base balance of the blood, which they execute through conserving or removing of hydrogen (H^+) and bicarbonate (HCO_3^-) ions with urine.

4. **Regulation of blood pressure.** The kidneys directly regulate blood pressure through the control of total blood volume, and indirectly by producing chemicals that affect blood volume and peripheral resistance.

5. **Regulation of red blood cells' production (erythropoiesis).** The kidneys release the hormone erythropoietin (EPO) that stimulates production of erythrocytes in red bone marrow.

6. **Metabolic functions** of the kidneys include conversion of toxic substances into nontoxic chemicals through processes collectively termed **detoxification**. The kidneys also activate vitamin D and participate in production of glucose from proteins through the process known as a **gluconeogenesis**.

CHECK YOUR UNDERSTANDING

- What are the six main functions of the kidneys?

- How do the kidneys control blood pH?

- How do the kidneys control red blood cells production?

21.2   Anatomy of the Kidneys

The kidneys occupy space on both latero-dorsal sides of the abdomen. They are bean-shaped organs found in the retroperitoneal space. Superiorly, they are attached to the dorsal abdominal wall. Ventrally, they lay above the peritoneal membrane, which separates them from the abdominal cavity. A membranous renal capsule covers kidney. Medially, the renal capsule has opening called the **hilum**. The hilum serves as a passage for blood vessels, lymphatic vessels, nerves, and the ureter.

Kidney Gross Anatomy

Vertebrate kidneys are a pair of compact masses of tubules located dorsal to the abdominal cavity. Urine produced in the nephron enters the **minor** and then the **major calyx**. There are a few major calyxes that fuse to form **renal pelvis**, a common chamber leading to the **urinary bladder** via the muscular tube called **ureter**. The kidneys are fastened to the dorsal surface of the abdominal wall on both sides to the vertebral column and are covered by three layers of connective tissue: 1) The outermost layer is called **renal fascia**. Renal fascia consists of an irregular dense connective tissue. It fastens kidney to the peritoneal membrane and to deep fascia that covers muscles in dorsal wall of abdomen; 2) **Adipose capsule** is a middle and thickest layer. It consists of adipose tissue, which protects kidneys from injuries. A prolonged starved organism uses this adipose tissue for a fuel. Adipose capsule loses its strength and kidneys can droop, which results in condition termed **nephroptosis**; 3) The very thin, but strong layer that directly covers

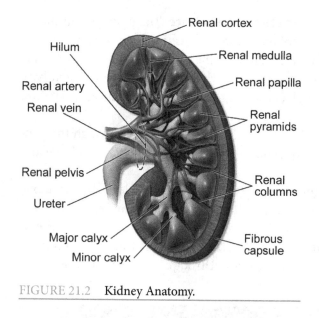

FIGURE 21.2   Kidney Anatomy.

kidneys is called **renal capsule**. Renal capsule consists of irregular dense connective tissue. It protects kidney from infections and physical trauma.

On the medial side, the renal capsule has an opening called the **hilum**. Through the hilum, kidneys receive their blood supply and innervation. The hilum opens into a central cavity called the **renal sinus**. Through the hilum, the renal capsule folds inside the kidneys. Here it lines the renal sinus. Inside the renal sinus, the renal capsule binds blood vessels and nerve fibers and holds them at their proper position. A system of tubes called calyxes collects urine and drains it into the renal sinus. A single funnel-shaped tube called the **ureter** receives this urine and takes it away from the renal sinus. It leaves the kidneys through the hilum.

The longitudinal section through the kidneys shows three distinct layers. The outermost layer just beneath the renal capsule is called the **renal cortex**. The renal cortex mostly contains small blood vessels and complex functional structures called **nephrons**. The middle layer is called the **renal medulla**. The renal medulla contains two main components: 1) **renal pyramids** are mostly composed of parallel tubes: **nephron loops**, **collecting tubules**, and **collecting ducts**; and 2) **renal columns** that contain major blood vessels. The inner area is a renal pelvis. It consists of system of tubules with progressively increased diameters. Collecting ducts in renal pyramids collect urine produced by nephrons. Collecting ducts open at the top of the renal pyramid, called the **renal papilla**. Urine enters the funnel shaped tubes (one tube per one renal papilla) called the **minor calyx**. The number of renal pyramids and minor calyces vary among different mammals. Minor calyces fuse and form three to five tubes of bigger diameters termed **major calyces**. Major calyces drain urine into the large collecting chamber called the **renal pelvis**, which leads into the ureter. Smooth muscles in the walls of the calyces and renal pelvis contracts to push urine into the ureter. The renal pelvis and all calyces are located in renal sinus (fig. 21.2).

CHECK YOUR UNDERSTANDING

- What are the connective tissues that cover the kidneys?

- What are the three regions of the kidneys, and what structures do they harbor?

- What is the functional unit of the kidneys?

Kidney Blood Supply

The kidneys receive approximately one-fourth of the total cardiac output. Renal arteries that supply kidneys with blood spring from the abdominal aorta. The renal artery is short and has a large diameter. This property allows it to maintain a comparatively high blood pressure inside the kidneys, which is important to maintain a healthy filtration rate in nephrons. The renal artery enters the kidneys through the hilum and then fans out into smaller **segmental arteries**. Segmental arteries divide into **interlobar arteries** that enter renal columns. On the border between the renal medulla and renal cortex, interlobar arteries make a right angle turn and become **arcuate arteries.** Arcuate arteries give rise to multiple **interlobular arteries**, which go deep inside the renal cortex. Interlobular arteries branch into tiny **afferent arterioles** that deliver blood to nephron. Thus, the kidneys have the following sequence of arteries: **renal artery** → **segmental artery** → **interlobar artery** → **arcuate artery** → **interlobular artery** → **afferent arteriole.** Afferent arterioles carry blood to a ball of tiny capillaries called a **glomerulus**. Glomeruli are sites of blood filtration. The **efferent arteriole** takes this blood from the glomerulus. The **peritubular capillaries** are the next capillary network on the blood's way through the nephron. The peritubular capillaries receive blood from the glomerulus. Thus, kidneys are one more organ in the mammalian body with a portal system. The afferent arteriole, glomerulus, efferent arteriole, and peritubular capillaries are parts of the kidneys' functional structure called the **nephron.** Thus, in the nephron blood travels through the **afferent arteriole** → **glomerulus** → **efferent arteriole** → **peritubular capillaries**. Peritubular capillaries drain their blood into the vein system of the kidneys. Venous vessels usually are parallel to the arteries. The **peritubular venules** receive blood from peritubular capillaries and transport it into veins with progressively increasing diameter. The total blood pathway out of the kidneys is next: **peritubular venules** → **interlobular vein** → **arcuate vein** → **interlobar vein** → **renal vein.** The renal vein leaves the kidneys through the hilum and empties into the posterior vena cava.

CHECK YOUR UNDERSTANDING

- Which major blood vessels are found on the border of renal cortex and medulla?

- What is the blood vessel that delivers blood to the nephron?

- What blood vessels are found in the portal system of the kidneys?

Nephron and Collecting System

Within the kidneys, the functional unit that forms urine is a microscopic **uriniferous** tubule. The uriniferous tubule consists of two parts: the **nephron** and the **collecting tubules**. The nephron is a major functional unit of the kidneys. It filters blood and from this filtrate forms urine. The nephron has two components: the **renal corpuscle** and **renal tubule.**

Two elements compose the renal corpuscle: the **renal** or **Bowman's capsule** and the **glomerulus.** The glomerulus is a ball-shaped loops of fenestrated capillaries. Fenestra in capillary walls makes them leaky for blood plasma and small molecules, such as glucose, but does not allow blood cells and big molecules, such as proteins (albumin, for example) to pass into filtrate.

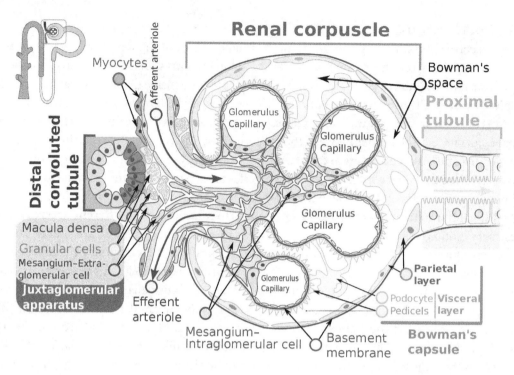

FIGURE 21.3   Renal Corpuscle.

The renal capsule is an extension of the nephron tubular system that has shape of a cap. The wall of the cap is made of a simple squamous epithelium. This sheet of simple squamous epithelium is folded and creates a cap with two parallel walls. A space between these walls is called the **capsular space**. The external fold of the wall is called the **parietal layer**. The inner fold is attached to the glomerulus and, by the analogy with serous membranes, is called the **visceral layer**. The space between the parietal and visceral layers forms the **capsular or Bowman's space**. The visceral layer of the glomerular capsule is composed of specialized epithelial cells called **podocytes** (fig. 21.3). Podocytes are octopus-like cells that have multiple extensions called **pedicels**. Podocytes wrap around capillary wall and their pedicels are incompletely interlocked like fingers of two hands around capillaries leaving tiny clefts called **filtration slits**.

A special group of modified smooth muscles called **mesangial cells** occupy space between the capillary loops of the glomerulus (fig. 21.3). These cells serve to 1) form an extracellular matrix that functions as a structural framework to support the glomerulus; 2) release growth factors for the development and main-tenance of glomerular capillaries; 3) secrete inflammatory factors; 4) phagocytize invading pathogens; and 5) contract to adjust filtration with blood pressure.

Two opposite sides of the renal capsule are called the **vascular pole** and **tubular pole**. The afferent and efferent arterioles enter and leave the nephron capsule through the vascular pole. The tubular pole opens into the proximal convoluted tubule (fig. 21.3).

The renal tubules are composed of simple epithelium resting on the basement membrane. It consists of three consecutive sections: the **proximal convoluted tubule**, the **distal convoluted tubule**, and the **nephron loop** or **loop of Henle** between them. The proximal convoluted tubule originates at the tubular pole of the renal capsule. It is composed of a simple cuboidal epithelium with tall, apical microvilli that significantly increase its surface area. The proximal convoluted tubule is main region of reabsorption and microvilli greatly elevates its reabsorption capacity.

The nephron loop is a middle region of the nephron tubular system. It begins with a sharp bend of the proximal convoluted tubule and extends toward the medulla. In medulla the nephron loop makes a U-turn, folds in two segments, and returns back into the renal cortex. The segment of nephron loop that conducts tubular filtrate toward or even inside the medulla is termed a **descending limb** and the segment that transports tubular filtrate back to the renal cortex is called an **ascending limb**. Both limbs are divided into thick and thin segments, which have different types of epithelial lining. The **thick segment** of each limb is composed of a simple cuboidal epithelium. The **thin segment** is made of a simple squamous epithelium.

The distal end of the ascending limb continues into the distal convoluted tubule. The distal convoluted tubule always lays within the renal cortex. Its wall is composed of simple cuboidal epithelium. The cells of

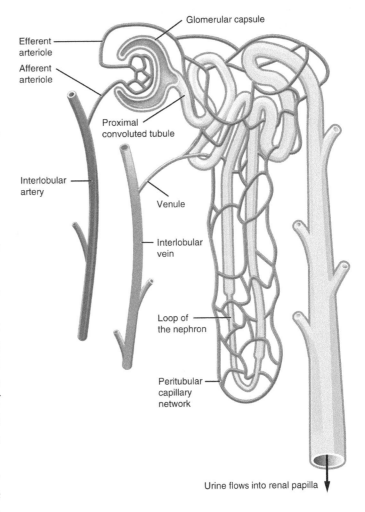

FIGURE 21.4 Nephron Anatomy.

distal convoluted tubule are small and have rare tufts of short apical microvilli. Because of that, the absorptive capacity of the distal convoluted tubules is lower than that of the proximal convoluted tubule. A group of distal convoluted tubules from adjacent nephrons merge and form a larger in diameter **collecting tubule** (fig. 21.4).

The collecting tubule receives urine from several nephrons and empties into a larger **collecting duct**. Each collecting duct receives input from a series of collecting tubules. The collecting ducts project through the renal medulla toward the renal papilla at the top of renal pyramid. On their way, they fuse to form **papillary ducts** that open into minor calyces. At their origin, collecting ducts are made of cuboidal epithelial cells, which at the end of the duct become longer and transform into columnar cells. Distal convoluted tubule, collecting tubule, and collecting duct contain two types of specialized epithelial cells called **principal** and **intercalated cells**. The principal cells have receptors to bind **aldosterone** and **antidiuretic hormone**. The intercalated cells are classified in **types A** and **B** cells. These cells play a key role in homeostasis of blood pH. The type A cell transports H⁺, and type B cell transports HCO_3^- ions from blood plasma into urine.

Types of Nephrons

Nephrons are categorized in two groups: **cortical nephrons** and **juxtamedullary nephrons**. Cortical nephrons make about 80 to 85 percent of all nephrons in mammalian kidneys. They received their name in recognition of the fact that they were found in the renal cortex. Their renal capsule is entirely housed in the outer renal cortex and only their short nephron loop sometimes is merged in the superficial area of the renal medulla. In most cases both the renal corpuscle and nephron loop are located within the renal cortex.

The juxtamedullary nephrons are less numerous. They constitute 15 to 20 percent of all nephrons in mammalian kidneys. Their renal corpuscle is located in close proximity or on the border between renal cortex and renal medulla. They have a very long nephron loop that dives deep into the renal medulla. The nephron loop is surrounded by an intensive ladder-like organized capillary network called the **vasa recta**, which arises from the efferent arteriole. Together with peritubular capillaries, the vasa recta empty into the interlobular vein. The tubules in the cortex are surrounded by peritubular capillaries from nearby cortical nephrons. This unique structure allows the juxtamedullary nephrons to function as a part of a system that controls volume and concentration of urine (fig. 21.5).

The juxtamedullary nephrons serve to regulate formation of urine and maintain normal systemic blood pressure. These functions are executed by a special structural organization of juxtamedullary nephron called **juxtaglomerular apparatus**. The

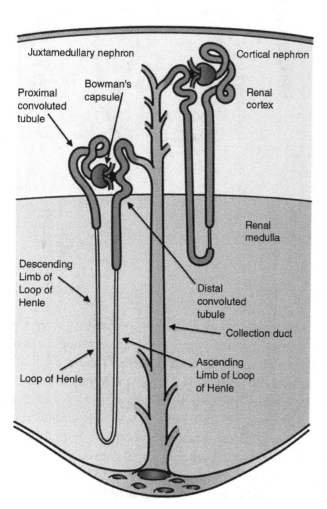

FIGURE 21.5   Cortical and Juxtamedullary Nephrons.

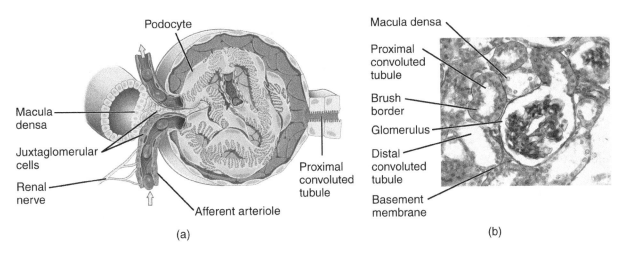

FIGURE 21.6   Juxtaglomerular Apparatus.

juxtaglomerular apparatus consists of three special types of cells termed **granular, macula densa**, and **extraglomerular mesangial cells**. Granular cells are modified smooth muscle cells. They are found in the wall of afferent arteriole near its entrance into the renal corpuscle. These cells serve two functions: 1) they contract when stimulated either by stretch or by the sympathetic neurons; and 2) they synthesize, store, and release the enzyme **renin**. Renin is enzyme that converts angiotensinogen into angiotensin I and, by that, triggers reactions in renin-angiotensin-aldosterone system (RAAS) (see chapter 14, page 409).

The macula densa is a group of modified epithelial cells in the wall of the distal convoluted tubule. They contact with granular cells. The macular densa cells have receptor proteins in their plasma membrane sensitive to sodium chloride (NaCl) within the lumen of the distal convoluted tubule. In response to varying concentration of NaCl, macula densa cells release paracrine signaling molecules, which stimulate granular cells to release renin.

The extraglomerular mesangial cells are located outside the glomerulus within a gap between afferent and efferent arterioles. They are also modified smooth muscle cells tightly bound with other cells of the juxtaglomerular apparatus by gap junctions. The function of extraglomerular mesangial cells is not well understood. It was found that they are associated with the secretion of **erythropoietin** and renin (fig. 21.6).

CHECK YOUR UNDERSTANDING

- What is the difference between the cortical and juxtamedullar nephron?

- What is the function of granular cells?

- What is the function of macula densa cells?

21.3   Renal Physiology

Urine is formed in the kidneys through three related processes: **filtration**, **reabsorption**, and **secretion**. The formation of urine begins in the nephron corpuscle with **ultrafiltration** (or very often, just a **filtration**).

Ultrafiltration occurs as a result of difference of hydrostatic pressure in glomerulus and lumen of the Bowman's capsule and proximal tubule. This difference in hydrostatic pressures drives fluid to enter the proximal tubule in **bulk flow** or **streaming**. Compounds of a large molecular size typically unable to pass through the pores in the capillary wall and **filtrate** accumulated in the tubule mostly consists of water and small solute molecules.

Filtration

Glomerulus is made of fenestrated capillaries. Their walls are tightly bound with the inner wall (visceral layer) of the nephron capsule. The walls of both structures are made of single layers of squamous epithelial cells. Thus, the blood in capillaries is separated from the nephron capsule only by two layers of squamous epithelial cells and porous incomplete basement membrane. This porous structure forms a **filtration membrane**. The visceral layer of the glomerular capsule is made of specialized epithelial cells called podocytes. These cells form the lining of the Bowman's capsule and play a special role in blood filtration (fig. 21.7).

Inorganic ions and small organic molecules, such as glucose, amino acids, and urea, freely move through the filtration membrane into the capsular space. The concentration of these solutes across the filtration membrane remains the same in the filtrate and in blood plasma. On the other hand, large organic molecules, such as albumins and other plasma proteins, are unable to cross this membrane and their concentration in filtrate normally is much lower than in blood. Thus, the filtrate or primary urine is very similar to the blood plasma in composition of inorganic ions and low-molecular-weight organic solute, but significantly different from blood plasma by high-molecular-weight organic solutes, such as proteins. This difference results in drastic difference in both solutions' osmotic pressure. The colloid osmotic pressure of blood normally is higher than that of filtrate.

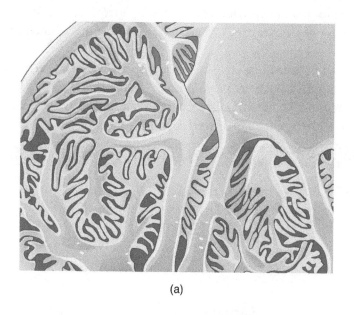

(a)

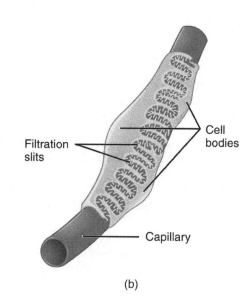

(b)

FIGURE 21.7   Podocytes with Pedicels.

- What is filtrate, and what is the relation between filtrate and blood plasma?

- What is the structure of a filtration membrane? How does it affect filtrate's osmotic pressure?

Glomerular Filtration Rate and Factors That Affect the GFR

Because proteins remain more concentrated in the blood plasma than in the filtrate, the osmotic pressure of the blood plasma is higher than the osmotic pressure of the filtrate. This difference in osmotic pressure is called the **colloid osmotic pressure** of the blood. Thus, there are two processes that drive fluids movement between blood and filtrate: 1) the gradient of the colloid osmotic pressure that drives capsular filtrate to move back into the glomerulus blood; 2) the gradient of the hydrostatic pressure between blood and Bowman's capsule. The latter generates fluid movement from the blood to the capsular filtrate. The net filtration is a trade between these two forces. Normally, hydrostatic pressure overruns the colloid osmotic pressure and fluid moves from the blood plasma into the capsular space. To maintain a healthy filtration rate in the kidney, blood pressure in the glomerular capillaries has to be higher than in other capillaries. Partially, this high blood pressure is due to the fact that the afferent arterioles have relatively large diameters and thus have relatively lower resistance.

The rate of primary urine formation by all of an animal's kidney tubules taken together is called the **glomerular filtration rate (GFR)**. It is defined as the rate at which the volume of filtrate is formed and it is expressed as a volume per unit time. Adult humans, for example, have a GFR of about 120 mL/min. At this rate, the equivalent of all the plasma water in the human body is filtered every half hour! This means that the GFR is greatly exceeds the rate of urine excretion and that most of the water from the filtrate is reabsorbed back into the blood. It also means that the kidneys play a crucial role in regulation of blood plasma composition.

Mammalians control urine formation via the regulation of the GFR. The rate of filtration into an individual nephron depends on the blood pressure in glomerulus, which can be modified by the vasomotor changes in the afferent arteriole diameter. This sort changes are initiated through 1) **intrinsic control** consisting of **renal autoregulation** that maintain the GFR at a normal level, and 2) **extrinsic control** based on nervous and endocrine systems influence on the GFR.

The renal autoregulation is based on negative feedback mechanism. It consists of the kidneys' intrinsic ability to maintain a constant blood pressure and glomerular filtration rate despite the variations in systemic arterial pressure. This autoregulation allows the kidneys to produce urine at a constant rate. Renal autoregulation functions through two mechanisms: 1) the **myogenic response** and 2) **tubuloglomerular feedback**.

The myogenic response involves contraction and relaxation of smooth muscle in the wall of the afferent arteriole in response to changes in stretch of afferent arteriole wall. A decrease in systemic blood pressure results in a lower volume of blood entering the afferent arteriole and reduction of tension in smooth muscles of the afferent arteriole wall. This causes relaxation of smooth muscles and dilation of arteriole wall. The increased influx of blood through arteriole with bigger diameter compensates the decrease of the systemic arteries blood pressure and the GFR remains on the regular normal level.

The increase in systemic blood pressure injects additional volume of blood to enter the afferent arteriole. Additional blood stretches smooth muscles in the arteriole wall. This stretch initiates smooth muscles contraction and causes vasoconstriction of the afferent arteriole. The constricted arteriole allows less blood to enter the glomerulus and the GFR decreases to normal.

The tubuloglomerular feedback mechanism is executed by the juxtaglomerular apparatus. It works through the regulation of NaCl levels in blood and urine. An increase of NaCl level in tubular fluid is detected by macula densa cells in the juxtaglomerular apparatus. The macula densa cells respond by releasing a signaling molecules that stimulate contraction of smooth muscle cells in the afferent arteriole wall. This paracrine stimulation results in further vasoconstriction of the afferent arteriole and a decreased volume of blood enters the glomerulus. Mesangial cells are also stimulated to contract, which decreases filtration membrane surface area. Both vasoconstriction of the afferent arteriole and smaller membrane surface area cause the GFR and the amount of filtrate formed to return to normal levels.

The mechanism of intrinsic control maintains the GFR within the normal homeostatic range. However, outside this range the renal autoregulation does not effective and the process of urine formation requires additional extrinsic factors for its control. The vasomotor changes can be executed via the autonomous nervous system and circulating hormones. Variation in the GFR is not the only mechanism that can control the rate of urine production. Animals can also regulate the rate at which the nephrons reabsorb filtrate back in blood. In fact, this is the preeminent process of urine volume control in mammals.

The sympathetic division of the nervous system influences vasoconstriction of both afferent and efferent arterioles. Strong vasoconstriction of the afferent arteriole greatly reduces blood flow into the glomerulus causing decrease of the GFR. Sympathetic stimulation also causes granular cells of the juxtaglomerular apparatus to release renin, with the subsequent production of angiotensin II. Angiotensin II stimulates myofilaments within the mesangial cells to contract. This contraction decreases surface area of the filtration membrane, and subsequently the GFR decreases. This adjustment is characteristic of a critical condition when an organism tries to stabilize fluid content at stress conditions, such as extensive hemorrhage.

Atrial natriuretic peptide (ANP) is a hormone released by the cardiac muscle cells in heart atria in response to stretch of cardiac muscle cells. It may happen when there is either an increase in blood volume or increase in blood pressure. ANP relaxes the afferent arteriole and inhibits release of renin from the granular cells relax the mesangial cells and filtration membrane surface area increases. The net result is an increase in the GFR. Thus, the ANP increases urine output and decreases blood volume and blood pressure to a normal value.

CHECK YOUR UNDERSTANDING

- What are the forces that drive filtration in the nephron corpuscle?

- What is the function of atrial natriuretic peptide?

- What are the mechanisms that control the glomerular filtration rate?

Tubular Reabsorption and Secretion

Two major processes that take place in the nephron tubular system are **tubular reabsorption** and **tubular secretion**. Tubular reabsorption is a process of removing water and important for organism substances, such as glucose and amino acids, from filtrate and return them back to the blood. Tubular secretion is a process of removing wastes, toxic, or accumulated above the healthy norm substances from the blood into the urine. The barrier that substances must cross is made of simple epithelium. Substance can pass this barrier via two ways: 1) through slits between epithelial cells called **paracellular transport** and 2) through epithelial cells called **transcellular transport**. The hydrostatic pressure in peritubular cap-

illaries is low because during glomerular filtration some fluid leaves capillaries for capsular filtrate. For the same reason, the colloid osmotic (**oncotic**) pressure is high, because the concentration of blood plasma proteins, especially albumins, with loss of solvent increases. These two important properties of the blood in peritubular capillaries facilitate reabsorption of substances from the filtrate within the renal tubule into the peritubular capillaries through bulk flow.

The maximum amount of substance that can be reabsorbed or secreted across the tubular epithelial lining in particular period of time is called the **transport maximum (T_m)**. Each transport protein is specialized on transportation of a particular chemical. The T_m depends upon the amount of transport protein in the membrane of epithelial cell. For example, the T_m for glucose reabsorption by the glucose transport proteins is approximately 375 mg/min. As far as the glucose concentration in tubular fluid exceeds this level the saturated transport proteins become unable to reabsorb more glucose and glucose shows up in urine. The maximum concentration of substance that can be transported is called the **renal threshold**. The renal threshold of glucose, for example, is 300 mg/dL.

Although reabsorption and secretion of substances occur along the entire length of the nephron tubule, collecting tubules, and collecting ducts, most reabsorption occurs in the proximal convoluted tubule, where the uptake processes are aided by the extensive microvilli on the cells' apical surfaces (fig. 21.8).

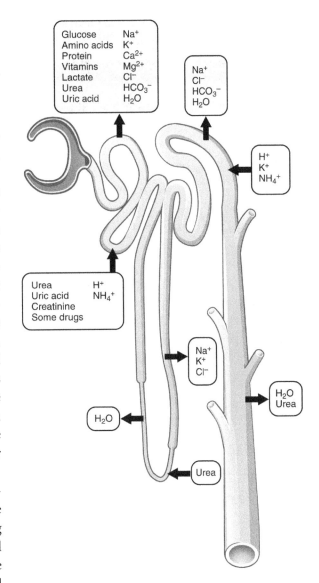

FIGURE 21.8   Tubular Reabsorption and Secretion.

Most of the water in the filtrate is normally reabsorbed and returned to the blood plasma. As the filtrate flows through the nephron tubular system, it undergoes transformations until it becomes urine and is excreted out of the body. Different regions of the nephron tubular system are lined by different types of epithelial cells. Within each region, the epithelial cells have distinctive characteristics in microvilli construction and membrane proteins, such as ion channels, transporters, and aquaporins. These properties give each region of the tubule distinctive abilities to reabsorb water and solutes from the tubular fluid, return it to the blood, and to secrete solutes from the blood into the tubular fluid. The processes carried out by each region of the nephron tubule, and the permeability properties of each region, are under endocrine control. The ability of mammals to concentrate their urine is one of their most important evolutionary achievements critical for life on land. The history of life reveals only three major groups of animals that have successfully mastered terrestrial life: mammals, birds, and insects.

CHECK YOUR UNDERSTANDING

- What are the two processes that proceed in the nephron tubular system?

- What is the difference between the paracellular and transcellular transports?

- What is the renal threshold?

Reabsorption and Secretion in the Proximal Convoluted Tubule

Water moves by osmosis. It is reabsorbed through both paracellular transport between cells and transcellular transport through aquaporins. The human body, for example, filters about 180 L of water daily. Of this water, only 1.5 to 2 L is voided with urine and 160 to 165 L is reabsorbed. Of this reabsorbed water, around 65 percent is recovered in the proximal convoluted tubules. The aquaporins here are a permanent component of the epithelial cell membrane. The water movement in the proximal convoluted tubules is combined with active transport of sodium ions. Na^+ pump in cellular membrane transports sodium from tubular filtrate into the interstitial space around the proximal convoluted tubule. The osmotic pressure of the filtrate drops, whereas the osmotic pressure of the nearby tissues grows. This colloid osmotic pressure across the wall of proximal convoluted tubules drives water to follow Na^+. Aquaporins facilitate water movement. This osmosis mechanism is called **obligatory water reabsorption** because it depends on the movement of sodium ions (fig. 21.9).

Nutrients are normally reabsorbed completely in the proximal convoluted tubules. Each particular nutrient has its own transporter. For example, glucose is transported by the Na^+/glucose symporter protein. It based on the usage of energy of moving down the gradient concentration sodium ions into the interstitial fluid. Glucose just follows sodium ions.

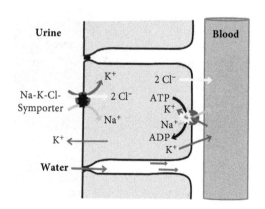

FIGURE 21.9 Na^+, Cl^-, and Water Reabsorption in Proximal Convoluted Tubule.

Normally, most large protein molecules cannot enter the capsule space with filtrate. However, some small and medium-sized peptides, such as insulin and angiotensin, may show up in the filtrate. In the proximal convoluted tubule, these compounds are completely reabsorbed. These molecules are transported across the tubular wall by pinocytosis and receptor-mediated endocytosis (see chapter 3, page 74). They enter the cell inside transport vesicles. In the cytoplasm of the cell, they are digested by the lysosomes into amino acids, and these amino acids move via facilitated diffusion into the surrounding interstitial space and then are returned into the blood flow.

The sodium movement plays a critical role for reabsorption of substances in the proximal convoluted tubules. The amount of reabsorbed Na^+ varies from 98 percent to 100 percent. Na^+ is reabsorbed along the entire length of nephron tubular system. However, the major amount of Na^+ (65 percent) is reabsorbed in the proximal convoluted tubule. Sodium is reabsorbed through transcellular transport. For that, it first enters the cell interior, and after that, it leaves the cell and moves into the interstitial space. Sodium concentration inside the cells of tubular walls is relatively low compared with both the tubular and interstitial fluids. The Na^+/K^+ pump maintains this low sodium concentration, constantly removing sodium out of the cell. Thus, following the gradient of concentration, Na^+ moves passively from the tubular fluid into the cell cytoplasm. From the cell into the interstitial space, sodium is pumped by the sodium-potassium pump. The pump transports Na^+ outside the cell in exchange for incoming K^+. This keeps Na^+ inside the cells always low. The Na^+ reabsorption is a very active process, and the Na^+/K^+ pump consumes about 80 percent of all energy invested in active transport within nephrons. The vasa recta pick up Na^+ from the interstitial space and return it into blood flow.

In the proximal convoluted tubule 60 to 80 percent of the K^+ in the tubular fluid is reabsorbed by paracellular transport. It is depended on movement of Na^+: 1) sodium is reabsorbed; 2) water follows the Na^+; 3) the concentration of the remaining solutes in the tubular fluid increases as water leaves it; 4) the higher than in the interstitial fluid solute concentration of tubular fluid is greater, which establishes a concentration gradient between the tubular fluid and interstitial fluid; 5) potassium moves down its concentration gradient from the tubular fluid by the paracellular route; and 6) these conditions also allow the passive reabsorption of other solutes, including cations Mg^{2+}, Ca^{2+}, phosphate ion PO_4^{3-}, fatty acids, and urea.

The levels of bicarbonate (HCO_3^-) and hydrogen (H^+) ions are critical for blood pH homeostasis. During filtration, bicarbonate ions move freely across the filtration membrane and its concentration in the filtrate is equal to that of blood plasma. Hydrogen ions in blood tend to bind large protein molecules. Attached to protein H^+ does not pass small pores in the filtration membrane and, consequently, presents in filtrate in a very small amount. Approximately 80 to 90 percent of HCO_3^- is recovered from the tubular fluid in the proximal convoluted tubules.

Nitrogenous wastes include **urea, uric acid**, and **creatinine**. The urea is a small organic molecule produced in protein catabolism in liver. The uric acid is a waste product of breakdown of nucleic acids in the liver. The creatinine is produced in muscles tissue. When accumulated in the body, these products become toxic and, thus, have to be removed. When urea and uric acid both are reabsorbed and secreted, the creatinine is only secreted. Urea is freely filtered and then is reabsorbed or secreted in different areas of the tubules. About 50 percent of urea is reabsorbed in the proximal convoluted tubules by the paracellular movement. Along with waste materials, the kidneys eliminate potentially harmful substances. These substances include drugs, antibiotics, aspirin, morphine, cannabinoids, and others. Most of them are secreted in the proximal convoluted tubules.

CHECK YOUR UNDERSTANDING

- What is the role of sodium reabsorption in transportation of other compounds?

- What is the relation between sodium and water reabsorptions in proximal convoluted tubules?

- What are the substances secreted in the proximal convoluted tubule?

Reabsorption in the Nephron Loop–Countercurrent Mechanism

The concentration gradient between the interstitial fluid and blood plays a leading role in tubular reabsorption. This concentration gradient is established and maintained through the mechanism called **countercurrent multiplier**. The countercurrent refers to the fact that fluids in descending and ascending limbs of the nephron loop move in opposite directions. It is called multiplier to demonstrate the fact that this opposite fluid movement increases concentrations of salts within the interstitial fluid. The long loop of the juxtamedullary nephrons plays a critical role in this process (fig. 21.10).

The walls of limbs of the loop of Henle are constructed from different epithelial cells. Thus, the wall of the descending limb is permeable to water but impermeable to salts, such as NaCl. In contrast, the wall of the ascending loop is impermeable to water, but salts can go out easily. As a result, the wall of the descending limb is leaky to water. Salts remain in the tubular fluid, and their concentration together with total osmotic pressure grows. Movement of the water into the interstitial space decreases the osmotic pressure of interstitial fluid. This creates osmotic pressure favorable to transport of salts from the tubular fluid into the interstitial space in the ascending loop. Most important, however, is that the salt concentration along the length of the nephron loop from the renal cortex to the depth of the renal medulla increases. This increased concentration of salts attracts more water. Additional water leaves fluid in the descending limb, which attracts more salt molecules to enter interstitial space. Thus, the salt concentration in the interstitial fluid is multiplied through this positive feedback.

The concentration gradient established in the interstitial fluid by the nephron loop is maintained by the vasa recta. The blood in the vasa recta moves in opposite to the tubular fluid direction. The blood flows deep into the medulla alongside the ascending limb, and then it flows back toward the cortex alongside the descending limb of the nephron loop. This opposite movement of fluids is termed the **countercurrent exchange system**. Countercurrent exchange facilitates effective exchange of solutes between nephron loop and capillaries of the vasa recta. As the blood flows through the vasa recta deep into the renal medulla, water moves by osmosis out of these capillaries into the more concentrated interstitial fluid. At the same time, salts in the interstitial fluid enter the vasa recta by diffusion down their concentration gradient. As a result, blood in vasa recta loses water, but loads with salts. Blood moves deeper and deeper into the medulla. Moving blood becomes more and more concentrated. When capillaries of vasa recta do the turn following the descending limb of the nephron loop and begin to ascend toward the renal cortex, the

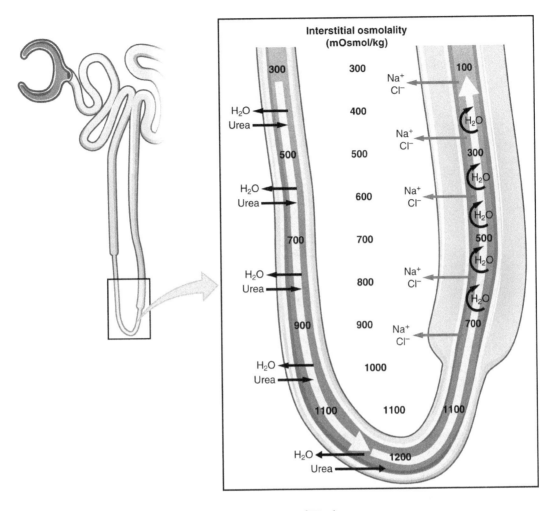

Countercurrent Multiplier in Loop of Henle.

movements of the salts and water are reversed. Now, salts diffuse back into the interstitial fluids and water back into the blood. As the blood moves closer to the renal cortex, it becomes less and less concentrated. When it returns back to the cortex its osmotic pressure is equal or almost equal to that of the blood vessels in the renal cortex (fig. 21.11).

An important solute that maintains high salt concentration in the interstitial fluid is urea. Recycled urea makes up about 50 percent of the solutes in the concentration gradient of interstitial fluid. The urea uniporter proteins remove urea from the tubular fluid in the collecting duct. It diffuses back into the tubular fluid in the thin segment of the ascending limb. Because both the thick segment of the ascending limb and the collecting tubules are not permeable to urea, it stays within the tubular fluid until it reaches the collecting duct, where it is removed from the tubular fluid. Thus, urea is cycled between the collecting duct and the nephron loop. Some amount of urea remains within the interstitial fluid and contributes to its concentration gradient.

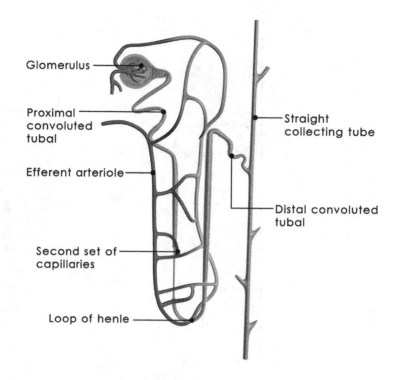

FIGURE 21.11   Countercurrent Exchange System in Nephron Loop.

CHECK YOUR UNDERSTANDING

- What is the principle of countercurrent multiplier?

- What is the principle of countercurrent exchanger?

Reabsorption and Secretion in the Distal Convoluted Tubule and Collecting Duct

The amount of sodium excreted in urine ranges from 0 to 2 percent of the total Na^+ filtered in the renal capsule. The reabsorption of this sodium in distal convoluted tubule, collecting tubule, and collecting duct is under the hormonal control. Two hormones: aldosterone and atrial natriuretic peptide (ANP) play the main role in this process. Aldosterone is a steroid hormone produced in the adrenal cortex (see chapter 14, page 409). It enters the principal cells and binds with receptor protein forming hormone-receptor complex. The complex triggers synthesis of Na^+ channel proteins and Na^+/K^+ pump. New channels and pump proteins are installed in the cell membrane, which increases reabsorption of the sodium. Water molecules follow the sodium out of the tubular fluid.

The ANP inhibits both reabsorption in the proximal convoluted tubule and collecting tubule. It also inhibits release of the aldosterone. It increases release of Na^+ and water in urine. Because ANP increases the GFR, it increases urine output. Thus, the secretion of ANP causes decreases of blood volume and blood pressure.

Water reabsorption in the distal convoluted tubule, collecting tubule, and collecting ducts is controlled by aldosterone and antidiuretic hormone (ADH). The aldosterone affects water reabsorption through the retention of the Na^+. The ADH supports to the water facilitated diffusion through aquaporins. ADH is produced in the hypothalamus and released via the posterior pituitary gland. The release of the ADH in the blood flow is controlled by the thirst center in the hypothalamus. ADH stimulates principal cells to manufacture and install aquaporins in the cellular membrane. As far as the osmotic pressure within the interstitial fluid is higher than in tubular fluid, water molecules are pulled out of the tubular fluid and aquaporins provide the means of its diffusion. Thus, the water reabsorption at the end of the tubular system is independent of Na^+ reabsorption (fig. 21.12).

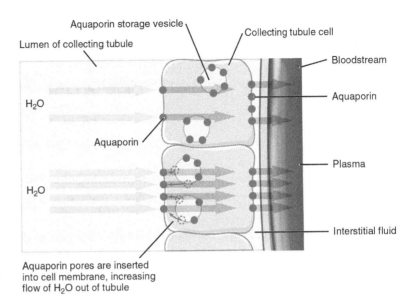

FIGURE 21.12   Role of Aquaporin in Water Reabsorption in the Distal Convoluted Tubule.

VETERINARY APPLICATION

Fanconi syndrome is a disease caused by abnormal function of the nephron tubular system. In Fanconi syndrome tubular system of nephron fails to reabsorb sodium, potassium, glucose, phosphate, bicarbonate, and amino acids. It was reported in several different dog breeds, but the vast majority of cases (75 percent) occurred in basenjis. Ten to 30 percent of basenjis in North America were affected. Affected individuals may exhibit signs of the syndrome as early as 11 weeks of age, but typically clinical signs emerge from four to seven years of age. Males and females are affected equally. The signs of Fanconi syndrome depends upon the severity of specific nutrients loss and whether kidney failure develops. Dogs with Fanconi syndrome may lose weight despite eating normally. Excessive drinking and urinating are the most common clinical signs. As the disease progresses, dogs may experience decreased appetite and lethargy. Very young dogs with Fanconi syndrome have abnormal bone development. Fanconi syndrome is characterized by the presence of glucose in urine, whereas blood glucose level is in the norm. About one-third of cases develop low blood potassium.

There is no way to reverse the abnormal reabsorption of solutes that occurs in Fanconi syndrome. Treatment may include potassium supplementation, nutritional management of kidney disease, and support of normal acid-base balance. Once, the values are stable, they have to be checked every two to four months. Some dogs remain stable for years, but others may develop rapidly progressing kidney failure. That is why most dogs with Fanconi syndrome die of end-stage kidney failure. However, many dogs with Fanconi syndrome who do not develop kidney failure can live close to a normal life.

In the collecting tubules and collecting ducts through the two cell types: principal and intercalated type A cells. Type A cells reabsorb K$^+$ continuously, whereas principal cells secrete K$^+$ at varying rates based on the aldosterone level. The aldosterone works through the negative feedback with potassium blood level. The increase of the K$^+$ in systemic blood flow triggers production and release of aldosterone, which stimulates secretion of K$^+$ into the collecting tubules and collecting ducts.

The Ca^{2+} balance is controlled by the parathyroid hormone (PTH). The PTH stimulates Ca^{2+} reabsorption in the distal convoluted tubule. At the same time, PTH inhibits reabsorption of PO$_4^{3-}$ in the proximal convoluted tubule and promotes its excretion in urine. The retained in the blood Ca^{2+} level increases and PO$_4^{3-}$ decreases. This prevents formation of calcium phosphate – a major component of the bone tissue ground matter. The level of blood Ca^{2+} increases, but its reposition into the bones as a calcium phosphate decreases.

The distal convoluted tubules regulate pH by absorbing bicarbonate and secreting H$^+$ into the filtrate, or by absorbing H$^+$ and secreting bicarbonate into the filtrate. These processes are executed by intercalated cells. The type A cells secretes hydrogen ions into urine and reabsorbs bicarbonate ions to the blood. The type B cells promote opposite process: H$^+$ is reabsorbed and HCO$_{3-}$ is secreted into urine. These intercalated cells' actions are critical components of a blood pH homeostasis and K$^+$ balance.

CHECK YOUR UNDERSTANDING

- What is the function of the antidiuretic hormone in water reabsorption in the distal convoluted tubule?

- What are the roles of intercalated A and B cells in K$^+$ balance and blood pH homeostasis?

- Which hormone regulates Ca^{2+} reabsorption in the distal convoluted tubule?

Urine Transport, Storage, and Elimination: Ureters, Urinary Bladder, and Urethra

The urinary tract consists of the ureters, urinary bladder, and urethra. These organs are responsible for transportation and storage of the urine. Urine collected by **minor** and **major calyces** enters the **renal pelvis** and then **ureter**.

The ureters are comparatively long contractile tubes that transport urine to the urinary bladder. Like kidneys, ureters have retroperitoneal position. The walls of ureters are composed of three concentric tunics: the **mucosa, muscularis,** and **adventitia** (fig. 21.13).

The ureter's mucosa is composed of a transitional epithelium (see chapter 5, page 136). Transitional epithelium is distensible, which allows ureter's wall to stretch to accommodate increased volume of urine, and impermeable to urine, which prevents its leaking back to body fluids. The lamina propria of the mucosal tunic is composed of thick irregular dense connective tissue. The middle muscular tunic contains two layers of smooth muscles: the inner longitudinal layer, and outer circular layer. Distention of the ureter wall by urine triggers rhythmic contraction of these muscles. Spatial organization of smooth muscles in ureter wall favor to synchronize their contractions into peristaltic waves of contractions that propel urine toward the urinary bladder. The adventitia is composed of areolar connective tissue rich with collagen and elastin fibers. Elastic flexible areolar tissue fastens ureter to the dorsal abdominal wall. The ureters project through the bladder wall obliquely. Because of the oblique course of the ureters through the bladder wall, the ureter walls are compressed as the bladder distends, decreasing the likelihood of urine backflow into the ureters from the bladder.

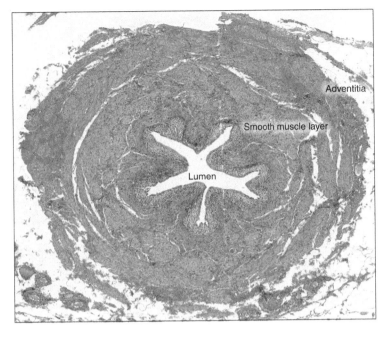

FIGURE 21.13   Histology of the Ureter.

The ureters are innervated by the autonomic nervous system. Sympathetic neurons extend from the T11–L2 segments of the spinal cord. That is why pain from the ureters is referred to the T11–L2 dermatomes. These dermatomes are distributed along a "loin-to-groin" region, and pain in this region typically signals about pathological process in the ureter or kidneys. The vagus nerve (CN X) innervates the anterior portion of the ureter. The splanchnic nerves in the pelvis innervates the posterior portion of the ureter.

The urinary bladder is an expandable, muscular organ that serves as a temporal reservoir of urine. It is located dorsally to the symphysis pubis. In mammalian females the urinary bladder is located ventrally to the uterus and vagina. Like kidneys and ureters, it has a retroperitoneal position. An internal posterior-dorsal area of the urinary bladder wall called **trigone**. It is formed by imaginary lines connecting the two ureter orifices and the urethral opening. The trigone is made of irregular dense connective tissue and remains immobile as the urinary bladder fills with urine and expands. Because the ureters and urethra form three points of this triangular region, infections are more common within this area (fig. 21.14).

The urinary bladder has four tunics: the mucosa, submucosa, muscularis, and adventitia. The mucosa is formed by the transitional epithelium and underlining it highly vascularized lamina propria. The distention of urinary bladder is supported by **mucosal folds** or **rugae**. Within the trigone region, the mucosa is smooth, thick, and lacking mucosal folds. The muscular tunic of the urinary bladder has three layers of smooth muscles called **detrusor muscle**. At the urethral opening, the urinary bladder forms a neck, which wall houses an involuntary **internal urethral sphincter**. The adventitia, the outer tunic is made of areolar connective tissue that covers the urinary bladder. A peritoneal membrane covers only the anterior surface of the urinary bladder.

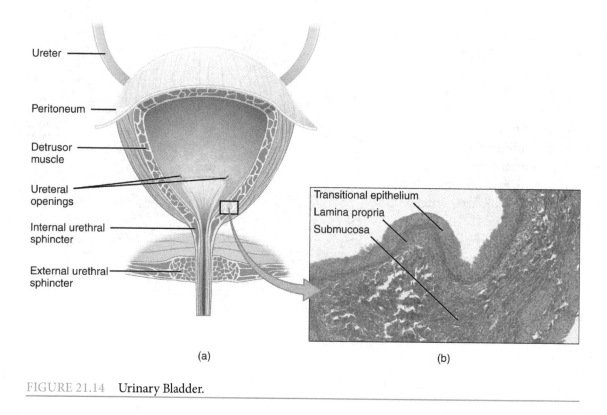

(a)

(b)

FIGURE 21.14   Urinary Bladder.

The urethra is a fibromuscular tube that extends from the ventro-caudal surface of the urinary bladder to the urethral opening. Two urethral sphincters secure the release of urine until the pressure within the urinary bladder becomes enough high. When the urinary bladder distends up to particular level, both sphincters are relaxed and allow the urine to move out. The internal urethral sphincter is considered an involuntary, superior sphincter. It is composed of smooth muscle and surrounds the neck of the urinary bladder. It is controlled by the sacral segment of the autonomic nervous system. The **external urethral sphincter** is inferior to the internal urethral sphincter and is composed of skeletal muscle of the pelvic diaphragm. This sphincter is considered to be voluntary and is under control of the frontal lobe of the cerebral cortex.

There is a significant difference between male and female urethra. The female urethra only conducts urine from the urinary bladder. It is comparatively short and lined by a stratified squamous epithelium. The male urethra is longer and serves two body systems: urinary for conduction of urine and reproductive for transport of semen. The male urethra is partitioned in three distinctive regions: **prostatic, membranous**, and the most distal, **penile** or **spongy urethra**. The prostatic urethra receives input from the urinary bladder and is contributed by many small prostatic ducts that enter it. This region of the urethra is lined by the transitional epithelium. Longitudinal and circular smooth muscles form its muscular tunic. The membranous urethra is the shortest. It is surrounded by skeletal muscle fibers that form the external urethral sphincter. The epithelium in this region is usually either stratified columnar or pseudostratified. The spongy urethra is the longest. It is located within the penis and encased by a cylinder of erectile tissue called the **corpus spongiosum**. It is lined by the pseudostratified epithelium (fig. 21.15).

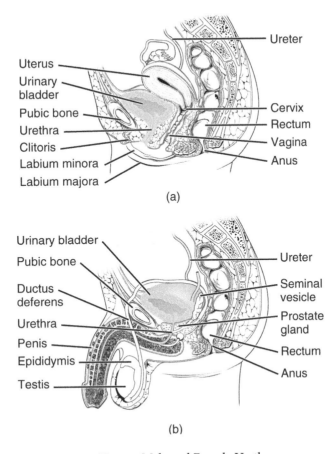

FIGURE 21.15   Human Male and Female Urethra.

CHECK YOUR UNDERSTANDING

- What type of epithelium lines the ureter and urinary bladder?

- What is the difference between male and female urethra?

- What is the trigone?

Micturition

The expulsion of urine from the urinary bladder is called **micturition**, **urination**, or **voiding**. Two reflexes control this process: the **storage reflex** and **micturition reflex**. Both are executed by the sympathetic and parasympathetic divisions of autonomic nervous system. The urinary bladder and urethral sphincters are innervated by the T11–L2 sympathetic nerves, which relax the detrusor muscle and contract the internal urethral sphincter. Thus, stimulation by the sympathetic division inhibits micturition and supports accumulation of urine in the urinary bladder. This process is referred to as a **storage reflex**. Pelvic splanchnic S2–S4 parasympathetic nerves trigger contraction of the detrusor muscle and relaxation of the internal sphincter muscle, which pushes urine out of the urinary bladder toward the urethral orifice. Thus, parasympathetic stimulation promotes micturition, whereas the parasympathetic nerves are parts of the **micturition reflex** arc. The reflex proceeds through three steps: 1) accumulation of urine in the urinary bladder causes its distention and baroreceptors in the bladder signal through the visceral sensory neurons to stimulate micturition center within pons; 2) the micturition center sends nerve signals down the spinal cord to the pelvic splanchnic nerves at the S2–S4 sections; and 3) parasympathetic stimulation causes the smooth muscle cells of the detrusor muscle to contract and the internal urethral sphincter to relax. The external urethral sphincter is composed of skeletal muscle and, thus, is under somatic nervous system (pudendal nerve) control. The pudendal nerve voluntary contracts this sphincter and prevents inconvenient urination.

CHECK YOUR UNDERSTANDING

- What is the storage reflex? What are the nerves that form the storage reflex arc?

- What is the micturition reflex? What are the nerves that form the micturition reflex arc?

CHAPTER SUMMARY

- The urinary system is composed of kidneys, ureters, urinary bladder, and urethra.

- Mammalian kidneys occupy **retroperitoneal** position. They receive blood from the abdominal aorta via **renal arteries** and discharged blood via **renal veins** to posterior vena cava.

- The kidneys 1) **eliminate metabolic wastes**; 2) **maintain homeostasis of body fluids and electrolyte balance**; 3) **regulate pH of body fluids**; 4) **regulate blood pressure**; 5) **regulate red blood cells' production (erythropoiesis)**; and 6) **metabolic functions** of the kidneys include conversion of toxic substances into nontoxic chemicals through processes collectively termed **detoxification**. The kidneys also activate vitamin D and production of glucose from proteins through the **gluconeogenesis**.

- Urine produced in nephron enters **minor**, then **major calyx**. Major calyxes fuse and form the **renal pelvis** leading to the **urinary bladder** via **ureter**. The kidneys are covered by 1) outermost **renal fascia**, 2) middle **adipose capsule**, and 3) **renal capsule**.

- Medially, the renal capsule has an opening called the **hilum**. The hilum opens in a central cavity called the **renal sinus**. It is a pathway for blood and lymph vessels, and nerves.

- The outermost layer of the kidneys is called the **renal cortex**. It contains blood vessels and **nephrons**. The middle layer is called the **renal medulla**. It contains 1) **renal pyramids** are composed of **nephron loops, collecting tubules**, and **collecting ducts**; and 2) **renal columns** contain interlobar blood vessels. The internal region is called renal sinus that houses minor and major calyces and renal pelvis. Ducts in the pyramid open in the **renal papilla** and urine enters the minor calyx.

- The kidneys receive approximately one-fourth of total cardiac output. The renal artery enters the kidneys through the hilum and splits into **segmental arteries**. The pathway of blood vessels is segmental arteries → **interlobar arteries** → **arcuate arteries** → **interlobular arteries** → **afferent arterioles** → **glomerulus** → **efferent arteriole** takes → **peritubular capillaries** → **peritubular venules** → **interlobular vein** → **arcuate vein** → **interlobar vein** → **renal vein**. The renal vein leaves the kidneys through the hilum and empties in the posterior vena cava.

- The nephron filters blood and produces urine. It consists of the **renal corpuscle** and **renal tubule**. The renal corpuscle has the **renal** or **Bowman's capsule** and **glomerulus**. The glomerulus is a ball-shaped loop of fenestrated capillaries. Fenestra make capillary leaky for blood plasma and small molecules, but do not allow blood cells and big molecules to pass.

- The renal capsule is an extension of the nephron tube. It has the shape of a cap. The wall of the cap is lined by simple squamous epithelium. Space between folds is called **capsular space**. The external fold makes the **parietal layer** and inner fold makes the **visceral layer**. The visceral layer is composed of epithelial cells called **podocytes**. Podocytes have multiple extensions called **pedicels**. Podocytes rap around capillary wall and their pedicels are incompletely interlocked like the fingers of two hands around capillaries leaving tiny clefts called **filtration slits**.

- A group of smooth muscles called **mesangial cells** occupies space between capillary loops of the glomerulus. They 1) form structural framework to support glomerulus, 2) release growth factors for development and maintenance of glomerular capillaries, 3) secrete inflammatory factors, 4) phagocytosis, and 5) regulate filtration according blood pressure.

- The renal tubules consist of 1) **proximal convoluted tubule**, 2) **distal convoluted tubule**, and 3) **nephron loop** or **loop of Henle**. Proximal convoluted tubule originates at the tubular pole of renal capsule. It is composed of a simple cuboidal epithelium with tall apical microvilli that significantly increase its surface area. It is a main region of reabsorption.

- The nephron loop is folded in **descending** and **ascending limbs**. The epithelial lining of both limbs divides them into thick and thin segments. **The thick segment** is composed of a simple cuboidal epithelium. **The thin segment** is made of a simple squamous epithelium.

- The distal convoluted tubule is within the renal cortex. It continues into a collecting tubule.

- The collecting tubule receives input from several nephrons and empties in the **collecting duct**. Collecting ducts project through the renal medulla toward the renal papilla. They fuse to form **papillary ducts** that open in the minor calyx. At their origin, collecting ducts are made of cuboidal epithelial cells. They become longer and at the end are replaced by columnar cells. The distal convoluted tubule, collecting tubule, and collecting duct contain **principal** and **intercalated cells**. Principal cells are sensitive to **aldosterone** and **antidiuretic hormones**. The intercalated cells are classified in **types A** and **B**. Type A cell excrete H^+ and type B – HCO_3^- ions into urine.

- There are two types of nephrons: **cortical** and **juxtamedullary**. Cortical nephrons are located entirely in renal cortex. Juxtamedullary nephrons constitute 15 to 20 percent. Their renal corpuscle is located in close proximity to renal medulla, but long nephron loop is in the renal medulla. It is surrounded by a capillary network called the **vasa**

recta, which arises from the efferent arteriole. Together with peritubular capillaries, the vasa recta empty into the interlobular vein.

- The juxtaglomerular apparatus consists of **granular, macula densa**, and **extraglomerular mesangial** cells. Granular cells are modified smooth muscle cells in the afferent arteriole wall near its entrance in renal corpuscle. These cells 1) contract when stimulated by stretching or by sympathetic neurons, and 2) release the enzyme **renin**.

- Macula densa are modified epithelial cells in the wall of distal convoluted tubule. These cells are sensitive to NaCl within fluid in distal convoluted tubule. High concentration of NaCl stimulates these cells to send paracrine signals that stimulate granular cells to release renin.

- Extraglomerular mesangial cells are outside of the glomerulus between afferent and efferent arterioles. They are modified smooth muscle cells that secrete **erythropoietin** and renin.

- Three processes create urine: **filtration, reabsorption**, and **secretion**. Urine formation begins in the nephron corpuscle with a process called **ultrafiltration** or **filtration**. Ultrafiltration is driven by the difference in hydrostatic pressure in the glomerulus and renal capsule. Large molecules are unable to pass, and **filtrate** mostly consists of water and small molecules.

- Ions and small organic molecules, such as glucose, amino acids, and urea, move freely with filtrate. Large organic molecules, albumins, and other plasma proteins are unable to cross the membrane, and their concentration in filtrate is lower than in blood. Filtrate or primary urine is very similar to the blood plasma in composition of inorganic ions and low-molecular-weight organic solute, but significantly different by high-molecular-weight organic solutes.

- Because proteins are more concentrated in blood than in filtrate, the osmotic pressure of the blood plasma is higher than of the filtrate. This difference in osmotic pressure is called **colloid osmotic pressure**.

- Processes that drive fluid movement between blood and filtrate are 1) gradient of the colloid osmotic pressure that drives capsular filtrate back into the blood; and 2) gradient of the hydrostatic pressure between blood and nephron capsule that drives fluid from blood into the filtrate. The net filtration is a compromise between these forces.

- Total urine formation is called the **glomerular filtration rate** (**GFR**). It is defined as the rate at which filtrate is formed and is expressed as a volume per time unit. The rate of filtration is initiated through 1) **intrinsic control** consisting in **renal autoregulation** that maintain the GFR at a normal level, and 2) **extrinsic control** based on nervous and endocrine control.

- Renal autoregulation is a negative feedback mechanism that consists of the kidneys' ability to maintain a constant blood pressure and glomerular filtration rate despite the variations in systemic arterial pressure. It proceeds via 1) **myogenic response** and 2) **tubuloglomerular feedback**.

- The myogenic response involves contraction and relaxation of smooth muscle in the wall of afferent arteriole. A decrease in systemic blood pressure reduces tension in smooth muscles and increases blood influx. An increase of blood pressure stretches smooth muscles in arteriolar wall. This stretch initiates muscles contraction and causes vasoconstriction of afferent arteriole.

- The tubuloglomerular feedback mechanism is executed by juxtaglomerular apparatus. An increase of NaCl level in tubular fluid is detected by macula densa cells that release signaling molecules. These signals stimulate contraction of smooth muscles in afferent arteriole causing its vasoconstriction and decrease of blood volume entering the glomerulus. Mesangial cells are also contract and decrease filtration membrane surface area.

- SNS has an influence on vasomotion of both afferent and efferent arterioles. Sympathetic stimulation also causes granular cells to release renin, with the subsequent production of angiotensin II. Angiotensin II stimulates myofilaments within the mesangial cells to contract, which decreases surface size of filtration membrane and, subsequently, the GFR decrease.

- **Atrial natriuretic peptide (ANP)** is a hormone released by cardiac muscle cells in response to stretch. ANP relaxes afferent arteriole and inhibits release of renin from the granular cells, which cause relaxation of mesangial cells and increase of filtration membrane surface area. The net result is an increase in the GFR.

- Tubular reabsorption is a process of returning of important substances back to blood. Tubular secretion is a process of removing wastes, toxic, or accumulated above the healthy norm substances from blood into urine. Substances are transported through 1) slits between epithelial cells called **paracellular transport** and 2) epithelial cells in **transcellular transport**.

- The maximum amount that can be reabsorbed or secreted in a unit of time is called **transport maximum (T_m)**. It depends on the number of transport proteins in membranes of epithelial cells. The maximum amount of substance that the kidneys can transport is called the **renal threshold**.

- Water moves via paracellular and transcellular transports. In proximal convoluted tubules, water reabsorption is associated with active transport of Na^+. Pumping Na^+ decreases filtrate osmotic pressure and increases it in a nearby tissue. This colloid osmotic pressure across the wall of proximal convoluted tubules drives water to follow Na^+ through aquaporins.

- Nutrients are reabsorbed completely in the proximal convoluted tubules. Each particular nutrient has its own transporter. Glucose is transported via a Na^+/glucose symporter.

- Sixty-five percent of Na^+ is reabsorbed in the proximal convoluted tubule. Sodium concentration inside tubule cells is relatively low compare with both the tubular and interstitial fluids. The Na^+/K^+ pump maintains this low sodium concentration inside the cell and Na^+ moves passively from tubular fluid inside the cell. From the interstitial fluid, Na^+ diffuses into vasa recta bloodstream.

- Sixty to 80 percent of K^+ is reabsorbed by paracellular transport in proximal convoluted tubule. It depends on movement of Na^+: Sodium is reabsorbed $\rightarrow$ water follows the Na^+ $\rightarrow$ concentration of remaining solutes in the tubular fluid increases as water leaves $\rightarrow$ solute concentration of tubular fluid becomes greater than in the interstitial fluid, creating a gradient between the tubular fluid and interstitial fluid $\rightarrow$ K^+ moves down concentration gradient by paracellular route $\rightarrow$ lower solute concentration in blood forces other solutes, including Mg^{2+}, Ca^{2+}, PO_4^{3-}, fatty acids, and urea diffuse to the blood.

- Nitrogenous wastes include **urea**, **uric acid**, and **creatinine**. Urea is produced in protein catabolism by the liver. Uric acid is a waste product of nucleic acid breakdown in the liver. Creatinine is produced in muscles. Whereas urea and uric acid are both reabsorbed and secreted, creatinine is only secreted. About 50 percent of urea is reabsorbed in the proximal convoluted tubules.

- The wall of the descending limb of the nephron loop is permeable to water but impermeable to salts. In contrast, the wall of ascending limb is impermeable to water, but salts are actively pumped out. As a result, water from descending loop moves into the interstitial space, but salts remain in the tubular fluid and its osmotic pressure grows. Water influx decreases osmotic pressure of interstitial fluid, which supports transport of salts from tubular fluid in the ascending limb. The salt concentration along the length of the nephron loop from the renal cortex to the depth of the renal medulla increases. This increase of salts' concentration attracts more water from descending limb, which encourage more salts left the ascending limb and salt concentration in interstitial fluid is multiplied through this positive feedback. This gradient is established through the positive feedback mechanism is called the **countercurrent multiplier**.

- Blood in the vasa recta moves in the opposite direction to the tubular fluid. It flows deep into the medulla alongside the ascending limb and then back to the cortex alongside the descending limb. This opposite movement of fluids is termed the **countercurrent exchange system**. As the blood flows through the vasa recta deep into the renal medulla, water by osmosis moves out of capillaries into the more concentrated interstitial fluid. At the same time, salts in the interstitial fluid enter the vasa recta. As a result, blood in vasa recta loses water, but loads with salts. When capillaries of vasa recta turn and begin to ascend toward the renal cortex, the movements of the salts and water are reversed.

- Urea makes up about 50 percent of the interstitial fluid concentration gradient. In collecting duct urea is removed from the tubular fluid by urea uniporters and is returned back into the thin segment of ascending limb. Both thick segments are not permeable to urea and it remains within the tubular fluid until it reaches the collecting duct again. Cycling between collecting duct and nephron loop urea within the interstitial fluid contributes to its concentration gradient.

- Na^+ reabsorption in distal convoluted tubule, collecting tubule, and collecting duct is controlled by hormones: 1) Aldosterone triggers synthesis of Na^+ channel proteins and Na^+/K^+ pump; 2) ANP inhibits Na^+ reabsorption in proximal convoluted and collecting tubules. It also inhibits release of aldosterone. This increases release of Na^+ and water in urine. Because ANP increases the GFR, it increases urine output, decreases blood volume and blood pressure.

- Water reabsorption in distal convoluted tubule, collecting tubule, and collecting ducts is controlled by aldosterone and antidiuretic hormone (ADH). The aldosterone affects water reabsorption through the retention of the Na^+. The ADH supports water facilitated diffusion via aquaporins. The release of the ADH is controlled by the thirst center in hypothalamus. ADH stimulates principal cells to manufacture and install aquaporins in cellular membrane. As far as the osmotic pressure within the interstitial fluid is higher than in tubular fluid, water molecules are pulled out of the tubular fluid and aquaporins provide the means of this diffusion.

- K^+ homeostasis is maintained through the principal and intercalated cells in collecting tubules and collecting ducts. Type A intercalated cells continuously reabsorb K^+. The principal cells secrete K^+ at varying rates based on aldosterone level. An increase of K^+ in blood triggers production and release of aldosterone, which stimulates its secretion into collecting tubules and collecting ducts and elimination from the body.

- Ca^{2+} balance is controlled by the parathyroid hormone (PTH). PTH stimulates Ca^{2+} reabsorption in distal convoluted tubule, inhibits reabsorption of PO_4^{3-} in proximal convoluted tubules and promotes its excretion with urine. Increases of blood Ca^{2+} and decrease of PO_4^{3-} results in decrease of Ca^{2+} deposition in bones, and increase its blood level.

- Distal convoluted tubules regulate pH by moving HCO_3^- and H^+ by intercalated cells. Type A cells secrete hydrogen ions and reabsorb bicarbonate ions. Type B cells do opposite: they reabsorb H^+ and secrete HCO_3^-.

- Ureters are long contractile tubes that transport urine to the urinary bladder. Walls of the ureters are composed of three concentric tunics: **mucosa**, **muscularis**, and **adventitia**.

- Sympathetic neurons from T11–L2 segments of spinal cord innervate ureters. The vagus nerve innervates superior region of the ureter. The splanchnic nerves innervate inferior ureter region.

- Urinary bladder has four tunics: mucosa, submucosa, muscularis, and adventitia. The mucosa is formed by the transitional epithelium and underlining it highly vascularized lamina propria. **Mucosal folds** or **rugae** allow urinary bladder to distend. Within the trigone, mucosa is smooth, thick, and has no folds. Muscular tunic has three layers of smooth muscles called detrusor muscle.

- Urethra is a fibromuscular tube extending from the urinary bladder. Smooth muscles form an internal urethral sphincter that encircles the urethral opening at the neck of the urinary bladder. **External urethral sphincter** is inferior to the internal urethral sphincter. It is composed of skeletal muscle of the pelvic diaphragm. It is under control of the frontal lobe of the cerebral cortex.

- The only function of the female urethra is conduction of urine out of the body. It is short and lined by a stratified squamous epithelium. The male urethra is longer and is part of the urinary and reproductive systems. It is partitioned into the **prostatic**, **membranous**, and **penile** or **spongy urethra**. The prostatic urethra receives urine from the urinary bladder. It is lined by the transitional epithelium. Longitudinal and circular smooth muscles form its muscular tunic. The membranous urethra is shortest part. It is surrounded by skeletal muscles that form an external urethral sphincter. The epithelium in this region is either stratified columnar or pseudostratified. The spongy urethra is the longest. It is located within penis and encased by a cylinder of erectile tissue called **corpus spongiosum**. It is lined by the pseudostratified epithelium.

- **Storage reflex** and **micturition reflex** regulate urination. Both are controlled by the autonomic nervous systems. The urinary bladder and urethral sphincters are innervated by the T11–L2 sympathetic nerves. They relax the detrusor muscle and contract internal urethral sphincter. Thus, the sympathetic nervous system inhibits micturition and supports of urine retention - a process referred to as a **storage reflex**. Pelvic splanchnic S2–S4 parasympathetic nerves trigger detrusor muscle contraction and internal sphincter muscle relaxation. This allows urine to flow out. Thus, parasympathetic stimulation promotes micturition, and parasympathetic nerves are parts of the **micturition reflex** arc.

CHECK YOUR KNOWLEDGE

LEVEL I. CHECK YOUR RECALL

1. What is the correct order of structures through which urine flows from the nephron?
    A. Calyx, renal pelvis, ureter, urinary bladder, urethra
    B. Renal pelvis, calyx, ureter, urinary bladder, urethra
    C. Renal pelvis, calyx, urethra, ureter, urinary bladder
    D. Renal pelvis, calyx, urinary bladder, ureter, urethra
    E. Calyx, urinary bladder, urethra, ureter, renal pelvis

2. What is the basic functional unit of the kidneys?
   A. Renal papilla
   B. Renal pyramid
   C. Renal pelvis
   D. Calyx
   E. Nephron

3. Which one of the following is the function of the urinary system?
   A. Regulate body water balance
   B. Control production of white blood cells
   C. Maintain homeostasis of body temperature
   D. Control blood flow in systemic circuit
   E. Convert toxins in nontoxic compounds

4. Which of the following correctly describes kidney function?
   A. Collecting duct are permeable to salts, but not to water.
   B. In the ascending limb of loop of Henle, Na^+ and Cl^- ions move into the tubular fluid.
   C. The descending limb of loop of Henle absorbs filtrate from the ascending loop.
   D. The distal convoluted tubule pumps water inside by an active transport.
   E. The proximal convoluted tubule reabsorbs glucose via the sodium symports.

5. Which of the following is the first to collect urine?
   A. Renal pelvis
   B. Minor calyx
   C. Major calyx
   D. Urinary bladder
   E. Ureter

6. The renal pyramids are within the:
   A. Renal column
   B. Renal cortex
   C. Renal medulla
   D. Renal sinus
   E. Renal pelvis

7. If the afferent arteriole constricts:
   A. Blood flow into the glomerulus increases.
   B. GFR decreases.
   C. GFR increases.
   D. The glomerular hydrostatic pressure rises.
   E. The secretion of proteins increases.

8. Which of the following is the correct sequence of the nephron with respect to fluid flow?
    A. Distal convoluted tubule → ascending limb → descending limb → proximal convoluted tubule → collecting tubule
    B. Ascending limb → descending limb → proximal convoluted tubule → distal convoluted tubule → collection tubule
    C. Proximal convoluted tubule → ascending limb → descending limb → distal convoluted tubule → collecting tubule
    D. Proximal convoluted tubule → descending limb → ascending limb → distal convoluted tubule → collecting tubule
    E. Collecting tubule → distal convoluted tubule → descending limb → ascending limb → proximal convoluted tubule

9. What effect does ADH have on urine's water content?
    A. It facilitates water permeability in the descending limb of loop of Henle.
    B. It decreases water permeability of the descending limb of the loop of Henle.
    C. It facilitates water permeability in the collecting tubule and collecting duct.
    D. It decreases water permeability in the collecting tubule and collecting duct.
    E. It decreases water filtration in the nephron corpuscle.

10. The compact ball-shaped capillary network in the nephron is called:
    A. Nephron loop
    B. Peritubular plexus
    C. Glomerulus
    D. Vasa recta
    E. Proximal convoluted tubules

11. What happens during glomerular filtration?
    A. Large protein molecules move from the capsular space into the capillary blood.
    B. Water and small molecules move from capillary blood into the capsular space.
    C. Water and small molecules move from the capsular space into the blood.
    D. Large protein molecules move from the capillary blood into the capsular space.
    E. Water and small molecules move from capillary blood into the capsular space, whereas large proteins move from capsular space into the capillary blood.

12. All the following are functions of the kidneys **except**:
    A. Gluconeogenesis—production of glucose from proteins
    B. Secretion of EPO to control erythrocyte production
    C. Production of plasma proteins to control blood volume
    D. Control of blood pressure through the secretion of renin
    E. Regulation of blood pH through reabsorption and secretion of H^+ and HCO_3^-

13. All are differences between the cortical and juxtamedullar nephrons **except**:
    A. Lengths of their nephron loops
    B. Structure of the capillary system around tubules
    C. Structure of their renal corpuscles
    D. Presence of granular cells and macula densa
    E. Ability to control blood pressure

14. All are correct about the glomerular filtration rate **except**:
    A. GFR increase when the afferent arteriole dilates.
    B. GFR increases when the efferent arteriole dilates.
    C. GFR decreases when the afferent arteriole constricts.
    D. GFR decreases when the efferent arteriole constricts.
    E. Both B and C

15. H_2CO_3 dissociates in the proximal tubule cells into H^+ and HCO_3^-. What happens to the H^+ when HCO_3^- is reabsorbed in the proximal tubule cells?
    A. It is secreted through a Na^+ antiporter to react with HCO_3^-.
    B. t is secreted through a Na^+ antiporter to react with CO_2.
    C. It is secreted through a Na^+ antiporter to react with H_2O.
    D. It is secreted through a Na^+ antiporter to react with O_2.

16. What does micturition mean?
    A. A kidney disease
    B. Pain while urinating
    C. Discharge of urine from urinary bladder
    D. Inability to urinate
    E. Accumulation of urine in the urinary bladder

17. The urine becomes diluted when the level of _____ is decreased.
    A. aldosterone
    B. ANP
    C. ADH
    D. PTH
    E. EPO

18. Which of the following structures is **not** a part of a nephron?
    A. Loop of Henle
    B. Renal pelvis
    C. Juxtaglomerular apparatus
    D. Bowman's capsule
    E. Proximal convoluted tubule

19. What type of epithelium lines the ureters and urinary bladder?
    A. Transitional
    B. Simple squamous
    C. Simple cuboidal
    D. Simple columnar
    E. Stratified squamous

20. Renal corpuscles are present in which part of the kidneys' structure?
    A. Renal pelvis
    B. Renal medulla
    C. Renal cortex
    D. Renal capsule
    E. Renal sinus

21. Which part of the nephron has receptors to aldosterone to stimulate Na+ reabsorption?
    A. The descending limb of the loop of Henle
    B. The glomerulus
    C. The proximal convoluted tubule
    D. The distal convoluted tubule and the collecting tubule
    E. The ascending limb of the loop of Henle

22. In the proximal convoluted tubule, water is reabsorbed via _____, whereas in the distal convoluted tubule, water is reabsorbed via _____.
    A. paracellular transport; transcellular transport through aquaporins
    B. transcellular transport through aquaporins; paracellular transport
    C. active transport through transporters; passive diffusion
    D. passive diffusion; active transport through transporters
    E. paracellular active transport via transporters; paracellular active transport via aquaporins

23. The renal medulla is composed of renal columns that contain _____, and renal pyramids are mostly composed of _____.
    A. nephrons; collecting and papillary ducts
    B. collecting and papillary ducts; nephrons
    C. collecting and papillary ducts; interlobar blood vessels
    D. interlobar blood vessels; collecting and papillary ducts
    E. interlobar blood vessels; nephrons

24. Intercalated type A cells _____ and type B cells _____.
    A. promote secretion of H^+ and reabsorption of HCO_3^-; secretion of HCO_3^- and reabsorption of H^+
    B. promote secretion of HCO_3^- and reabsorption of H^+; secretion of H^+ and reabsorption of HCO_3^-
    C. promote secretion of Na^+ and reabsorption of K^+; secretion of K^+ and reabsorption of Na^+
    D. promote secretion of K^+ and reabsorption of Na^+; secretion of Na^+ and reabsorption of K^+
    E. promote secretion of H^+ and reabsorption of K^+; secretion of K^+ and reabsorption of H^+

25. True or false: The micturition reflex is executed through the parasympathetic vagus and pudendal nerves.

26. True or false: Aldosterone facilitates water retention through reabsorption of sodium in distal convoluted tubules, whereas ADH facilitates water retention through aquaporins in collecting tubules.

27. True or false: Macula densa cells produce and release renin and erythropoietin.

28. True or false: Glucose is reabsorbed in the distal convoluted tubules via paracellular diffusion.

29. Match the term with its description:

_____ Paratubular mesangial cell   a.   Sensitive to tubular fluid NaCl concentration

_____ Principal cells   b.   Produce renin

_____ Intercalated cells type A   c.   Produce EPO

_____ Intercalated cells type B   d.   Have receptors to aldosterone and ADH

_____ Macula densa cells   e.   Reabsorb H^+ and secrete HCO_3^-

_____ Granular cells   f.   Reabsorb HCO_3^- and secrete H^+

_____ Podocytes   g.   Cytoplasmic extension of cell

_____ Pedicel   h.   Create visceral layer of nephron capsule

LEVEL 2. CHECK YOUR UNDERSTANDING

1. The condition known as metabolic acidosis is characterized by a low blood pH from accumulation of metabolic acids. How does it affect urine pH?

2. How will low blood pressure (hypotension) affect glomerular filtration?

3. Why do urinary tract infections, which involve the urethra and urinary bladder, more often affect females than males?

4. After a meal rich with carbohydrates, why does urine have some glucose?

LEVEL 3. APPLY YOUR KNOWLEDGE TO REAL LIFE

1. Which of the following hormones could be administered to decrease blood pressure: ADH, aldosterone, or ANP?

2. In the disease diabetes insipidus, the posterior pituitary gland does not release ADH. Why does this condition lead to dehydration of the organism?

Chapter 22

The Reproductive System

LEARNING OBJECTIVES

In this chapter you will find information on anatomy and physiology of reproduction and the reproductive system. When you have read this chapter, you will be able to:

1. Explain the basic difference between mitosis and meiosis.

2. Describe special characteristics of meiosis in males and females.

3. Compare the anatomy of male and female reproductive organs.

4. Understand the physiology of reproduction and hormonal control of reproductive cycles.

INTRODUCTION

The reproductive system includes the primary sex organs: gonads (testes and ovaries); their products: hormones and gametes (sperm cells and oocytes); and accessory organs: ducts and external reproductive organs that facilitate the reproductive process. The principal function of the reproductive system is directed not on the individual well-being, but on the well-being of populations and species in general. Reproduction facilitates the survival and evolution of species. Reproduction is based on production of haploid gametes, usage of anatomic structures, and behavioral adaptations.

22.1   Overview of Male and Female Reproductive Systems

Development of the Reproductive System

Both male and female gonads are paired structures. Both arise from the genital ridge—a swelling on the dorsal wall of the embryo abdominal cavity. At that period of their development, gonads have no specific male or female characteristics and, because of that, are called **indifferent gonad**. From the very beginning, gonads contain **germ cells**: future sperm or eggs. As a matter of fact, germ cells develop outside of gonads. They arise outside the embryo in the extraembryonic endoderm of the yolk sac and migrate to the genital ridge (fig. 22.1). In females they populate the cortex of the genital ridge. In males they take up residency in the

Primordial germ cells – gonocytes – appear among endoderm in dorsal wall of yolk sac. Gonocyte migrate along dorsal mesentery of hindgut into the gonadal ridges and induce (!) gonad development.

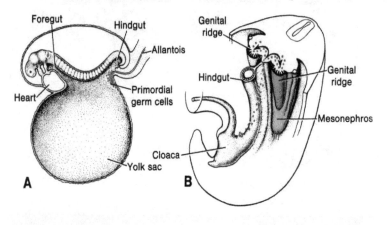

FIGURE 22.1   Development of the Reproductive System. A. An Embryo with Primordial Germ Cells in the Wall of the Yolk Sac Close to the Attachment of the Allantois. B. Migration Pathway of the Primordial Germ Cells along the Wall of the Hindgut and Dorsal Mesentery into the Genital Ridge.

medulla. Later in males the medulla of the genital ridge develops into the seminiferous tubules inside the testes. Testes migrate outside of the body through the inguinal canal at the bottom of the abdominal wall to the scrotum. The temperature in the scrotum is around 5–8°C lower than inside the body. When the testes fail to descend (a condition called cryptorchidism), sperm production decreases or even completely ceases. Why some mammals have a scrotum whereas others do not is not understood. When germ cells populate the genital ridge cortex, they become oogonia. Ovaries remain inside the abdominopelvic cavity. Oogonia become completely surrounded by the connective tissue cells called pregranulosa cells. The **primordial follicle** is a structure composed of the oogonia at the center surrounded by pregranulosa cells. They remain in the cortical layer of the ovary, whereas the center of the ovary or its medulla connects the ovary with the rest of the organism through the blood vessels, lymph vessels, and nerve fibers. As seen in fig. 22.1.A, there are orange primordial germ cells at the base of the yolk sac. Primordial germ cells arise from a layer of cells in the inner cell mass of the blastocyst, which is located near a yolk sac. During the next step of embryo development, called gastrulation, they migrate through the area called primitive streak into the hindgut and continue to move until they reach the genital ridge that later develops into gonads: ovaries or testes. The passage of migration germ cells to the genital ridge in fig. 22.1.B is an example of programmed body development driven by activity of so-called morphogens. These genes code production and release of special protein signaling molecules. Primordial germ cells driven by positive chemotaxis move towards the source of these proteins' secretion in the genital ridge.

Overview of Meiosis

The major event of the reproductive process is a fusion of gametes: sperm and egg cells, called **fertilization**. At fertilization, a new diploid cell known as a **zygote** emerges. To create a diploid zygote, both gametes have to be haploid; that is, have a single set of chromosomes. The possessing of only a single set of chromosomes is a principal difference among gametes (sperm and ova) and other cells of the body, which are called **somatic cells**. Somatic cells have diploid set of chromosomes: one set came from mother and the other from the father. Both paternal and maternal chromosomes are matched in pairs: every maternal chromosome with a particular set of genes has a complementary paternal chromosome with the same set of genes. These complementary chromosomes are known as **homologous chromosomes**. Thus, every diploid somatic cell has a set of two pairs of homologous chromosomes. Even when the set of genes in homologous chromosomes remains the same, the genes may carry different states of the same character (for example, eye color may be brown or blue, or hair color may be black or white). These different states of the gene are called **alleles**. Somatic cells reproduce through the cell division that guarantees an absolutely identical diploid set of chromosomes to all daughter cells. This type of cellular division is called mitosis (see chapter 3, page 90). At the same time, gametes are haploid cells; that is, they have a single set of unpaired chromosomes. In opposite to somatic cells, the production of gametes requires a special type of cell division that both sperm and egg cells have a haploid set of chromosomes, which are not required to be genetic identical. The cell division that makes it possible is called **meiosis**.

VETERINARY APPLICATION

Cloning of organisms is the procedure of creating a new organism that is genetically identical to the prototype. This process is an asexual method of reproduction, where fertilization is absent. For reproductive cloning, a nucleus from the somatic cell is transferred inside an egg whose own nucleus has been removed. If the nucleus transplantation is successful and the egg begins to divide, it is transferred into the uterus of the surrogate mother. The first successful clone was Dolly, a Finn-Dorset ewe. Dolly was formed from a cell from the udder of her six-year old biological mother. It took 434 attempts before an embryo was successful. She was born on July 5, 1996, but only announced to the world on February 22, 1997. The modern cloning techniques have been successfully performed on the following species: northern leopard frog, carp, mice, rhesus monkey, pig, gaur, cattle, cat, rat, mule, horse, dog, wolf, Pyrenean ibex, camel, goat, and macaque monkey.

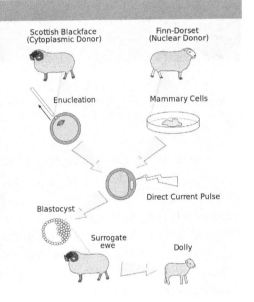

Both divisions require that cell be prepared. During S phase of interphase, the cell doubles structures that have to be distributed between daughter cells. First of all, the cell makes second copies of all DNA molecules. Originally, every chromosome has only one DNA molecule. In S phase the cell makes absolutely identical copies of each DNA (see chapter 3, page 88). These DNAs are bound with proteins. The complex of DNA and nuclear proteins is called **chromatin**. Every chromatin contains only one DNA molecule. The chromatins that have identical DNAs are called **sister chromatids**. After duplication of DNA, all chromosomes possess two chromatids. Until the cell division sister chromatids remain bound to each other by a special complex protein structure called **kinetochore** at a region known as **centromere**. That is why, when at the beginning of cell division chromosomes condense and become visible under the light microscope, you can see that they have the shape of the letter *X*. Two arms of this letter are two sister chromatids bind at centromere (fig. 22.2). When DNAs, centrosomes, and some other important structures are duplicated, the cell is ready to divide.

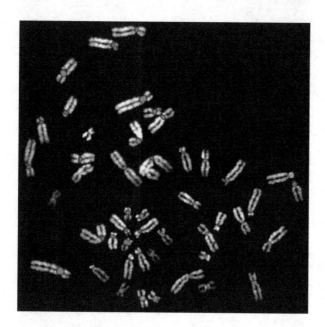

FIGURE 22.2   Orangutan Chromosomes. Each Chromosome Contains Two Sister Chromatids Bound at Centromere.

Meiosis consists of two consecutive divisions: **meiosis I** and **meiosis II**. By the analogy to mitosis, particular steps of both divisions are called: Prophase, Metaphase, Anaphase, and Telophase. Thus, there are **prophase I**, **metaphase I**, **anaphase I**, **telophase I**, and **prophase II**, **metaphase II**, **anaphase II**, and **telophase II**. Remember that at the beginning of the meiosis the germ cell (oogonia) is diploid; that is, it has two sets (2n) of homologous chromosomes. At the end of the meiotic division it is haploid or it has only one set (1n) of chromosomes.

Prophase I. The first phase of meiosis I is a prophase I. It begins with condensation of chromatin. The threads of chromatin fold many times, which makes them thick and short. Nucleoli disappear and the nuclear envelope defragments. Centrioles become visible. They move in opposite directions and project spindle fibers. Prophase I does not exactly repeat what happened in mitotic prophase. In the middle of prophase I, homologous chromosomes organize in pairs and firmly stick to each other side by side. This process is called **synapsis**. Two synapsis homologous chromosomes create a **tetrad**. As you can see, every tetrad has four chromatids: two chromatids represent maternal chromosome, and two other chromatids are from paternal chromosome. In place of the strongest attachment, chromatids may exchange segments of their chromatin. Both chromosomes break down at the synapsis and then reconnect again. The reconnection happens accidentally, and part of the maternal chromosome may reconnect with the paternal chromosome and vice versa. This process is known as **crossing over**. Crossing over does not create new genes, but it creates a new gene combinations. If you take into account that every gene may have a few alternate states or alleles, you will see that crossing over may create new combinations of characters that did not exist together in the parents (fig. 22.3). For example, chromosome may have a combination of black hair and blue eyes, whereas the father has black hair and brown eyes and the mother is blond with blue eyes. The crossing over makes sister chromatids genetically different and, because of that, every gamete is unique. At the end of the prophase I nuclear envelop disappears, centrosomes reach opposite sides (poles) of the cell, and spindle fibers from centrosomes are attached to centromeres of tetrads.

Metaphase I. In metaphase I tetrads line up along the equatorial or metaphase plane. Spindle fibers connect centromeres of homologous chromosomes with centrosomes (fig. 22.4).

Anaphase I. In anaphase I spindle fibers shorten and pull homologous chromosomes to opposite poles. After separation of homologous chromosomes, every pole of the cell gets only one set of chromosomes (1n). Another very important detail is that because in tetrads homologous chromosomes occupy their position accidentally, the combination of these haploid sets of chromosomes is also an accident. This random

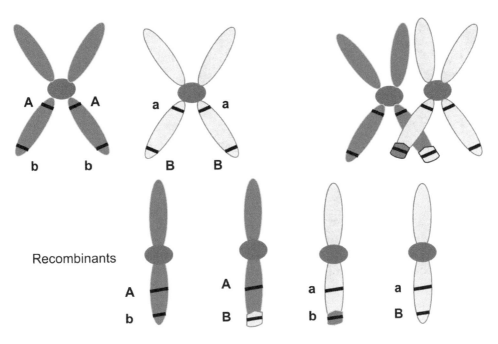

Recombinants

FIGURE 22.3   Tetrad Formation and Crossing Over.

tossing of homologous chromosomes is called **independent assortment**. Independent assortment, like crossing over, does not create new characters, but produces a new combination of chromosomes. Thus, independent assortment and crossing over lead to production of gametes with unique combination of characters. That is why all offspring (except monozygotic siblings) of the same parents are different in one or another way. As you can see the reduction of total number of chromosomes from 2n to 1n happens in anaphase I. That is why meiosis I is also called **reduction division**. Remember that every chromosome still has two sister chromatids!

Telophase I. In telophase I, chromosomes aggregate around poles. Two nuclear envelopes reorganize around them (very often this process does not end by a complete reconstruction of the nuclear membrane). The phase ends by the division of the cytoplasm and separation of two daughter cells called **cytokinesis**. The cytokinesis begins with development of the circular groove on the surface of the maternal cell called a **cleavage furrow**. The cleavage furrow deepens inside the cell until the two daughter cells split. These cells have a single (haploid) set of chromosomes and are genetically different from each other and from the maternal cell because of the crossing over and independent assortment.

Prophase II. There is not another DNA duplication before meiosis II. Two cells begin meiosis II with a haploid set of chromosomes. Every chromosome has two sister chromatids. Prophase II is very similar to prophase of mitosis. During this phase, the nuclear membrane degrades again, chromosomes condense, centrosomes begin their travel to poles, and spindle fibers' aster develops (fig. 22.4).

Metaphase II. At metaphase II centrosomes occupy their polar positions and spindle fibers connect them with centromeres. A haploid set of chromosomes lined the metaphase plate.

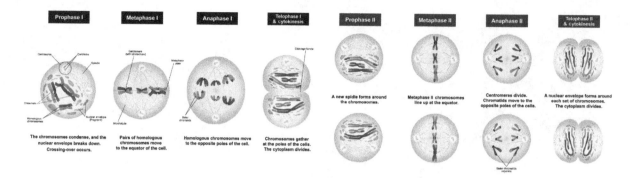

FIGURE 22.4   Meiosis.

Anaphase II. In anaphase II spindle fibers shorten and every chromosome splits into two sister chromatids. Pulled by the spindle apparatus, sister chromatids move towards opposite poles. From the moment when sister chromatids separate, they become chromosomes and begin independent life. Note, that these are sister chromatids (not homologous chromosomes, like in anaphase I) that are separated in anaphase II.

Telophase II. Telophase II accomplishes the process. Chromosomes concentrate around poles. A new nuclear membrane forms around them. Cytokinesis separates daughter cells. Centrosomes and chromosomes become invisible. The original germinal cell with diploid set of chromosomes (Tasmanian devil has 2n = 14, American mink has 30, cat has 38, horse and guinea pig have 64, dog has 78 chromosomes) divides into 4 daughter cells with haploid set of chromosomes (Tasmanian devil 1n = 7, American mink has 15, cat has 19, horse and guinea pig have 32, and dog has 39).

The process of meiosis, described above, outlines production of sperm cells, called **spermatogenesis**, and egg cells, called **oogenesis**. However, there are very important differences between these two processes. Spermatogenesis beginning at puberty continues through the whole male life without significant break or hold between phases; that is, once beginning meiosis continuously proceeds to the end with development of four daughter cells that later develop in sperm cells (fig. 22.5). In oogenesis, as a rule, only one

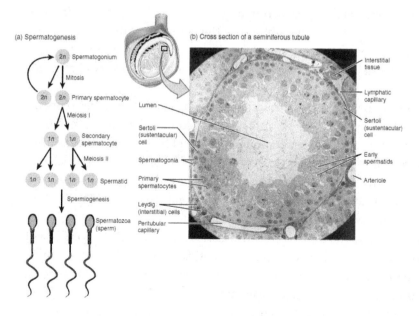

FIGURE 22.5   Spermatogenesis.

cell survives and develops in the ovum, whereas other daughter cells create so-called **polar bodies** that later degrade. Oogenesis proceeds with breaks, it is not a continuous process. It begins during the female prenatal period of development. At that time all oogonia undergo meiosis. The first time the process is arrested at prophase I before the female birth. The second arrest occurs at the stage of secondary oocyte in metaphase II during the female adulthood before the ovulation. In females meiosis completes only after fertilization. The entrance of the sperm cell inside the ovum triggers accomplishment of the meiosis.

CHECK YOUR UNDERSTANDING

- Describe the difference between prophase of mitosis and prophase I of meiosis.

- What processes make all gametes genetically different?

- How do somatic cells differ from gonads?

- At which moment of meiosis do cells become haploid?

22.2   Anatomy of the Male Reproductive System

Testes

Testes are male primary sex organs. They are paired and have two major roles: production of sperm cells and secretion of hormones (fig. 22.6). In most mammals the testes are located outside the abdominopelvic cavity. In this case, they are suspended in a pouch called **scrotum**, but remain connected to the abdominal cavity via an **inguinal canal**. Some mammals have testes descended into the scrotum temporary only during the breeding period (chipmunks and squirrels, for example). In sirenians, elephants, sloths, and armadillos, the testes remain inside the body cavity.

Scrotum is composed of skin, connective tissue membranes, and smooth muscles. Smooth muscles of scrotum are known as **dartos muscles**. Together with smooth muscles of the **spermatic cord** called **cremaster muscles** they maintain temperature inside testes around 5–8°C below the body temperature. A tonus of this muscles is responsible for the wrinkled (rugose) appearance of the scrotum. Two membranes or tunics surround testes. The external membrane is called the **tunica vaginalis**. Serous membrane underlines the skin. Like all serous membranes, it is folded. The external fold attaches to the walls of scrotum and is called the **parietal vaginal tunic**. The internal fold

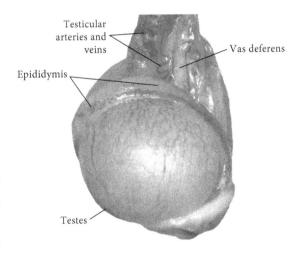

Testicular arteries and veins

Vas deferens

Epididymis

Testes

FIGURE 22.6   Cat Testicle.

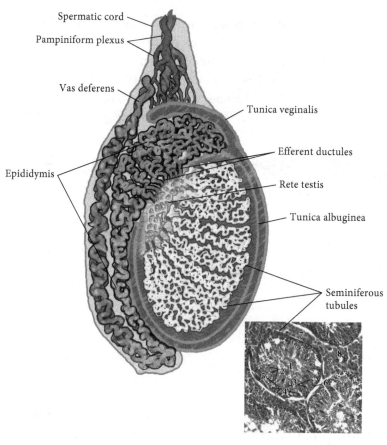

Spermatic cord
Pampiniform plexus
Vas deferens
Tunica veginalis
Efferent ductules
Rete testis
Tunica albuginea
Epididymis
Seminiferous tubules

FIGURE 22.7   Testes.

covers testes and is called the **visceral vaginal tunic**. The **vaginal cavity** is a space between the parietal and visceral layers. The cavity is filled with film of serous fluid, which provides smooth frictionless movement of testes inside the scrotum. The second tunic is called the **tunica albuginea**. It is a strong connective tissue membrane. Its folds invaginate deep inside the testes and there separates internal space into chambers or **lobules**. Every lobule contains one to four tightly coiled **seminiferous tubules**. The walls of seminiferous tubules are made of **spermatogenic** and **sustentacular cells**, surrounded by **myoid cells**. Spermatogenic cells, as their name suggests, are germinal cells that produce sperm cells by meiosis. Sustentacular cells support sperm cell production and direct sperm development. These cells produce testicular fluid, which nourish developing sperm. The myoid cells

are contractile cells. Their contraction pushes sperm cells and testicular fluid off the seminiferous tubules and out of the testes into the epididymis. The space between seminiferous tubules inside the lobules is populated by **interstitial** or **Leydig cells** that produce male sex hormones. All hormones produced by testes are steroids and collectively are named **androgens**. The principal androgen of testes is **testosterone**. This hormone controls the development and facilitates activity of the secondary male sex organs. At the end seminiferous tubules are organized in a tubular network called the **rete testis**. Sperm cells leave the rete testis through the **efferent ductules** and accumulate in a long, convoluted tube called the **epididymis** (fig. 22.7).

Scrotum gets blood supply from the blood vessels in the spermatic cord. The **testicular artery** takes blood from the abdominal aorta just behind renal artery and carries it to the testes. The venous blood vessels create a complex network—the **pampiniform venous plexus**—that drains blood back into the **testicular vein** and then the posterior vena cava. Pampiniform venous plexus surrounds incoming warm blood in testicular artery and cool it. When arterial blood enters testes, it has a lower temperature than blood inside the body. This mechanism helps maintain a low temperature in the testes.

Cryptorchidism is a result of abnormal development, when the testes are retained in the **abdomen** or inside the **inguinal canal**. The testes develop near the kidneys within the abdomen and normally descend into the scrotum by two months of age. In certain dogs it may occur later, but rarely after six months of age. Cryptorchidism occurs in all breeds, but the toy breeds, including toy poodles, Pomeranians, and Yorkshire terriers, are at higher risk. Approximately 75 percent of the cases of cryptorchidism involve only one retained testicle and 25 percent involve failure of both testicles to descend into the scrotum. The right testicle is more than twice as likely to be retained as the left testicle. Cryptorchidism affects approximately 1.2 percent of all dogs. If both testicles are retained, the dog may be infertile. The retained testicles continue to produce testosterone, but generally fail to produce sperm. Frequently, a retained testicle become cancerous. The congenital abnormalities associated with cryptorchidism include patellar luxation (dislocated kneecap), shortened or kinked tail, tetralogy of fallot (a life-threatening heart defect), tarsal deformity (abnormal legs), microphthalmia (abnormally small eyes), and upper eyelid agenesis (eyelids that don't develop), and spermatic cord torsion (twisting onto itself).

Neutering and removal of the retained testicle(s) are recommended as soon as possible. There are several good reasons for neutering a dog with cryptorchidism. The first is to remove the genetic defect from the breed line. Cryptorchid dogs should never be bred. Second, dogs with a retained testicle are more likely to develop a testicular tumor (cancer) in the retained testicle. Finally, dogs with a retained testicle typically develop the undesirable characteristics associated with intact males like urine marking and aggression.

Ducts and Glands

From testes sperm cells travel through a long system of ducts. At first, they enter the epididymis, than move along **vas deferens, ejaculatory duct, prostatic urethra, membranous urethra, penile** or **spongy urethra**, to the **external urethral orifice**. Epididymis is a long, convoluted tube. Inside, the ductus epididymis is lined by a mucous membrane: a pseudostratified ciliated epithelium with long immovable microvilli called **stereocilia**. Sperm cells that enter the epididymis from the rete testis and efferent ductules are immature. At that time they are still incapable of independent movement and cannot fertilize the egg. In the epididymis sperm cells are accumulated and maturate. Ciliated cells of mucous membrane absorb excess of the testicular fluid and release in the lumen of ductus epididymis nutrients to maintain sperm cells' life and stimulate their development. Fluid in the long epididymis moves slowly, and sperm cells have enough time to become mature sperm, when they leave the epididymis and enter the next duct, the **vas deferens**.

The vas deferens extends through the spermatic cord and enters inside the pelvic cavity through the inguinal canal. It passes along the latero-dorsal sides of the urinary bladder and on the dorsal side of the urinary bladder enlarges in a wide sac called **ampulla**. The organization of the walls of the vas deferens is similar to the other ducts. The lumen of the duct is lined with three layers or tunics. The innermost layer is a mucous tunic or mucosa. It is composed of pseudostratified columnar epithelium resting on the areolar connective tissue that binds mucosa with middle layer. The middle layer or tunica muscularis is made of smooth muscles. Muscles are organized in three layers: internal and external muscular layers have a longitudinal position of muscle fibers, whereas middle muscular layer has circular muscle fibers. When muscles of all three layers contract together, their contraction creates wave-like movement or peristalsis of the walls of the vas deferens. Peristalsis pushes sperm cells along the duct. The external layer is a fibrous tunic or adventitia. It is made of fibrous connective tissue. This layer gives strength to the walls of the vas deferens and binds it with other internal structures. Sperm in the vas deferens are already mature, but

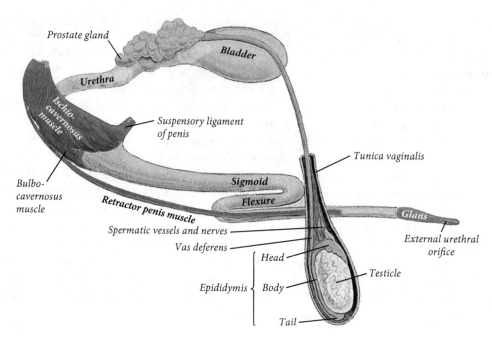

FIGURE 22.8 Bull Reproductive Organs.

are still remain immovable. The peristaltic movement of the walls of the vas deferens propel them toward the ampulla and to the ejaculatory duct (fig. 22.8).

The ejaculatory duct is short. It receives input from the ducts of the **seminal vesicle**. The seminal vesicle is an exocrine gland located on the dorsal side of the urinary bladder. The gland secretes **seminal fluid**, a yellowish secretion that constitutes 60 to 70 percent of the total semen volume. The principal components of the seminal fluid are:

1. Fructose that nourishes sperm cells and provides fuel for ATP production.
2. Prostaglandins, which stimulate smooth muscle contractions in male and female reproductive organs during intercourse. Prostaglandins also stimulate sperm cells movement.
3. Proteins and enzymes that together with proteins of the prostate gland create a temporary clot of semen inside the female reproductive organs.
4. Electrolytes that increases alkalinity of the semen to neutralize acids inside male and female reproductive tracts.

After receiving secretion of the seminal vesicle, ejaculatory duct travels through the wall of the prostate gland and falls into the urethra. In the urethra the secretion of the seminal vesicles receives the secretion of the **prostate gland** and **bulbourethral** or **Cowper's glands**. The secretion of the prostate gland constitutes about 20 to 30 percent of the semen and contains the following:

1. Citrate is a component of the Crab's cycle. Sperm need it to manufacture ATP.
2. Prostatic specific antigen (PSA) and other enzymes that dissolve the semen clot in the female reproductive tract and free sperm to move to the meeting with the egg.

3. Bactericide enzymes that prevent bacterial growth inside the female reproductive system.
4. Electrolytes that bind hydrogen ions and neutralize acids in the male urethra and female reproductive tract.

The prostatic gland surrounds the urethra. It is covered by a fibrous capsule. The smooth muscles in the walls of the prostate gland contract during ejaculation and eject prostatic secretion into the urethra.

Cowper's glands are pared compound tubule-alveolar glands. They empty their secretion into the membranous urethra just at the base of the penis. Glands produce alkaline fluid with mucoproteins that neutralizes acids in urethra prior to ejaculation and lubricates **glans penis** during copulation. They are composed of several lobules held together by a fibrous capsule. Each lobule has a number of small alveolar sacs with secretory cells, lined by columnar epithelial cells. The sacs are open into a duct that joins with the ducts of other lobules to form a single excretory duct. Glands are surrounded by the sphincter urethrae muscle. During the ejaculation sphincter urethrae muscle contracts and empties glands' secretion. At the same time, its contraction closes urethra and traps urea inside the urinary bladder (fig. 22.10). Dogs have no Cowper's glands (fig. 22.9).

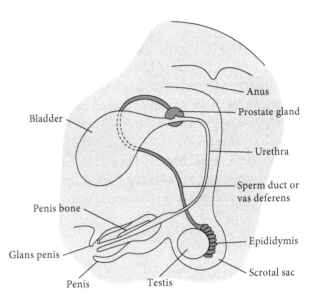

FIGURE 22.9   Male Reproductive System of Dog.

VETERINARY APPLICATION

Testicular torsion is a rare pathological disorder of the male testis characterized by mechanical torsion of the spermatic cord and consequent testicular necrosis and infertility.

Mechanical torsion usually results in constriction of blood flow to the affected testis, edema, and venous congestion. Ischemia longer than six hours usually results in azoospermia and permanent testicular atrophy. In dogs, this is commonly associated with Sertoli cells tumor and seminoma or germ cells' tumor. Among other breeds, boxers with testicular torsion have the highest predisposition to the cryptorchidism. A retained testis is more susceptible than a scrotal testis to spermatic cord torsion, and the risk of this condition is increased even more with progressive enlargement of the neoplastic organ. Clinically affected dogs usually present with acute testicular and inguinal pain. The testis is often enlarged and tender. Dogs are frequently anorectic and display locomotory difficulty. A definitive diagnosis usually requires exploratory surgery. Bilateral or unilateral orchidectomy is usually curative in dogs.

Penis

Three regions of the penis are: root, body or shaft, and **glans penis**. The skin surrounding the penis is loose and forms circular folds around the glans penis called **prepuce**. The penile urethra passes the length of the penis and opens at the top of the glans penis by the external urethral orifice. An erectile tissue called **corpus spongiosum** wraps around the urethra. That is why the penile urethra is also called the **spongy urethra**. There are three cylindrical bodies in the penis made of erectile tissue: a single corpus spongiosum that surrounds the urethra, and two dorsally located **corpora cavernosa**. In the root of the penis, corpora cavernosa split and form two **crura** that anchor the penis in the pelvis by attaching it to the rami of ischium bone. The erectile tissue has a dense network of blood vessels with small vascular sections. At sexual arousal, increased blood flow fills these sections and erectile bodies engorge, expand, and become stiff. The blood supply comes from the pudendal arteries, branches of the internal iliac arteries. Pudendal arteries branch on **dorsal** and **deep penile arteries**. Dorsal arteries serve to the skin of the penis and corpus spongiosum. Deep arteries carry their blood to both corpora cavernosa. Groups of **superficial** and **deep dorsal veins** drain blood from the penis. Superficial veins take blood from the skin, whereas deep veins receive blood from spongy bodies. Remember that veins have comparatively week muscular layer in their walls and cannot keep their shape effectively, like arteries. When spongy bodies expand during intercourse, they press on the veins, veins collapse, and blood is locked inside spongy bodies (22.10).

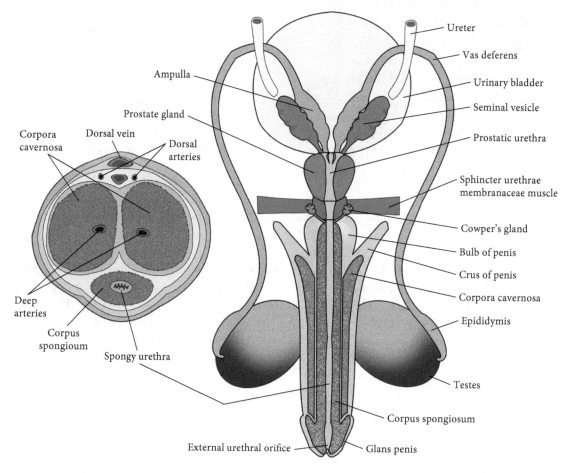

FIGURE 22.10   Human Male Reproductive Organs.

Most of placental mammals have **os penis** or **baculum**. The bone is located above the urethra (fig. 22.11). It is absent in humans, but present among other primates (gorilla and chimpanzee, for example).

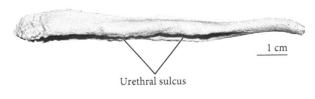

FIGURE 22.11   Os Penis of Dog.

Marsupials (like a kangaroo), carnivores (like a dog), bovines, and deer have a long S-shaped curve of the root of their penis. A retractor penis muscle is attached to this curve. When the penis is not erected, this muscle retracts it inside the body (fig. 22.8). During the sexual arousal retractor muscle relaxes and penis expands outside. In most mammals the penis is single, but in marsupials it is divided to fit into two female lateral vaginas (fig. 22.12).

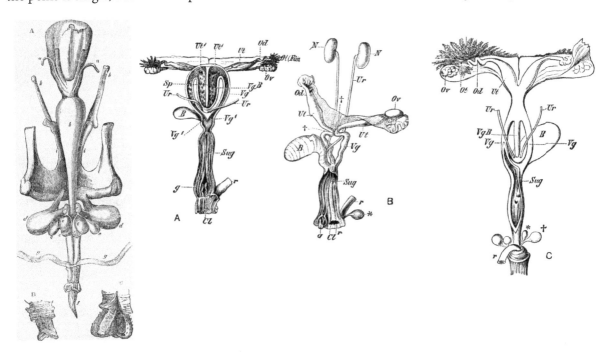

FIGURE 22.12   Reproductive System of Kangaroo (Marsupials).

CHECK YOUR UNDERSTANDING

- Where are sperm cells produced?

- What is the principal role of the epididymis?

- Describe the pathway of sperm from the place of their production to outside during ejaculation.

- What is the major function of the corpus spongiosum and corpora cavernosa?

- Describe glands of the male reproductive system and their function.

22.3   Physiology of the Male Reproductive System

Spermatogenesis

Spermatogenesis is the process of sperm production. It begins at puberty and continues throughout the whole male life. The process begins from the **spermatogonia**, a stem cells with diploid set of chromosomes (2n) inside the seminiferous tubules. When the male becomes mature, some of these cells develop in **primary spermatocytes**. Primary spermatocytes are still diploid. Primary spermatocytes are pushed by other spermatogonia cells toward the center of the seminiferous tubule. When the primary spermatocyte lost connection with the membranous walls of the seminiferous tubules, it undergoes meiosis I and becomes a **secondary spermatocyte**. Secondary spermatocytes are haploid. Two secondary spermatocytes come through the meiosis II. The final result of this division is the four haploid cells called **spermatids**. Spermatids continue their travel toward the lumen in the center of the seminiferous tubules. They lost most of their cytoplasm and organelles, grow a long tail (flagellum) and acrosome. When they reach the lumen, they eventually become sperm cells. However, they are still not active and cannot move. For that, they have to complete their maturation in epididymis and are activated by fluids from the seminal vesicles.

For normal development, sperm cells need help from supporting sustentacular cell, also called **nurse** or **Sertoli cell**. Sertoli cells are long and extend from the basement membrane of the wall to the lumen of the seminiferous tubules. Tight junctions bind sustentacular cells in a continuous network that separates developing sperm cells from the male immune system. Sperm cells has a unique haploid set of chromosomes. As a result, recessive traits that are never expressed in somatic diploid cells may be presented in haploid gametes. That is why sperm cells often have surface proteins that cannot be recognized by the male immune system as a "self-cells." The blood-testis barrier created by sustentacular cells prevents attack of white blood cells on the sperm. Sustentacular cells also create a structural frame for the stem cells and secrete testicular fluid that makes a media and delivers nutrients for sperm.

Hormonal Control of Male Reproduction

The hormonal regulation of the spermatogenesis and male sexual behavior is based on multilevel organized negative feedback mechanisms. The hypothalamus, anterior pituitary gland, and interstitial cells of the testis play principal role in this process. The relationship of these glands in the male reproductive function creates so called hypothalamic-pituitary-gonadal axis. The hypothalamus in this axis is a master gland that also connects sensory input with production and release of sexual hormones. The gonadotropin-releasing hormone (GnRH) from hypothalamus stimulates the anterior pituitary gland to secrete gonadotropins: follicle stimulating and luteinizing hormones (in males, this hormone is also called interstitial cell-stimulating hormone or ICSH, to emphasize its effect on interstitial cells in testes). In males LH stimulates interstitial cells to produce and release testosterone. FSH stimulates sustentacular cells in seminiferous tubules to release **androgen binding protein (ABP)** and hormone **inhibin**. Testosterone and inhibin have negative impact on hypothalamus and anterior pituitary gland. Inhibin decreases the release of FSH. The testosterone inhibits secretion of GnRH. In adult male level of the testosterone remains comparatively stable during the whole life with a slow steady decrease with aging. However, we know that most mammals reproduce seasonally or have another type of reproductive cycles. Studies demonstrate that such factors as temperature and body weight may influence these cycles; but it seems that the female reproductive cycle has a principal impact on male sexual activity. Seasonal production and release of pheromones and change of behavior are among these principal factors.

Testosterone is a well-known hormone that identifies male behavior together with stimulation of sperm production (fig. 22.13). Other hormones that influence male behavior are oxytocin and vasopressin. Oxytocin is produced by the hypothalamus and released through the posterior pituitary gland. It has been shown that in rats and guinea pigs, interstitial cells secrete testicular oxytocin. The hormone causes smooth muscles contraction. In males during the copulation the hormone triggers smooth muscles of vas deference and urethra to contract and causes ejaculation. In males it also decreases anxiety and stress, facilitates social behavior and inhibits avoidance. Oxytocin also increases empathy. In wild chimpanzees, when they shared food with a non-kin-related chimpanzee, the oxytocin level increases as were measured through their urine. Oxytocin affects social distance between adult males and females, and may be responsible, at least in part, for romantic attraction and monogamous pair formation. The researchers suggested that oxytocin may help promote fidelity within monogamous relationships. For this reason, it is sometimes referred to as the "bonding hormone." Vasopressin regulates salt and water balance that results in blood pressure. In males this hormone also initiates aggression and is a foundation of male behavior in family protection and fighting with invaders.

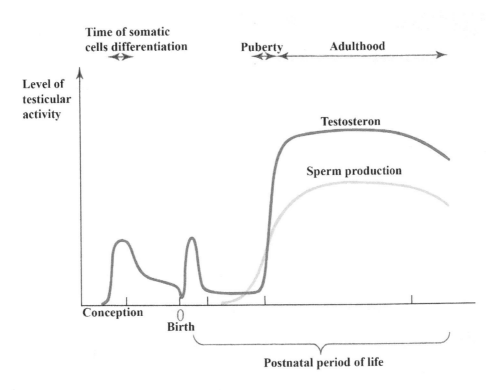

FIGURE 22.13   Relation between Sperm Production and Level of Testosterone at Male Adulthood.

CHECK YOUR UNDERSTANDING

- Which cells produce male sex hormones?

- What is the function of semen?

- Describe the role of the sustentacular cells.

- Describe role of the hypothalamus-anterior pituitary gland-testes axis.

VETERINARY APPLICATION

Studies of two different rodent species—the prairie vole (*Microtus ochrogaster*) and mountain vole (*Microtus montanus*)—show that vasopressin and oxytocin control social and monogamy behaviors. The prairie vole is a monogamous species. The animals form family bond during mating. Over a 24-hour period, a pair copulates 15 to 30 times. Their behavior significantly changes and they demonstrate strong preference of each other's company. The male becomes aggressive toward other males. Both parents care for their young even several weeks after weaning. In contrast to that, montane voles do not form family bonds after mating. They breed promiscuously and the male leaves the female after copulation. He does not care about their young. Even the female abandons her offspring two to three weeks after the birth.

The hormones vasopressin and oxytocin control vasoconstriction and smooth muscles contraction respectively. They also play role of neurotransmitters in the CNS. The study demonstrates that injection of the oxytocin into the cerebral ventricles of the brain of unmated prairie vole female causes her to form a pair bond with a male without mating. An injection of the vasopressin into the cerebral ventricles of an unmated prairie vole male makes him aggressive toward other males. The study of distribution of postsynaptic receptors for oxytocin and vasopressin the brain of two vole species show that monogamous prairie voles have a high density of oxytocin receptors in the nucleus accumbens and a high density of vasopressin receptors in the ventral pallidum. The promiscuous montane voles do not have both receptors in these areas. Both areas are part of the rewarding brain system associated with reinforcement and conditioning of particular behavior. A current hypothesis states that mating stimulates release of an increased amount of oxytocin and vasopressin, which activates the brain rewarding system and reinforces the formation of family bonds. The absence of receptors in the brain of montane voles explains their inability to create stable pairs.

22.4 Anatomy of the Female Reproductive System

Ovaries

Female primary sex organs are ovaries. Ovaries produce eggs and sex hormones. They are located on the lateral walls of the pelvic cavity. Ovaries are covered by the membranes that protect them and anchor their position inside the body. Three of these ligaments play a major role. The **broad ligament** is a large flat membrane that binds together ovaries, **uterine tubes**, and **uterus**, and attaches them to the pelvis. The **ovarian ligament** connects ovaries to the uterus near the entrance of uterine tubes. The **suspensory ligament** binds ovaries with wall of the pelvic cavity and carries **ovarian arteries**, **ovarian veins** and nerve fibers (fig. 22.14).

The superficial structures of ovaries constitute **ovarian cortex**. All follicles are located in this area. The internal region of ovaries is called **ovarian medulla**. Ovarian medulla houses blood vessels, lymphatic vessels, and nerves (fig. 22.15).

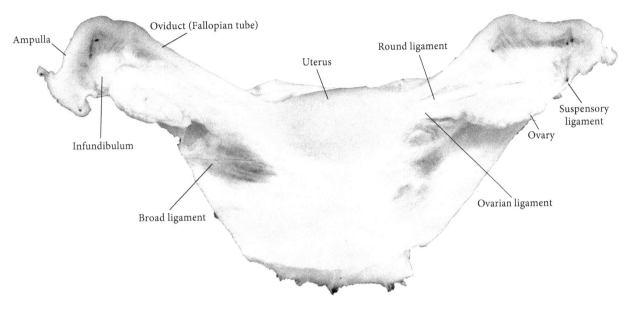

FIGURE 22.14 **Human Ovary.**

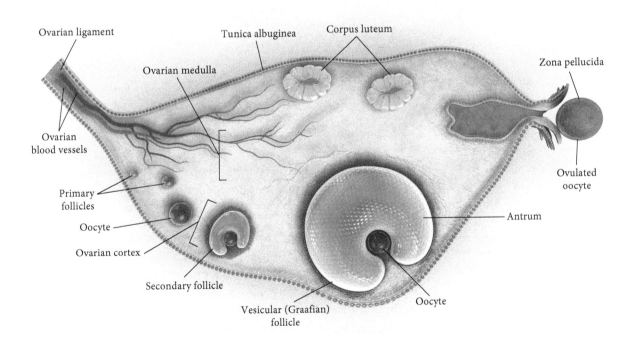

FIGURE 22.15 **Ovary.**

Oviducts

Oviducts also are called **fallopian tubes** or **uterine tubes**. Oviducts occupy retroperitoneal position. They lay on the lateral walls of the pelvic cavity and ventrally covered by the peritoneum. The broad ligament binds them with ovaries and walls of body cavity. Oviducts develop as lateral projections of the uterus. The region of oviduct connected with uterus is narrow and is known as **isthmus**. The enlarged opposite end of the oviduct is called **ampulla**. Ampulla turns around ovary and continues into the funnel-shaped **infundibulum** that opens nearby ovary. The opening of infundibulum is known as **ostium**. Oviduct does not physically connect with ovary. The ostium opens into the peritoneal cavity. The boarder of the ostium has finger-like projections called **fimbriae**. Fimbriae drape around the ovary (fig. 22.16).

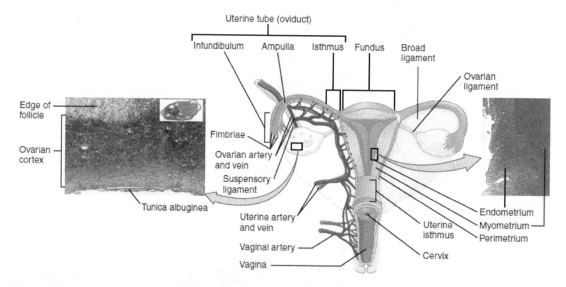

FIGURE 22.16   Human Female Reproductive Organs.

VETERINARY APPLICATION

Follicular cystitis may develop if the dog demonstrates a prolonged secretion of estrogen and continuous signs of estrus (heat) and attractiveness to males. Ovulation may not occur during such abnormal estrous cycles. Follicular cysts should be suspected in any dog showing signs of heat for more than 40 days. The condition is diagnosed through ultrasonography and laboratory tests. The treatment of choice is removal of the ovaries and uterus, which is curative. If the dog is to be bred, administration of drugs that cause ovulation might resolve the condition. However, these dogs must be monitored closely for uterine disease.

A wall of oviduct has four distinct layers: serosa, subserosa, lamina propria, and mucosa. Mucosa is made of a simple columnar epithelium. Ciliated columnar cells are dominate throughout the tube, but are most numerous in the infundibulum and ampulla. The rhythmic beat of the cilia creates a fluid flow along the oviduct. Estrogen increases the production of cilia on these cells. Between the ciliated cells there are **peg cells**, which secrete tubular fluid. This fluid contains nutrients for spermatozoa, oocytes, and zygotes. The secretion of the peg cells also promote capacitation of the sperm. Progesterone increases the number of peg cells, while estrogen increases their secretory activity. Lamina propria is a vascular connective tissue. Subserosa is composed of loose connective tissue, blood and lymphatic vessels, and two layers of smooth muscles. Smooth muscles in outer layer have longitudinal direction, whereas inner smooth muscles are circular. Contraction of these smooth muscles generates peristalsis. Serosa is a thin, outermost covering of the oviducts. Its major components are simple squamous epithelium and areolar connective tissue. Thin serous fluid secreted by the serosa lubricates the oviducts and prevents friction with neighboring organs. Fig. 22.17 shows ventral view of cat pelvis. In this figure, you can see a bicornuate uterus of the cat. The body of the uterus is located between urinary bladder on the ventral side and rectus on dorsal side. The uterine horns are long. Fallopian tubes are short ends of uterine horns. Fimbria of the fallopian tubes looks as enlarged clamps of pink tissue on the top of ovaries. The embryo implantation may occur along all length of uterine horns. Pink-colored suspensory ligaments above the ovaries carry blood and nerve fibers.

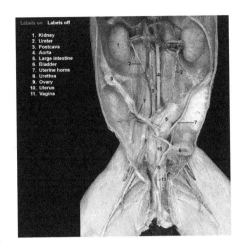

FIGURE 22.17   Female Cat Reproductive Organs.

During **ovulation**, when an immature **oocyte** leaves the ovary, a gentle beat of fimbriae pushes the oocyte inside the infundibulum. The further travel of oocyte inside the oviduct is facilitated by a rhythmic beating of the cilia together with peristaltic contraction of uterine tube. The **fertilization**, a process of fusion of egg and sperm cells, usually takes place in ampulla. A new diploid cell resulted from the fertilization is called **zygote**. Very soon the zygote divides. Divisions follow, and the zygote develops into a multicellular hollow inside ball. At this stage of development, it is called a **blastocyst**. During the process of transformation of the zygote into blastocyst a new organism continues its travel along the oviduct. Finally, the blastocyst enters the uterus through the isthmus. The further embryo development continues inside the uterus.

Uterus

The uterus is located in the pelvis between the rectum and urinary bladder. It is a hollow muscular organ. In many mammals it divides in two **uterine horns** that receive blastocysts from the oviducts. Its position is maintained by ligaments. **Lateral cervical ligament** extends from the cervix and vagina to the lateral wall of the pelvic cavity. **Uterosacral ligament** connects uterus to the sacrum; and **round ligament** binds uterus with ventral walls of the pelvic cavity (figs. 22.14 and 22.16).

VETERINARY APPLICATION

Metritis is an inflammation of the uterus that occurs after pregnancy. It is usually caused by bacterial infection. Factors such as prolonged delivery and retained fetuses or placentas may cause metritis. *Escherichia coli* bacteria are a common cause of infection of the uterus. The primary sign of infection is a pus-like discharge from the vulva. Female dogs with metritis are usually depressed, feverish, and may neglect their offspring. Pups may become restless and cry incessantly. The infection is diagnosed through physical examination, ultrasonography, and laboratory tests. Treatment includes a course of antibiotics.

A narrow opening of the uterus into the vagina is called the **cervix**. Cervix glands secrete mucus, which lubricates the vagina during intercourse. The biggest part of the uterus is called body. Uterine horns are extensions of the uterine body. There are four types of eutherian uteri. In the **duplex uterus**, there are two uteri and two cervixes. The duplex uterus is found in the lagomorphs and rodents. In the **bipartite uterus**, there are two uteri and one cervix. The bipartite uterus is found in the cetaceans and carnivores. In the **bicornuate uterus**, there is one single uterine body that on its distal end splits into two uterine horns. The bicornuate uterus is found in insectivores, some bats, perissodactyls, and artiodactyls. In the **simplex uterus**, the uterine horns are absent. The single uterus body opens into the vagina through a single cervix. (fig. 22.18). The simplex uterus is found in primates, some bats, and edentates.

Three layers compose the walls of the uterus: the **perimetrium**, **myometrium**, and **endometrium**. The outer layer, the perimetrium, is an extension of the parietal peritoneum. The thick myometrium is composed of smooth muscles. The innermost endometrium lines the uterine cavity. It is a mucous membrane, composed of simple columnar epithelium and lamina propria.

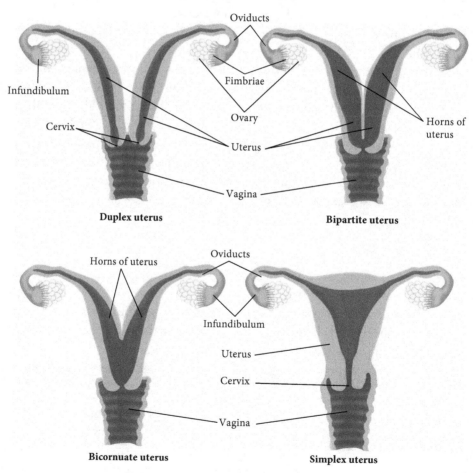

FIGURE 22.18   Four Types of Female Eutherian Mammals' Reproductive Organs.

Vagina

The vagina is an elastic muscular canal located between urethra and rectum. It extends from the cervix to **vulva**. Vulva is an external structure surrounded by **labia minora**. Vagina and urethra separately open into the vulva through **vaginal** and urethral **orifice**. Vaginal canal creates folds around the cervix called **fornix**. Transvers ridges of the vaginal wall are called **rugae** (fig. 22.16). Rugae increase stimulation of the penis during intercourse. The vaginal wall from the lumen outwards consists of a mucosa: a not keratinized stratified squamous epithelium and underlying connective tissue of lamina propria. A middle layer consists of two layers of smooth muscle: circular fibers above longitudinal fibers. An outer layer of connective tissue is called adventitia. Epithelial cells of mucosa secrete glycogen. Bacteria that live in vagina consume this glycogen by glycolysis and produce lactic acid. This helps maintain the acidic pH that keeps the vagina healthy and free of infection.

External Genitalia

External genitalia or vulva includes **labia majora**, **labia minora**, **clitoris**, and secretory glands. The **labia majora** (singular: **labium majus**) are two longitudinal cutaneous folds. The labia majora are homologous to the male scrotum. An outer surface of labia majora is covered by skin. It is keratinized pigmented with strong pubic hair stratified squamous epithelium. An inner wall of labia majora is a nonkeratinized smooth with large sebaceous follicles stratified squamous epithelium. Areolar tissue lays beneath epithelium and binds it with underlying adipose tissue and a tissue resembling the dartos muscles of the scrotum, besides vessels, nerves, and glands. Anteriorly the labia majora fuse and form the **anterior labial commissure**. Posteriorly, they are not joined, but appear to become lost in the neighboring integument, ending close to, and nearly parallel to, each other. Between the labia majora and the inner thighs are the **labiocrural folds**. Interlabiar sulcus separates the labia majora and labia minora. The labia minora extend from the clitoris obliquely downward, laterally, and backward on either side of the vulval vestibule, ending between the bottom of the vulval vestibule and the labia majora. The posterior ends of the labia minora are usually joined across the middle line by a fold of skin, named the **frenulum of labia minora** or **fourchette**. Lips of labia minora surround the clitoris. Both lips above the clitoris form a fold, which overhangs the **glans clitoridis** (head of the clitoris). This fold is named the **clitoral hood**. The clitoral hood is analogous to the prepuce of the male penis. The walls of labia minora are made of nonkeratinized stratified squamous epithelium with numerous sebaceous glands not associated with hair follicles (fig. 22.19).

The **clitoris** is a mammalian female secondary sex organ, also presented in some other animals. It is a homologue of male penis. The clitoris usually lacks a reproductive function. However, some animals urinate through the clitoris and use it for reproduction. For example, the spotted hyena, which has an especially large clitoris, urinates, mates, and gives birth via clitoris. The clitoris develops from a genital tubercle as penis does. The development of the genital tubercle into either a penis or clitoris depends on the presence or absence of the **protein tdf**, which is codified by a single gene on the Y chromosome. The clitoris is a complex structure. Like a penis it has erectile tissue and may expand during the sexual arousal. It also has a bone—**os clitoris** or **baubellum**—which is a homologue to the male baculum.

The **Bartholin's glands** or **greater vestibular glands** are two compound glands located on both sides of the vaginal orifice. They secrete mucus to lubricate the vagina and are homologous to bulbourethral glands of the males. The ducts of the gland are paired and open on the surface of the vulva.

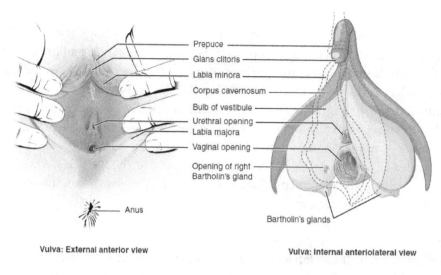

Vulva: External anterior view

Vulva: Internal anteriolateral view

FIGURE 22.19   Human External Genitalia.

Mammary Glands

A **mammary gland** is an exocrine gland in mammals that produces milk to feed offspring. Mammals get their name from the Latin word *mamma*, meaning "breast." The majority of specialists agree that they are a specialized type of apocrine sweet glands. The mammary glands are arranged in organs such as the breasts in primates (for example, humans and chimpanzees), the udder in ruminants (for example, cows, goats, and deer), and the dugs of other animals (for example, dogs and cats). Lactorrhea is an occasional production of milk. It can occur in any mammal, but in most mammals lactation occurs only among females during **gestation**. In a few mammalian species where observed male lactation. The basic structures of a mature mammary gland are the alveoli lined with milk-secreting cuboidal cells surrounded by myoepithelial cells. These alveoli join to form groups known as **lobules**. Each lobule has a **lactiferous duct** that drains into openings in the nipple. The myoepithelial cells contract under the oxytocin stimulation and eject the milk into the lobule lumen. The structure with one single lactiferous duct is called a **simple mammary gland**. A cluster of many lactiferous ducts (simple mammary glands) is called **complex mammary gland**. Humans, for example, have two complex mammary glands, one in each breast, and each complex mammary gland consists of 10–20 simple glands (fig. 22.20). The

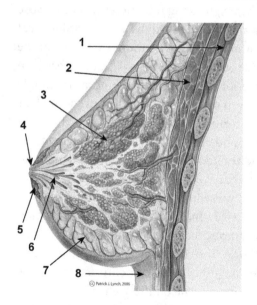

FIGURE 22.20   Human Mammary Gland. 1. Chest Wall (Intercostal Muscles); 2. Pectoralis Major Muscle; 3. Lobules; 4. Nipple; 5. Areola; 6. Lactiferous Duct; 7. Adipose Tissue; 8. Skin.

presence of more than two nipples is known as **polythelia** and the presence of more than two complex mammary glands as **polymastia**.

VETERINARY APPLICATION

Mastitis is an inflammation of the mammary gland(s) that occurs in dogs after giving birth. It is caused by a bacterial infection. Risk factors for developing mastitis include poor sanitary conditions, trauma inflicted by offspring, and whole-body infection. Mastitis may involve a single gland or multiple glands. Milk is usually abnormal in color or consistency. The affected glands are hot and painful. If mastitis progresses to a generalized infection, signs of illness such as fever, depression, poor appetite, and lethargy may be seen. The disease is diagnosed based on the physical examination and the dog's medical history. A test for bacteria to determine which antibiotic to use in cases of infective mastitis has to be performed. Warm compresses should be applied to the affected glands four to six times daily, and the puppies should be encouraged to nurse from these glands. An abscessed mammary gland should be lanced, drained, and treated as an open wound. At the time of weaning, there may be an abundance of milk and glands that are warm, swollen, and painful to touch, but the dog should remain alert and healthy. Lactation can be diminished by reducing food and water intake.

CHECK YOUR UNDERSTANDING

- Which three ligaments support ovary position?
- Describe the difference between the ovarian cortex and ovarian medulla.
- Which ovarian structures produce eggs?
- Name three layers of the uterus and their function.

22.5 Physiology of the Female Reproductive System

Oogenesis

Oogenesis or **ovogenesis** is the process of the ovum or egg development. It begins from the **oogonia**, a diploid germ cell at the center of primordial follicles. Oogonia mitotically divides and produces **primary oocytes**, a diploid cell that is determined to divides by meiosis. Oogenesis has three steps: **oocytogenesis**, **ootidogenesis**, and **oogenesis proper**—a final step of ovum maturation (table 22.1).

TABLE 22.1   Steps of Oogenesis

Cell Type	Ploidy or Number of Chromosomes	Number of Chromatids	Process
Oogonium	Diploid (2n)	2C	Oocytogenesis (mitosis)
Primary oocyte	Diploid (2n)	4C	Ootidogenesis (meiosis I)
Secondary oocyte	Haploid (1n)	2C	Ootidogenesis (meiosis II)
Ootid	Haploid (1n)	1C	Ootidogenesis (meiosis II)
Ovum	Haploid (1n)	1C	

Oocytogenesis starts with development of primary oocytes. Oocytogenesis is complete either before or shortly after birth. After oocytogenesis is complete, no additional primary oocytes are created. It means that primary oocytes reach their maximum development during gestation. Recent publications, however, have challenged the belief that a finite number of oocytes are set around the time of birth. The renewal of ovarian follicles from germline stem cells (originating from the red bone marrow and peripheral blood) has been reported in the postnatal mouse ovary.

The next phase ootidogenesis begins after primary oocyte divides by meiosis and becomes an **ootid**. This process begins at prenatal age, but stops at prophase I. In late fetal life and childhood, all oocytes, are primary oocytes. Only when female reach puberty the process of ootid development continues. As a result of meiosis I, the primary oocyte develops into the secondary oocyte and the first polar body. Immediately after meiosis I, the haploid secondary oocyte initiates meiosis II. However, this process is also halted at the metaphase II stage until fertilization, if such should ever occur. If fertilization happen, then meiosis II completes. The meiosis II produces an ootid and a second polar body. Synchronously with ootidogenesis, the ovarian follicle surrounding the ootid develops from a primordial follicle to a preovulatory one. Both polar bodies disintegrate at the end of meiosis II, leaving only the ootid, which then eventually undergoes maturation into a mature ovum.

Parallel to the oogenesis another process called **folliculogenesis** takes place. The folliculogenesis is the process of development of densely packed pocket of somatic cells surrounded an immature oocyte. This group is called **follicle**. The folliculogenesis consists in development of small **primordial follicle** into large **preovulatory follicle** (fig. 22.21). The sequence of folliculogenesis event is next: Primordial follicle – (Oocytogenesis/Mitosis) → Primary follicle – (Ootidogenesis/Meiosis I) → Secondary follicle – (Ootodogenesis/Meiosis I) → Graaphian follicle – (Ootidogenesis/Meiosis II) → Yellow body – (Oogenesis proper/Meiosis II). The primordial follicle consists of primary oocyte surrounded by a single layer of squamous follicular cells. The next stage of folliculogenesis is a **primary follicle**. In primary follicle the follicular cells change shape from squamous to cuboidal. At that time they are referred to as **granulosa cells**. A zona pellucida–glycoprotein layer around the primary oocyte is formed. The secondary follicle is characterized by thick follicular wall and follicular fluid collected in small pockets. The granulosa cells enlarge and form **thecal cells** around the follicle. Granulosa cells produce estrogens from the secretions of the thecal cells. The preovulatory, tertiary, or Graafian follicle is characterized by development of large cavity called **antrum** from merged small pockets. The primary oocyte rests on the stock of granulosa cells called cumulus oophorus. The primary oocyte completes meiosis I and forms secondary oocyte and first polar body (fig. 22.21).

Female Reproductive Cycles

Females of most mammal species advertise fertility to males with visual behavioral cues, pheromones, or both. This period of advertised fertility is known as **oestrus, estrus,** or **heat**. In species that experience estrus, females are generally receptive to copulation only while they are in heat (dolphins are an exception). In the estrous cycles of most placental mammals, if no fertilization takes place, the uterus reabsorbs the endometrium. This breakdown of the endometrium without vaginal discharge is called **covert menstruation**. **Overt menstruation** characterizes by blood flow from the vagina and occurs primarily in humans and close primates such as chimpanzees. Some species, such as domestic dogs, experience small

(a) Stages of Folliculogenesis

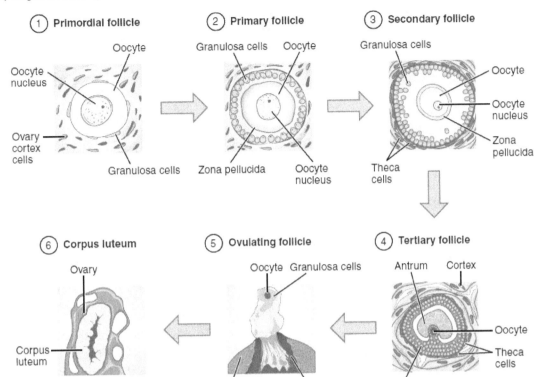

(b) A Secondary Follicle

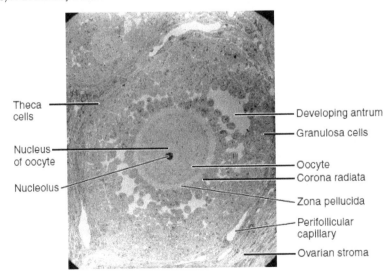

FIGURE 22.21   Folliculogenesis.

amounts of vaginal bleeding while approaching heat. However, this discharge has a different physiologic cause than menstruation. Thus, there are two types of female reproductive cycles: **menstrual** and **estrous**.

The menstrual cycle includes the production of eggs and preparation of the uterus to pregnancy. The cycle can be divided into three phases based on events in the ovary (ovarian cycle) or in the uterus (uterine cycle). The ovarian cycle consists of the follicular phase, ovulation, and **luteal phase**, whereas the uterine cycle is divided into menstruation, **proliferative phase**, and **secretory phase**. Stimulated by gradually increasing amounts of estrogen in the follicular phase, discharges of blood (menses) flow stop, and the lining of the uterus thickens. With the increase of FSH secretion, follicles grow and after several days one or more depending on species become dominant. All nondominant follicles shrink and die. When the luteinizing hormone (LH) reach specific threshold level, the dominant follicle releases an oocyte, in an event called ovulation. After ovulation, the emptied dominant follicle becomes a corpus luteum. Corpus luteum produces progesterone. The progesterone prepares the uterus lining to potential embryo implantation. If implantation does not occur within some period, the corpus luteum degrades. It stops to produce hormones, connective tissue fills corpus luteum inside, and corpus luteum transforms into **corpus albicans**—a scar that remains after corpus luteum degradation. Degradation of corpus luteum causes dramatic decrease of levels of both progesterone and estrogen. The drop of secretion of both hormones initiates the uterus to shed its lining in a process that is termed menstruation (fig. 22.23). Beside human and primates, menstruation also occurs in some other animals including shrews and bats.

Estrus is derived from the Latin *oestrus*, which means "gadfly." This name refers to the ancient Greek myth about a human woman named Io, who got attention from Zeus. His wife, the goddess Hera, sent a gadfly to punish Io for her love affair with Zeus. There are four phases in the estrous cycle: **proestrus**, **estrus**, **metestrus**, and **anestrus** (fig. 22.22).

In proestrus one or several follicles of the ovary start to grow. Their number is species specific. Typically, this phase can last as little as one day or as long as three weeks, depending on the species. Under the influence of estrogen, the endometrium of the uterus grows. Some animals, like dogs, may experience vaginal secretions that could be bloody. At that time female is not yet sexually receptive. The old corpus luteum, which remains from the previous ovulation, degenerates. The uterus and vagina distend and fill with fluid, become contractile and secrete a clear light-yellow fluid. The vaginal epithelium proliferates, and the vaginal smear shows a large number of noncornified nucleated epithelial cells.

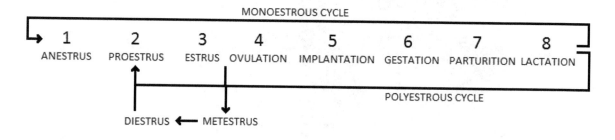

FIGURE 22.22   A Four-Phase Terminology to Describe Animal Estrous Cycle.

Estrus refers to the period when the female is sexually receptive. Ovarian follicles mature and estrogen reaches maximum level. In some species labia become red and swollen. Females of many species demonstrate the lordosis reflex, when female spontaneously elevates her hind body parts.

The metestrus phase follows ovulation (fig. 22.22). It is characterized by the activity of the corpus luteum, which produces progesterone. The estrogen influence decreases and the corpus luteum forms. The endometrium lining of the uterus grows to prepare for possible embryo implantation. In the absence of pregnancy the diestrus phase (also called pseudo-pregnancy) terminates with the regression of the corpus luteum. The lining in the uterus is not shed, but is resorbed without vaginal discharge until the next cycle.

Anestrus refers to the phase when female is at rests. This is typically a seasonal event and controlled by light exposure through the melatonin released by the pineal gland. Melatonin inhibits reproduction in long-day breeders and stimulates reproduction in short-day breeders. Melatonin regulates the hypothalamic pulse secretion of the gonadotropin-releasing hormone. Anestrus is influenced by time of year, pregnancy, lactation, significant illness, chronic energy deficit, and possibly age. Continuous exposure to anabolic steroids may also induce a persistent anestrus due to negative feedback on the hypothalamus-pituitary-gonadal axis. After completion (or abortion) of a pregnancy, some species have **postpartum estrus**. It begins with ovulation, forming of new corpus luteum, and the offspring birth. For example, the mouse has a fertile postpartum estrus that occurs 14 to 24 hours following parturition. The estrous cycle varies in length among species. Estrous cycles are typically more frequent in smaller animals. Even within species, significant variability can be observed; thus, cats may undergo an estrous cycle of three to seven weeks.

Some species, like cats, cows, and domestic pigs, are **polyestrous**. They have heat several times per year. Seasonally polyestrous animals or seasonal breeders have more than one estrous cycle during a specific time of the year and can be divided into short-day and long-day breeders. Short-day breeders: sheep, goats, deer, and elk are sexually active in fall or winter. Long-day breeders like horses, hamsters, and ferrets are sexually active in spring and summer. Species that go into heat twice per year are called **diestrous**. **Monoestrous** species—bears, foxes, and wolves—have only one breeding period, typically in spring. A few mammalian species: rabbits, do not have an estrous cycle and are able to conceive at almost every arbitrary moment. In general, the time of estrus is organized to maximize the offspring survival.

The female cat in heat has an estrus of 14 to 21 days and is generally characterized as an induced ovulator. The ovulation in cat is induced by coitus. However, various incidents of spontaneous ovulation have been documented in the domestic cat and various nondomestic species. Cats are polyestrous, but experience a seasonal anestrus in autumn and late winter.

A female dog is usually diestrous. The proestrus is relatively long at 5 to 9 days, while the estrus may last 4 to 13 days, with a diestrus of 60 days followed by about 90 to 150 days of anestrus. Female dogs bleed during estrus, which usually lasts from 7 to 13 days, depending on the size and maturity of the dog. Proestrus bleeding in dogs is common and is believed to be caused by diapedesis of red blood cells from the blood vessels due to the increase of the estradiol-17β hormone. Ovulation occurs 24–48 hours after the luteinizing hormone reach its peak. Usually, it happens somewhere around the fourth day of estrus. It is the best time for breeding.

A horse female or mare can be in heat for 4 to 10 days and about 14 days in diestrus. Thus, a mare cycle may be short, around 3 weeks. Horses mate in spring and summer, autumn is a transition time, and anestrus rules the winter. Horses and other large herd animals are usually affected by the seasons. At short daylight hours these animals are anestrous. As days grow longer, the hormones initiate beginning of the breeding cycle. This prevents newborn animals from a risk of the cold of winter.

The estrus frequency of rats is 4 to 5 days; sheep is 18 days; cattle, goat, and pigs is 21 days; donkeys from 13 to 31 days; elephants is 112 days; whereas rabbits have a variable frequency.

Hormonal Control of Female Reproductive Cycles

The female reproductive cycle consists of two complementary processes: **ovarian cycle** and **uterine cycle**. The ovarian cycle describes the process of ovum development from primary oocyte to release of the secondary oocyte from the ovary called **ovulation**. The uterine cycle describes changes in uterus. Both processes are controlled by sexual hormones. The trigger hormone is a gonadotropin-releasing hormone (GnRH) produced by the hypothalamus. At childhood this secretion is very low. At puberty it increases. The GnRH is released in pulses. A negative feedback from androgens and estrogens regulates production. Low-frequency GnRH pulses triggers FSH release, whereas high-frequency GnRH pulses stimulate LH pulses. There is a difference in GnRH secretion between females and males. In males GnRH is secreted in pulses at a constant frequency. In females the frequency of the pulses varies during the menstrual cycle, and there is a large surge of GnRH just before ovulation. FSH and LH are produced by the anterior pituitary gland. FSH initiates follicular growth, specifically affecting granulosa cells. At the end of the luteal phase, there is a slight rise in FSH level that seems initiates the start of the next ovulatory cycle. LH stimulates the ovaries to produce androgens and hormonal precursors for estradiol. The fast rising of LH level leads to an "LH surge" that triggers ovulation. LH also initiates conversion of the residual follicle into a corpus luteum.

Generally, estrogen has a negative feedback effect on the release of GnRH by the hypothalamus and inhibits production by the anterior pituitary gland gonadotropins (FSH and LH), reducing their sensitivity to GnRH. Rupture of the ovarian follicle at ovulation causes a drastic reduction in estrogen synthesis and increase in secretion of progesterone by the corpus luteum.

VETERINARY APPLICATION

Ovarian remnant syndrome is a condition that occurs when ovarian tissue remains inside the body after a female cat is spayed. This tissue can produce estrogen, triggering signs of heat in the cat. In an unspayed cat, the ovaries produce a number of hormones, including estrogen. It is this estrogen that triggers the cat to go into heat. When the cat is spayed, the entire reproductive tract (including both ovaries and the uterus) is surgically removed. The spayed cat no longer goes into heat. If a previously-spayed animal shows signs of going into heat, this may indicate that functioning ovarian tissue (known as an ovarian remnant) is still present and producing estrogen. The continued presence of estrogen predisposes cats to mammary gland tumors (breast cancer), pyometra (infection of the uterus), and ovarian tumors. Ovarian remnant syndrome is treated by surgically removing the remaining ovarian tissue. This surgery should be performed while your pet is in heat, in order to maximize the chances of being able to visualize the remaining ovarian tissue.

The ovarian cycle includes both folliculogenesis and oogenesis. Follicular phase is the first part of the ovarian cycle. The follicle stimulating hormone (FSH) produced by anterior pituitary gland stimulates ovarian follicles to maturate. The process of maturation includes growth of oocyte in size, a layer of glycoprotein called **zona pellucida** covers the oocyte, and supporting cells of the follicle known as **granulosa cells** multiply. Inside the follicle forms a space filled with fluid (**atrium**). When FSH reach its peak level, oocyte sit on the top of cells called **cumulus oophorus** and granulosa cells surround zona pellucida to form **corona radiata**. The follicle that reaches this state is called a tertiary or **Graafian follicle**. It contains a "ready to go" ovum. LH level at this period continues to grow, but still remains low inhibited by increasing production of estradiol.

Ovulation is the second phase of the ovarian cycle. At this phase a mature egg is released from the ovarian follicle. During the follicular phase, estradiol suppresses release of luteinizing hormone (LH) by the anterior pituitary gland. When the egg becomes nearly mature, the estradiol level reaches a threshold above which its effect on the LH secretion is reversed and estrogen begins to stimulate the production of a large amount of LH known as the LH surge. In animals, a gonadotropin-releasing hormone (GnRH) surge has been shown to precede the LH surge. The LH surge causes final maturation of the egg. The wall of the follicle weakens, raptures, and secondary oocyte is released. The secondary oocyte fast transforms into an ootid and then becomes a mature ovum. Species, whose ovaries release many eggs in one cycle, are called **multiparous**. Their offspring is called **litter**. Here belong cats, dogs, and sows. In horses, cattle, and humans, ovaries produce only one egg per cycle. These species are called **uniparous**. Which of the two ovaries of uniparous species releases this single ovum, left or right, appears random. So far, no known process that coordinates left and right ovulation has been discovered. Sometimes both ovaries release an egg simultaneously. If both these eggs are fertilized, the result is fraternal twins. After being released from the ovary, the egg is swept into the fallopian tube by the fimbria. After about a day, if the fertilization does

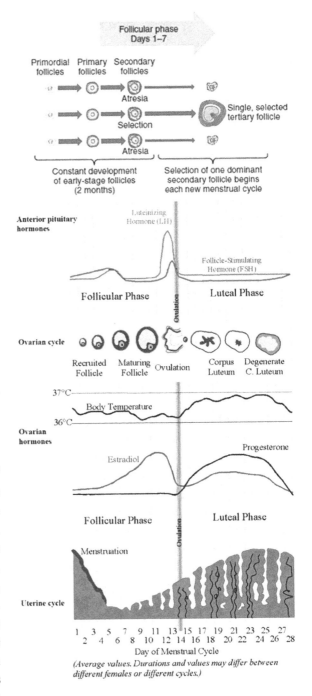

FIGURE 22.23 Hormonal Regulation of Human Menstrual Cycle.

not happen, the egg will disintegrate or dissolve in the fallopian tube. Fertilization by a spermatozoon, when it occurs, usually takes place in the ampulla, the widest section of the fallopian tubes. The surge of LH causes a decrease of the estradiol secretion below the threshold level and negative effect of estradiol on production of LH and FSH returns back. Levels of all three hormones fall.

The luteal phase is the final phase of the ovarian cycle, and it correlates with the secretory phase of the uterine cycle. During the luteal phase, the FSH and LH cause the remaining parts of the dominant follicle to transform into the **corpus luteum**. The corpus luteum produces **progesterone**. The primary role of the progesterone is to maintain thickness of the proliferative endometrium. It is necessary for embryo implantation and normal development at the first embryo stages. The increased progesterone continues to suppress production of the FSH and LH. The levels of both hormones quickly fall, and the corpus luteum subsequently atrophies.

The corpus luteum atrophy causes a decrease in progesterone level. Low progesterone cannot maintain thick endometrium in the uterus. And the proliferative endometrium shades with menstruation. A low estradiol level allows the anterior pituitary to increase production of FSH and LH. A new cycle begins. The other scenario happens if sperm fertilizes the egg. Fertilization results in fusion of haploid egg and sperm cells and emerging of a new diploid cell called a **zygote**. In a short time, the zygote divides and after a dozen divisions develops into a multicellular structure called a **blastocyst**. The outer layer of the blastocyst is called the **syncytiotrophoblast**. Cells of the syncytiotrophoblast secrete **chorionic gonadotropin** (CG): a hormone similar to LH. The release of CG preserves the corpus luteum and it continues to secrete progesterone to maintain thickness of the endometrium (fig. 22.24).

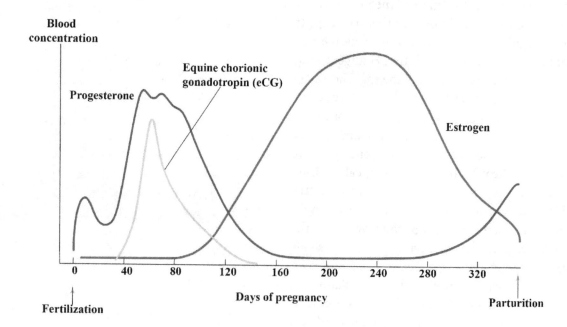

FIGURE 22.24   Equine Chorionic Gonadotropin (eCG) Maintains Corpus Luteum at First Days of Pregnancy.

The uterine cycle has three phases: **menses**, **proliferative**, and **secretory**. Menstruation or menses is the first phase of the uterine cycle. The flow of menses normally serves as a sign of absence of pregnancy and beginning of a new cycle. This cycle is primarily under control of the estrogens and progesterone.

The proliferative phase is the second phase of the uterine cycle when estrogen causes the lining of the uterus to grow, or proliferate. Maturating ovarian follicles secrete increasing amounts of estrogens, first of all estradiol. The estrogens initiate the formation of a new layer of endometrium in the uterus, histologically identified as the **proliferative endometrium**. The estrogens also stimulate the cervix to produce fertile cervical mucus.

The secretory phase is the final phase of the uterine cycle. It correlates with the luteal phase of the ovarian cycle. During the secretory phase, the corpus luteum produces progesterone, which plays a vital role in making the endometrium receptive to implantation of the blastocyst and supports the early period of pregnancy. Progesterone increases blood flow to the endometrium, stimulates uterine secretions, and reduces the contractility of smooth muscle in the uterus. It also increases the basal body temperature.

The fig. 22.25 demonstrates bovine estrous cycle. Bovines' follicular phase continues from 17 to 19 days. Progesterone declines with degrading of the corpus luteum. The decrease of progesterone secretion results in rapid increase of estrogen and FSH secretion. The estrogen level reaches a threshold level. It triggers massive release of LH called the LH surge, and LH surge stimulates ovulation.

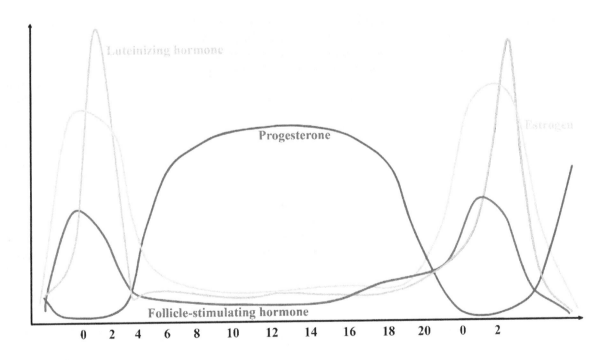

FIGURE 22.25   Bovine Estrous Cycle.

CHECK YOUR UNDERSTANDING

- Compare ovarian and uterine cycles.

- Which hormones control ovarian cycles and which control uterine cycles?

- What is the corpus luteum?

- What is the role of chorionic gonadotropin hormone?

CHAPTER SUMMARY

- Male and female gonads are paired structures that originated from the genital ridge. Precursors of gametes are germ cells that develop outside of gonads. They arise in extraembryonic endoderm and migrate to the indifferent gonads. In females they populate cortex. In males they reside in medulla, which later develops in seminiferous tubules.

- Fusion of gametes, called **fertilization**. creates a new diploid cell called a **zygote**. Gametes have one single set of chromosomes called haploid. Somatic cells have diploid set: complementary chromosomes from the mother and father are known as **homologous chromosomes**. Somatic cells reproduce via mitosis, whereas gametes reproduce via **meiosis**.

- Meiosis proceeds through two consecutive divisions: **meiosis I** and **meiosis II**, each divided in: **prophase I, metaphase I, anaphase I, telophase I**, and **prophase II, metaphase II, anaphase II**, and **telophase II**. In prophase I chromatin condenses, the nucleus defragments, and centrioles move in opposite directions. The most remarkable event of prophase I is organization of homologous chromosomes in **tetrads**. In tetrad chromosomes exchange segments of chromatin known as **crossing over**. Crossing over does not create new genes, but it creates new combinations. In metaphase I tetrads line up metaphase plane, spindle fibers connect centromeres and centrosomes. In anaphase I spindle fibers shorten and pull homologous chromosomes to opposite poles. In telophase I, two nuclear envelopes reorganize around two haploid groups of chromosomes. The phase ended by the division of the cytoplasm and separation of two daughter cells. There is no another DNA duplication before the meiosis II. Two cells begin meiosis II with haploid set of chromosomes, where every chromosome made of two sister chromatids. In anaphase II spindle fibers shorten and chromosomes split in two sister chromatids. Pulled by the spindle apparatus, sister chromatids move towards opposite poles. Telophase II and cytokinesis accomplish the process.

- Production of sperm cells is called **spermatogenesis**; production of eggs is called **oogenesis**. Spermatogenesis begins at puberty and continues through the whole male life. Meiosis continuously proceeds and ends by four daughter cells. In oogenesis only one cell develops in oocyte, whereas other daughter cells become **polar bodies** and degrade. Oogenesis proceeds with stops. The first stop is prophase I occurred before female's birth. The second stop occurs at the stage of secondary oocyte in metaphase II during female adulthood. The process completes only after fertilization: fusion with sperm triggers its accomplishment.

- Male primary sex organs are testes. They produce sperm and secrete sex hormones. In most mammals testes are in the **scrotum**, but remain connected to the abdominal cavity via the **inguinal canal**. In some mammals testes descend into the scrotum temporary only during the breeding period. Sirenians, elephants, sloths, and armadillos have testes inside the body all the time.

- Scrotum is composed of skin, connective tissue membranes, and dartos smooth muscles. Dartos muscles together with cremaster muscles in the spermatic cord maintain temperature in testes below the body temperature. Testes are surrounded by external membrane called the **tunica vaginalis**. The second tunic is called the **tunica albuginea**. It is a strong connective tissue membrane. It folds inside testes and separates internal space in **lobules**. Every lobule contains one to four tightly coiled **seminiferous tubules**. Walls of the seminiferous tubules are made of **spermatogenic** and **sustentacular cells**, surrounded by **myoid cells**. Spermatogenic cells produce sperm. Sustentacular cells support and direct their development. Myoid cells are able to contract and push sperm cells off the seminiferous tubules into epididymis. Space between seminiferous tubules is populated by **interstitial** or **Leydig cells** that produce sex hormones, collectively named **androgens**. The principal androgen is **testosterone**. It controls development and facilitates activity of the secondary male sex organs. At the end seminiferous tubules are organized in a network called the **rete testis**. Sperm cells leave the rete testis trough the **efferent ductules** and accumulate in the **epididymis**. The **testicular artery** carries blood from the aorta. Veins are organized in a network—the **pampiniform venous plexus**—that drains blood in the **testicular vein** that falls in the posterior vena cava.

- The male reproductive system includes the epididymis, vas deferens, ejaculatory duct, prostatic urethra, membranous urethra, and spongy urethra ended by the **external urethral orifice**. The epididymis is a long, convoluted tube lined by a pseudostratified epithelium with immovable microvilli called **stereocilia**. Sperm cells that enter the epididymis are immature and cannot fertilize an egg. The vas deferens extends through the spermatic cord and enters the pelvic cavity through the inguinal canal. It passes along the latero-dorsal sides of the urinary bladder. The end of the vas deferens is a large sac called the **ampulla**. Sperm in the vas deferens are already mature, but still immovable. The peristaltic movement of the vas deferens wall propels sperm toward the ampulla and to the ejaculatory duct. The ejaculatory duct receives input from the **seminal vesicle**. The gland secretes **seminal fluid** that constitutes 60 to 70 percent of the semen volume. Semen passes the ejaculatory duct, prostate gland, and enters the urethra. In the urethra semen receives secretion of the **prostate** and **bulbourethral (Cowper's)** glands. Prostate secretion constitutes 20 to 30 percent of semen. Cowper's glands produce alkaline fluid that neutralizes acids in the urethra prior to ejaculation and lubricates **glans penis** during copulation.

- The penis has three regions: root, shaft, and **glans penis**. Skin that surrounds penis is loose and forms folds around the glans penis called **prepuce**. Penis contains cylindrical erectile bodies: single corpus spongiosum that surrounds urethra, and two dorsally located **corpora cavernosa**. In the root of penis, the corpora cavernosa diverges and form two **crura** that anchor the penis in the pelvis by attaching it to the ischium bone. The erectile tissue has a dense network of blood vessels with small vascular sections. Internal iliac arteries through the pudendal arteries branch in **dorsal** and **deep penile arteries**. Dorsal artery carry blood to skin and corpus spongiosum. Deep arteries carry blood to both corpora cavernosa. Groups of **superficial** veins take blood from the skin. **Deep dorsal veins** drain blood from spongy bodies. Most of placental mammals have **os penis** or **baculum**. It is located above the urethra. Penis root of marsupials, carnivores, bovines, and deer have a long S-shaped curve. A retractor penis muscle is attached to this curve. At sexual arousal retractor muscle relaxes and penis expands outside of the body.

- Spermatogenesis begins from **spermatogonia**—diploid stem cells in seminiferous tubules. Some of these cells develop in **primary spermatocytes**. After meiosis I primary spermatocytes become haploid **secondary spermatocytes**. Meiosis II produces four haploid **spermatids**. They lost most of cytoplasm and organelles, grow flagellum and acrosome, and become sperm cells.

- **Nurse** or **Sertoli cell** is long extended from basement membrane to the lumen of seminiferous tubule. They are bound by tight junctions in a continuous network that separates developing sperm cells from male immune system and prevents them from immune reaction. Sustentacular cells secrete testicular fluid that deliver nutrients to sperm cells.

- Gonadotropin-releasing hormone (GnRH) from hypothalamus stimulates anterior pituitary gland to secrete follicle stimulating (FSH) and luteinizing (LH) hormones. LH stimulates interstitial cells to produce testosterone. FSH stimulates sustentacular cells in seminiferous tubules to release **androgen binding protein** and hormone **inhibin** that decreases production of FSH. Testosterone inhibits secretion of GnRH. In adult male testosterone level is stable during male life slow decreasing with aging. Oxytocin stimulates smooth muscles contraction during ejaculation, increases empathy, initiates romantic attraction and monogamous pair formation. Vasopressin initiates aggression and stimulates male to protect family.

- Ovaries produce eggs and sex hormones. Three ligaments anchor the ovary to other organs and walls of the pelvic cavity: 1) **broad ligament** is a large flat membrane bound ovaries, **uterine tubes**, and **uterus**, and pelvis; 2) **ovarian ligament** connects ovaries to the uterus; 3) **suspensory ligament** bound ovaries with the pelvic cavity wall, carries **ovarian arteries** and **veins**, and nerves. Superior layer of ovaries is called **ovarian cortex**. Follicles are located in this area. The core of ovaries is called **ovarian medulla**. It houses blood and lymphatic vessels, and nerves.

- **Oviducts, fallopian tubes**, or **uterine tubes** have retroperitoneal position. The broad ligament binds them with ovaries and walls of body cavity. The region of oviduct fails in uterus is narrow and is called **isthmus**. The opposite side of oviduct is enlarged and called **ampulla**. Ampulla continues into the funnel-shaped **infundibulum** that opens by ostium close to ovary. It opens in peritoneal cavity. Finger-like projections called **fimbriae** surround ostium and drape around the ovary. During **ovulation** a gentle beat of fimbriae pull oocyte inside the infundibulum. The **fertilization** usually takes place in ampulla.

- Uterus is located in the pelvis between rectum and urinary bladder. **Lateral cervical ligament** attaches cervix and vagina to the lateral wall of pelvic cavity. **Uterosacral ligament** connects uterus to the sacrum. **Round ligament** binds it with ventral walls of the pelvic cavity. The narrow opening of the uterus into the vagina is called **cervix**. Cervix glands secrete mucus, which lubricates the vagina during intercourse. There are four types of eutherian uteri. **Duplex uterus** has two uteri and two cervixes. The **bipartite uterus** has two uteri and one cervix. The **bicornuate uterus** has a single uterine body that distally splits in two horns. The **simplex uterus** has no uterine horns. Its single body opens in vagina through a single cervix. Three layers compose walls of the uterus: **perimetrium, myometrium**, and **endometrium**. The perimetrium is an extension of the parietal peritoneum. The myometrium is a thick layer of smooth muscles. The endometrium is a mucous membrane, made of simple columnar epithelium and lamina propria.

- The vagina is an elastic muscular canal. The vaginal canal creates folds around the cervix called **fornix**. Ridges of the vaginal wall are called **rugae**.

- External female genitalia or vulva includes **labia majora, labia minora, clitoris**, and **Bartholin's** or **greater vestibular glands** located on both sides of the vaginal orifice.

- **Mammary gland** produces milk to feed offspring. They are arranged in breasts in primates, udder in ruminants, or dugs of dogs and cats. Mammary gland consists of alveoli made of milk-secreting cuboidal cells surrounded by myo-epithelial cells. Alveoli are organized in **lobules**. Each lobule has a **lactiferous duct** that carries milk to the nipple. The structure with one single lactiferous duct is called a **simple mammary gland**. A cluster of many lactiferous ducts is called **complex mammary gland**. Presence of more than two nipples is known as **polythelia**, and the presence of more than two complex mammary glands as **polymastia**.

- **Oogenesis** or **ovogenesis** is a process of egg development. It begins from **oogonium** that produces **primary oocytes** by mitosis. Oogenesis has three steps: **oocytogenesis**, **ootidogenesis**, and **oogenesis proper**. The sequence of events is next: Oogonium — (Oocytogenesis) → Primary Oocyte — (Meiosis I) → First Polar Body (Discarded afterward) + Secondary oocyte — (Meiosis II) → Second Polar Body (Discarded afterward) + Ovum. The development of follicles is called folliculogenes. It begins from a small **primordial follicle** and ends by a large **preovulatory follicle**.

- Oocytogenesis starts with primary oocytes and completes either before or shortly after birth. After oocytogenesis is complete, no additional primary oocytes are created. The next phase—ootidogenesis—begins when primary oocyte divides by meiosis in **ootids**. This process occurs at prenatal period, but stops at prophase I. In late fetal life and childhood, all oocytes, are primary oocytes. Their development continues only in puberty. After meiosis I, primary oocyte gives secondary oocyte and first polar body. Secondary oocyte undergoes meiosis II, which is halted at the metaphase II and is finished after fertilization. Meiosis II produces an ootid and second polar body. Synchronously, ovarian follicle around the ootid develops from primordial follicle. Both polar bodies disintegrate at the end of meiosis II and ootid becomes ovum.

- The period when female advertises her fertility is known as **oestrus**, **estrus**, or **heat**. Females are generally receptive to copulation only while they are in heat. Resorption of endometrium without vaginal discharge is called **covert menstruation**. **Overt menstruation** characterizes by vaginal blood flow. There are two types of female reproductive cycles: **menstrual** and **estrous**.

- The menstrual cycle has three phases based on events in the ovary (ovarian cycle) and uterus (uterine cycle). The ovarian cycle consists of 1) follicular, 2) ovulation, and 3) **luteal** phases. The uterine cycle is divided in 1) menstruation, 2) **proliferative**, and 3) **secretory** phases.

- The estrous cycle proceeds through: **proestrus**, **estrus**, **metestrus**, and **anestrus**. In proestrus one or several follicles in the ovary start to grow. Their number is species specific. Under the influence of estrogen, the endometrium grows. The old corpus luteum, remaining from previous ovulation, degenerates. The uterus and vagina distend, fill with fluid, and begin to contract. Estrus is a phase when a female is sexually receptive. Her ovarian follicles mature, and estrogen reaches a maximum level. The metestrus begins after ovulation. At that time, the corpus luteum produces progesterone. The endometrium lining grows to prepare for embryo implantation. At the absence of pregnancy, the diestrus phase (also called pseudo-pregnancy) terminates with the regression of the corpus luteum. The lining in the uterus is not shed, but is resorbed until the next cycle. In anestrus female is at rests. It is typically a seasonal event controlled by light exposure. Melatonin from pineal gland inhibits reproduction in long-day breeders and stimulates reproduction in short-day breeders. It regulates the hypothalamic pulse secretion of the GnRH. Completion (or abortion) of pregnancy in some species results in **postpartum estrus**. Some species are **polyestrous** and have heat several times per year. Short-day breeders are sexually active in fall or winter. Long-day breeders are sexually active in spring and summer. Species that go into heat twice per year are called **diestrous**. **Monoestrous** species have one breeding period. Some mammals do not have an estrous cycle and are able to conceive at almost every arbitrary moment.

- **Ovarian** and **uterine** cycles are complementary processes triggered by the GnRH. It is released in pulses. Low-frequency pulse triggers FSH release, whereas high-frequency GnRH pulse stimulates LH pulses. In females the frequency of the pulses varies during the menstrual cycle, and there is a large surge of GnRH just before ovulation. FSH initiates follicular growth, specifically affecting granulosa cells. At the end of the luteal phase, there is a light rise in FSH level that initiates the start of the next ovulatory cycle. LH stimulates the ovaries to produce androgens and estradiol precursors. Fast rise of LH level called an "LH surge" triggers ovulation. LH also initiates conversion of residual follicle into a corpus luteum. Estrogen has negative feedback effect on the release of GnRH, FSH, and LH. Ovulation causes a drastic reduction in estrogen synthesis, but increases secretion of progesterone by the corpus luteum.

- The follicular phase is the first phase of the ovarian cycle. FSH stimulates development of follicles. A layer of glycoprotein called **zona pellucida** covers the oocyte, and supporting **granulosa cells** multiply. The follicle forms atrium filled with fluid. When FSH reaches a peak level, oocyte sits on the top of **cumulus oophorus** and granulosa cells form **corona radiata**. Follicle at this time is called a tertiary or **Graafian follicle**. It contains a "ready to go" ovum.

- Ovulation is the second phase of the ovarian cycle. At this phase an egg is released from the follicle. During the follicular phase, estradiol suppresses release of LH. When the egg becomes nearly mature, the estradiol level reaches a threshold level and its effect on the LH secretion is reversed. Now it stimulates production of a large amount of LH (LH surge). Wall of the follicle weakens, raptures, and secondary oocyte is released. The secondary oocyte transforms into an ootid and then becomes a mature ovum. Species whose ovaries release many eggs in one cycle are called **multiparous**. Their offspring is called **litter**. Species that release only one ovum are called **uniparous**. The surge of LH causes a decrease in the estradiol secretion and negative effect of estradiol on production of LH and FSH returns back. Levels of all three hormones fall.

- The luteal phase is final phase of ovarian cycle. It correlates with the secretory phase of the uterine cycle. During the luteal phase, the remaining parts of the dominant follicle becomes **corpus luteum** that produces **progesterone**. Progesterone secures thickness of the proliferative endometrium. It suppresses production of FSH and LH. The levels of both hormones fall, which results in corpus luteum atrophy. Atrophy of corpus luteum causes decrease of progesterone level, which now unable to maintain thick endometrium and it shades with menstruation. A low estradiol level allows anterior pituitary increase FSH and LH production and a new cycle begins. If sperm fertilize the egg, a new diploid cell called a **zygote** emerges. After some divisions, the zygote develops into a **blastocyst**. Syncytiotrophoblast—an external layer of cells in a blastocyst—secretes **chorionic gonadotropin** (CG). Release of CG preserves the corpus luteum, and it continues to secrete progesterone to maintain endometrium.

- The uterine cycle has three phases: **menses**, **proliferative**, and **secretory**. Menstruation or menses is the first phase of the uterine cycle. The proliferative phase is the second phase, characterized by growth of a **proliferative endometrium**. The secretory phase is final in the cycle. It correlates with the luteal phase of the ovarian cycle. During the secretory phase, the corpus luteum produces progesterone. Progesterone increases blood flow to the endometrium, stimulates uterine secretions, and reduces contractility of smooth muscles.

CHECK YOUR KNOWLEDGE

LEVEL 1. CHECK YOUR RECALL

1. The uterine type with two uterus and two cervixes is called:
   A. Bipartite uterus
   B. Bicornuate uterus
   C. Duplex uterus
   D. Simplex uterus

2. Which of the following structures is the site of sperm production?
   A. Seminiferous tubules
   B. Epididymis
   C. Vas deferens
   D. Ejaculatory duct
   E. Prostatic urethra

3. Which of the following structures is the site of sperm maturation?
   A. Seminal vesicles
   B. Epididymis
   C. Seminiferous tubules
   D. Vas deferens
   E. Ejaculatory duct

4. What is the role of interstitial cells in testes?
   A. Production of sperm cells
   B. Control and support of developing sperm cells
   C. Creation of blood-sperm barrier
   D. Production of seminal fluids
   E. Production of androgens, primarily testosterone

5. Tetrads are:
   A. A complex of fused-together homologous chromosomes
   B. A place where a chromosome is attached to the spindle fiber
   C. A complex of DNA molecule and proteins
   D. Chromosomes with a new combination of alleles that is absent in both parents

6. The separation of homologous chromosomes that results in development of haploid sex cell takes place at:
   A. Prophase I
   B. Prophase II
   C. Anaphase I
   D. Anaphase II

7. Meiosis results in the _____, whereas mitosis results in the _____.
   A. production of four genetically identical cells; production of two genetically identical cells
   B. production of four genetically different cells; production of two genetically different cells
   C. production of four genetically identical cells; production of two genetically different cells
   D. production of four genetically different cells; production of two genetically identical cells

8. Which hormone is **not** produced in the ovaries?
   A. Oxytocin
   B. Progesterone
   C. Estrogen
   D. Relaxin

9. Which of these ligaments does **not** support the ovaries?
   A. Round ligament
   B. Lateral cervical ligament
   C. Broad ligament
   D. Ovarian ligament
   E. Suspensory ligament

10. A surge of which hormone plays a primary role in ovulation?
    A. Estrogen
    B. Gonadotropin-releasing hormone
    C. Follicle stimulating hormone
    D. Luteinizing hormone
    E. Oxytocin

11. _____ initiates functional endometrium development, whereas _____ maintains thickness and prevents its shading.
    A. FSH; LH
    B. LH; FSH
    C. FSH; progesterone
    D. Progesterone; estrogen
    E. Estrogen; progesterone

12. True or false: Spermatogonia are diploid stem cells that begin the process of spermatogenesis and divide by mitosis.
13. True or false: Scrotum contains the testes and maintains the temperature of testes higher than body temperature, which is optimal for spermatogenesis.
14. True or false: Testosterone and inhibin both control hypothalamus production of GnRH through the negative feedback.
15. True or false: Oogenesis begins before a female is born.
16. True or false: Progesterone inhibits release of gonadotropins and continues to do this during pregnancy.

17. Match the term with its description:

_____ Prophase I
_____ Metaphase I
_____ Anaphase I
_____ Telophase I
_____ Prophase II
_____ Metaphase II
_____ Anaphase II
_____ Telophase II

a. Homologous chromosomes aggregates around opposite poles.
b. Tetrads line up along the equatorial plate.
c. Chromosomes line up along the equatorial plate.
d. Sister chromatids remain bound together.
e. Sister chromatids aggregate around opposite poles.
f. Crossing over occurs.
g. Homologous chromosomes are separated and pull apart.
h. Sister chromatids are separated and pull apart.

18. Match the term with its description:

_____ Spermatogenic cell
_____ Sustentacular cell
_____ Interstitial cell
_____ Myoid cell
_____ Secondary spermatocyte

a. A cell that secretes testosterone
b. A cell that secretes testicular fluids
c. A stem cell that can produce sperm cells
d. A haploid cell after meiosis I
e. A contractile epithelial cell.

19. Match the follicle stage with its description:

_____ Primordial follicle
_____ Primary follicle
_____ Secondary follicle
_____ Graafian follicle
_____ Corpus luteum

a. Several layers of granulosa cells with pockets of follicular fluid surrounding the primary oocyte
b. Yellow-colored endocrine gland that secretes progesterone
c. A single layer of squamous follicular cells surrounding the primary oocyte
d. One or two layers of granulosa cells around the primary oocyte secrete zona pellucida
e. A secondary oocyte rests on top of cumulus oophorus. Antrum is filled with follicular fluid.

LEVEL 2. CHECK YOUR UNDERSTANDING

1. Explain why meiosis I is also called reduction division.
2. Explain why the blood-sperm barrier is so important for normal sperm production.
3. Which anatomical structures of male and female reproductive organs are homologous? What characteristics make them similar?

LEVEL 3. APPLY YOUR KNOWLEDGE TO REAL LIFE

1. Kartagener's syndrome is characterized by ciliary dyskinesia, which manifests in all systems using cilia. Explain why females with this syndrome are at risk of an ectopic pregnancy.
2. What do you expect to see on the contrast dye salpingogram image, if the patient fallopian tubes are patent?

Figure Credits

Fig. 1.1A: Copyright © by Giovanni Maki (CC BY-SA 3.0) at https://commons.wikimedia. org/wiki/File:Amphioxus.png.

Fig.1.1B: Copyright © by Silke Baron (CC BY 2.0) at https://commons.wikimedia.org/wiki/ File:Sea_Squirt.jpg.

Fig. 1.1C: Copyright © by Fredlyfish4 (CC BY-SA 4.0) at https://commons.wikimedia.org/ wiki/File:Lampetra_aepyptera_UMFS_2.JPG.

Fig. 1.2A: Copyright © 1999 by Degan Shu. Reprinted with permission.

Fig. 1.2B: Copyright © by Talifero (CC BY-SA 3.0) at https://commons.wikimedia.org/wiki/ File:Haikouichthys_3d.png.

Fig. 1.2C: Copyright © by Harsh Awasthi99 (CC BY-SA 4.0) at https://commons.wikimedia. org/wiki/File:Carassius_auratus_at_Kanpur_Zoo_(2015).jpg.

Fig. 1.2D: Copyright © by Dmitry Bogdanov (CC BY 3.0) at https://commons.wikimedia. org/wiki/File:Panderichthys12DB.jpg.

Fig. 1.3: Source: https://commons.wikimedia.org/wiki/File:Spindle_diagram.jpg.

Fig. 1.4: Source: https://commons.wikimedia.org/wiki/File:Bilayer_scheme.svg.

Fig. 1.5A: Source: https://commons.wikimedia.org/wiki/File:Deux_ours_Regourdou.jpg.

Fig. 1.5B: Source: https://commons.wikimedia.org/wiki/File:Farmer%27s_cyclopedia_of_ live_stock_BHL23726732.jpg.

Fig. 1.5C: Source: https://commons.wikimedia.org/wiki/File:The_new_book_of_the_horse_ (Pl._25)_(8536501755).jpg.

Fig.1.5D: Source: https://commons.wikimedia.org/wiki/File:Farmer%27s_cyclopedia_of_ live_stock_BHL23726732.jpg.

Fig. 1.5E: Source: https://commons.wikimedia.org/wiki/File:Anatomischer_anzeiger_ Baum_Hund.PNG.

Fig. 1.5F: Copyright © by Bryan Brandenburg (CC BY-SA 3.0) at https://commons.wikimedia. org/wiki/File:Respiratory_function_by_Bryan_Brandenburg.jpg.

Fig. 1.5G: Source: https://commons.wikimedia.org/wiki/File:Farmer%27s_cyclopedia_of_ live_stock_BHL23726584.jpg.

Fig. 1.5H: Copyright © by National Human Genome Research Institute (CC BY 2.0) at https://commons.wikimedia.org/wiki/File:Dog_Bladder_(26990477411).jpg.

Fig. 1.5I: Source: https://commons.wikimedia.org/wiki/File:The_new_book_of_the_horse_ (Pl._27)_(8536503249).jpg.

Fig. 1.6A: Copyright © by Rainer Klute (CC BY-SA 3.0) at https://commons.wikimedia. org/wiki/File:Stylised_atom_with_three_Bohr_model_orbits_and_stylised_nucleus.svg.

Fig. 2.6: Copyright © by Michal Maňas (CC BY-SA 3.0) at https://commons.wikimedia.org/wiki/File:3D_model_hydrogen_bonds_in_water.jpg.

Fig. 2.7: Copyright © by Manzurur Rahman Khan (CC BY 3.0) at https://commons.wikimedia.org/wiki/File:HouseLizard.JPG.

Fig. 2.8: Source: https://commons.wikimedia.org/wiki/File:Hex_ice.GIF.

Fig. 2.9: Copyright © 2013 Depositphotos/thomasmales.

Fig. 2.10: Copyright © by OpenStax College (CC BY 3.0) at https://commons.wikimedia.org/wiki/File:214_Dissociation_of_Sodium_Chloride_in_Water-01.jpg.

Fig. 2.11: Copyright © by OpenStax College (CC BY 4.0) at https://commons.wikimedia.org/wiki/File:0307_Osmosis.jpg.

Fig. 2.12: Copyright © by OpenStax College (CC BY 3.0) at https://commons.wikimedia.org/wiki/File:216_pH_Scale-01.jpg.

Fig. 2.15: Source: https://commons.wikimedia.org/wiki/File:Glycogen.png.

Fig. 2.16: Source: https://commons.wikimedia.org/wiki/File:AminoAcidball.svg.

Fig. 2,17: Source: https://commons.wikimedia.org/wiki/File:Peptidformationball.svg.

Fig. 2.18: Copyright © by OpenStax College (CC BY 3.0) at https://commons.wikimedia.org/wiki/File:225_Peptide_Bond-01.jpg.

Fig. 2.19: Source: http://science.halleyhosting.com/sci/ibbio/chem/notes/chpt3/triglyceride.htm.

Fig.2.20A: Source: https://commons.wikimedia.org/wiki/File:Gamma-Linolenic-acid-3D-balls.png.

Fig2.20B: Source: https://commons.wikimedia.org/wiki/File:Palmitelaidic-acid-3D-balls.png.

Fig. 2.22: Copyright © by OpenStax (CC BY 4.0) at https://commons.wikimedia.org/wiki/File:0322_DNA_Nucleotides.jpg.

Fig. 2.23: Copyright © by Zephyris (CC BY-SA 3.0) at https://commons.wikimedia.org/wiki/File:DNA_Structure%2BKey%2BLabelled.pn_NoBB.png.

Fig. 3.1: Copyright © by Kgerow16 (CC BY-SA 4.0) at https://commons.wikimedia.org/wiki/File:Louis_Pasteur_Experiment.svg.

Fig. 3.2: Copyright © by OpenStax (CC BY 4.0) at https://commons.wikimedia.org/wiki/File:0312_Animal_Cell_and_Components.jpg.

Fig. 3.3: Source: https://commons.wikimedia.org/wiki/File:Phospholipids_aqueous_solution_structures.svg.

Fig. 3.4: Copyright © by Dhatfield (CC BY-SA 3.0) at https://commons.wikimedia.org/wiki/File:Cell_membrane_detailed_diagram_4.svg.

Fig. 3.5: Source: https://commons.wikimedia.org/wiki/File:Cell_membrane_detailed_diagram_en.svg.

Fig. 3.6: Copyright © by OpenStax College (CC BY 3.0) at https://commons.wikimedia.org/wiki/File:2705_Sodium_Potassium_Pump.jpg.

Fig. 3.7: Source: https://commons.wikimedia.org/wiki/File:Porters.PNG.

Fig. 3.8: Source: https://commons.wikimedia.org/wiki/File:Endocytosis_types.svg.

Fig. 3.9: Copyright © by OpenStax (CC BY 4.0) at https://commons.wikimedia.org/wiki/File:0313_Endoplasmic_Reticulum.jpg.

Fig. 3.10: Copyright © by OpenStax (CC BY 4.0) at https://commons.wikimedia.org/wiki/File:0314_Golgi_Apparatus.jpg.

Fig. 3.11: Source: https://commons.wikimedia.org/wiki/File:Animal_mitochondrion_diagram_en.svg.

Fig. 4.12: Source: https://commons.wikimedia.org/wiki/File:Connective_Tissue_Adipose_(41066513704).jpg.

Fig. 4.13: Source: https://commons.wikimedia.org/wiki/File:Connective_Tissue_Reticular_(40885194425).jpg.

Fig. 4.14: Copyright © by Nephron (CC BY-SA 3.0) at https://commons.wikimedia.org/wiki/File:Tendon_-_very_high_mag.jpg.

Fig. 4.15: Source: https://commons.wikimedia.org/wiki/File:Normal_Epidermis_and_Dermis_with_Intradermal_Nevus_10x.JPG.

Fig. 4.16: Source: https://commons.wikimedia.org/wiki/File:Connective_Tissue_Human_Elastic_Tissue_(41813163682).jpg.

Fig. 4.17: Source: https://commons.wikimedia.org/wiki/File:Connective_Tissue_Human_Blood_(39982278130).jpg.

Fig. 4.18: Copyright © by OpenStax College (CC BY 3.0) at https://commons.wikimedia.org/wiki/File:412_Types_of_Cartilage-new.jpg.

Fig. 4.19: Copyright © by OpenStax College (CC BY 3.0) at https://commons.wikimedia.org/wiki/File:624_Diagram_of_Compact_Bone-new.jpg.

Fig. 4.20: Copyright © by BruceBlaus (CC BY 3.0) at https://commons.wikimedia.org/wiki/File:Blausen_0672_NeuralTissue.png.

Fig. 5.1: Copyright © by OpenStax College (CC BY 3.0) at https://commons.wikimedia.org/wiki/File:2313_The_Lung_Pleurea.jpg.

Fig. 5.2: Copyright © by OpenStax College (CC BY 3.0) at https://commons.wikimedia.org/wiki/File:2311_Lung_Tissue.jpg.

Fig. 5.3: Source: https://commons.wikimedia.org/wiki/File:Normal_Epidermis_and_Dermis_with_Intradermal_Nevus_10x.JPG.

Fig. 5.4: Copyright © by OpenStax College (CC BY 3.0) at https://commons.wikimedia.org/wiki/File:504_Melanocytes.jpg.

IMG 5.1: Copyright © by Michel Milinkovitch.

Fig. 5.5: Copyright © by BruceBlaus (CC BY 3.0) at https://commons.wikimedia.org/wiki/File:Blausen_0353_Epidermis.png.

Fig. 5.6: Copyright © by Madhero88 and M.Komorniczak (CC BY-SA 3.0) at https://commons.wikimedia.org/wiki/File:Skin_layers.svg.

Fig. 5.7: Copyright © by BruceBlaus (CC BY 3.0) at https://commons.wikimedia.org/wiki/File:Blausen_0438_HairFollicleAnatomy_02.png.

Fig. 5.8: Copyright © by Joel Mills (CC BY-SA 3.0) at https://commons.wikimedia.org/wiki/File:Anal_gland_abscess.JPG.

Fig. 5.9: Copyright © by Uwe Gille (CC BY-SA 3.0) at https://commons.wikimedia.org/wiki/File:Viol-Gland-dog.jpg.

Fig. 5.10: Copyright © by BruceBlaus (CC BY 3.0) at https://commons.wikimedia.org/wiki/File:Blausen_0406_FingerNailAnatomy.png.

Fig. 5.11A: Source: https://commons.wikimedia.org/wiki/File:The_topographical_anatomy_of_the_limbs_of_the_horse_(Page_83)_BHL23953839.jpg.

Fig. 9.2: Copyright © by OpenStax (CC BY 4.0) at https://commons.wikimedia.org/wiki/File:1023_T-tubule.jpg.

Fig. 9.3: Copyright © by OpenStax (CC BY 4.0) at https://commons.wikimedia.org/wiki/File:1022_Muscle_Fibers_(small).jpg.

Fig. 9.4A: Source: angelfire.com/sc3/toxchick/physiology/physiology18.html.

Fig. 9.4B: Erin C. Amerman, from Human Anatomy & Physiology. Copyright © 2016 by Pearson.

Fig. 9.5: Copyright © by OpenStax (CC BY 4.0) at https://commons.wikimedia.org/wiki/File:1003_Thick_and_Thin_Filaments.jpg.

Fig. 9.6: Adapted from Copyright © by David Giganti, et al. (CC BY 4.0) at https://commons.wikimedia.org/wiki/File:Titin_IG_Domains.jpg.

Fig. 9.7: Copyright © by David Richfield (CC BY-SA 3.0) at https://commons.wikimedia.org/wiki/File:Sarcomere.svg.

Fig. 9.8A: Source: angelfire.com/sc3/toxchick/physiology/physiology18.html.

Fig. 9.8B: Erin C. Amerman, from Human Anatomy & Physiology. Copyright © 2016 by Pearson.

Fig. 9.8C: Copyright © by JeeJee~commonswiki (CC BY-SA 3.0) at https://commons.wikimedia.org/wiki/File:Sarcomere.jpg.

Fig. 9.9: Copyright © by BruceBlaus (CC BY 3.0) at https://commons.wikimedia.org/wiki/File:Blausen_0818_Sodium-PotassiumPump.png.

Fig. 9.10: Source: https://www.thinglink.com/scene/722914716149612545

Fig. 9.11A: Copyright © by Hlj55567516 (CC BY-SA 3.0) at https://commons.wikimedia.org/wiki/File:%E8%BF%90%E5%8A%A8%E7%BB%88%E6%9D%BF.JPG.

Fig. 9.11B: Source: https://i.stack.imgur.com/qD1Xn.jpg.

Fig. 9.12: Copyright © by OpenStax (CC BY 4.0) at https://commons.wikimedia.org/wiki/File:1009_Motor_End_Plate_and_Innervation.jpg.

Fig. 9.13: Adapted from https://www.austincc.edu/apreview/PhysText/PNSefferent.html. Copyright © by Thomson Learning.

Fig. 9.14A: Adapted from https://www.austincc.edu/apreview/PhysText/PNSefferent.html. Copyright © by Thomson Learning.

Fig. 9.14B: Source: https://www.slideshare.net/BradleyChristman/myasthenia-gravispptnew.

Fig. 9.15: Source: https://www.slideshare.net/BradleyChristman/myasthenia-gravispptnew.

Fig. 9.16: from "Physiology of Skeletal Muscle Contraction." Copyright © by Earth's Lab.

Fig. 9.17: Adapted from http://www.supplementshop.lk/product/2922/

Fig.9.18A: Source: https://commons.wikimedia.org/wiki/File:Capillaries.jpg.

Fig. 9.22: Copyright © by OpenStax CNX (CC BY 3.0) at https://commons.wikimedia.org/wiki/File:2017abc_Cardiac_Muscle.jpg.

Fig. 9.24: Adapted from: Copyright © by Boumphreyfr (CC BY-SA 3.0) https://commons.wikimedia.org/wiki/File:Actin_myosin_filaments.png.

Fig. 10.1: Copyright © by Nsdiagram (CC BY-SA 3.0) at https://commons.wikimedia.org/wiki/File:NSdiagram.png.

Fig. 10.2: Copyright © by Fabuio (CC BY 4.0) at https://commons.wikimedia.org/wiki/File:Piramidal_cell.svg.